THE ROUTLEDGE HANDBOOK OF SEMIOSIS AND THE BRAIN

This *Handbook* introduces neurosemiotics, a pluralistic framework to reconsider semiosis as an emergent phenomenon at the interface of biology and culture.

Across individual and interpersonal settings, meaning and communication are influenced by external and internal processes bridging phenomenological and biological dimensions. Yet, each of these dyads has been segregated into discipline-specific topics, with attempts to chart their intersections proving preliminary at best. Bringing together perspectives from world-leading experts, this volume seeks to overcome these disciplinary divides at both the empirical and theoretical levels. Its various chapters chart the foundations of neurosemiotics; characterize linguistic and interpersonal dynamics as shaped by neurocognitive, bodily, situational, and societal factors; and examine other daily neurosemiotic occurrences driven by faces, music, tools, and even visceral signals.

This comprehensive volume is a state-of-the-art resource for students and researchers interested in how humans and other animals construe meaningful experience, informing such fields as cognitive neuroscience, biosemiotics, philosophy of mind, neuropsychology, neurolinguistics, and evolutionary biology.

Adolfo M. García specializes in the neuroscience of language and communication. He serves as Director of the Cognitive Neuroscience Center (UdeSA, Argentina), Senior Atlantic Fellow at the Global Brain Health Institute (UCSF, USA), Associate Researcher at USACH (Chile), Director of Language Science at Redenlab, and Researcher at CONICET (Argentina). Dr García leads research projects in more than ten countries across the globe. He has more than 200 publications, including works in top-ten journals. His scientific contributions have been recognized by various awards and distinctions.

Agustín Ibáñez works on global approaches to dementia and social, cognitive, and affective neuroscience. He is Director of the Latin American Brain Health Institute (BrainLat) and Full Professor at the CSCN (Universidad Adolfo Ibáñez, Chile); and Associate Research Professor and Group Leader of Predictive Brain Health Modelling Group (Trinity College Dublin, Ireland). Dr Ibáñez has over 300 publications, including works in top-ten journals. His intense work has helped Latin American translational neuroscience by establishing a framework to engage scientists through internships, workshops, master's and PhD programs, organizing educational activities for the health community, and focusing on cognitive neuroscience, among others.

ROUTLEDGE HANDBOOKS IN LINGUISTICS

Routledge Handbooks in Linguistics provide overviews of a whole subject area or subdiscipline in linguistics, and survey the state of the discipline including emerging and cutting-edge areas. Edited by leading scholars, these volumes include contributions from key academics from around the world and are essential reading for both advanced undergraduate and postgraduate students.

The Routledge Handbook of Language and Science
Edited by David R. Gruber and Lynda Walsh

The Routledge Handbook of Language and Emotion
Edited by Sonya E. Pritzker, Janina Fenigsen, and James M. Wilce

The Routledge Handbook of Language Contact
Edited by Evangelia Adamou and Yaron Matras

The Routledge Handbook of Pidgin and Creole Languages
Edited by Umberto Ansaldo and Miriam Meyerhoff

The Routledge Handbook of Cognitive Linguistics
Edited by Xu Wen and John R. Taylor

The Routledge Handbook of Theoretical and Experimental Sign Language Research
Edited by Josep Quer, Roland Pfau, and Annika Herrmann

The Routledge Handbook of Language and Persuasion
Edited by Jeanne Fahnestock and Randy Allen Harris

The Routledge Handbook of Semiosis and the Brain
Edited by Adolfo M. García and Agustín Ibáñez

Further titles in this series can be found online at www.routledge.com/series/RHIL

THE ROUTLEDGE HANDBOOK OF SEMIOSIS AND THE BRAIN

Edited by Adolfo M. García and Agustín Ibáñez

Routledge
Taylor & Francis Group
NEW YORK AND LONDON

Cover image: Getty Images

First published 2023
by Routledge
605 Third Avenue, New York, NY 10158

and by Routledge
4 Park Square, Milton Park, Abingdon, Oxon, OX14 4RN

Routledge is an imprint of the Taylor & Francis Group, an informa business

ISBN: 9780367509163 (hbk)
ISBN: 9781032355610 (pbk)
ISBN: 9781003051817 (ebk)

DOI: 10.4324/9781003051817

Typeset in Bembo
by Newgen Publishing UK

CONTENTS

FIGURES

TABLES

ACKNOWLEDGMENTS

We extend our gratitude to all the authors for joining this project and enriching it beyond our original vision. The excellent material they produced was harmonized and streamlined by our local proofreading and copy-editing team: Catalina González Santibáñez, Ignacio Peña Jorquera, Matías Calderón Pena, Rafael Badillo, and Sebastián Requena Cancino. We thank them for their diligence and professionalism in this task.

We are also indebted to the several colleagues who reviewed the chapters and provided critical insights. May this alphabetical list serve as recognition for their insightful contributions: Aaron Newman, Alexei Sharov, Annabelle Lukin, Antoni Rodríguez-Fornells, Arjen Stolk, César Meurer, David Beltrán, Enrique García-Marco, Enzo Tagliazucchi, Georg Northoff, Giovanni Buccino, Hans van Hateren, Hernando Santamaría-García, Kalevi Kull, Konrad Lehmann, Lisa Quadt, Manuel de Vega, Maya Visser, Michael Kaschak, Michael Trimble, Philipp Kanske, Riccardo Dalla Volta, Rutvik Desai, Sandra Baez, Sergio Salvatore, Sladjana Lukic, Valentina Borghesani, Virginia Sturm, and Yogi Hendlin.

Finally, we acknowledge the support of our affiliations and funders. Adolfo M. García thanks the Cognitive Neuroscience Center at Universidad de San Andrés (Argentina), the Global Brain Health Institute (GBHI) at University of San Francisco, California (United States) and Trinity College Dublin (Ireland), the National Scientific and Technical Research Council (Argentina), and the Faculty of Humanities at Universidad de Santiago de Chile (Chile). He is supported by funding from GBHI, Alzheimer's Association, and Alzheimer's Society (Alzheimer's Association GBHI ALZ UK-22-865742); ANID, FONDECYT Regular (1210176); and Programa Interdisciplinario de Investigación Experimental en Comunicación y Cognición (PIIECC), Facultad de Humanidades, USACH. Agustín Ibáñez expresses his gratitude to the Latin American Brain Health Institute (BrainLat) at Universidad Adolfo Ibáñez (Chile), the Global Brain Health Institute (GBHI) at University of San Francisco, California (United States) and Trinity College Dublin (Ireland), the Cognitive Neuroscience Center at Universidad de San Andrés (Argentina), and the National Scientific and Technical Research Council (Argentina). He is supported by grants from Alzheimer's Association GBHI ALZ UK-20-639295; Takeda CW2680521; ANID/FONDECYT Regular (1210195, 1220995); ANID/FONDAP 15150012; ANID/PIA/ANILLOS ACT210096; Sistema General de Regalías (BPIN2018000100059); Universidad del Valle (CI 5316); BrainLat seed funds; and the Multi-Partner Consortium to Expand Dementia Research in Latin America (ReDLat), funded by the National Institutes of Aging (NIA) of the National Institutes of Health (NIH) under award number R01AG057234, an Alzheimer's Association grant (SG-20-725707-ReDLat), the Rainwater Foundation, and the Global Brain Health Institute. The content is solely the responsibility of the authors and does not represent the official views of these institutions.

CONTRIBUTOR INFORMATION

Editors

Adolfo M. García specializes in the neuroscience of language and communication. He serves as Director of the Cognitive Neuroscience Center (UdeSA, Argentina), Senior Atlantic Fellow at the Global Brain Health Institute (UCSF, USA), Associate Researcher at USACH (Chile), Director of Language Science at Redenlab, and Researcher at CONICET (Argentina). Dr. García leads research projects in over ten countries across the globe. He has more than 200 publications, including works in top-ten journals. His scientific contributions have been recognized by awards and distinctions from various relevant entities.

Agustín Ibáñez works on global approaches to dementia and social, cognitive, and affective neuroscience. He is Director of the Latin American Brain Health Institute (BrainLat) and Full Professor at the CSCN (Universidad Adolfo Ibáñez, Chile); and Associate Research Professor and Group Leader of Predictive Brain Health Modelling Group (Trinity College Dublin, Ireland). Dr. Ibáñez has over 300 publications, including works in top-ten journals. His intense work has helped Latin American translational neuroscience by establishing a framework to engage scientists through internships, workshops, Masters and PhD programs, organizing educational activities for the health community, focusing on cognitive neuroscience, among others.

Contributors

Jubin Abutalebi is a cognitive neurologist and Associate Professor of Neuropsychology at the Faculty of Psychology, University Vita Salute San Raffaele, Milan, Italy. He is the Director of the Centre for Neurolinguistics and Psycholinguistics (CNPL) at the same university. From 2014, he is the editor-in-chief of *Bilingualism: Language and Cognition* (Cambridge University Press). He is also an Adjunct Professor at the Arctic University of Tromsø, Norway.

Sandra Baez holds a PhD in psychology. She serves as Professor of Psychology and Neuroscience at the University of Los Andes (Colombia). Her interests and research experience are focused on neuropsychological aspects as well as neurophysiological and neuroanatomical correlates of social cognition processes in patients with neurological and psychiatric disorders. She has more than 80 publications, including books, chapters, and articles in top-ten journals on neuropsychiatric research and cognitive neuroscience (e.g., *Nature Reviews Neurology, JAMA Neurology, Neurology, Brain, Scientific Reports, SCAN, Philosophical Transactions of the Royal Society B, Neuroscience & Biobehavioral Reviews, Nature Human Behavior*).

Jana Bašnáková investigates how people use context in communication to arrive at the meaning of even highly indirect utterances. She obtained her PhD at the Max Planck Institute for Psycholinguistics (Nijmegen, the Netherlands) under the supervision of Jos van Berkum and Peter Hagoort. After researching scientific literacy and decision-making at the Institute for Experimental Psychology (Bratislava, Slovakia), she joined the Donders Institute in Nijmegen as director of the Synergy Group investigating context-dependent communication in autism.

Josselin Baumard is a professor and researcher in neuropsychology at the University of Rouen, France, where he has been managing a Master's in Neuropsychology since 2017. He earned his PhD at the University of Angers, France, in 2015. He is the author of some 25 scientific publications on higher-order motor disorders (i.e., apraxia and optic ataxia). His work has focused on patients with either stroke or dementia. Some of his most recent publications address the role of multisensory integration in bodily experience, imitation skills in normal aging, the role of memory, planning, and reasoning in tool use.

Amy M. Belfi is an assistant professor in the Department of Psychological Science at Missouri University of Science and Technology. She received her BA in psychology from St. Olaf College, her PhD in neuroscience from the University of Iowa, and completed postdoctoral training in neuroaesthetics at New York University. Her work covers a broad range of topics relating to music perception and cognition, including music and autobiographical memory, lexical and conceptual knowledge of musical objects, aesthetic judgments of music, and musical anhedonia.

Giovanni Buccino is Professor of Human Physiology at the University San Raffaele, Milan. He graduated in Medicine and Surgery at the University of Parma, where he also completed a neurology residency and obtained his PhD in neuroscience. He is involved in studying the relationships between the motor system and higher cognitive functions such as language, empathy, and motor learning. Over the last decade, he has focused on the neural mechanisms sub-serving language processing. Dr Buccino also developed a novel approach known as Action Observation Treatment (AOT), which has been shown to be effective in the rehabilitation of several neurological and non-neurological diseases.

David Butt works with textual evidence, in particular grammatical evidence, in social, institutional, literary, and medical contexts. His focus includes "latent patterning" in text – namely, the consistencies that are semantically consequential, but unconscious and difficult to make explicit, as they are marked configurations of otherwise habitual semiotic choices. His publications include works on the fields of psychotherapy in psychiatry; interaction in surgical teams and other institutional contexts; patterning in literary texts; and the role of semiosis in human evolution. Following the work of his teachers in systemic functional linguistics, he has devised practical network representations to capture salient differences between social contexts.

Ruth Campbell is an experimental psychologist and neuropsychologist, with interests in the psychology of language and communication, and in developmental aspects of cognition. She was a founder and co-director of the Deafness, Cognition and Language Centre at University College London (UK) from 2005 until her retirement in 2008. She has special interests in understanding lipreading (speechreading), and co-edited *Hearing by Eye* with Barbara Dodd and *Hearing by Eye II* with Barbara Dodd and Denis Burnham.

Valentina Cuccio is Assistant Professor of Philosophy of Science at the Department of Ancient and Modern Civilizations, University of Messina. She received a PhD in Philosophy of Language from the University of Palermo. She has done postdoctoral research at the University of Parma, Johns Hopkins University, the University of Amsterdam, the University of Palermo, and Humboldt University. She is interested in the cognitive neurosciences of language and the philosophy of neuroscience. In recent years, she has published on language and embodied cognition, the embodiment of metaphor, and the embodiment of abstract concepts and negation.

Manuel de Vega is Professor of Psychology at the University of La Laguna. He founded the University Institute of Neurosciences (IUNE) and worked as its director until 2021. His main line of research deals with the neurophysiology and neuroanatomy of language from an embodiment approach. Specifically, he studies how the brain reuses the neural networks of action, inhibition, visual-spatial perception, and emotion for the understanding of language. Dr de Vega has served as principal investigator of more than a dozen competitive projects, published around 100 articles in international journals, and written or edited six books on cognitive neuroscience.

Terrence Deacon has held faculty positions at Harvard University, Harvard Medical School, Boston University, and the University of California, Berkeley, where he is currently Professor of Biological Anthropology and Cognitive and Brain Sciences. His laboratory research includes comparative neuroanatomy and cross-species fetal neural transplantation. His 1997 book *The Symbolic Species: The Co-evolution of Language and the Brain* explored the evolution of the human brain supporting language abilities. His 2012 book *Incomplete Nature: How Mind Emerged from Matter* explored the interrelationships between thermodynamic, self-organizing, and evolutionary processes underlying the emergence of life, mind, and other teleological causal processes.

Nicola del Maschio is Assistant Professor at the Faculty of Psychology, University Vita-Salute San Raffaele, Milan, Italy. His research focuses on the organization of the brain mechanisms supporting language in monolingual and bilingual speakers, a topic he investigates with healthy individuals and using behavioral and neuroimaging techniques.

Rutvik H. Desai is a Professor of Psychology at the University of South Carolina. He has broad training in cognitive science, and currently studies neural basis of word meaning. His work has contributed to our understanding of embodiment of concepts, speech processing, reading, metaphors, and effects of neurological disorders on language processing.

Claus Emmeche is a theoretical biologist and philosopher of science. He is associate professor in the Section for the History and Philosophy of Science at the Department of Science Education, University of Copenhagen, Denmark. He worked for many years with Jesper Hoffmeyer, one of the founders of biosemiotics. He teaches courses in the philosophy of science for students in chemistry, biochemistry, and biology programs. His research interests are biosemiotics, the philosophy of science, and more recently, the philosophy of interdisciplinarity with friendship studies as a case.

Donald Favareau has been teaching biosemiotics at the National University of Singapore since 2004. His background is in philosophy of mind, neurobiology of language, interaction analysis, and the history of science. He is editor of the volumes *Essential Readings in Biosemiotics* (2010), *Co-operative Engagements in Intertwined Semiosis* (2018) and *A More Developed Sign: Interpreting the Work of Jesper Hoffmeyer* (2012).

Karl Friston is a theoretical neuroscientist and authority on brain imaging. He invented statistical parametric mapping (SPM), voxel-based morphometry (VBM), and dynamic causal modelling

(DCM). These contributions were motivated by schizophrenia research, formulated as a dysconnection hypothesis. Mathematical contributions include variational Laplacian procedures and generalized filtering for hierarchical Bayesian model inversion. Dr Friston currently works on models of functional integration in the brain and the principles that underlie neuronal interactions. His main contribution to theoretical neurobiology is a free-energy principle for action and perception (active inference).

Bruno Galantucci is a Professor of Psychology at Yeshiva University. His domain of expertise is human communication, which he has investigated from a number of perspectives. His earlier research focused on the psychology of spoken language, with an emphasis on speech perception. He then investigated the emergence and evolution of non-linguistic forms of human communication in the laboratory, contributing to the development of experimental semiotics. Over the last few years, he has expanded his research interests to the investigation of miscommunication in spontaneous interactions, which he has studied through experiments involving textual exchanges as well as face-to-face conversations.

Diego Gorini is a PhD candidate in Philosophy at the University of Salento, Italy. He holds a BA in Classics and an MA in Philosophy from the University of Florence. He has worked as a computational linguist developing semantic models for natural language processing and understanding.

Philipp Kanske is Chair of Clinical Psychology and Behavioral Neuroscience at the Faculty of Psychology at Technische Universtität Dresden, Germany. He is a licensed psychotherapist in cognitive behavioral therapy. His research aims to understand the cognitive and affective processes underlying social interactions, their neural underpinnings, alterations in psychopathology and plasticity through interventions.

Sahib S. Khalsa is a psychiatrist and neuroscientist focused on studying the role of interoception in mental health. He is the Director of Clinical Operations at the Laureate Institute for Brain Research and a tenured Associate Professor in the Oxley College of Health Sciences at the University of Tulsa.

Kalevi Kull teaches biosemiotics at the University of Tartu, Estonia. He has studied biology and worked in ecophysiology, theoretical biology and semiotics. His research focuses on general semiotics, primary mechanisms of meaning-making, and history of ideas. His work includes *Jakob von Uexküll: A Paradigm for Biology and Semiotics* (2001), *Towards a Semiotic Biology: Life is the action of Signs* (2011), and *On Theoretical Biology: Life Science Between Mathematics and Semiotics* (2019).

Konrad Lehmann is a researcher and doctoral candidate at the Faculty of Psychology, Clinical Psychology and Behavioral Neuroscience at Technische Universität Dresden, Germany. His research aims to understand the cognitive and neural mechanisms that underwrite and enable dynamic social interaction.

Mathieu Lesourd is Assistant Professor of Neuropsychology at the University of Bourgogne Franche-Comté, France. He works on the cerebral correlates of representations that support the production of gestures. His studies involve healthy subjects as well as brain-damaged individuals and persons with neurodegenerative diseases. He has participated in roughly 30 scientific publications in the field of apraxia and tool use, including works on effect tool use despite defective hand posture and neural correlates of imitation of intransitive gestures.

Annabelle Lukin is Associate Professor of Linguistics at Macquarie University in Sydney. She researches on ideology in diverse contexts of human experience, including politics and media, clinical settings, and literary text. She teaches functional grammar, discourse analysis, and general linguistic theory. Her major publication is *War and Its Ideologies: A Social-Semiotic Theory and Description* (Springer, 2019), based on over a decade of research into media reporting of the 2003 invasion of Iraq. She is a regular contributor to the Australian media, including *The Conversation*, on language issues.

Catherine Merck is a neuropsychologist in the Memory Unit of Rennes University Hospital, specializing in contributing to the diagnosis and the follow-up of patients with semantic dementia. She works on residual semantic knowledge in patients with semantic dementia and has published relevant papers based on neuropsychological and eye-tracing evidence.

Antoine Milette-Gagnon is a graduate student in philosophy at Université du Québec à Montréal (UQAM). Trained in cognitive science at McGill University in Montreal, Canada, his background is marked by interdisciplinarity, having worked in experimental neuroscience, philosophy, and journalism. The main theme driving his research is the problem of the naturalization of meaning, approached from both a philosophical and scientific point of view. To address this problem, he is studying the possibility of integration of multiple frameworks, notably biosemiotics, enactivism, and the active inference framework.

Jonas Nölle is a cognitive scientist studying meaning-making in interaction. He has used experimental semiotics approaches, including silent gesture and iterated learning, to study how communication systems evolve culturally in response to cognitive, communicative, and environmental factors. During his PhD studies at the Centre for Language Evolution at the University of Edinburgh, he innovated the use of virtual reality to study these phenomena in ecologically more valid lab settings. Currently, he investigates how speech, facial expressions and gesture integrate to create complex multimodal signals in social interactions as part of the FACESYNTAX project at the University of Glasgow.

Georg Northoff is a philosopher, neuroscientist, and psychiatrist. He works in Ottawa, Canada, holding the Canada Research Chair for Mind, Brain Imaging, and Neuroethics. His research focuses on brain–mind connection. The question driving him is "Why and how can our brain construct mental features like self and consciousness?" He is a leading figure in linking philosophy, psychiatry, and neuroscience, having developed non-reductive neurophilosophy. He has authored over 300 journal articles and 18 books, which have been translated into several languages, including *Neurophilosophy and the Healthy Mind* (2016) and *Code of Time* (2021).

François Osiurak is Professor of Psychology at the University of Lyon, France. He earned his PhD at the University of Angers, France in 2007. He is the author of over 130 scientific publications on the neurocognitive origins of human tool use and cumulative technological culture. His published articles include works on the understanding of affordances and the links between cognition and cumulative technological culture. He was appointed a Junior Member of the French University Institute in 2014.

Hannah I. Pearson is a social psychology graduate student at the University of Hawai´i at Mānoa. She uses an experimental and socio-cultural approach in her focus on how religion and culture impact identity, thoughts, social interactions, and behavior.

Daniela Perani is a neurologist and radiologist, and Full Professor of Neuroscience at the Faculty of Psychology, University Vita-Salute San Raffaele, Milan, Italy. She is the Coordinator of the Doctoral Course in Cognitive Neuroscience and the Director of the School of Specialization in Neuropsychology in the same university, and Chief Coordinator of Nuclear Medicine Neurology in the Nuclear Medicine Unit at IRCCS Ospedale San Raffaele. Her research deals with in vivo neuroimaging studies of neurological diseases, in particular neurodegenerative dementias, and with cognitive neuroscience.

Maxwell Ramstead is the Director of Research at the VERSES Research Lab. He is also an Honorary Fellow at the Wellcome Centre for Human Neuroimaging in Imaging Neuroscience. His research focuses on the free-energy principle, Bayesian mechanics, multiscale active inference, and computational phenomenology.

Nicholas Riccardi is a graduate student in the Department of Psychology at the University of South Carolina. He uses lesion-symptom mapping and neuroimaging to investigate the neural bases of language and concepts. His work has shown the importance of action-perception systems in concept representation and shed light on the role of semantic hubs.

Bruno Rossion is a cognitive neuroscientist at the CNRS and Université de Lorraine in Nancy (France) and the founder and head of the Face Categorization Lab, investigating human face recognition with a wide variety of methods and populations. He introduced the gaze-contingency approach with face stimuli to demonstrate holistic over analytic visual recognition modes, and made significant contributions to the understanding of prosopagnosia as a category-selective face identity recognition disorder. Over the last decade, he has developed original frequency-tagging approaches in EEG, fMRI, and especially human intracerebral recordings to characterize (face) recognition and its neural basis.

Joni Y. Sasaki is an Associate Professor of Psychology at the University of Hawai`i at Mānoa. She uses an integrated biological and socio-cultural approach to conduct basic psychological research on multiple forms of diversity – including ethnic, religious, and biological diversity – in the areas of social cognition and social behavior.

Leonhard Schilbach is Professor of Psychiatry at the Ludwig-Maximilians-Universität in Munich and Deputy Medical Director and Head of the Department for General Psychiatry II at the LVR-Klinikum Düsseldorf. His work has led to an "interactive turn" in social neuroscience and opened up new avenues for the transdiagnostic investigation and treatment of psychiatric disorders construed as "disorders of social interaction." He has published more than 100 peer reviewed articles in the domain of social neuroscience and psychiatry and been the recipient of several awards in recognition of the relevance of his scientific work for psychiatry.

Ryan Smith holds a PhD in psychology. He serves as a Principal Investigator at the Laureate Institute for Brain Research (LIBR) and as a Research Associate Professor at the University of Tulsa. His interests and research experience are focused on the neural, cognitive, and computational processes underlying interactions between interoception, emotion, and cognition in patients with psychiatric disorders. He currently has more than 100 publications, including book chapters and articles in leading journals on psychiatric research and cognitive neuroscience (e.g., *Neuroscience & Biobehavioral Reviews, Progress in Neurobiology, Journal of Psychiatry & Neuroscience, Scientific Reports, NeuroImage, and Biological Psychiatry*).

Arjen Stolk investigates how human minds meet during social interaction, including how that conceptual ability is altered in disorders of communication, such as those seen in autism. He studied human movement sciences in Groningen (Netherlands) before joining the Donders Institute in Nijmegen (Netherlands) for his PhD in cognitive neuroscience. After working with Ivan Toni at the Donders Institute, and Bob Knight at UC Berkeley (USA), he joined the Department of Psychological and Brain Sciences at Dartmouth as director of the Mutual Understanding Lab.

Enzo Tagliazucchi is a professor at Universidad de Buenos Aires (Argentina) and Universidad Adolfo Ibáñez (Chile), and a researcher at the Latin American Brain Health Institute (BrainLat) and CONICET, where he leads the interdisciplinary Consciousness, Culture and Complexity Lab. He has published over 100 articles and a book on the neuroscientific bases of human consciousness, in particular on how different brain states support distinct altered states of consciousness.

Ivan Toni investigates the neurobiological and cognitive mechanisms that allow the motor system to generate behavior adapted to rules, percepts, and social constructs, using neurophysiological techniques in neurotypical, neurological, and psychopathological groups. He studied Biology in Bologna before joining the Institute of Human Physiology (Parma, Italy) and INSERM Unité 94 (Lyon, France) for his PhD in neuroscience. After working with Dick Passingham at the Functional Imaging Laboratory (London), and with Karl Zilles (Jülich, Germany), he joined the Donders Institute in Nijmegen (Netherlands) as principal investigator of the Intention and Action Research Group.

Morten Tønnessen is a Professor of Philosophy at the University of Stavanger (UIS), Norway, and chair of the steering group for Cognitive and behavioral neuroscience lab (UIS). He has previously served as an Editor-in-Chief of *Biosemiotics* (2013–2020). His publications include "Beyond Sentience: Biosemiotics as Foundation for Animal and Environmental Ethics" (with Jonathan Beever, in Hadley and Aaltola (Eds.), *Animal Ethics and Philosophy: Questioning the Orthodoxy*, 2014), "The Search Image as a Link Between Sensation, Perception and Action" (2017), and *Semiotic Agency: Science Beyond Mechanism* (with Alexei Sharov, 2021).

Samuel Veissière is Assistant Professor of Psychiatry, co-director of the Culture, Mind, and Brain Program, and an associate member of the Department of Anthropology at McGill University, Canada. He has worked with varied populations, examining social and evolutionary dimensions of cognition, mental health, and human wellbeing through a variety of projects including placebo effects and hypnosis, social polarization, gender and mental health, among others. Dr Veissière has published broadly on novel theories and experimental findings on the social nature of attention, cognition, mental health, and healing, and on the impact of the internet and new technologies on human sociality and wellbeing.

Maya Visser has worked on several neuroimaging projects at international research centers in the Netherlands (Maastricht University), the United Kingdom (University of Manchester), and Spain (University Pompeu Fabra and University Jaume I). By using neuroimaging techniques, her PhD project (2010) was able to construct a model of how the neural language system forms semantic concepts. After a postdoctoral position, she was able to set up her own research project on semantic memory impairments in temporal lobe epilepsy patients funded by the Spanish Government and the University Jaume I. She is currently setting up a new research project at the University Jaume I on the role of semantic processing in social behaviors.

INTRODUCTION

Semiosis, brain, and context: The unmet need for a transdisciplinary framework

Adolfo M. García and Agustín Ibáñez

Neurosemiotics: What, how, why?

The human organism is typified by an unyielding drive towards sensemaking (Cosmelli & Ibáñez, 2008; Deacon, 1997; Halliday, 1978; Hodge, 2014; Ibáñez, 2022; Ibáñez & Cosmelli, 2008; Ibáñez & García, 2018; Peirce, 1998; Van Leeuwen, 2005). Anchored in the humanities, classical semiotics first studied this phenomenon focusing on sign properties (e.g., indication, reference, symbolism, analogy, metaphor), with later perspectives tracing links among signs, body processes, and cultural niches in interpersonal communication. More recently, new insights have stemmed from the natural sciences, including predominantly biological approaches, such as biosemiotics (Emmeche et al., 2000; Hoffmeyer, 2015, Kosoy & Kosoy, 2018; Sharov et al., 2016; Sharov, 2016; van Hateren, 2015), alongside contributions from neuropsychology (Faust, 2012; Shallice, 1988), the behavioral sciences (Carey, 2011; Mareschal et al., 2010; Murphy, 2004), and social cognitive and affective neuroscience (Amoruso et al., 2013; Falk & Scholz, 2018; Fiske & Taylor, 2013; Pessoa et al., 2022; Pezzulo et al., 2018, 2019). Nevertheless, integrative efforts across cultural and biological traditions have been preliminary at best, failing to track the convergences of the neurological, cognitive, sensorimotor, visceral, perceptual, and social processes that jointly shape our individual and social semiotic experiences (Brier, 2015; Cosmelli & Ibáñez, 2008; Ibáñez, 2022; Ibáñez & García, 2018). Understanding this convergence requires a new framework that surpasses the "two cultures" divide (Ibáñez et al., 2017; Snow, 2012) by consolidating a third culture – one that effaces methodological and theoretical boundaries, foregrounds epistemological continuities among traditions, and leads to applicable innovations in theory building, basic research, clinical science, data analytics, and diverse applied arenas. In other words, a new theoretical and empirical space must emerge that captures semiosis as codetermined by brain, body, and culture. We will refer to this field as neurosemiotics – embracing the convenient synecdoche of the prefix "neuro" while rejecting any reductionism or popular hype that may be attached to it.

Early on, a field bearing this name was envisioned as an "epistemological domain which includes the scientific investigation of the neurological processes underlying communicative behavior in all its forms as well as the prerequisites for such behavior," including "the perception of the environment as meaningful, both globally and discretely, and the general capacity to engage in symbolic interactions" (Bouissac, 1986: 204–206). Even when metatheoretically and empirically simplistic, this initial proposal goes beyond the study of signs as abstract entities, enabling new outlooks to integrate socio-biological perspectives on meaning and communication. The topics potentially targeted by

DOI: 10.4324/9781003051817-1

neurosemiotics are thus manifold, multidimensional, and informed by a variety of methods, including tools from neuroscience (e.g., brain imaging, brain stimulation), neuropsychology (e.g., anatomo-clinical correlations), behavioral science (assessments of outward performance), cognitive science (e.g., behavioral and kinetic measures), linguistics (e.g., text analysis), biology (e.g., animal communication), and social sciences (e.g., sociopolitical analysis). On account of its conceptual breadth and plurality, neurosemiotics can inspire theoretical, epistemological, methodological, and translational breakthroughs.

However, neurosemiotics is far from a consolidated field. For all its potential, the research program it inspires has been notoriously underexploited. Granted, the field has been acknowledged in encyclopaedias of semiotics (Bouissac, 1998) and neuroscience (Jorna, 2009), and a few books devoted to related topics have offered initial insights in circumscribed chapters (Baggio, 2018; Deacon, 1997; Plebe & De La Cruz, 2016). However, no single work has yet formulated an overarching framework for a holistic understanding of the phenomena at hand, which deprives several disciplines of major opportunities for cross-fertilization. In fact, without knowing so, numerous scholars in neuroscience have long been nurturing the neurosemiotics agenda in a compartmentalized manner, through segregated studies on language, emotion, gesture, and social interaction (Ibáñez & García, 2018). In line with recent calls (Deacon & Rączaszek-Leonardi, 2019; Falk & Scholz, 2018; Ibáñez, 2019; Ibáñez, 2022; Ibáñez & Schulte, 2020; Ibáñez & García, 2018; Ibáñez et al., 2017), such fragmentary developments can and must be integrated towards creating a pluralistic view of human semiotics that is both biologically and socially grounded. Similarly, semiotically oriented trends in cultural studies have begun to consider their crucially social explananda as influenced by cognitive, genetic, and biological factors, offering multilevel and pluralistic explanations (Alexandrov, 2000; Armstrong, 2019; Blackman et al., 2008; Kleinman, 1987; Mendoza-Collazos, 2020; Tamm & Torop, 2022). Yet, these approaches lack common theoretical horizons and they are extremely heterogeneous. A first step to combine both realms is to collect, organize, and interrelate available insights from neuroscience, behavioral studies, neuropsychology, cognitive science, social sciences, and biosemiotics, as well as experimental psychology, linguistics, pragmatics, sociopolitical approaches, cultural studies, and philosophy, among other fields.

That is precisely our pragmatic strategy in this book. We aim to efface transdisciplinary borders via bona fide examples. In targeting different semiotic processes, each contribution combines metatheoretical and empirical moves from both sides, including theoretical synergies, methodological expansions, multilevel approaches, and pluralistic explanations. The evidence presented in a given chapter may be *hatched* within a particular field, but that does not mean that it is *relevant* only to such a field. This premise teems with opportunities to create novel pluralistic theorizations and empirical foundations for neurosemiotics. The hyper-specialization and compartmentalistic nature of scientific fields have hindered the pursuit of the above goals, and they speak more to the structure of academia than to the structure of semiotic processes. Neurosemiotics is a deliberate, albeit preliminary, attempt to subvert this segregationist tradition. This book incarnates a timely, informed hope for disciplinary reorganization.

As previously stated, the prefix "neuro" in "neurosemiotics" should be understood as an abridgement and not as an attempt for neuroscience to conquer the domains of semiotics. Neurosemiotics is not concerned mainly with the examination of neural signatures of classical semiotic or semiological constructs. We pursue epistemic intersections between semiotic capacities beyond the classical divide between biology and culture. Yet, the scope of the field is not to be confounded with that of other disciplines, such as biosemiotics, zoosemiotics, experimental semiotics, or social cognitive affective neuroscience. Although no clear delimitations can be established among these disciplines, neurosemiotics calls for transdisciplinary openness, multilevel explanations, and empirical innovations beyond specific disciplines. As such, neurosemiotics foregrounds a major gap in our academic demarcations of semiotic explananda. No complete theory, definite empirical methodology, or well-established topics should be expected from current neurosemiotics. Neither should one anticipate a unitarian, Carnapian theoretical structure. From academic schisms, to enduring dichotomies between reductionism and transcendentalism, as well as scientific attentional blindness to holistic phenomena, neurosemiotics is not free of classical problems. However, we believe transdisciplinary efforts will provide truly innovative steps enabling us to move forward from current preliminary approaches to an ever stronger field.

The *Handbook* at a glance

This *Handbook* is organized in four parts. Part I (Prolegomena to Neurosemiotics) describes historical, epistemological, theoretical, and methodological foundations of neurosemiotics. Part II (Language and Its Pathways to Meaning) addresses neurocognitive aspects of language and their interplay with bodily, situational, and experiential mechanisms. Part III (The Neurosemiotics of Social Dynamics) is devoted to the biology of social interaction, including insights on spectatorial processes, interpersonal dynamics, and broader societal phenomena. Part IV (Further Semiotic Domains) reaches into other fundamental dimensions of daily semiosis, driven by external signs (faces, music, tools) and internal phenomena (including interoception and the very construal of self).

Part I opens with seminal insights by Kalevi Kull and Donald Favareau. In Chapter 1, the authors provide a historical overview of the discipline and discuss its scope, approaches, and principal problems. They also address key issues for delineating biological accounts of semiosis, such as the process-relation duality, the role of the spatial *Umwelt*, and the importance of codes overall. This work provides basic epistemological anchorage for present and future developments in the field.

Additional core notions are offered by Terrence Deacon in Chapter 2, which charts a fertile theoretical territory at the crossing of semiotics and neuroscience. After expounding the limitations of classical computational approaches to cognition, Deacon draws from Peircean theory to outline an alternative framework articulating the notions of semiosis, sign vehicles, objects, and interpretants. He further argues for a reconsideration of the icon–index–symbol triad, framing the relation among these signs as hierarchical rather than horizontal. Distinct neural mechanisms are postulated as correlates of these constructs, from single neurons to more complex dynamical systems. Overall, this chapter illustrates the profound implications of conceiving human communication, cognition, and experience from an explicit neurosemiotic stance.

A different viewpoint is offered by Antoine Milette-Gagnon, Samuel P. L. Veissière, Karl J. Friston, and Maxwell J. D. Ramstead in Chapter 3. Their work traces connections between Peircean semiotics and active inference, a recent creature-centered framework stemming from Bayesian predictive coding approaches. Peirce's notion of interpretant and the icon/index/symbol triad, the authors propose, can be formulated in terms of active inference and the free-energy principle due to their conceptual analogies (e.g., the notion of abductive inference in living systems). This account invites novel interdisciplinary investigations at the crossing of semiotics, life sciences, and cognitive science to shed light on meaning-making phenomena.

Next, in Chapter 4, Jonas Nölle and Bruno Galantucci introduce experimental semiotics as a framework to investigate communicative interactions with a neurosemiotic spirit. Achievements and challenges of this approach are described across theoretical, methodological, and translational dimensions. A call is made (and shown to have been partly met) for more ecological designs capturing the inception, deployment, and adaptability of human semiotic skills. Progress in this direction proves fundamental for the consolidation of neurosemiotics at large.

Part I concludes with Chapter 5 by Morten Tønnessen, which tackles a broad neurosemiotic question: How much can we learn about other animals by solely comparing them with humans? In his reply, the author adopts von Uexküll's *Umwelt* theory and complements it with insights into the neural code, described as a set of rules that mediate sensory signals and mental images. Emphasis is placed on subject–object relations, including distinctions among species and conspecifics. Such differences are predicated in terms of the *Umwelt* (the outer subjective world) and the *Innenwelt* (the inner subjective world), delimited by a subject's body and intersecting as individuals relate to objects in their surroundings. Finally, Tønnessen ponders on the consequences that the anthropocentric perspective has had for neurobiology studies, limiting our knowledge about animals' inner worlds. *Umwelt* theory, the author concludes, can circumvent this bias.

Part II encompasses eight contributions on a human-specific semiotic faculty: language. We begin with Chapter 6, in which Maya Visser discusses a mainstream account of conceptual processing: the hub-and-spoke model. Visser summarizes evidence from clinical and healthy populations showing that verbal and non-verbal concepts, stemming from the integration of modality-specific systems distributed across the brain, hinge on the integrity and functionality of the bilateral anterior temporal lobe (especially including its ventral portions). Specifications are offered concerning this hub's lateralization, functional particularities, and interaction with executive networks. The model incarnates the non-compartmentalist philosophy of neurosemiotics, adding core constraints towards a full-fledged picture of semantic systems.

Complementary insights are gleaned by Giovanni Buccino in Chapter 7, which posits that language comprehension involves re-enacting the experiences evoked by particular words. Specifically, Buccino focuses on the reactivation of sensorimotor mechanisms during processing of action-related verbs and object-related nouns, and of socio-affective circuits during processing of emotion-laden words. Such evidence supports the role of embodied mechanisms in semantic processing, as proposed by prominent (though hotly debated) neurolinguistic models. By tracing continuities between bodily, neural, and communicative dimensions of human experience, this proposal incarnates some of the core premises of neurosemiotics.

Another distinguishing property of language is the possibility of conveying meanings that exceed literal interpretations. Such is the target of Valentina Cuccio in Chapter 8. Focusing on metaphors, the author delineates key distinctions between literal and figurative language use, contemplating neuroanatomical and electrophysiological aspects. This serves as input for a discussion of competing hypotheses on the nature of figurative language processing. Given its ubiquity in human communication, Cuccio concludes, the study of non-literal language should be central to the neurosemiotics agenda.

Zooming further in, Enzo Tagliazucchi devotes Chapter 9 to discussing neurochemical aspects of semantic processes. He proposes that dopamine and serotonin contribute differentially to salience attribution and semantic meaning attribution, respectively. Relevant neuroscientific findings are introduced alongside novel views on psychiatric symptoms as deficits in these domains. Finally, a neurosemiotic account is set forth with implications for psychological and psychiatric models and treatments.

Reaching beyond word-level approaches to semantics, in Chapter 10 Manuel de Vega challenges mainstream conceptions and posits that syntax, too, fulfils semantic and pragmatic functions during communication. Specifically, diverse grammatical elements are shown to convey meaningful situational information and to help specify reference across interlocutors. Moreover, syntactic patterns and negation markers are proposed to recycle neural networks originally devoted to sensorimotor functions, thus mirroring the embodied dynamics supporting word-level processing. These views help to reconceptualize grammar as a meaning-making neurosemiotic domain, rather than a collection of mere sequencing regularities.

The evidence compiled in the previous chapters comes mainly from tasks employing isolated words, phrases, or sentences. Yet, how often do we actually face such units in a textual vacuum? In Chapter 11, Nicholas Riccardi and Rutvik H. Desai lay the groundwork for a neurosemiotics of naturalistic language processing. The authors survey text-level neuroimaging studies on well-established effects (word frequency, surprisal and entropy, as well as semantic phenomena), considering their modulation by co-textual factors. Moreover, they outline the neuroanatomy of discourse processing, proposing distinct roles for regions such as the anterior temporal lobe, the angular gyrus, the precuneus, and the posterior cingulate. To conclude, the chapter offers critical considerations of the contributions, limitations, and challenges of a neurosemiotic account of discourse-level processing.

Incarnating a different research tradition, Chapter 12, by Nicola del Maschio, Jubin Abutalebi, and Daniela Perani, reminds us that processing language is not always tantamount to processing *only one* language. This piece delves into the intricacies of bilingualism as a window into the interplay among neurocognition, communication, and experiential factors. The authors focus on the organization, dynamicity, and control of the bilingual lexico-semantic system, considering its reconfigurations depending on the age of second-language appropriation as well as the degree of proficiency in, and exposure to, such a language. These views are embedded within an emergentist embodied account, fleshed out by reference to a particular phenomenon: iconicity in bimodal bilinguals. The integrative framework thus outlined opens exciting avenues for a neurosemiotics of bilingual (and, more broadly, multilingual) communication.

Of course, verbal communication is not restricted to oral and written modalities. In Chapter 13, Ruth Campbell analyzes the functioning of deaf people's brains during communication, *vis-à-vis* those of hearing individuals. The author distinguishes between homesign users and sign language users, affirming that the former rely more on iconicity. She then describes the structural and semantic properties of sign languages. In particular, sign language users are proposed to activate the same core language regions implicated in oral language, with differential engagement of the ventral pathway (to process discrete entities) and the dorsal pathway (to process dynamic actions). The chapter concludes with a neurosemiotic reading of the interplay between body and brain in sign languages and beyond.

Part III is concerned with interpersonal and sociocultural dynamics. A central observation is that, to a large extent, communication hinges on resonating with others. Therein lies a central claim of Konrad Lehmann and Philipp Kanske in Chapter 14. The authors sketch a neurosemiotic account of empathy, distinguishing between affective and cognitive dimensions that jointly shape inferences about others' inner states. They discuss the neural bases of these dimensions, their integration during real-life interactions, and the mechanisms through which they influence meaning-making processes. Briefly, this work delineates a neurosemiotic agenda to characterize situated socio-affective dynamics.

Next, in Chapter 15, Sandra Baez provides a multidimensional overview of another critical interpersonal skill: the passing of moral judgments. Baez argues for a neurosemiotic outlook on moral mechanisms. Semiotic, cultural, and psychological insights are integrated with neural, hormonal, and genetic evidence to delineate a socio-biological account of the domain. Through a synergistic view across methods and traditions, this contribution invites a reconceptualization of moral cognition.

The research informing the previous chapters mainly employs single-person paradigms, in which participants face predefined stimuli unaffected by their own behavior. Yet, as Leonhard Schilbach shows in Chapter 16, alternative approaches have emerged in recent years. Schilbach integrates neurosemiotics with second-person neuroscience, a burgeoning field that aims to capture neural signatures of actual interpersonal events. Existing evidence warrants new insights on how people interact, highlighting the role of the mentalizing network as a key neural mechanism supporting dyadic communication. Moreover, the author outlines applied implications for psychiatry and the study of mental disorders in general, laying the groundwork for more ecological translational research on social cognition.

This theme also cuts across Chapter 17, by Arjen Stolk, Jana Bašnáková, and Ivan Toni. Joint epistemic engineering is introduced as a neurosemiotic account of interactive communication. The framework focuses on actual communicative tokens (as opposed to types) while integrating three types of signals: Shannon-signals (deployed to reduce uncertainty over the identity of its referent); Grice-signals (ostensive marks of communicative value); and Peirce-signals (cues aligning possible interpretations across interactants). The authors then argue against a fixed-code view of language and communication, underscoring the import of contextual factors supporting disambiguation, strategic reasoning, and mutual coordination. This is followed by illustrations of the framework's descriptive potential, including insights on relevant neural mechanisms and the consequences of their disruption across disparate disorders. The agenda laid out here enables fruitful reflections on dialogue, negotiation, and other forms of communicative interaction.

In Chapter 18, Claus Emmeche begins by describing the requisites for such a goal, before dissecting a widely publicized study on neural homophily – namely, the detection of greater neurocognitive similarities between friends than between non-related individuals. The critique spans notional, methodological, and epistemic levels, leading to observations on the role of common sense and ethics in the interpretation of neuroscientific results. Overall, Emmeche argues for a multidimensional account of friendship, which integrates semiotic and biological considerations while avoiding strong conclusions from fragmentary data.

Socio-semiotic phenomena are tackled through broader lenses in Chapter 19. Specifically, Anabelle Lukin and David Butt face the challenge of conceiving of ideology in in neurosemiotic terms. The authors criticize traditional neuroscientific studies on the topic, arguing for a new theoretical view informed by linguistic and neurocognitive theories. In particular, ideology is proposed to arise through the evolution of language and to hinge on distinct brain properties, including the size, extent, complexity, metastability, and degeneracy of the brain. Lukin and Butt's interdisciplinary position illustrates how large-scale societal phenomena can productively be reframed on neurosemiotic premises.

Socio-historical considerations also figure prominently in Chapter 20, by Joni Y. Sasaki and Hannah I. Pearson. The authors maintain that, in construing meaning, we are influenced by cultural forces, with religion playing a vital role for myriad individuals. These interactions, they further contend, are modulated by biological factors. As such, insights derived from social science alone will be necessarily partial. Against this background, the authors describe behavioral, neurocognitive, and genetic correlates of distinct cultural and religious profiles, highlighting their impact on daily semiosis.

Part IV covers other semiotic dimensions shaping our daily life. In Chapter 21, Bruno Rossion conceives of human faces as ideal stimuli to understand whole–part relationships and categorization skills. Relying on neurocognitive evidence, he further argues that, beyond sensory processes, face identity recognition also recruits semantic mechanisms. Moreover, this domain is deemed central to reveal important neurocognitive differentiations between people and non-human animals. With a thorough treatment of these issues, Rossion demonstrates the relevance of face processing research for the core agenda of neurosemiotics.

No less central is the role of music, another semiotic realm that sets us apart from multiple species. This is the focus of Amy M. Belfi in Chapter 22. In particular, Belfi integrates behavioral and neurocognitive findings on musical semantics. Pitch, tonality, and rhythm are described as sources of meaning. Moreover, their integration in actual musical pieces can evoke particular emotions, concepts, and cross-modal associations, involving cortico-subcortical networks that mediate more general affective and cognitive processes. The author then summarizes neurophysiological studies showing that particular semantic experiences can emerge quite swiftly upon music perception. In short, this chapter further demonstrates the pervasive role of music in our situated experiences.

In Chapter 23, François Osiurak, Josselin Baumard, Catherine Merck, and Mathieu Lesourd address a deceptively simple question: How do we know how to correctly manipulate a tool? The authors reject the classical hypothesis that ascribes this capacity primarily to semantic knowledge. Conversely, they advance a more complex view involving *both* semantic knowledge and technical reasoning. While semantic knowledge would provide socio-contextual information regarding specific tools, technical reasoning would help us overcome associated mechanical constraints. This account has translational implications, as it illuminates, for example, why people with semantic memory deficits can still properly use a tool. Briefly, Osiurak and colleagues set forth a context-sensitive, enactive account of a key trait in human evolution.

It has not escaped our attention that, in addition to external stimuli, semiotic processes are crucially shaped by inner bodily signals. Such is the focus of Ryan Smith and Sahib S. Khalsa in

Chapter 24. Through an original reconsideration of multidimensional evidence, the authors describe how interoceptive information is signaled, integrated, and interpreted within and across individuals. Disruptions of these processes, they further show, may impact physical and mental health, and with them daily semiosis at large. These insights lay the foundations for a neurovisceral view of our meaning-making capacities.

The volume concludes with Chapter 25, in which Georg Northoff and Diego Gorini propose that the very emergence of self is in constant interplay with semantic phenomena. The authors distinguish among the interoceptive self, the extero-proprioceptive self, and the mental self, which are respectively associated with self-relatedness, self-prediction, and self-referential processing. Original links are proposed between these constructs and the notions of semantic similarity and relatedness, with the former comprising paradigmatic relations (substitutability) and the latter accounting for syntagmatic relations (co-occurrence) in language. Specifically, lower layers of self would be mediated by the brain's short timescales, arguably critical for capturing semantic similarity, whereas higher layers of self would hinge on longer timescales that are also implicated in processing semantic relatedness. These mappings incarnate the transdisciplinary ethos of neurosemiotics, with implications for consciousness studies, linguistics, and cognitive neuroscience.

Looking forward

Traditional approaches have historically tried to domesticate meaning, sensemaking, and other semiotic phenomena via academic demarcations. However, we believe that proper explanations of these issues must overflow disciplinary frontiers. Despite multifarious progress, conceiving these phenomena as purely cultural or purely neurocognitive is epistemically sterile. We hope that current neurosemiotic approaches will not only foreground this caveat, but also provide starting points for its transdisciplinary subversion, with breakthroughs across theoretical, methodological, and translational levels.

Before the development of astrophysics in the nineteenth century, the sun was believed to be made of coal. Different disciplinary approaches then struggled to understand how oxygen and combustion could make that star as durable as it is. Attempts to answer "Why does the sun shine?" continually drew from inadequate approaches to the combustion of an equal mass of coal. This core dilemma was resolved only through transdisciplinary synergy and reorganization, triggered by dialogue among astronomy, psychics, gravitational approaches, geology, and nuclear insights. Present-day neurosemiotics is still made of coal, but we have learned how to move beyond that stage. With its transdisciplinary openness and ongoing theoretical and empirical efforts, this book may provide initial steps for a humbler yet necessary revolution in the study of semiosis.

Funding

Adolfo García is a Senior Atlantic Fellow at the Global Brain Health Institute (GBHI) and is supported with funding from GBHI, Alzheimer's Association, and Alzheimer's Society (Alzheimer's Association GBHI ALZ UK-22-865742); ANID, FONDECYT Regular [1210176]; the Latin American Brain Health Institute (BrainLat), Universidad Adolfo Ibáñez, Santiago, Chile (#BL-SRGP2021-01); and Programa Interdisciplinario de Investigación Experimental en Comunicación y Cognición (PIIECC), Facultad de Humanidades, USACH.

Agustín Ibáñez is supported by grants of Alzheimer's Association GBHI ALZ UK-20-639295; Takeda CW2680521; ANID/FONDECYT Regular (1210195, 1220995); ANID/FONDAP 15150012; ANID/PIA/ANILLOS ACT210096; Sistema General de Regalías (BPIN2018000 100059); Universidad del Valle (CI 5316); BrainLat seed funds; and the Multi-Partner Consortium to Expand Dementia Research in Latin America (ReDLat), funded by the National Institutes of Aging (NIA) of the National Institutes of Health (NIH) under award number R01AG057234, an

Alzheimer's Association grant (SG-20-725707-ReDLat), the Rainwater Foundation, and the Global Brain Health Institute. The content is solely the responsibility of the authors and does not represent the official views of these institutions.

References

Alexandrov, V. (2000). Biology, semiosis, and cultural difference in Lotman's semiosphere. *Comparative Literature, 52*, 339–362. doi: 10.1215/-52-4-339

Amoruso, L., Gelormini, C., Aboitiz, F., Alvarez Gonzalez, M., Manes, F., Cardona, J. F., & Ibáñez, A. (2013). N400 ERPs for actions: Building meaning in context. *Frontiers of Human Neuroscience,* 7, 57. doi: 10.3389/fnhum.2013.00057

Armstrong, P. B. (2019). Neuroscience, narrative, and narratology. *Poetics Today, 40*(3), 395–428. doi: 10.1215/03335372-7558052

Baggio, G. (2018). *Meaning in the Brain*. Cambridge, MA: MIT Press.

Blackman, L., Cromby, J., Hook, D., Papadopoulos, D., & Walkerdine, V. (2008). Creating subjectivities. *Subjectivity, 22*(1), 1–27. doi: 10.1057/sub.2008.8

Bouissac, P. (1986). Semiotics in Canada I. In T. A. Sebeok, & D. J. Umiker-Sebeok (Eds.), *The Semiotic Web* (pp. 191–252). Berlin: Mouton de Gruyter.

Bouissac, P. (1998). *Encyclopedia of Semiotics*. Oxford: Oxford University Press.

Brier, S. (2015). Can biosemiotics be a "science" if its purpose is to be a bridge between the natural, social and human sciences? *Progress in Biophysics and Molecular Biology, 119*(3), 576–587. doi: 10.1016/j.pbiomolbio.2015.08.001

Carey, S. (2011). *The Origin of Concepts*. Oxford: Oxford University Press.

Cosmelli, D., & Ibáñez, A. (2008). Human cognition in context: on the biologic, cognitive and social reconsideration of meaning as making sense of action. *Integrative Psychology and Behavioral Science, 42*(2), 233–244. doi: 10.1007/s12124-008-9060-0

Deacon, T. (1997). *The Symbolic Species*. New York: W.W. Norton.

Deacon, T. W., & Rączaszek-Leonardi, J. (2019). Abandoning the code metaphor is compatible with semiotic process. *Behavioral Brain Sciences, 42*, e224. doi: 10.1017/s0140525x19001419

Emmeche, C., Koppe, S., & Stjernfelt, F. (2000). Levels, emergence, and three versions of downward causation. In P. B. Andersen, C. Emmeche, N. O. Finnemann, & P.V. Christiansen (Eds.), *Downward Causation* (pp. 322–348). Aarhus: University of Aarhus Press.

Falk, E., & Scholz, C. (2018). Persuasion, influence, and value: Perspectives from communication and social neuroscience. *Annual Review of Psychology, 69*, 329–356. doi: 10.1146/annurev-psych-122216-011821

Faust, M. (2012). *The Handbook of the Neuropsychology of Language*. New York: Wiley.

Fiske, S. T., & Taylor, S. E. (2013). *Social Cognition: From Brains to Culture*. Thousand Oaks, CA: Sage.

Halliday, M. A. K. (1978). *Language as a Social Semiotic: The Social Interpretation of Language and Meaning*. Baltimore, MD: University Park Press.

Hodge, B. (2014). Social semiotics. In T. Miller (Ed.), *The Routledge Companion to Global Popular Culture* (pp. 58–66). London: Routledge.

Hoffmeyer, J. (2015). Semiotic individuation and Ernst Cassirer's challenge. *Progress in Biophysics and Molecular Biology, 119*(3), 607–615.

Ibáñez, A. (2019). Insular networks and intercognition in the wild. *Cortex,* 115, 341–344. doi: 10.1016/j.cortex.2019.01.024

Ibanez A. (2022). The mind's golden cage and the cognition in the wild. *Trends in Cognitive Sciences*, https://doi.org/10.1016/j.tics.2022.07.008

Ibáñez, A., & Cosmelli, D. (2008). Moving beyond computational cognitivism: understanding intentionality, intersubjectivity and ecology of mind. *Integrative Psychology and Behavioral Science, 42*(2), 129–136. doi: 10.1007/s12124-007-9045-4

Ibáñez, A., & Schulte, M. (2020). Situated minds: Conceptual and emotional blending in neurodegeneration and beyond. *Brain, 43*(12), 3523–3525.

Ibáñez, A., & García, A. M. (2018). *Contextual Cognition: The Sensus Communis of a Situated Mind*. Heidelberg: Springer.

Ibáñez, A., Sedeño, L., & García, A. M. (2017). *Neuroscience and Social Science: The Missing Link*. Heidelberg: Springer.

Jorna, R. J. (2009). Neurosemiotics. In M. D. Binder, N. Hirokawa, & U. Windhorst (Eds.), *Encyclopedia of Neuroscience* (pp. 2830–2833). Heidelberg: Springer.

Kleinman, A. (1987). Anthropology and psychiatry: The role of culture in cross-cultural research on illness. *British Journal of Psychiatry, 151*(4), 447–454. doi: 10.1192/bjp.151.4.447

Kosoy, M., & Kosoy, R. (2018). Complexity and biosemiotics in evolutionary ecology of zoonotic infectious agents. *Evolutionary Applications, 11*(4), 394–403. doi: 10.1111/eva.12503
Mareschal, D., Quinn, P. C., & Lea, S. E. G. (2010). *The Making of Human Concepts*. Oxford: Oxford University Press.
Mendoza-Collazos, J. C. (2020). On the importance of things: A relational approach to agency: Review article of Malafouris, L. 2013. How things shape the mind: A theory of material engagement. *Cognitive Semiotics, 13*(2). doi: 10.1515/cogsem-2020-2034
Murphy, G. (2004). *The Big Book of Concepts*. London: Bradford.
Peirce, C. S. (1998). *Charles S. Peirce: The Essential Writings*. Amherst, NY: Prometheus Books.
Pessoa, L., Medina, L., & Desfilis, E. (2022). Refocusing neuroscience: Moving away from mental categories and towards complex behaviours. *Philosophical Transactions of the Royal Society B: Biological Science, 377*(1844), 20200534. doi: 10.1098/rstb.2020.0534
Pezzulo, G., Donnarumma, F., Dindo, H., D'Ausilio, A., Konvalinka, I., & Castelfranchi, C. (2018). The body talks: Sensorimotor communication and its brain and kinematic signatures. *Physics of Life Reviews*. doi: 10.1016/j.plrev.2018.06.014
Pezzulo, G., Donnarumma, F., Dindo, H., D'Ausilio, A., Konvalinka, I., & Castelfranchi, C. (2019). The body talks: Sensorimotor communication and its brain and kinematic signatures. *Physics of Life Reviews, 28*, 1–21. doi: 10.1016/j.plrev.2018.06.014
Plebe, A., & De La Cruz, V. M. (2016). *Neurosemantics: Neural Processes and the Construction of Linguistic Meaning*. Berlin: Springer.
Shallice, T. (1988). *From Neuropsychology to Mental Structure*. Cambridge: Cambridge University Press.
Sharov, A., Maran, T., & Tonnessen, M. (2016). Comprehending the semiosis of evolution. *Biosemiotics, 9*(1), 1–6. doi: 10.1007/s12304-016-9262-7
Sharov, A. A. (2016). Evolutionary biosemiotics and multilevel construction networks. *Biosemiotics, 9*(3), 399–416. doi: 10.1007/s12304-016-9269-0
Snow, C. P. (2012). *The Two Cultures*. Cambridge: Cambridge University Press.
Tamm, M., & Torop, P. (2022). *The Companion to Juri Lotman: A Semiotic Theory of Culture*. London: Bloomsbury.
van Hateren, J. H. (2015). The natural emergence of (bio)semiosic phenomena. *Biosemiotics, 8*(3), 403–419. doi: 10.1007/s12304-015-9241-4
Van Leeuwen, T. (2005). *Introducing Social Semiotics*. London: Routledge.

PART I

Prolegomena to neurosemiotics

1
NEUROSEMIOTICS
A brief history of its development and key concerns

Kalevi Kull and Donald Favareau

Introduction

Semiotics is the study of sign processes and sign relations. What are the processes and structures, the systems and mechanisms that are necessary for meaning-making? How are different features and types of interpretation related to different features and types of meaning-making mechanisms? These are the central questions being addressed by biosemiotics. Neurosemiotics is the area that asks these questions in an explicit relationship to the neural components of animals. Bouissac (1998: 446) writes that "neurosemiotics has come to designate a wider subdomain of biosemiotics, including most of the field of inquiry covered by the cognitive neurosciences" (see also Andrews, 2019).

Neurosemiotics – and particularly the neurosemiotics of the human brain – is probably not the right area of semiotics for finding answers to the fundamental questions of biosemiotics *per se*. However, with its particular attention to the *mechanisms* and to the empirical knowledge of the processes that make neural meaning-making possible, neurosemiotics is critically important to every semiotician. Likewise, the importance of neurosemiotics lies in providing the fundamental models of meaning production that are necessary for any neurobiological or neuropsychological study of cognition and consciousness (Favareau, 2002a). Müller and Wolff (2003: 2670) concur: "Interestingly, there is still an obvious theoretical deficit regarding the mechanisms involved in the assignment of meaning on the various organizational levels of the nervous system and in their interaction with the organismic environment." Paradoxically, the majority of neurosemiotic research has been done on humans, while it would obviously be easier to begin with animals whose semiotic repertoire is less diverse.[1]

In 2012, one of founders of the Tartu-Moscow School of semiotics, Vyacheslav V. Ivanov, who wrote about neurosemiotics in the 1970s, was asked: "What are the most pressing problems of contemporary semiotics and the ways of their possible solution?" Ivanov responded:

> In my opinion, one of the most important tasks consists in the development and experimental verification of the basic principles of neurosemiotics, the science of the sign activity of the brain. Its main ideas were outlined long ago, by … psychologist Lev S. Vygotsky and his friend and collaborator Alexander R. Luria, with whom I happened to work together. Neurosemiotics, which develops along with closely related cognitive neuropsychology, explores the division of functions between the brain hemispheres and other parts of the brain, as a person grows up and develops in a cultural sense, taking hold of an increasing

DOI: 10.4324/9781003051817-3

> number of different sign systems and memorizing a significant number of sign texts. The development of neurosemiotics seems to be the key to solve the basic problem of the development of knowledge and the noosphere in the 21st century, that is, a deep understanding of the basic mechanisms of the historical evolution of humanity and an overcoming of difficulties that are increasing along this path.
>
> *(Ivanov, quoted in Velmezova & Kull, 2020: 28)*

In this chapter, drawing mainly from biosemiotic and general semiotic perspectives, we: (1) provide a brief account of the history of neurosemiotics; (2) review the overall scope and aims of neurosemiotic research; (3) list some general problems of neurosemiotics; (4) specify some features of neural systems that are relevant for semiosis; and (5) describe some general features of neurosemiosis.

A brief history of neurosemiotics

Some embryonic neurosemiotics can be found in early medical semiotics (e.g., Sprengel, 1815: 384). An important step was made by Johannes Müller, who formulated the law of specific nerve energies. The modality of sensation, according to Müller (1826), cannot be found in the external causes bringing about the neural excitation. This is an important statement about the arbitrariness that fundamentally characterizes the relation between the internal and external world of neural organisms.

Some pioneers of biosemiotics were also pioneers for neurosemiotics. Among them we find Jakob von Uexküll (1864–1944), whose work on neuromuscular regulation in marine invertebrates in the laboratories of Heidelberg and Naples (e.g., Uexküll, 1905) led to the formulation of a neurosemiotic model of the functional circle (see Berthoz & Christen, 2008). Neurologist Kurt Goldstein (1878–1965) is also considered a pioneer of biosemiotics and neurosemiotics (Andersch, 2016). Friedrich Rothschild (1899–1995) studied the phenomena of hemispheric asymmetry in the 1930s. In the introduction to his work, he wrote that "the starting point, which is far from what is traditional and customary in the natural sciences, is precisely the prerequisite for freeing oneself from the fetters of mechanistic and teleological thinking and finding a new way in *symbolic* thinking" (Rothschild, 1935: x).

In the 1960s, and even more so in the 1970s, language and code metaphors became rather widely used as an approach for conceptualizing life and brain processes (e.g., Perkel & Bullock, 1968; Pribram, 1971). This seemed appropriate because "language" was then often defined in a very general way (e.g., structural elements plus syntax). At that time, semiotics was also seen to be related to cybernetics and neuropsychology (e.g., Deacon, 1976; Ivanov, 1979).

The term "neurosemiotics" appears in print at least as early as 1971. In his review of psychology programs in Canada, Arthur Z. Arthur (1971: 59) writes that the University of Windsor had a course entitled "Neurosemiotics and neurological diagnosis." Since Arthur's survey was carried out in 1969, the term was seemingly already in use in Canada by then.

"Neurosemiotics" is used also by Vyacheslav V. Ivanov (1979) in the title of his article "Neurosemiotics of oral speech and functional asymmetry of the brain." Later, he described the history of the Russian branch of neurosemiotics, with an emphasis on the works of Lev Vygotsky and Alexander Luria (Ivanov, 2014).[2] An influential work on language and the brain was at that time published by Roman Jakobson (Jakobson & Santilli, 1980). On this topic, a symposium entitled "Functional Parallelism Between the Asymmetry of Functions of the Cerebral Hemispheres and the Semiotic Asymmetry of Culture as a Mechanism of Collective Consciousness" was held in 1981 in Tartu, organized as a meeting between neurophysiologists Lev Balonov, Vadim Deglin, and Tatjana Chernigovskaja from St Petersburg and semioticians from Tartu (Balonov & Deglin, 1976; Chernigovskaja, 1995; Lotman, 1981).

Paul Bouissac uses the term "neurosemiotics" in a 1979 paper, writing: "[Y]et there is no doubt that his [Peirce's] rich theoretical contribution, which is now irrigating the semiotic field, is a stimulant to fruitful reflection and could contribute to the formulation of testable hypotheses, possibly in the field of neurosemiotics" (Bouissac, 1979: 49).

Bouissac (1987: 204) later noted that the term "neurosemiotics" was coined in interactions between the Toronto Semiotic Circle (established in 1973) and the research team of the Université de Montréal, headed by André Roch Lecours.

In 1985, a special issue of *Recherches sémiotiques/Semiotic Inquiry (RS/SI)* on the topic of neurosemiotics appeared, edited by Justine Sergent. That issue contained Bouissac's paper on the definition of neurosemiotics (Bouissac, 1985), while the next issue of *RS/SI* published a position paper on neurosemiotics by Jean-Luc Nespoulous (1985).

Additionally, as of this writing, chapters on neurosemiotics have appeared in several handbooks and encyclopedias of semiotics and neuroscience: in Bouissac's *Encyclopedia of Semiotics* (Bouissac, 1998); in the second edition of Nöth's *Handbook of Semiotics* (Nöth, 2000: 258, as a small paragraph on "Neurologische Semiose und Neurosemiotik"); in Posner's et al. *Handbook* (Müller & Wolff, 2003); in a Danish encyclopedia of semiotics (Wallentin, 2007; Brier, 2007); in the *Encyclopedia of Neuroscience* (Jorna, 2009); in Cobley's *Companion to Semiotics* (Favareau, 2010); and in Trifonas's *Handbook of Semiotics* (Cariani, 2015).

Until now, however, only a couple of books have been published that have used the word "neurosemiotics" in their titles (Grzybek, 1993a; Tsvetkov & Pereguda, 2019), along with the special journal issue of *RS/SI* (Sergent, 1985).[3]

Some aspects of neurosemiotic research appear labeled with different terms. The term "neurosemantics" was used already by Alfred Korzybski (1941: xliv) and described by Plebe and Cruz (2016: 4) as the study of "how neural circuits can carry representations of the world … how brain circuits capture knowledge of the external world." We should also not forget the project of "neuropragmatics" as an integral part of neurosemiotics (Schumann 1999; Solymosi & Shook, 2014). According to Bambini and Bara (2012: 1),

> neuropragmatics revolves around the mind/brain processes underlying the construction of context-appropriate meanings for the purpose of the communicative exchange. By taking into account the contextual dimension, neuropragmatics focuses on the activity of communicating, and deals with how communicative agents' minds brains represent and share intentions, beliefs, situations and the various components of context in order to construct a shared meaning and to engage in successful communication.

Neurosemiotics also overlaps with neurolinguistics (e.g., Andrews, 2011; Chernigovskaya & Arshavsky, 2007; Tymoczko, 2021) and its various branches (e.g., neurosyntactics) as well as with biolinguistics and cognitive linguistics.

Also of interest here is the usage of the close term "neurosemiology" in medicine (Lamer, 2002), which follows an old tradition of medical semiotics. Thus, we can see that the development of a proper "neurosemiotics" discipline has been a long time in the making.

Characteristics of research in neurosemiotics

As the study that integrates semiotics and neurobiology, neurosemiotics may be distinguished from psychosemiotics, which is the semiotic study of psychic phenomena without there necessarily being any neurobiological considerations, as well as from the many investigations into mind and brain (e.g., Jean-Pierre Changeux, Gerald Edelman, Antonio Damasio, Joseph LeDoux) that assume a basic underlying semiotic relationship but are not explicitly informed by any prior semiotic theorizing.[4] In practice, of course, all these areas overlap extensively.[5]

Watt (1984: 4) notably predicted that "the future science of 'neurosemiotics' … will study how the cognitive realities demonstrated by psychosemiotics are physically represented in the brain." According to Bouissac (1987: 204):

> [Neurosemiotics] refers to the study of the neurophysiological substrata of the production (encoding) and understanding (decoding) of signs, the perception of the environment as meaningful, both globally and discretely, and the general capacity to engage in symbolic interactions. Neurosemiotics attempts to correlate neurophysiological processes with well-defined aspects of semiotic behavior in order to better understand them and therefore to be able to devise appropriate remedial semiotic strategies when these capacities become impaired because of disease or injury.

Bouissac also added:

> It seems obvious … that neurolinguistics can only be a part, albeit an essential one, of a more inclusive program of scientific inquiry. The term "neurosemiotics" appears to be particularly qualified for the designation of an epistemological domain which includes the scientific investigation of the neurological processes underlying communicative behaviour in all its forms as well as the prerequisites for such behaviour – namely, the capacity for categorizing, structuring, combining, encoding and decoding, etc., that is to say the capacity for making sense out of the environment and for acting vicariously upon it.
>
> *(Bouissac, 1987: 206)*

Favareau, who has written a couple of articles on neurosemiotics (Favareau, 2002a, 2002b), defines the field as

> the study of neuronal sign processes taking place in the central nervous system of organisms, especially the brain, where such processes are thought to enable and coordinate the semiotic accomplishments of perception, representation, categorization and the species-specific varieties of cognition that emerge therefrom.
>
> *(Favareau, 2010: 275)*

Identifying neurosemiotics as a part of biosemiotics (and, within it, endosemiotics), Favareau observes that

> a fully developed neurosemiotics would seek to empirically examine the ways in which individual and collective neuronal events 'stand for' something other than themselves, so as to engender the phenomena of understanding and thought. Given the inability of contemporary neuroscience to bridge the divide between the physical and the mental naturalistically, the future of development research projects such as neurosemiotics seems assured.
>
> *(Favareau, 2010: 275)*

In his review article, Larangé (2010) says neurosemiotics is a new ideological bridge between biological sciences and humanities.[6] The same view was held by Ivanov (2008: 235), who claimed that

> the continuation of neurosemiotic studies promises a breakthrough in understanding those parts of the work of the brain that are most intimately connected to culture. From this point of view semiotics may play an outstanding role in the synthesis of biological science and humanities.

Or, as Weir (1990: 7) points out, "our task is to generate new models of text-processing and of discourse analysis mapped onto neurosemiotic and neurophilosophical schemes."

Relatedly, Jorna (2009: 2830) writes:

> Neurosemiotics is about the sign or signal related aspects of synapses, neurons and neural nets. Because neurons are the physiological tissue within which the brain or mind resides, neurosemiotics is also about cognition or about humans as information processing and connectionist systems.

For their part, van Leeuwen et al. (1992: 979) maintain that:

> Meaning as perceived within the context of neurosemiotics would be a result of classification activities within the brain ... What we propose is to reframe the search for meaning within the language-system, divorced from a material substrate, by an approach wherein the signification processes are studied as embodiments.

Cariani (2015: 918) describes the research program of neurosemiotics as follows:

> If mind is regarded as the functional, informational organization of the brain, then an elaborated neurosemiotic framework that deals in terms of neural codes and signal processing operations becomes in effect a general semiotics of psychological process and mental function. Additional neurophenomenological bridge laws beyond this may be needed in order to account for conscious states and their experiential contents.

A brief account of a neurosemiotic research project was sketched by Brandt (2011: 285). Elkouch (2017) demonstrates the close relationship between neurosemiotics, biosemiotics and cognitive semiotics. A neurosemiotic analysis of hand gestures was provided by Givens (2016) and one of alarm calls was advanced by Queiroz and Ribeiro (2002). Roepstorff (2004) made an interesting attempt to apply the concept of an "actant" in neurosemiotics.

Research on artificial intelligence, starting with its early works (McCulloch & Pitts, 1943), also attempts to solve largely the same problems as neurosemiotics. However, beyond some exceptions (e.g., Cariani, 1995; Emmeche, 2001; Erasmus & Bodenstein, 2004; Jorna et al., 1993; Steels, 2006; Ziemke & Sharkey 2001), explicit links between these approaches have not been made frequently.

Finally, neurosemiotics is not only a scientific discipline, but now also an applied field, used for commercial purposes in marketing, advertising, and consumer studies (Bresinsky et al., 2017; Marques dos Santos, 2018), and for developing the methods of text and picture analysis (e.g., Grzybek, 1993b).

Preconditions for neural semiosis

For a histologist, every tissue is a version or variety of the living structure. The nerves and brain are organs that were primarily discovered and defined on the basis of anatomical, not functional, studies of organisms' bodies – as is the case with many other tissues and organs. Neural tissue exists in a majority of organisms in the animal kingdom, and it appears in rather early stages of their ontogeny. Neural tissue consists of neurons (nerve cells) and neuroglia (glia cells), and it builds the nervous system, which has its peripheral and central parts – the latter including brain in many animals.

Clarifying the specificity of neural tissue in the context of semiosis and ascertaining whether its morphology (certain features of its form) and physiology (the mechanisms of its dynamics and behavior) have some relationship to a particular type of semiosis are the fundamental problems of neurosemiotics. A brain is not a necessary condition for semiosis – as extensively evidenced in biosemiotics, semiosis can obviously occur in living systems without nervous systems. Cognitive (i.e., semiotic) functions have been described in non-neural cells (e.g., Bechtel & Bich, 2021, but see Barandiaran & Moreno, 2006). Likewise, following Thomas A. Sebeok, Nöth (1994: 48–50) lists genetic, immunological, and neurological semiosis. Thus, one of our problems here – and perhaps the central problem for neurosemiotics – is to understand why and how the semiosis in or with neural cells differs from that of its other forms. That this problem is not trivial and that the differences are ill-established has been well demonstrated by Godfrey-Smith (2016).

In a review article for a semiotics *Handbook*, Müller and Wolff (2003: 2667) explain the specificity of nervous systems for semiotic phenomena:

> Nervous systems are characterized by the fact that they build up *internal representations* of all other organs, functional structures and their mediating functional dynamics in the respective organism and of its environment, insofar as these affect the organism via receptors or the organismic effectors modify the perceptible environment. Organ representations include "functional-morphological features" of all sensory systems (sensory organs or dissociated receptor cell systems) and effector organs (muscles, glands) that are connected to the respective nervous system via input and/or output "channels" and allow a "mediated" interaction with the organismic environment. The function of the nervous system is therefore inextricably linked with the ability of this special organ to assign a functionally adequate meaning to phenomena outside and inside the organism, including its own subsystems.

We do not address the phenomenon of consciousness here; instead, we address semiosis, which we believe is a precondition for consciousness (Emmeche, 2004).[7] Thus we start from a more fundamental level, or from more general questions of neurosemiotics, than do the studies that focus on the neural correlates of various mental or psychological or linguistic phenomena.

Assuming that neural tissue is largely and uniquely responsible for enabling animal semiosis, we should specify which of its features make it possible. For this, we first need to ask what is functionally or qualitatively unique to this "animal type" of semiosis.[8]

Semiosis in general – which we describe as *interpretation* – creates *optionality*, makes *choices*, and produces *habits*.[9] Interpretation includes active perception, which requires the use of a search pattern – if only a very simple one. Another necessary condition for interpretation (i.e., semiosis) is the formation of the temporal whole, the finite moment of the present, which we call the "subjective present." Decision-making takes place within this instantaneous, though finite, moment, and its existence is the necessary and sufficient condition for the emergence of the dimension of sign relations.

Primary animal semiosis examines choices that are based on spatial distinctions, which means that more than one point is distinguished simultaneously within the perceptual field. In order for there to be *spatial optionality*, *simultaneous* spatial distinctions must exist, thus requiring the contribution of more than one receptor into the simultaneous perceptual field. In other words, this animal type of semiosis creates subjective *space* – a cognitive map, however simple, wherein decision-making agency can manifest. The primary vegetative *Umwelt* is non-spatial, while the primary animal *Umwelt* is spatial (Kull, 2018a). There is certainly much more than this involved in animal semiosis, but this allows us to specify one aspect of its uniqueness.

Another universal aspect of semiosis is learning – and learning is what produces habits. Habits are based on interpretants, and habits are of two large types: category-related and association-related. Accordingly, learning that deals with pattern recognition can form categories, or re-categorize existing ones; and learning that deals with associations can form and modify the relations between categories.

Thus, we conclude that in order to carry out animal semiosis, the nervous system should be capable of (1) generating at least simple categorical (iconic) cognitive representations (maps), and

Table 1.1 Three broad types of learning made possible by animal nervous systems

Interpretant-based habit types	*Producing and modifying*
Category-generating	Iconic mappings
Association-generating	Associations between mappings
Symbol-generating	Virtual mappings between mappings

(2) establishing indexical associations. Perhaps it is only in the more complexly recursive nervous systems that we see the capacity for (3) human-like symbolic reference (Table 1.1).

Some features of neural cells that are relevant for semiosis

Neurons are very diverse, and glia cells are more so. Simple neurocytes may not be radically different from many other eukaryotic cells; however, the majority of neurons have some peculiar features that may contribute significantly to the uniqueness of animal semiosis.

The branched morphology of neurons – the existence of dendrites and axons – results in very diverse *connectivity* potential. If a cell in a regular parenhymal tissue has in average of 14 immediate neighbors (Thompson, 1942), a neuron, via its synaptic connections, may be in active connection with hundreds or more (10^5 for Purkinje cells), many of which are situated a long distance from each other in a variety of organs and sub-systems. Moreover, the size of the group of cells in which each cell is the immediate neighbor of each other can reach tens in the case of neurons, while no more than five in other tissues – and, of course, the synaptic network of cells of which any neuron may be a part of at any given moment can be vast. Such distributed and intense cell interaction may contribute to the complexity of coherent pattern in the "subjective present."

In addition to the distributed system of neuronal cells, however, a large part of neuroglia the astrocytes – forms a reticulate syncytium (Kiyoshi & Zhou, 2019). The coexistence of discrete (cellular) and continuous (reticulate) cell populations in the same nervous tissue may give rise to a particular type of analog-digital semiosis that Hoffmeyer and Emmeche (1991) call "code-duality."[10]

On the aspect of connectivity, the connections between neurons can be modified by synaptic interaction. High diversity and flexible connectivity make it possible to have large numbers of cellular subgroups that can develop equally flexible synchronicity of state and "representational" power. Crucial in terms of semiosis – and an area in which neural tissue remarkably distinguishes from most other tissues – is its capacity for *plasticity*, which is the ability to actively modulate and change cellular connectivity, both by synaptogenesis and pruning in development, and by the processes of long-term potentiation and depression throughout the lifespan. Such plasticity of connectivity is a precondition for learning and habituation. The quasi-stability of synaptic states (Ballintyn et al., 2019; Citri & Malenka, 2008) may, in turn, be a precondition for the animal-specific phenomenon of decision-making (Kull, 2018b).

Such malleable synaptic connectivity allows for the differentiation of states by synaptic patterns, taking into account that "a neuron with several thousand synapses segregated on active dendrites can recognize hundreds of independent patterns of cellular activity even in the presence of large amounts of noise and pattern variation" (Hawkins & Ahmad, 2016, para. 1). Together with the capacity for pattern differentiation on the level of the groups of synapses, such connectivity provides an infrastructure for the various levels of semiosis in its flexibility of association-making and (at least functional) "labelling" of increasingly complex differentiated states.

The most noted specific feature of neural cells, of course, is their capacity to generate the all-or-nothing conduction of the electrical impulse received. This includes the capacity to modify the impulse, and to either change or not change its own state as a result. Such features have often allowed the neuron to be modelled as if it were a logic gate.

A remarkable feature of such neural excitability is its high *speed*, in comparison with other modes of transfer in organisms, as nerve cells conduct electric impulses extremely well. However, it is obviously not necessary for semiosis to be based solely on electric impulses. Where speed may have a decisive semiotic role, however, is in the creation of the field of synchronous options – that is, of the option-negotiating behavior that characterizes animal semiosis. For options, in order to *be* options, should be presented simultaneously, in the subjective present. While it is not clear what the temporal limit of the "subjective present" is – it certainly varies between species, as shown experimentally by Jakob von Uexküll – in most known cases it is no more than a few seconds or considerably less. Thus, the animal-specific "simultaneity" of option presentation and decision-making must be understood in this sense.

We should mention here that several features of neural tissue can be found also in some other tissues, and not only in the animal kingdom (e.g., Baluška, 2010). Concluding their study on plant movements (e.g., shoot and root tips), for instance, Charles and Francis Darwin wrote that:

> Two, or perhaps more, of the exciting causes often act simultaneously on the tip, and one conquers the other, no doubt in accordance with its importance for the life of the plant. The course pursued by the radicle in penetrating the ground must be determined by the tip; hence it has acquired such diverse kinds of sensitiveness. It is hardly an exaggeration to say that the tip of the radicle thus endowed, and having the power of directing the movements of the adjoining parts, acts like the brain of one of the lower animals; the brain being seated within the anterior end of the body, receiving impressions from the sense-organs, and directing the several movements.
>
> *(Darwin & Darwin, 1880: 573)*

Such phenomena have given rise to arguments that one may even speak about "the neurobiology of plants" (Brenner et al., 2006). However, while phenomena such as the above certainly refer to semiosis in plants, such plant movements can be explained without assuming the kind of spatial *Umwelt* proper to animal semiosis (Kull, 2018a).

Thus, we can conclude that neural tissue has some histological peculiarities that allow for the formation of a variety of temporally coherent subpopulations of cells – similar to the "transient functional clusters" posited by Edelman and Tononi (2000) – wherein the size of these subpopulations can also change. According to our hypothesis, the internal diversity of the network of cells that participate in any given "moment of semiosis" is a contributing factor to the logical and phenomenological richness of semiosis.

Neurosemiosis, or the neural processes that are responsible for the creation of sign-relations

The main scientific task of neurosemiotics is to demonstrate which neural mechanisms are responsible for the particular features of semiosis and sign relations. This research also clarifies what semiosis and sign relations *are*, and in particular what is unique about animal semiosis. Below we offer some remarks that may be especially important for further research.

Process–relation duality

It is important to specify as clearly as possible what we mean by semiosis. Semiosis is the *process* that is responsible for the existence of *sign relations*. Or, less technically, semiosis is the *process of meaning-making*, and thus responsible for the existence of particular *meanings*. Meaning or *sign-relation* is the foundation of knowledge, and a "sign" is an entity of a *logical* kind – that is, accordingly, atemporal and non-local. The *process* that creates the relation, however, belongs to the realm of the empirical, and thus has a duration and locus. This distinction between the sign process (semiosis) and the sign-relation is important and universal. We may call it the *process-relation duality* that characterizes every sign.

A principal feature of the sign *relation* is *aboutness* – the property of a sign *being about* something other than itself. This is the feature that characterizes the phenomenal world and all knowledge. Sign relations were described by Ferdinand de Saussure as binary, by Charles Peirce as triadic, and by Charles Morris as pentadic. Most of semiotics is thus a study of sign relations – for example, types of relations, conditions for various types of relations, systems of relations, etc.

But a sign also has another side, namely the *process* that brings into being the relation, or rather the complex of relation-generating processes. These include the physiological processes and mechanisms needed for the relation to appear – indeed, these are what create and support the relation within and between organisms, and without which such relations could never occur. Some research has attempted to discover these processes – for example, in neurosemiotics, neurolinguistics, neuropsychology, psychosemiotics – and from the biosemiotic evidence we also know that sign-creation is not specific to language or humans, nor even the possession of a brain.

Thus, the sign proper consists of atemporal relations, and of the temporal mechanisms that generate such relations. Accordingly, *every complete model of signs should describe both the relation and the relation-generator*, as depicted in Figure 1.1.

The *relation-generating process* or mechanism is sometimes described as an *interpreting agent*. But here an additional distinction is required. An interpreting agent is commonly understood as an organism,

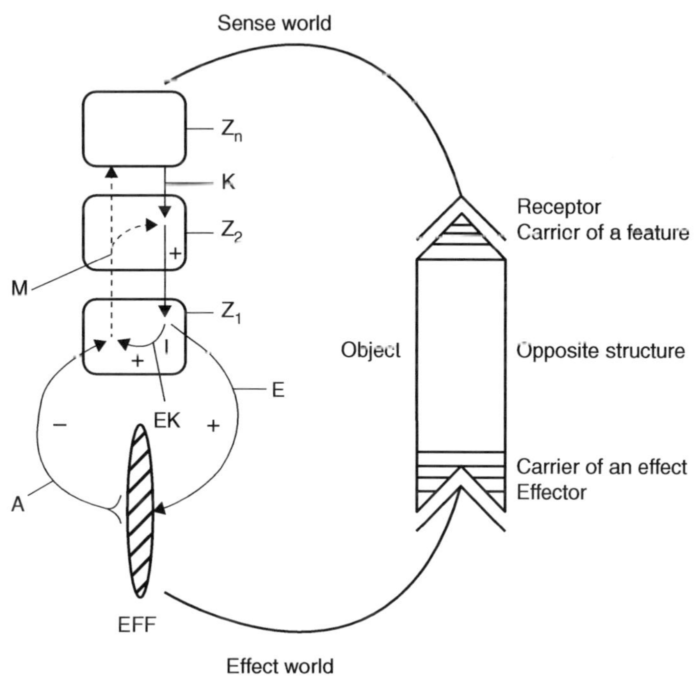

Figure 1.1 Relations and relation-generators

Explicating the process aspect of the process-relation duality is where neurosemiotics can advance of our understanding of sign processes, such as by joining the reafference model of Erich von Holst and Horst Mittelstaedt with the functional circle of Jakob von Uexküll (illustration adapted by the authors).

a cell for instance, that can repeatedly carry on semiosis – that is, the constant negotiation of many signs. Yet, the relation-generator as a part of the sign's nature can be specific and unique for each sign, as much as each sign is specific and unique from any other sign. Indeed, we can say that the relation-creator (or interpretant- or sign-creator) is working precisely at that moment when a relation "becomes" a sign. Thus, the relation-creator is the minimal individual interpreting agent, or sub-agent. It is not the whole brain (or the whole body) that is taking part in the generation of any particular sign-relation. Only some parts of the organism are included in the sign-generating process in the case of each particular sign, and these may not always be exactly the same parts, even in the case of each particular sign.

Thus, in order to provide the complete description of a particular sign, in addition to the sign relation, the relation-generating process should be *localized*, and its *duration* estimated. That is not often done in semiotics, while it is precisely one of the aims of neurosemiotics. It should be understood that the relation-generators are always web-like, which means to some extent distributed. The relation-generator can be modelled as dialogic (or rather polylogic) complex process that may include several organisms, whose contributions are united into the subjective present.

Thus, we suggest accepting the fundamental duality of signs: the relation-process duality.[11] The relation (which is triadic, according to Peirce)[12] is a-temporal and a-spatial, has no locus, and is in-between. At the same time, the process and the mechanisms that manifest the relation anew each time are localizable in the living system (again, no matter how widely distributed), occur exclusively in the subjective present, and have a measurable duration.

Semiosis is the process that creates the simultaneous presence of multiple options

As argued earlier, semiosis is the process that brings together possibilities (options) and choice (Kull, 2018b). The extraordinary, as well as characteristic, property of semiosis is *the state of being confronted with multiple possibilities* – of having more than one way to proceed, with this multiplicity being available for the system to actively negotiate. This state – the space of possibilities (options) – is formed by a complex of processes, which bring the separate channels of acting (including mental action) into a state of ambiguity in which a deliberate reduction of those possibilities, or choice, has to be made under conditions of incomplete regulation, or in the absence of an algorithm determining how to behave.

The state of simultaenous multiple options – the state of indeterminacy – requires a finite duration in order to include the simultaneity of the multiple in one. This is the state of incompatible habits – incompatible in the sense that these cannot be executed simultaneously. Making a choice in such a situation is inescapable. The absence of a controlling algorithm means that the choice itself is free – that is, arbitrary – while more or less motivated. This is where the act of semiosis is different from a logic gate.

Understanding the emergence of the state of simultaneous multiple options is deeply related to the aspect of time (see Schmidgen, 2014). The duration of semiosis is a characteristic that therefore deserves much more serious attention in neurosemiotics, and in semiotics in general.

Codes are the building blocks of semiosis

The history of neurosemiotics reveals that semiosis itself has been imagined or modelled or defined by prior thinkers in at least two very different ways:

1. Neurosemiosis is essentially the encoding and decoding of phenomena. This leads to the model of neuron as a logic gate and, from there, to a computational theory of mind and to algorithmic models of neuronal networks. In this view, semiosis would be a rather complex but deterministic process of the type that modern computers use.
2. Neurosemiosis is based on the active negotiation of simultaneously incompatible options. According to this understanding, all elementary semiotic systems have a certain degree of

freedom (or indeterminacy) in their interpretative (or choosing) processes, mind is essentially non-computational, and semiosis itself is non-algorithmic.

Initially, the distinction between these two views was obscured, as the concept of neural coding may have been thought of as including both possibilities: "The problem of neural coding is defined as that of elucidating the transformations of information in the nervous system, from receptors through internuncials to motor neurons to effectors" (Perkel & Bullock, 1968: 307). However, the critical distinctions soon became more evident with the development of information technologies based on (1), but in which (2) was excluded.[13]

The difference between algorithmic computation and semiosis lies in their relation to choosing. In case of an algorithm, the result is determinate, while in the case of semiosis, possibilities or options exist, action upon which is at least to some extent freely chosen and indeterminate. This implies that the computational view of the brain does not yet tell us much about semiosis. Therefore, we are using the terminology according to which semiosis always corresponds to (2).

Indeed, despite the divide between (1) and (2) seeming rather fundamental, the boundaries between them may often be fuzzy and almost continuous because, in living systems, the extent of freedom can be very small, habituation may have become canalized to the point that it is almost automatic, incompatibility between the codings may be very minimal, or choice may be so strongly motivated that it is extremely predictable. Semiotic freedom always falls along a continuum.

For example, neural codes have been divided into rate codes (if information about the stimulus is encoded by the firing rate of the neuron), temporal codes (which utilize the timing information of spike discharges to signal stimulus identity), or other types of codes (Cariani, 1995; Li & Tsien, 2017; Murphy 2016). It is clear from the definitions that such encodings are components of, and thus preconditions for, interpretative semiosis, and that (1) is thus a mechanized case of (2), i.e., in the majority of cases, such encodings, moreover, are themselves the products of prior semiosis (Figure 1.2).

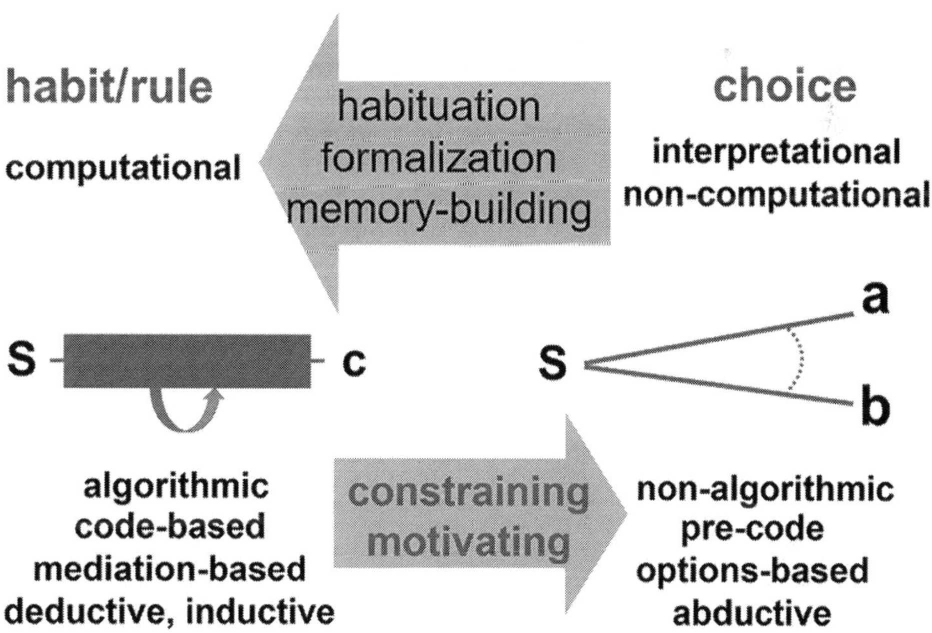

Figure 1.2 Computational and interpretational aspects of neural processes

S: agent; c: action; a, b: possibilities / possible actions. See e-book for a full-color version of this figure.

Neural habituation can thus be seen as canalization of semiosis, but to the extent that it is so automated (i.e., algorithmically determinable) that it does not yet rise to the level of "interpretation," which always requires the agentive negotiation of indeterminacy made possible by the availability of simultaneously incompatible possibilities (options) and choice (Kull, 2020).

To conclude, semiosis as we understand it is non-algorithmic and, accordingly, non-computational – even while including computational algorithmic components.[14]

Habituation quasi-stabilizes the neural structure

From the semiotic perspective, far more important than the particular method of neural encoding is the fact of the code itself – the code as a mediator – because the code provides, and is the means to make, an arbitrary link. This is a principal function of the neural system: to make the links between the organs of perception and organs of action. Moreover, the organs of perception and organs of action could not even exist without such codes – the codes are what necessarily provide functionality to the organs and the cells, the ability to coordinate so as to create singular coherent "actions" (Godfrey-Smith, 2016: 791).

Accordingly, the increasing complexity of nervous systems provides increasing degrees of freedom in making new (arbitrary) sensorimotor links, as well as increasing both their diversity and complexity. The development and modification of such links is integral to *learning* (see, e.g., Shingarov, 1978, as an early work on the semiotic interpretation of "conditioning"), and thus the brain, as well of the rest of the animal nervous system, is also a repository of learned connections, conventions, habits, and codes.

Accordingly, for most organisms, the external environment is much poorer and more homogenous than the internal environment. Therefore, the majority of communication in multicellular organisms is intraorganismal. Neurosemiotics is thus largely endosemiotics, and the relevant categories that are distinguished in cognition (e.g., phonemes, words, concepts, figures, patterns, qualities or their changes) all exhibit signature activation patterns in the brain, as has been demonstrated by brain imaging studies. While these studies are usually semiotically under-informed (but see Cuccio & Gallese, 2018; Deacon, 1997), a good potential use in them exists in establishing the specific temporal and localization aspect of the process side of semiosis's process-relation duality.

The brain, in this sense, provides living space for the ongoing establishment and association of these categories. It is obviously not so important where exactly in the brain the neural assemblies underlying any particular category appear – the more important aspect is that each category requires some space for such assemblies, and the richer the state of simultaneous options, the more space is needed for the synchronous activation of a set of categories.

Conclusion

A fuller explication of a model of semiosis *per se* is necessary in order to be able to identify and understand all the various instances of semioses in a living system – including those manifesting in the brain. While most of semiotics has studied sign relations and their products (sign systems, types of meaning, and meaning-making behavior), the core of neurosemiotics is to study the physiological processes that are responsible for creating sign relations on the neural level. In the context of semiotics as a whole, neurosemiotics occupies a key position in the linking of biosemiotics and anthroposemiotics.

Under the label "neurosemiotics" – a term appearing in print since the 1970s – the research linking neurobiology and semiotics deserves special attention since, in its models, some of the major problems of the emergence of meaning are formulated in a rather minimal and effective way. We thus share the enthusiasm of neurosemiotics expressed by Sarti and Barbieri (2018) when they state:

> The added value of this conception of systemics is dual: with respect to classic semiotic studies, the knowledge about material (physical, electrical, and biochemical) neural fluxes will offer a new complex substance to which to apply semiotic modulation, allowing to rethink semiosis not anymore on a structural basis but as an embodied process. On the other side with respect to classical cognitive neuroscience studies, a post-cognitive dimension is added, where the subject is not anymore generic but this time is situated, singular, social. In any case, we find ourselves at the beginning of a new era of fruitful cooperation between the natural sciences and human studies, in which the interpretative dimension becomes an integral part of modeling practices.
>
> *(Sarti and Barbieri, 2018: 71)*

The richness of animal (including human) semiosis as distinct from the varieties of semiosis found in other living beings is largely dependent on neurosemiotic mechanisms. As we have described, neuronal organization has some relevant peculiarities that contribute to the emergence of a spatial *Umwelt* and a diversity of distinctions accessible to animal semiosis. The next steps in understanding the holism of neuro-sensory-motor systems require the modelling of meaning-making that includes both the physiological sign-creating processes and the specific sign-relations emerging in semiosis. The development of a rigorous and semiotically informed discipline of neurosemiotics will play a key role in this expansion of our understanding of animal life and mind.

Acknowledgements

We thank the biosemiotics group of the Department of Semiotics of the University of Tartu for helpful discussion, and a reviewer and the editors of this volume for good suggestions. The research was supported by the grants PRG314 (Estonia) and National University of Singapore AcRF A-0003116-00-00.

Notes

1 Arguably, neuroscientist Eric Kandel's work on learning and memory in *Aplysia*, which recall Jakob von Uexküll's earlier work on *Echinoidea* and *Ophioglypha*, is a notable exception here – although, like most such work, it is not informed by any rigorous conceptualization of semiosis *per se*.

2 On V.V. Ivanov's work in neurosemiotics, see Grzybek (1991). See also Ivanov (1993).

3 Cf. Sendlmeier, 1996.

4 An interesting exception to this would be the work of neuroscientist Joaquin Fuster (2003), which develops the notion of a minimal representation-bearing neuronal unit that he calls a *cognit,* and that is based directly on Uexküll's concept of the *Funktionskreis* or "perception-action cycle" understood as a neural circuit.

5 See more on the definitions of psychosemiotics and neurosemiotics in Grzybek (1993c).

6 See also García et al. (2020).

7 N. Katherine Hayles (2017) uses the term "non-conscious cognition" in a similar sense.

8 See more on this topic in Kull (2018b). Note, too, that this distinction between what we are calling "animal semiosis" and "vegetative semiosis" may not precisely coincide with the boundary of the kingdom *Animalia.*

9 This can be seen as corresponding to the Peircean triadic model of sign: optionality being first, choice-making second, and habituation third.

10 The code duality principle has several independently developed parallels – for instance, Allan Paivio's dual coding theory, Fred Dretske's analog and digital encoding, and Juri Lotman's principle of multiple coding.

11 This relation–process duality of sign *is not* what has been described as the wave–particle duality or the signifier–signified duality or the type–token duality or the code–duality or the dual process theory. However, it is analogical to these.

12 Such sign relations are sometimes described instead as affordances; we could rather say that affordances *are* sign relations, and may be examined and defined more precisely as such.

13 The distinction between (1) and (2) has some correlation with the differences between structuralism and post-structuralism. Views corresponding to (1) were rather widespread in the semiotics of 1960s and 1970s, when cybernetics and semiotics were developing hand in hand. Since the 1980s, however, (2) has become more frequent in semiotic research. We can see a shift from (1) to (2) at around the same time in the works of Umberto Eco and Juri Lotman. The code duality principle of Hoffmeyer and Emmeche (1991) is a version of (2). It is remarkable that there exist both (1)-type and (2)-type readings of Peirce's semiotics.

14 This view is shared by biosemiotics and enactivism – see, for instance, De Jesus (2018).

References

Andersch, N. (2016). Kurt Goldstein – ein Pionier der Neurosemiotik? *Schriftenreihe der DGGN, 22*, 93–112.

Andrews, E. (2011). Language and brain: Recasting meaning in the definition of human language. *Semiotica, 184*, 11–32. doi: 10.1515/semi.2011.020

Andrews, E. (2019). Semiotic principles in cognitive neuroscience. In M. Silvera-Roig, & A. López-Varela Azcárate (Eds.), *Cognitive and Intermedial Semiotics* (pp. 1–10). New York: IntechOpen.

Arthur, A. Z. (1971). Applied training programmes of psychology in Canada: A survey. *Canadian Psychologist/ Psychologie Canadienne, 12*(1), 46–65. doi: 10.1037/h0082074

Ballintyn, B., Shlaer, B., & Miller, P. (2019). Spatiotemporal discrimination in attractor networks with short-term synaptic plasticity. *Journal of Computational Neuroscience, 46*, 279–297. doi: 10.1007/s10827-019-00717-5

Balonov, L. J., & Deglin, V. L. (1976). *Sluh i rech dominantnogo i nedominantnogo polusharij*. Saint Petersburg: Nauka.

Baluška, F. (2010). Recent surprising similarities between plant cells and neurons. *Plant Signaling and Behavior, 5*(2), 87–89. doi: 10.4161/psb.5.2.11237

Bambini, V., & Bara, B. G. (2012). Neuropragmatics. In J.-A. Östman, & J. Verschueren (Eds.), *Handbook of Pragmatics* (pp. 1–22). Amsterdam: John Benjamins.

Barandiaran, X., & Moreno, A. (2006). On what makes certain dynamical systems cognitive: A minimally cognitive organization program. *Adaptive Behavior, 14*(2), 171–185. doi: 10.1177/105971230601400208

Bechtel, W., & Bich, L. (2021). Grounding cognition: Heterarchical control mechanisms in biology. *Philosophical Transactions of the Royal Society B*, 376: 20190751, 1–11. doi: 10.1098/rstb.2019.0751

Berthoz, A., & Christen, Y. (Eds.) (2008). *Neurobiology of* "Umwelt": *How Living Beings Perceive the World*. New York: Springer.

Bouissac, P. (1979). Semiotics and surrealism. *Semiotica, 25*(1/2), 45–58. doi: 10.1515/semi.1979.25.1-2.45

Bouissac, P. (1985). Neurosemiotics, a definition. *Recherches sémiotiques/Semiotic Inquiry, 5*(3), 223–224.

Bouissac, P. (1987). Semiotics in Canada I. In T. A. Sebeok, & J. Umiker-Sebeok (Eds.), *The Semiotic Web 1986* (pp. 191–252). Berlin: Mouton de Gruyter.

Bouissac, P. (1998). Neurosemiotics. In P. Bouissac (Ed.), *Encyclopedia of Semiotics* (pp. 446–447). Oxford: Oxford University Press.

Brandt, P. A. (2011). CogSem notes: Studies and issues in cognitive semiotics. *Chinese Semiotic Studies, 5*(1), 281–286. doi: 10.1515/css-2012-0124

Brenner, E, D., Stahlberg, R., Mancuso, S., Vivanco, J., Baluška, F., & von Volkenburgh, E. (2006). Plant neurobiology: An integrated view of plant signaling. *Trends in Plant Science, 11*(8), 413–419. doi: 10.1016/ j.tplants.2006.06.009

Bresinsky, P., Schießl, M., & von den Brincken, C. (2017). Nerven – Zeichen – Wege: Erkenntnisse der Neurosemiotik für erfolgreiche Außenwerbung. *Transfer: Werbeforschung & Praxis, 4*, 39–44.

Brier, S. (2007). Neurosemiotik II. In: T. Thellefsen, & B. Sørensen (Eds.), *Livstegn: Encyklopædi semiotik.dk* (pp. 219–223). Copenhagen: Haase Forlag.

Cariani, P. (1995). As if time really mattered: Temporal strategies for neural coding of sensory information. *Communication and Cognition – Artificial Intelligence, 12*(1/2), 161–229.

Cariani, P. (2015). Sign functions in natural and artificial systems. In P. P. Trifonas (Ed.), *International Handbook of Semiotics* (pp. 917–949). New York: Springer.

Chernigovskaya, T. (1995). Cerebral asymmetry: A neuropsychological parallel to semiogenesis. In U. Figge (Ed.), *Language in the Würm Glaciation: Acta Coloquii* (55–66). Heidelberg: Universitätsverlag.

Chernigovskaya, T. V, & Arshavsky, V. V. (2007). Olfactory and visual processing and verbalization: Cross-cultural and neurosemiotic dimensions. In M. Plümacher, & P. Holz (Eds.), *Speaking of Colors and Odors* (pp. 227–238). Amsterdam: John Benjamins.

Citri, A., & Malenka, R. C. (2008). Synaptic plasticity: Multiple forms, functions, and mechanisms. *Neuropsychopharmacology, 33*(1), 18–41. doi: 10.1038/sj.npp.1301559

Cuccio, V., & Gallese, V. (2018). A Peircean account of concepts: Grounding abstraction in phylogeny through a comparative neuroscientific perspective. *Philosophical Transactions of the Royal Society B*, 373: 20170128. doi: 10.1098/rstb.2017.0128

Darwin, C., & Darwin F. (1880). *The Power of Movement in Plants*. London: Murray.

Deacon, T. (1976). Semiotics and cybernetics: The relevance of C. S. Peirce. In System and Structure Study Group (Eds.), *Sanity and Signification: Essays in Communication and Exchange*. Washington, DC: Fairhaven College Press.

Deacon, T. (1997). *The Symbolic Species: The Co-evolution of Language and the Brain*. New York: W.W. Norton.

De Jesus, P. (2018). Thinking through enactive agency: Sense-making, bio-semiosis and the ontologies of organismic worlds. *Phenomenology and the Cognitive Sciences*, *17*, 861–887. doi: 10.1007/s11097-018-9562-2

Edelman, G., & Tononi, G. (2000). *A Universe of Consciousness: How Matter Becomes Imagination*. New York: Basic Books.

Elkouch, H. (2017). Semiotics of living systems: From neural signs to genotext. *Ansaq*, *1*(2), 143–163.

Emmeche, C. (2001). Does a robot have an *Umwelt*? Reflections on the qualitative biosemiotics of Jakob von Uexküll. *Semiotica*, *134*(4), 653–693. doi: 10.1515/semi.2001.048

Emmeche, C. (2004). Causal processes, semiosis, and consciousness. In J. Seibt (Ed.), *Process Theories: Crossdisciplinary Studies in Dynamic Categories* (pp. 313–336). Philadelphia, PA: Kluwer.

Erasmus, L. D., & Bodenstein, C.P. (2004). RealNeurons, artificial intelligence based on the mechanisms of biological intelligence. *IEEE Africon*, 423–428. doi: 10.1109/AFRICON.2004.1406708

Favareau, D. (2002a). Constructing representema: On the neurosemiotics of self and vision. *S.E.E.D. Journal*, *2*(4), 3–24.

Favareau, D. (2002b). Beyond self and other: On the neurosemiotic emergence of intersubjectivity. *Sign Systems Studies*, *30*(1), 57–100. doi: 10.12697/SSS.2002.30.1.05

Favareau, D. (2010). Neurosemiotics. In P. Cobley (Ed.), *The Routledge Companion to Semiotics* (pp. 275–276). London: Routledge.

Fuster, J. M. (2003). *Cortex and Mind: Unifying Cognition*. Oxford: Oxford University Press.

García, A.M., Franco-O'Byrne, D., & Ibáñez, A, (2020). Neurosemiotics: Blurbing a field beyond the "two cultures divide." In: L. Lacková, C.J. Rodríguez Higuera, & K. Kull (Eds.), *Gatherings in Biosemiotics XX* (pp. 92–97). Tartu: University of Tartu Press.

Givens, D. B. (2016). Reading palm-up signs: Neurosemiotic overview of a common hand gesture. *Semiotica*, *210*, 235–250. doi: 10.1515/sem-2016-0053

Godfrey-Smith, P. (2016). Individuality, subjectivity, and minimal cognition. *Biology & Philosophy*, *31*, 775–796. doi: 10.1007/s10539-016-9543-1

Grzybek, P. (1991). Neurosemiotik – Kultursemiotik: Farbwahrnehmung und Farbbezeichnung als Beispiel eines integrativen Konzepts. In L. Eimermacher, & P. Grzybek (Eds.), *Zeichen – Text – Kultur* (pp. 97–186). Bochum: Universitätsverlag Brockmeyer.

Grzybek, P. (Ed.) (1993a). *Psychosemiotik – Neurosemiotik: Psychosemiotics – neurosemiotics*. Bochum: Universitätsverlag Brockmeyer.

Grzybek, P. (1993b). A neurosemiotic perspective on text processing. In H. H. Brownell & Y. Joanette (Eds.), *Narrative Discourse in Neurologically Impaired and Normal Aging Adults* (pp. 47–74). San Diego, CA: Singular Publishing Group.

Grzybek, P. (1993c). Psychosemiotics – neurosemiotics: What could/should it be? (Introduction). In P. Grzybek (Ed.), *Psychosemiotik – Neurosemiotik: Psychosemiotics – neurosemiotics* (pp. 1–14). Bochum: Universitätsverlag Brockmeyer.

Hawkins, J., & Ahmad, S. (2016). Why neurons have thousands of synapses: A theory of sequence memory in neocortex. *Frontiers in Neural Circuits*, *10*(23), 1–13. doi: 10.3389/fncir.2016.00023

Hayles, N. K. (2017). *Unthought: The Power of the Cognitive Nonconscious*. Chicago: University of Chicago Press.

Hoffmeyer, J. & Emmeche, C. (1991). Code-duality and the semiotics of nature. In M. Anderson & F. Merrell (Eds.), *On Semiotic Modeling* (pp. 117–166). Berlin: Mouton de Gruyter.

Ivanov, V. V. (1979). Nejrosemiotika ustnoj rechi i funkcionalnaja asimmetrija mozga. In M. A. Šeljakin (Ed.), *Lingvisticheskaya semantika i semiotika 2* (pp. 121–142). Tartu: Tartu State University.

Ivanov, V.V. (1993). Neurosemiotics and neurobiology. *Semiotica*, *94*(1/2), 103–121. doi: 10.1515/semi.1993.94.1-2.0

Ivanov, V. V. (2008). Semiotics of the 20th century. *Sign Systems Studies*, *36*(1), 185–244. doi: 10.5840/signsystems200836151

Ivanov, V.V. (2014). Cultural-historical theory and semiotics. In A. Yasnitsky, R. van der Veer, & M. Ferrari (Eds.), *The Cambridge Handbook of Cultural-Historical Psychology* (pp. 488–516). Cambridge: Cambridge University Press.

Jakobson, R., & Santilli, K. (1980). *Brain and Language: Cerebral Hemispheres and Linguistic Structure in Mutual Light*. Bloomington, IN: Slavica.

Jorna, R. J. (2009). Neurosemiotics. In M. D. Binder, N. Hirokawa, Nobutaka, & U. Windhorst (Eds.), *Encyclopedia of Neuroscience* (pp. 2830–2833). New York: Springer.

Jorna, R.J., van Heusden, B., & Posner, R. (Eds.) (1993). *Signs, Search, and Communication: Semiotic Aspects of Artificial Intelligence*. Berlin: Mouton de Gruyter.

Kiyoshi, C. M., & Zhou, M. (2019). Astrocyte syncytium: A functional reticular system in the brain. *Neural Regeneration Research, 14*(4), 595–596. doi: 10.4103/1673-5374.247462

Korzybski, A. (1941). *Science and Sanity: An Introduction to Non-Aristotelean Systems and General Semantics* (2nd ed.). New York: Institute of General Semantics.

Kull, K. (2018a). On the logic of animal *Umwelten*: The animal subjective present and zoosemiotics of choice and learning. In G. Marrone, & D. Mangano (Eds.), *Semiotics of Animals in Culture: Zoosemiotics* 2.0 (pp. 135–148). New York: Springer.

Kull, K. (2018b). Choosing and learning: Semiosis means choice. *Sign Systems Studies, 46*(4), 452–466. doi: 10.12697/SSS.2018.46.4.03

Kull, K. (2020). Codes: Necessary, but not sufficient for meaning-making. *Constructivist Foundations, 15*(2), 137–139.

Lamer, A. J. (2002). *A Dictionary of Neurological Signs: Clinical Neurosemiology*. New York: Springer.

Larangé, D. S. (2010). La neurosémiotique: Un nouveau pont idéologique entre les sciences humaines et la biologie. *Protée, 38*(3), 39–52. doi: 10.7202/045615ar

Li, M., & Tsien, J. Z. (2017). Neural code – neural self-information theory on how cell-assembly code rises from spike time and neuronal variability. *Frontiers in Cellular Neuroscience, 11*(236), 1–9. doi: 10.3389/fncel.2017.00236

Lotman, J. (1981). Doklad 13 marta 1981 goda. Manuscript in *Juri Lotman Semiotics Repository*. Tallinn: Tallinn University.

Marques dos Santos, J. P. (2018). Social and cultural consumer neuroscience getting insights into consumers' brain function (and other people too). *Livro Actas, 3*, 14–34.

McCulloch, W. S. & Pitts, W. (1943). A logical calculus of the ideas immanent in nervous activity. *Bulletin of Mathematical Biophysics, 5*, 115–133. doi: 10.1007/BF02478259

Müller, A., & Wolff, J. R. (2003). Semiotische Aspekte der Neurophysiologie: Neurosemiotik. In R. Posner, K. Robering, & T.A. Sebeok (Eds.), *Semiotics: A Handbook on the Sign-theoretic Foundations of Nature and Culture* (pp. 2667–2698). Berlin: Walter de Gruyter.

Müller, J. (1826). *Zur vergleichenden Physiologie des Gesichtssinnes des Menschen und der Thiere: Nebst einem Versuch über die Bewegungen der Augen und über den menschlichen Blick*. Leipzig: C. Cnobloch.

Murphy, E. (2016). Evolutionary monkey oscillomics: Generating linking hypotheses from preserved brain rhythms. *Theoretical Linguistics, 42*(1/2), 117–137. doi: 10.1515/tl-2016-0005

Nespoulous, J.-L. (1985). Neurosemiotics: Structures, processes and strategies. *Recherches sémiotiques/Semiotic Inquiry, 5*(4), 383–392.

Nöth, W. (1994). Opposition at the roots of semiosis. In W. Nöth (Ed.), *Origins of Semiosis: Sign Evolution in Nature and Culture* (pp. 37–60). Berlin: Mouton de Gruyter.

Nöth, W. (2000). *Handbuch der Semiotik*. Stuttgart: Metzler.

Perkel, D.H., & Bullock, T.H. (1968). Neural coding. *Neurosciences Research Program Bulletin, 6*(3), 221–348.

Plebe, A., & Cruz, M. de la V. (2016). *Neurosemantics: Neural Processes and the Construction of Linguistic Meaning*. New York: Springer.

Pribram, K. H. (1971). *Languages of the Brain: Experimental Paradoxes and Principles in Neuropsychology*. Englewood Cliffs, NJ: PrenticeHall.

Queiroz, J., & Ribeiro, S. (2002). The biological substrate of icons, indexes, and symbols in animal communication: A neurosemiotic analysis of vervet monkey alarm calls. In M. Shapiro (Ed.), *The Peirce Seminar Papers 5* (pp. 69–78). New York: Berghahn Books.

Roepstorff, A. (2004). Cellular neurosemiotics: Outline of an interpretive framework. In J. Schult (Ed.), *Biosemiotik – praktische Anwendung und Konsequenzen für die Einzelwissenschaften* (pp. 133–154). Berlin: VWB Vlg. F. Wissenschaft.

Rothschild, F. S. (1935). *Symbolik des Hirnbaus: Erscheinungswissenschaftliche Untersuchungen über den Bau und die Funktionen des Zentralnervensystems der Wirbeltiere und des Menschen*. Basel: Karger.

Sarti, A., & Barbieri, D. (2018). Neuromorphology of meaning. In D. Compagno (Ed.), *Quantitative Semiotic Analysis* (pp. 55–74). New York: Springer.

Schmidgen, H. (2014). *Hirn und Zeit: Die Geschichte eines Experiments 1800–1950*. Berlin: Matthes & Seitz.

Schumann, J. H. (1999). A neurobiological basis for decision making in language pragmatics. *Pragmatics & Cognition*, 7(2), 283–311. doi: 10.1075/pc.7.2.03sch

Sendlmeier, W. F. (Ed.) (1996). Mentale Repräsentation von Zeichen. *Zeitschrift für Semiotik, 18*(2/3), 163–313.

Sergent, J. (Ed.) (1985). Special issue on Neurosemiotics. *Recherches Sémiotiques/Semiotic Inquiry, 5*(3), 221–335.

Shingarov, G. K. (1978). *Uslovnyy refleks i problema znaka i znacheniya*. St Petersburg: Nauka.
Solymosi, T. & Shook, J. R. (Eds.) (2014). *Neuroscience, Neurophilosophy, and Pragmatism: Brains at Work with the World*. London: Palgrave Macmillan.
Sprengel, K. (1815). *Handbuch der Semiotik*. Runkel: Till Verlag.
Steels, L. (2006). Semiotic dynamics for embodied agents. *IEEE Intelligent Systems*, *5*(6), 32–38. doi: 10.1109/MIS.2006.58
Thompson, D'A. W. (1942). *On Growth and Form*. Cambridge: Cambridge University Press.
Tsvetkov, A. V., & Pereguda, S. N. (2019). *Nejrosemiotika: Mozg, simvol i kontekst*. St Petersburg: Knig Kom.
Tymoczko, M. (2021). *Neuroscience and Translation*. Tartu: University of Tartu Press.
van Leeuwen, E., Dillmann, R., & Broekman, J. (1992). Neurosemiotics – the loss of reference. In M. Balat, J. Deledalle-Rhodes, & G. Deledalle (Eds.), *Signs of Humanity, Vol. 2: Semiotics in Action* (pp. 969–980). Berlin: Mouton de Gruyter.
Velmezova, E. & Kull, K. (2020). Vyacheslav Vsevolodovich Ivanov o semiotike. *Kritika i semiotika*, *2*, 9–33.
von Uexküll, J. (1905). *Leitfaden in das Studium der experimentellen Biologie der Wassertiere*. Kalundborg: Bergmann.
Wallentin, M. (2007). Neurosemiotik II. In T. Thellefsen & B. Sørensen (Eds.), *Livstegn: Encyklopædi semiotik.dk* (pp. 216–219). Copenhagen: Haase Forlag.
Watt, W. C. (1984). As to psychosemiotics. In R.P. Fawcett, M.A. K. Halliday, S.M. Lamb, & A. Makkai (Eds.), *The Semiotics of Culture and Language* 2 (pp. 3–28). Mineola, NY: Dover.
Weir, L. (1990). Neurophilosophy and text semiotics. *The Semiotic Review of Books*, *1*(1), 7.
Ziemke, T., & Sharkey, N. (2001). A stroll through the worlds of robots and animals: Applying Jakob von Uexküll's theory of meaning to adaptive robots and artificial life. *Semiotica*, *134*(4), 701–746. doi: 10.1515/semi.2001.050

2

STEPS TO A SEMIOTIC COGNITIVE NEUROSCIENCE

Terrence W. Deacon

Cognition explained away

Semiosis: The missing link

Breakthroughs in neuroscience have accelerated at an incredible rate. This has been aided by new tools for observing brain activity *in vivo* during all manner of cognitive tasks. Using animal models to analyze neural function at the cellular and molecular level has provided incredible detail concerning the function of neurons and the connections between them. Cognitive science has also expanded to become one of the fastest growing areas of experimental research. It has revolutionized what once was a largely qualitative science by taking advantage of the logic of computer algorithms to precisely analyze, simulate, and test models of mental processes. Thus, both at the molecular-cellular and the functional levels, cognitive neuroscience seems poised to uncover some of the deep mysteries of brain function. Yet, this accumulation of ever-increasing detail about brain functions and cognitive processes still seems no closer to bridging a critical explanatory gap: the link between neural activity and mental experience.

In many respects, the promise of cognitive science has been predicated on the assumption that the computational metaphor could either explain or explain away this experiential feature of cognition. Nevertheless, there has always been a dilemma lurking at the very heart of this paradigm. Computation is ultimately just a re-description of a machine's operation, in which each machine state is assigned a representational interpretation and each distinct semiotic operation is mapped to a machine operation. From a computational perspective, each representational relation is simply assigned by fiat. It is the product of a separate extrinsic re-description assigned by a designer/user, and not anything intrinsic to the machine. Therefore, applying this metaphor to brain function passes the explanatory buck to an already assumed interpretive perspective. Following this to its logical implications can only result in an eliminative conclusion (i.e., that representation is epiphenomenal) or a pan-psychic/pan-semiotic conclusion (i.e., that all physical processes are also semiotic processes). Both effectively collapse the mind/matter distinction and successfully pass the explanatory buck.

Cognitive neuroscientists widely use the term "representation" in the literature, but without a clear definition (Vilarroya, 2017). Worse, by setting aside the messy issues involved in understanding the nature of representational relationships, cognitive explanations tend to alternate between and combine two alternative computational paradigms, often characterized as algorithmic (symbolic)

 DOI: 10.4324/9781003051817-4

processes and neural network (sub-symbolic) processes. This distinction, based on a generic conception of symbolic representation, has a long prehistory that is entangled with the history of logic, mathematics, and linguistics. One aim of the present analysis is to re-complexify this conception of "symbol," and thus expose the hidden infrastructure that computational approaches ignore.

Nevertheless, treating cognition algorithmically and in terms of connectional networks has had a pragmatically valuable effect: cognitive neuroscience has been remarkably productive precisely because it did not need to confront underlying semiotic issues. So long as the problem of explaining representation could be provisionally set aside and treated as an unanalyzed mapping relation, the correlations between brain processes and cognitive activities could be studied with the same sorts of analytical tools as used by other physical sciences. Within this framework, identifying a correlation between engaging in a particular cognitive task and observing heightened neural activity in an anatomically distinct brain region has become the gold standard of cognitive neuroscience. How the neural activity is causally related to the phenomenal experience of that process remains for philosophers to ponder.

However, this amounts to a methodological dualism. Is this unavoidable? I do not think so. It is just that studying the relationship between neural processes and mental experiences has been impeded by lack of a bridging language in which both physical and semiotic attributes can be co-defined. In this respect, semiotic theories might have the potential to help overcome this methodological dualism, since it is the goal of semiotic analysis to characterize different modes of representational relationship and explain the processes that give rise to them. In other words, semiotic theories directly address the very issues that cognitive neuroscience has bracketed. Unfortunately, semiotic theory has mostly been explored within the humanities, debated in philosophy and employed in the arts. What might be described as "semiotic science" is for the most part undeveloped. Hence, until now, this potential has mostly gone unrealized.

If we are to have any hope of reversing this trend and to develop tools that are useful for analyzing neurocognitive functions in semiotic terms, we must, on the one hand, deconstruct some of the non-semiotic assumptions that have become the unspoken foundation of contemporary cognitive neuroscience and, on the other hand, find ways to ground semiotic theory in physical processes.

The non-semiotic framing of cognitive science

In a computational framework, any inferential process that can be completely described in terms of the manipulation of sign-tokens can be instantiated by the operations of a machine. This is often described as the Church-Turing conjecture (for a review, see Copeland, 2020) and became the default assumption of computational cognitive science after Newell and Simon (1972, 1976). The idea was that machine operations could substitute for the corresponding human mental operations to manipulate representational tokens or their equivalents. Presumably, all that would be required would be an appropriate mapping between meaningful sign-token manipulations and transformations between machine states that preserve sufficient isomorphism.

An advantage of the computational paradigm, which enabled it to eclipse the behavioristic paradigm that preceded it during the first half of the twentieth century, was that algorithms were structures interpolated between inputs and outputs that could be of indefinite complexity. Unlike introspective descriptions or behavioral input-output mappings, algorithms can be described and analyzed precisely to any arbitrary level of detail. If any act of cognition can be modeled as the manipulation of representational states according to some algorithm, then it would seem that cognition can be studied empirically by just analyzing the syntax of the algorithm.

Yet, like behaviorism, this algorithmic conception of cognition effectively bypasses any need to explain the experience of mental representation ("aboutness"), and therefore is agnostic about the semiotic aspects of cognition. In many respects, the computational model of cognition can be conceived as an extension of behavioristic logic into the hidden structures that mediate between inputs and outputs. This is nicely exemplified by the recently popular "neural net" approaches to cognition.

Consider, for example, a typical neural net classifier that can be trained to recognize spoken English words as distinct from nonword sounds. The system is "trained" by providing the analogues of rewards and punishments in the form of strengthening and weakening connection strengths with respect to their correlated involvement in contributing to correct or incorrect classifications. A fully trained neural net is effectively an algorithm that is structured to produce the desired input-output mapping given complex input data. Representation is reduced to a mapping relation that is implicitly prefigured in the pattern of extrinsically assigned correct and incorrect correspondence relations.

A recently attractive alternative to computationalism is provided by dynamical systems approaches to cognition (e.g., Ward, 2001), but they, too, are largely antagonistic to any theory of mental representation. They instead invoke the "structural coupling" of brain dynamics with environmental dynamics. Although few would disagree with the view that the immediate neurological correlate of sensory experience is a change in the dynamical activity of certain brain structures, the fact is that some dynamical "coupling" alone has little explanatory value. The challenge is to determine what specific complex sort of dynamical relationship constitutes the neurological competence to recognize and act with respect to the only partially predictable constraints and dynamics of the environment. Dynamical coupling does not distinguish simple efficient causal relationships from representation relationships, yet it is precisely the *non-efficient aspects* of semiotic relationships that demand explanation. Therefore, like the computational metaphor, this too evades rather than addresses the problem of explaining mental representation.

The remainder of this chapter sketches the outlines of a theory that reinterprets semiotic theory in neurophysiological terms and reanalyzes brain functions in semiotic terms. The second section begins by shifting the focus of semiotic analysis to the process of generating interpretants – mental sign production – and away from treating sign vehicle properties as the basis for their referential function. It focuses on iconic interpretation as the basic neurosemiotic operation from which all higher order semiotic relations are derived. The chapter takes up the challenge of mapping this semiotic interpretive logic to the neurological processes that support them. It argues that iconic interpretant generation involves evoking dynamical attractor patterns of neural activity within distinct cortical areas, and explores the relationship between cortical architecture, interpretant differentiation, and the restructuring of mnemonic processes by symbolic language.

Semiotic preliminaries

Semiosis: The process of interpreting

In many respects, semiotic theory is the complement to computational theory. Its primary concern is to explain the nature of representational relationships and to make sense of the different modes of representation and how they are interrelated. Central to this approach has been the reframing of representation in terms of the concept of "sign." This shift in emphasis was introduced by the father of modern semiotic theory, Charles Sanders Peirce (1839–1914), in part to avoid the psychologism of the late nineteenth century, in which the concept of mind was taken as an unanalyzed container of ideas and assigner of meaning. For Peirce, sign relations are discrete phenomena that can be characterized by distinctive physical and relational properties, which determine their relationships with one another and how this constitutes their referential and pragmatic effects. Yet, what is most relevant for cognitive science is the way this shift of emphasis breaks down the distinction between communication and thought. A central claim of Peircean semiotics is that "We think only in signs" (CP 2.302).[1] This implies that there should not be a different set of concepts used for studying minds and studying communication.

From this perspective, cognition *is* semiosis: the process of producing and interpreting signs. In this way, Peirce described the process of mental interpretation in terms that did not invoke the actions of a mind, but rather only as a process involving the production of signs. In these terms, interpretation is a physical process with a specific form. Signs are not reducible to mere tokens, as in computational paradigms, and interpretation is not reducible to the mere manipulation of tokens. The physical tokens are not signs in themselves, but are sign vehicles (the term I will use here instead of Peirce's neologism "representamena"). A sign, for Peirce, is a complex relation among three components: a sign vehicle; what it refers to (which he called its *object*); and another sign that establishes this link (which he called an *interpretant*; about which more will be said below). But the physicality of all of these phenomena, their relationships to one another, and their production in the interpretive process suggest that a bridge between the physical and representational aspects of mental processes might be possible in these terms.

According to this perspective, the process of interpretation is the second-by-second development and differentiation of sign relations that emerge with the generation of signs in response to other signs. It is a process that can be observed both outside and inside interpreters. In this respect, the signs that are labeled in our various taxonomies are not abstract categorical types. From a cognitive point of view, they should rather be understood as transient phases in a process of interpretation. This suggests a departure from the way semiotic terminology is most commonly used. In the analysis of semiotic relationships in the arts or humanities, for example, it is common to label certain events or tokens as signs of a particular type. But when the focus turns to the interpretive process, as is necessary to adapt semiotic analysis to mental processes, this structuralist tendency is unhelpful. For if semiotic theory is to be useful for cognitive neuroscience, semiotic classification must ultimately be regulated by a theory of the generation of semiotic relationships in which the homunculus of an interpreter is replaced by a process analysis. The necessity of this approach is implicit in Peirce's introduction of the concept of an interpretant.

An interpretant is a sign generated in the process of interpreting another sign. It is a mediating sign that is necessary to endow a given sign vehicle with its link to something it can thereby represent. Thought is in this sense a physical sign-generation process, which may be confined entirely within the brain, coupled to muscular activity, or involve the interactions of agents. The central role played by interpretant production makes semiotic relationships retrospective in an important sense. Although the presence of a sign vehicle precedes the generation of its interpretant in time, its semiotic function (i.e., that which makes it a sign rather than a mere event or artifact) is assigned *post hoc* by this process of interpretant generation. In other words, the semiotic function of a given sign vehicle only comes into existence after the process of interpretant generation is completed. Although superficially it might appear that the interpretant necessarily follows the sign in time, this way of phrasing things makes the mistake of assuming that a given sign vehicle is already a sign *of something* before it is interpreted. This does not imply, as is sometimes suggested, that because an interpretant is also a sign vehicle, interpretation is indefinitely postponed. The interpretant is not the interpretation. Rather, it is the physical process of interpretant generation itself that transforms a non-efficient possible relationship into an efficient actual relationship. The semiotic process is a normal physical process, but one that introduces new efficient causal relationships into the world.

Semiotic affordances

Iconic reference depends on shared formal properties between the sign vehicle and what it refers to. For example, with a bit of imagination, a face can be discerned on the full moon or in a cloud formation, and this experience might even remind you of someone you know. Yet, there are often innumerable similarities between any two phenomena. The fact of shared form, therefore, cannot determine iconism. It is the interpretive use of a particular similarity that matters. Moreover, simply failing to notice a distinction can be sufficient to ground iconic reference, as when a color-blind person confuses unripe and ripe fruit. This shows us that it is not the similarity in the sign vehicle and object that matters, but rather whether the interpretations given to them differ. The determinative role of interpretive competence is particularly evident in the case of highly complex and abstract forms of iconism. Consider, for example, a mathematical equation. Peirce argues that an equation refers iconically, but only once you know how to discern its symbol-mediated isometry (e.g., between the structure of the equation and a corresponding geometric or dynamical relationship). It can only be interpreted to be iconic (e.g., of a parabolic trajectory) if one knows how to discern the way progressive differences in the results of operations on the various symbolic elements of the equation correspond to progressive differences in the positions of points constituting the geometric object of reference. Thus, recognizing its holistic iconicity is the conclusion of a multistep interpretive process that may extend over a considerable period of time. It is necessarily preceded by a number of iconic, indexical, and symbolic interpretive stages in the process of constructing this final complex interpretant.

Indices refer by correlation in space, time, or contiguity deriving from a common substrate. A simple correlation can therefore be the ground for indexical reference. For example, a lipstick smear on a man's shirt collar can be a troublesome indication to his wife, a urine scent on a branch can be a sexual index to a female lemur, and the mobbing call of a small bird can indicate the present of a raptor. What gets correlated and how (physical, cultural, or evolutionary, respectively) is arbitrary, but the *fact of correlation* is not. A rat in a Skinner box that has been trained to press a bar in response to a bell in order to get a water reward has learned that the bell is an index of the state of the apparatus even though this pairing was the whim of an experimenter. The arbitrary pairing does not make the one a symbol of the other. For the rat, what matters is discovering this correlation so it can use the bell to indicate the availability of water. Although the particular physical properties of the bell sound have no intrinsic relationship to water, learning the reliable temporal correlation with the water reward makes it an index. Analogously, repeated pairing over the course of generations in the evolution of a species can similarly be the basis for an innate tendency to interpret something indexically. This is the case for the indexicality of a vervet monkey alarm call sound, its correlation with the presence of a type of predator, and the urge to engage in an appropriate defense activity or escape behavior (such as climbing a tree to avoid a leopard).

What matters, then, is the interpretive process and how it makes use of selected sign vehicle attributes. In the terms of ecological psychology (e.g., Gibson, 1966), the attributes of sign vehicles that are selected to bring to mind a given object of reference are merely "affordances." Depending on the interpretive process, they can be used or ignored.

Deconstructing the code analogy

Since the beginnings of philosophy, human cognition has been analyzed in terms of our most familiar publicly available aid to thought: language. Not only did linguistics contribute critically to the initial development of cognitive science, along with computational theory, but many cognitive theories have been explicitly framed in linguistic terms. This is only natural since language is the principal means by which we convey our thoughts to one another.

Yet, treating language as a generic mode of cognition inverts the developmental and evolutionary relationships between language and other communicative and mental functions. In evolutionary terms, language is an unprecedented, most recent, most divergent, most highly differentiated form of animal communication, and its role in organizing cognition is likely also a recent overlay on much more ancient and basic mental processes. In semiotic terms as well, language is dependent on a complex infrastructure of more basic semiotic processes.

Ironically, the study of language and its neurological underpinnings is an area of cognitive science research that has long suffered from a lack of semiotic sophistication. A major reason for this is that the unprecedented symbolic mode of referring is often treated as though it is self-evident and simple, when it is in fact the most distinctive and atypical mode of reference to have evolved in the animal kingdom. Failure to recognize that symbolization is not just generic representation collapses a critical distinction that obscures its dependence on a vast infra-symbolic foundation.

In most linguistics texts, symbolization tends to be treated as an arbitrary (unconstrained) mapping relation between two classes of objects: signifiers (e.g., words) and what they signify (e.g., concepts). From this perspective, linguistic reference appears to be as simple as possible, involving minimal defining criteria compared with other forms of reference. When conceived in these terms, symbolic reference tends to be defined negatively, as a reference that does not depend on either iconic or indexical criteria and that is thus arbitrary. From this point of view, symbolic reference seems primary, while both iconic and indexical reference forms are treated as the more complex and derived forms.

Nonetheless, this superficial characterization is deeply flawed. This negative way of defining symbols only tells us that neither formal likeness nor factual correlation is used as the basis for symbolic reference. This fails to specify exactly how the symbolic referential relation is established. It merely passes the buck, so to speak, to some assumed and unexplained means by which reference is established, often described as convention (discussed in more detail below).

First, consider the nature of "arbitrariness." All semiotic relationships include some degree of arbitrariness because those attributes that are taken as the ground for the sign–object linkage can be chosen from many dimensions, and only some will be utilized. In this respect, anything can be chosen as a sign vehicle to represent anything else by any mode, depending on the interpretive process involved. For example, depending on the interpreter and social context, the same facial grimace can be interpreted as a sign of pain, a neurological disorder, or the communication of social censure. By the same token, the sight of smoke can be seen to resemble a cloud, to indicate a fire, or to signal the election of a pope. The relevant property is selected by the interpreter and what is being referred to depends on the capacity of the interpreter to use that property in a particular way.

Hence, although it has become common to call conventional sign vehicles *symbols*, this shorthand terminology has obscured a critical distinction. The current vernacular that calls alphanumeric characters *symbols* only reflects the fact that these characters have been developed explicitly over millennia to express symbolic relations. When your computer begins randomly spewing alphanumeric characters onto your screen, they are interpreted as indications of a malfunction, not as symbolizing anything.

Equating symbolic reference with mere conventional correspondence also ignores a complex semiotic infrastructure, since convention itself is a consequence – not a cause – of semiotic processes. Conventions do not just exist by fiat: they are shared interpretive habits that must be created or discovered. Social conventions in particular need to be created semiotically – that is, by communicating. To avoid circularity, then, we need to understand how conventional forms of communication are created using nonconventional semiotic processes.

As Charles Peirce pointed out over a century ago, we must distinguish properties of a sign vehicle (e.g., a drawing or spoken word) from properties taken to link it to its object of reference. Symbolic reference involves a conventional type of sign vehicle that additionally represents its object of reference in a conventionally mediated way. Something can be considered symbolic, then, only if the property determining its relationship to what it refers to is also due to a shared rule or convention. Symbols are in this sense doubly conventional. They are conventionally derived sign vehicles that refer to things via conventionally determined means. Yet this implies they must be derived from other sorts of referential relationships that are involved in the creation of these two levels of conventionality, and these must ultimately rest on a nonconventional foundation.

So, instead of using the term "symbol" to refer to a conventional sign vehicle, as is common in a computational paradigm, semiotic theory reserves the term "symbol" for sign forms that are doubly conventional. This helps distinguish symbolic reference from conventional iconic (e.g., the typographical smiley face) and conventional indexical reference (e.g., a military salute), as well as from nonconventional iconic (a face in the clouds) or indexical (a loud bang) relations. Because of this doubly conventional aspect, symbolic reference is necessarily more complex and more demanding of interpretive work than iconic and indexical relations. To construct these conventional frameworks presupposes antecedent semiotic work in which prior iconic and indexical processes are required. This means that to explain the neurological basis of symbolic interpretive competence, it is necessary to have already explained how brains interpret things iconically and indexically.

Nested interpretive dependencies

Probably the most important contribution of semiotic theory to the analysis of mental functions will derive from recognizing the hierarchically nested dependency of the three canonical modes of representation relationships: icon, index, and symbol. They are most often treated as mutually distinct sign categories defined by the relationship between the properties of the sign vehicle and the properties of its objects (described above). However, this taxonomic classification ignores a deeper constructive relationship between these modes of reference. This is because these defining affordances are not what determines the mode of reference. As noted above, anything can be taken as a sign representing anything else in any respect (e.g., icon, index, or symbol) if an appropriate interpretation process is generated. Neither the intended interpretation of a produced sign nor any intrinsic properties of a given sign vehicle determine its semiotic function. Intrinsic sign vehicle features can at best constrain and bias interpretation. It is the form of the interpretive process that matters. Yet, as noted above, the interpretation process also consists in the production of other signs – interpretants – and it is the pattern of this interpretive sign production process that determines how a given sign relation is differentiated.

As an example of this hierarchic interpretive process, consider how one might go about interpreting the significance of a windsock (Figure 2.1). Imagine, if you will, a naive traveler observing a windsock through a window, having never seen one before. What interpretive steps would be necessary for the traveler to recognize that it indicates the strength and direction of the wind? Her interpretive competence will depend on knowing that fabric and similar materials (e.g., clothing, umbrellas, palm trees, sails) will tend to hang vertically unless something lifts them. It will also depend on the experience of seeing flags being blown horizontal by a strong wind. Observing the windsock stretched out will thus tend to bring the memory of these experiences to mind, if only dimly and vaguely. These remembered experiences are initial interpretant signs invoked by their similarity in form to that of the extended windsock. Although invoked spontaneously without effort, their generation is the recognition of an iconism (maybe only experienced as a sense of vague familiarity). Nevertheless, each of these memories also has something else in common with the others: an association with the experience of wind. This is an additional secondary iconism shared between these initial interpretants. It might be described as an *insight* because it is effectively a perception of features of the perceptual process itself. Hence, this additional iconism among the invoked memories comprises a higher order iconism, which is the interpretant that must be generated in order to infer that the windsock indicates something not currently experienced: the strength and direction of wind. Without recognizing an initial iconism between the windsock and these remembered experiences, and without recognizing the additional iconism also shared by these remembered experiences – the presence of wind in each instance – there could be no such inference and no indexical interpretation of this invisible inferred correlate of the windsock's behavior.

Of course, this interpretive capacity can also be made more complex. Discovery of the indexicality of a windsock can be augmented with additional iconic and indexical features. The distinctive tubular form of the cloth-like material and its placement on a pole so it can rotate freely can be given an additional interpretation. Whereas the initial recognition of this indexical relation is merely a unique instance, these other features of the windsock can be seen as non-incidental to its intended semiotic function. The windsock might therefore also be recognized as a conventional device designed specifically for this indicative purpose. Its distinctive form and its presence in a context where wind

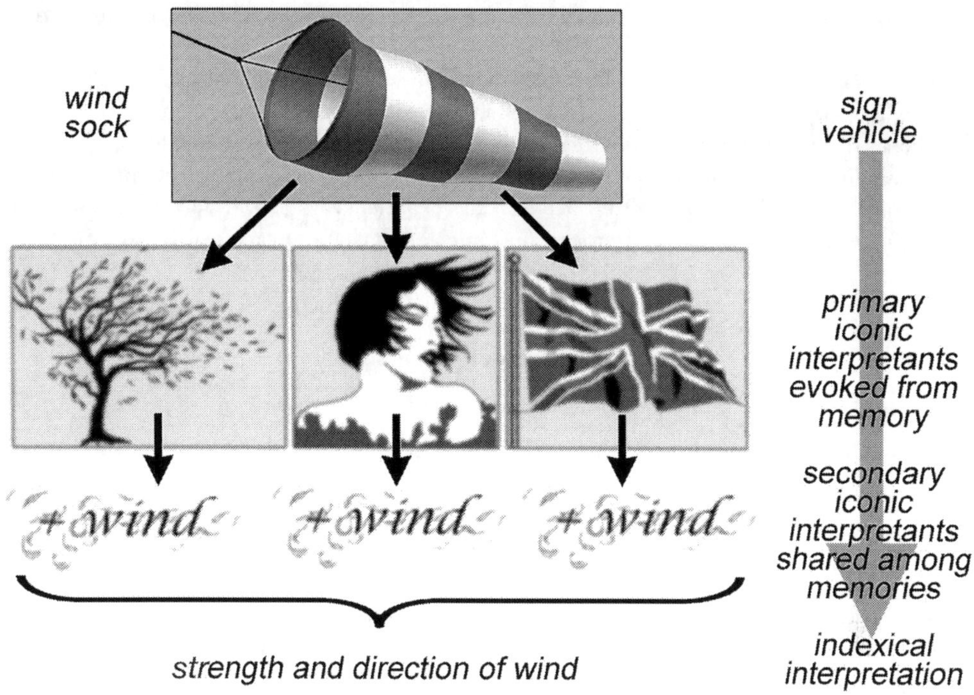

Figure 2.1 Example of an index interpretation process

Schematic depiction of the two-phase process of interpreting a windsock to be an index of the strength and direction of wind. A two-phase two level interpretant generation process is depicted. The three images shown are intended to represent "mental images" serving as initial iconic interpretants invoked from memory by the sight of the windsock. The second phase is the recognition of an additional iconism linking all these memories that becomes the basis for inferring the unobserved indicated feature: the wind.

strength and direction might have special relevance (e.g., an airport) can now further contribute to interpreting the windsock as a conventional type of sign rather than as merely an accidental one-of-a-kind occasion that provides this information.

Of course, all this mental activity necessary to achieve this indexical inference can take place in a fraction of a second. The memories do not need to be rendered in any detail, just barely differentiated to the point that their higher order iconism is thereby evoked. With experience, as this interpretive habit is developed, the entire process will be distilled by a kind of least-work tendency to strip away all unnecessary detail so this interpretive infrastructure becomes automatic and nearly unconscious. Yet, without recognizing an initial iconism between features of the windsock and these remembered experiences, and without recognizing the additional iconism between these remembered experiences (i.e., that wind was also part of each experience), there can be no such implicit inference and no indexical interpretation.

Notice that, in this example, interpreting the windsock as an index was a function of generating multiple levels of iconic interpretants – icons in response to the windsock and higher order icons in response to certain similarity relationships among these icons. In this sense, the indexical interpretation is a sign relation of a higher order than the iconic interpretations upon which it is based. This logic can be generalized as follows: *interpretation involves the production of lower-order signs that bring a more developed sign into existence, with iconic signs representing the lowest order.* Thus, every sign is the result of a developmental progression through a series of recursive phases of increasing semiotic complexity until the process stops because of its sufficiency for a given pragmatic end. Both where the process starts and where it stops determine a level of iconism – the point at which further distinctions can be ignored.

To generalize the point of this example, the transition from one interpretive phase to the next higher phase is made possible by the generation of lower-order signs (mentally generated interpretants) along with their relationships to one another. This additional multiple sign-generation process required to interpret a newly experienced sign comprises a complex interpretant (which may involve many steps) that mediates between the experienced sign and what it refers to. Thus, an internal mental sign-production process (interpretant generation) can create increasingly more developed signs.

Semiotic neuroscience

A dynamical basis for cortical iconism

Understanding the hierarchical logic of interpretant generation has two important neurosemiotic implications: first, it suggests that the fundamental neurosemiotic process is iconic interpretation;[2] second, it suggests that the generation of higher order forms of sign relations (like indexicality) is the result of recursively generating iconic interpretations of other iconic interpretations. In neurological terms, this suggests that the basic neurological operation is the generation and recognition of iconic relationships and that there need not be any neural structures specialized for indexical and symbolic functions. These higher order semiotic processes are instead a function of differences in the interrelationships between different modalities and levels of iconic interpretation processes. It also suggests that the process of generating iconic interpretants is at the same time both a perceptual and behavioral activity because generating a pattern of neural activity can both interpret sensory input and be linked to extrinsic effectors. For this reason, it should not surprise us that the basic cellular architecture of the cerebral cortex does not differ radically from sensory-specialized to motor-specialized cortical areas, except in the relative numbers of cell types in the different layers and patterns of afferent innervation and efferent targets. It also suggests that, in many respects, perception is a form of action and action is a form of perception.

To claim that the fundamental semiotic function of a cortical area is iconic is only partly helpful. Even if we accept this hypothesis, it begs what is still one of the most fundamental questions of neuroscience: How is this iconism realized neurologically?

In the 1960s, David Hubel and Torsten Wiesel used single cell recordings to demonstrate that individual neurons in the cat's visual cortex were differentially responsive to distinct features in distinct positions within the visual field. By 1981, when Hubel and Wiesel were awarded the Nobel Prize in Medicine for this work, single neuron recording was considered the gold standard for understanding neural function. Currently, there still is a tendency to look to the correlations between single neuron activity and extrinsic phenomena to explain how the brain represents the world.[3] In part, this is consistent with a computational conception of brain function, in which discrete structures with precise "memory addresses" comprise the fundamental unit of information storage. Yet, critics have long suspected that this attribution of high-level function to individual neurons is too simple (Brette, 2019; Yuste, 2015). It is often caricatured as a *reductio ad absurdum* by imagining a specialized "grandmother neuron" that encodes the appearance of one's grandmother.

An alternative to a single neuron approach was provided by the work of the University of California, Berkeley neuroscientist Walter Freeman, beginning in the 1980s – see Freeman & Skarda (1990) and, more recently, Cossert et al. (2003) as well as Breakspear (2017). Recording from distributed extracellular sources on the olfactory bulb of rabbits, he found that recognition of distinctive odors was associated with distinctive dynamical patterns of activity. In the terminology of dynamical systems theory, these patterns of activity are called "attractors" because they are not precise but just highly internally redundant and distinct from each other and from the more chaotic background from which they emerge. This led him to propose a distributed population-level approach to memory retrieval and perception, and to reject single neuron representational approaches.

Although this approach is still not mainstream, this is due in part to the fact that we currently lack technology capable of analyzing the complex attractor dynamics generated in networks of thousands of interacting neurons. Recent challenges to what can be described as neuron-level function have come from a number of sources. Two kinds of evidence are typical. The first type of evidence comes from long-train stimulation studies that suggest that complex distributed and highly coordinated patterns of neural activity can produce complex naturalistic behaviors in experimental animals – see the recent study and review by Halley et al. (2020). This is reminiscent of cortical stimulation effects reported by the neurosurgeon Wilder Penfield in the 1950s (e.g., Penfield & Rasmussen, 1950). He reported that stimulation of the exposed cortex of neurosurgery patients could sometimes elicit complex memories and percepts (Penfield, 1958). The second type of evidence comes from long-term or repeated recordings from single neurons. Contrary to the expectations of neuron-level theories, these studies demonstrate that neurons do not retain correlated response tendencies despite stable retention of the function attributed to them (Schoonover et al., 2021). This suggests that individual neurons are merely playing a supportive role in a larger collective function, and that their correlations with extrinsic features merely reflect their particular position and contribution to the collective activity.

A musical melody is a useful metaphor for a dynamical attractor. Moreover, it provides a useful way to conceive dynamical iconicity. A musical motif can be recognized by its distinctive harmonic modes and patterns of tonal transitions even when it is subject to considerable variation, ornamentation, fractionation, and juxtaposition with countermelodies. A neurological dynamic attractor would be subject to similar variations on an underlying theme, and be able to be superimposed with other similar attractors or induce resonant patterns of activity in linked areas. In addition, the presence of ongoing activity would not be particularly surprising in a system where representations are created and retrieved dynamically via the correlation of spatiotemporal patterns and resonant themes. Ongoing background activity would also facilitate entrainment of similar or complementary attractors that tend to resonate with each other dynamically. Moreover, an attractor forming from "noisy" ongoing activity can be analogized in such a way that a complex melody can be formed by resonance with simpler incessantly playing melodies. In contrast, from a neuron-centric conception, ongoing activity is considered noise because it has no recognized function in systems where representations are statically encoded.

Although these considerations do not offer definitive support for a distributed dynamical theory of cortical recognition and memory, they are consistent with it and inconsistent with the neuron-level alternative. From a neurosemiotic point of view, then, distributed dynamical attractors provide ideal models for cortical iconic interpretant production, as well as being suggestive of a resonance-like model for the generation of higher order iconic interpretive processes.

Counter-current information processing

An important property of iconism, which is also consistent with a dynamical attractor perspective, is that iconism is a graded phenomenon. Any two patterns can be judged to be more or less iconic of one another in some respect. This is a critical feature enabling the massive parallelism of brain functions. Such a distributed parallelism is most evident in large mammal brains.

Consider visual cortical areas. In macaque monkey brains, over a dozen distinct cortical areas have been identified and each appears to be specialized to respond to distinct aspects of visual input. This fractionation of visual analysis enables areas to be specialized to discriminate some distinct class of features, such as colors, contours, topology, relative location, direction of movement, and so forth. Fractionation and parallel processing of visual features are facilitated both by "vertical" input–output connections with subcortical systems and by "horizontal" input–output connections with other

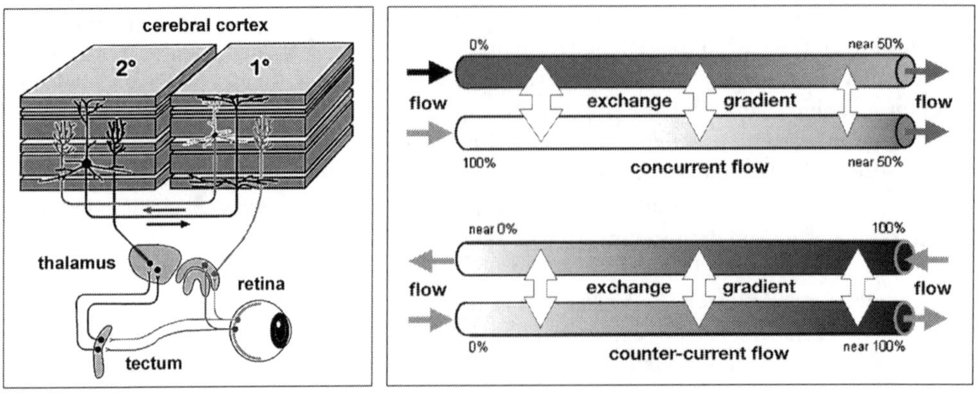

Figure 2.2 Illustration of inter-areal connections in the brain

Left panel: Adjacent cortical areas within a modality are connected reciprocally by cortico-cortical connections that originate and terminate in different layers depending on their relative direction in a gradient with respect to how directly connected the area is to peripheral receptors (or effectors). Connections from more peripherally specialized (1°) areas to less peripherally specialized (2°) areas originate from pyramidal neurons in superficial layer III and have axons terminating in a columnar pattern within layers IV and III. Reciprocal connections tend to originate from pyramidal calls in deeper layer V and terminate in a sheet-like patter in layers I and VI. Right panel: Two alternative models of dynamical exchange processes, such as in molecular or heat exchange, are shown; generally described as concurrent and counter-current exchange processes. It is hypothesized that the reciprocal connection pattern that links adjacent cortical areas functions analogous to counter-current exchange. In thermodynamic and physiological processes counter-current exchange can drive diffusion processes far beyond equilibrium by virtue of the way it optimizes the gradient between juxtaposed media originating from sources with highly divergent values. Neuro-semiotically this is analogous to optimizing similarity between divergently structured signal patterns (e.g., interacting iconic interpretants). Redrawn from Deacon (2016).

cortical areas. Vertical connection differences between cortical areas are reflected in differences in thalamic input. At one extreme is the cortical area that is often (misleadingly) described as "primary visual cortex" because it receives fairly direct, minimally processed inputs related from the retina via the lateral geniculate nucleus. Yet, the majority of functionally distinct visual cortical areas receive relatively indirect preprocessed visual information from midbrain structures. These area-specific functional discontinuities are integrated with one another by virtue of cortico-cortical connections. Each visual cortical area is reciprocally connected with adjacent visual cortical areas. To make things even more complicated, these cortico-cortical connections are organized in ways that reflect each area's relative "position" in an iconic differentiation hierarchy.

This connectional asymmetry between cortical areas is reflected in differences in the source and target cortical layers of neuron cell bodies and their projections, respectively (Figure 2.2). The basic asymmetric geometry of these connection patterns can be described as linking peripherally specialized areas at one extreme (receiving minimally preprocessed input) to arousal and motivationally specialized areas at the other extreme (receiving input from limbic and paralimbic sources). Depending on the species, there may be as many as five or six interconnected areas bridging between these cortical extremes. In general terms, this reflects a flow of sensory information "inward" toward brain systems mediating generalized arousal and an inverse flow of attentional-arousal information "outward" toward peripherally specialized areas – for a recent analysis of this counterstream connectional architecture, see Vezoli et al. (2021).

Using a physics metaphor, I describe the central-to-peripheral direction *centrifugal* connections, and the peripheral-to-central direction *centripetal* connections (Deacon, 1989). These two opposed directions of reciprocal connections are also distinguished by their source and target cortical layers. Centrifugal connections originate from neuron cell bodies in layer V (by convention, cortical layers are designated using roman numbers I to VI, from surface to depth of cortex) and have outputs terminating in neighboring, more peripherally specialized areas in sheet like patterns in layers I and VI. In contrast, in the reverse direction, centripetal connections originate from neuron cell bodies in layer III and have outputs terminating in neighboring, more centrally specialized areas in a columnar pattern in layers IV and III. This pattern is shown in Figure 2.2.

This pattern, in which multiple cortical areas within a modality span between peripherally specialized and central arousal systems, is characteristic not just of vision, audition, and tactile senses but is also of motor cortical areas. The so-called "primary" motor cortex is in this respect analogous to a "primary" sensory area in terms of its extreme centrifugal position and fairly direct connections with peripheral systems. This parallelism of connectional organization confronts us with the question: In what way is the generation of a behavior analogous to the generation of a perception? The short answer is that both involve the stage-by-stage differentiation of iconic neural interpretants (generated centrifugally), which become stage-by-stage selectively fine-tuned by peripheral information (flowing centripetally). Elsewhere (Deacon, 1989, 2016a), I have compared this process with counter-current exchange processes found in a variety of physiological processes from fish gills to bird lungs and engineered systems from multistage flash distillation to multistage ultra low-temperature freezers.

In physical systems, the countervailing flows are capable of driving exchange processes far beyond equilibrium. For example, fish can extract far more oxygen from water than would be possible from passive diffusion to equilibrium (Figure 2.2, right panel). By analogy, the cerebral cortex can generate iconic interpretants that are differentiated in stages from central to peripheral areas and fine-tuned moment by moment to adapt to the sensory and behavioral affordances encountered in the environment.

In semiotic terms, this complex pattern of interconnected areas generates a simultaneously nested set of iconic interpretants. Each cortical area contributes a parallel more or less differentiated iconic interpretant with respect to the same object of reference. Because they are reciprocally interconnected in constant counter-current relation to each other, they will also remain optimally complementary and minimally dissonant with their adjacent neighbors. The result is that many parallel iconic interpretants with different degrees of differentiation are linked and simultaneously superimposed to produce a single holistic percept (Figure 2.3).

Recursive interpretation

Let us now return to the example of interpreting a windsock as an index of the strength and direction of the wind. As we saw above, this requires the generation of multiple iconic interpretants (evoked memories) and then interpreting a higher order iconic relationship that each one shares with the others. In other words, it is a two-step, two-level interpretive process in which the initial interpretants are taken together as a (mental) sign vehicle requiring further interpretation of this implicit iconic relationship between them. To interpret this higher order iconism, which will provide the object of the indexical inference, a subsequent and separate neurological process must be involved. For this to occur, the initial interpretants (memories) need to be differentiated to the point where this nonvisual feature (the "feeling" of the wind) becomes salient. In this process, the memories of past similar experiences that constitute the initial interpretants are likely rendered with minimal differentiation in the visual counter-current hierarchy, probably only to the point where they begin to evoke mnemonic responses in other cortical areas responding to different sensory modalities. This cross-modal "resonance" is probably mediated by long cortico-cortical connections between different modalities at fairly early levels of differentiation.

In the case of the windsock, this higher order iconic feature is likely interpreted in a nonvisual sensory modality (tactile and possibly auditory cortex). This transfer (which need not be across modalities) will also be correlated with a shift of attention, as this new secondary iconicity becomes active

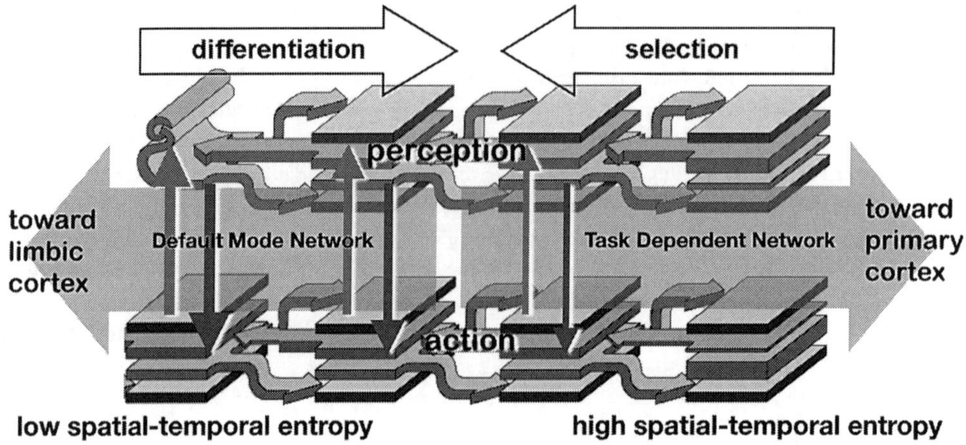

Figure 2.3 Global counter-current organization of cortico-cortical connections

Depiction of the distinctive laminar asymmetry of connection patterns (see Figure 2.2, left panel) with respect to the gradient from peripherally driven (toward primary cortex) to arousal driven (toward limbic cortex) areas. These extremes of cortical specialization are also sometimes described as comprising task dependent networks versus default mode cortical networks, respectively. Only one sensory modality is depicted for simplicity. Long projections linking modalities are also depicted (vertical arrows) and tend to be more extensive between areas that are less directly connected to the periphery.

and the prior activity fades. This shift of attention is probably additionally facilitated by cortical areas within the prefrontal cortex that enhance or inhibit activity in sensory areas thereby shifting from one modality to another or from one level of iconic differentiation to another.

Symbolic interpretation

Every act of cognition is thus a potentially complex multistep semiotic interpretive process. Even a simple indexical interpretation is the result of a developmental progression of signs interpreting signs. Furthermore, the more indirect the relation between sign and reference, the more complex the underlying interpretive process must be. This is particularly relevant for understanding the cognitive difficulty underlying the competence to communicate symbolically. This interpretive complexity likely explains why symbolic communication has not evolved in species other than humans, and why it is so difficult for other species to be trained to exhibit even a rudimentary symbolic interpretive competence.

As discussed above, interpreting something iconically is essentially automatic since the only mental interpretant necessary is a pattern of neural activity that is similar in some vague respect. Interpreting something indexically, as in the windsock example, only requires a slightly more complex set of iconic processes operating on lower-level iconic processes. In both cases, the relevant semiotic affordances are intrinsic sign vehicle properties, just hierarchically embedded. In contrast, the sign vehicles that are used to convey symbolic reference typically have been chosen irrespective of exhibiting any intrinsic iconic or indexical clues to what they refer. As a result, the only cues available to aid interpretation are iconic and indexical relationships between the sign vehicles (e.g., word–word relations) and the conventional interpretive habits shared among speakers of a common language.

Therefore, although this same semiotic constructive logic is involved in the interpretation of symbolic reference, it requires interpretant generation at a level higher than indexical interpretation. Symbolic interpretation additionally requires the generation of multiple indexical interpretants and interpreting the higher order relations between them, just as indexical interpretation requires. This symbolic dependency on indexicality can be intuitively grasped when pointing behavior helps to fix the reference of a name or declaration, but it is also implicit in the way words in a language effectively point to one another. One could, for example, consider a dictionary or thesaurus to be a kind of vast network of words pointing to other words or phrases, and a sentence as a way for words to constrain how neighboring words are to be interpreted. Indeed, the constructive importance of indexicality for the symbolic interpretation of words in a sentence is exemplified by the centrality of contiguity in syntax, whether expressed in agglutination, inflection, word order restrictions, or the special means required to signal long-distance dependencies.

Ungrounding symbolic reference

A consideration of the complex interpretive infrastructure of symbols is particularly important for explaining why language is so radically different from non-symbolic forms of communication observed in animals and humans. Because symbolic reference is determined irrespective of the physical properties of individual sign vehicles, symbolic sign vehicles can be combined and manipulated with respect to their intrinsic properties without undermining their referential associations. This allows the iconic and indexical relationships between the sign vehicle properties themselves to now become useful. However, this poses a problem. How can their referential links to the world outside of symbols be established and maintained despite the lack of clues provided by sign vehicle properties?

In a now-famous paper, cognitive scientist Steven Harnad (1990) articulated a worry that had long puzzled philosophers of language and cognitive scientists in general. He called it the "symbol grounding problem." The mystery was how arbitrary marks, such as the sounds of speech or the states of a brain, could reliably become correlated with specific referents so that symbolic communication is possible. In other words, without determining this mapping extrinsically (i.e., by using symbolic communication to negotiate the establishment and sharing of these correspondences), how could these mappings ever be established in the first place. If it takes communication with symbols to establish this shared mapping convention between symbols and their referents then we are faced with a vicious regress. In that paper, he speculates that symbol grounding must therefore be achieved using non-symbolic means.

To understand how symbols are grounded cognitively, we need to invert this perspective. We must ask how iconic and indexical forms of communication – which are intrinsically "grounded" due to the sign vehicles sharing properties with their referents – can be used to support representation using ungrounded sign vehicles (i.e., words/symbols). This is, of course, the challenge faced by every human toddler. From a semiotic perspective, there is a rich and complex set of social semiotic skills being acquired during the first year of life and significantly prior to the early stages of explicit language acquisition. Seen from this semiotic perspective, the explosive growth of language during the second and third years of life is a process in which these earlier iconic and indexical capabilities aid the child's discovery of how to use words and word combinations symbolically (Deacon, 2018).

This is an ungrounding process to the extent that the toddler has to discover how to transfer from using intrinsically grounded to using ungrounded sign vehicles, all the while maintaining referential continuity. This can only be maintained if these iconic and indexical relations are in some way preserved in the transition to symbolic communication. Since properties that could provide referential grounding are absent from linguistic sign vehicles, reference can only be preserved by means extrinsic to them – that is, in iconic and indexical relations between them, provided by grammar and syntax.

From index to symbol

Every child navigates this challenge of semiotic ungrounding and eventually replaces interpreting words as indices for interpreting them symbolically. To do this, the child must recapitulate the semiotically implicit icon(index[symbol]) interpretive hierarchy. During language acquisition, the child begins by acquiring a prelinguistic repertoire of intrinsically grounded iconic and indexical communications (Raczaszek-Leonardi et al., 2018). This will become the scaffold upon which symbolic competence is built. In this process, early word uses are indexically correlated with objects of reference by virtue of regular co-occurrence. This is aided by the uniquely evolved human adaptation for pointing to coordinate joint attention. When pointing behavior is correlated with the utterance of a word and linked to a type of object, a two-component transitive form of indexicality results. This is critical for learning to differentiate which aspect of a given object is being referred to. Repeated uses of the same word sound are iconic of one another, whereas each instance of its correlation with a physical object or event may be different in many respects. The iconism of a repeated word sound coupled with the expected constant correlation of indexical reference motivates an abductive search for the possibly cryptic feature that is shared in common with the many different objects. In the process, the child begins to build a repertoire of indexical associations between words and objects, but this is not symbolic.

The transition from indexical to symbolic use of words begins as many new words are acquired and the use of word-word relations begins to eclipse their indexical use. This is driven by a mnemonic problem. Indexical associations are one-to-one associations. Because word sounds are conventional the association lacks any iconic support for remembering the association. The only iconism is provided by repeated pairing. Yet, as the size of the word repertoire grows, the mnemonic load increases, while the regularity of constant sound–object pairing decreases. As is well known, maintaining simple associations depends on reliable stimulus pairing. When this physical co-occurrence becomes unreliable (as it does in the case of language use), these learned indexical associations should tend to be extinguished. Thus, if word reference was merely the result of indexical correlation, we should expect that word reference would regularly fade. Of course, it does not, and even modest vocabularies tend to include tens of thousands of words. This is because words are mnemonically supported by their iconic and indexical associations with other words. These associations are stably maintained in the language community and are reflected in their content association in everyday usage in sentences and so on. Unlike simple physical correlations, they are not subject to extinction. In one sense, then, the shift to the systemically supported symbolic reference is in part driven by a mnemonic least-work principle (although this does not explain why other species exposed to language do not do this).

This is an important clue for understanding the neurological basis for symbolic interpretive processes, and why there are not new language-specific structures in the human brain. Rather, the distinctive symbolic nature of language has recruited cortical and subcortical systems that evolved in response to otherwise unrelated sensory and behavioral adaptive needs. Moreover, it requires that these otherwise distinctive functional systems work together in novel synergistic ways. This is because of the way symbolic reference is supported by distributed indexical interpretive processes. But in this case, the indexicality is between symbolic sign vehicles (e.g., words) themselves on the basis of their sound iconicity and indirectly by their implicit but displaced referential indexicality. Recall the above description of indexical interpretant generation as second-order iconicity facilitated by an attentional shift mediated by prefrontal cortex intervention. To the extent that symbolic interpretant generation involves second-order indexical relationships between sign vehicles that are themselves indexically correlated with their referents, there needs to be an iconic representation of this word–word, meaning–meaning network of relations. This necessarily requires a complex functional synergy between frontal and posterior cortical systems.

Interestingly, an early suggestion regarding this necessary semiotic neurological synergy was provided by the structuralist-linguist Roman Jakobson. In his analysis of sentential structure, Jakobson suggested that there were two orthogonal dimensions of sentence processing, which he termed the syntagmatic and paradigmatic dimensions (Figure 2.4). Syntagmatic mental operations are diachronic, involving alternating shifts between functionally exclusive sentential units, such as metonymic associations (e.g., tree–squirrel), whereas paradigmatic mental operations are synchronic, involving

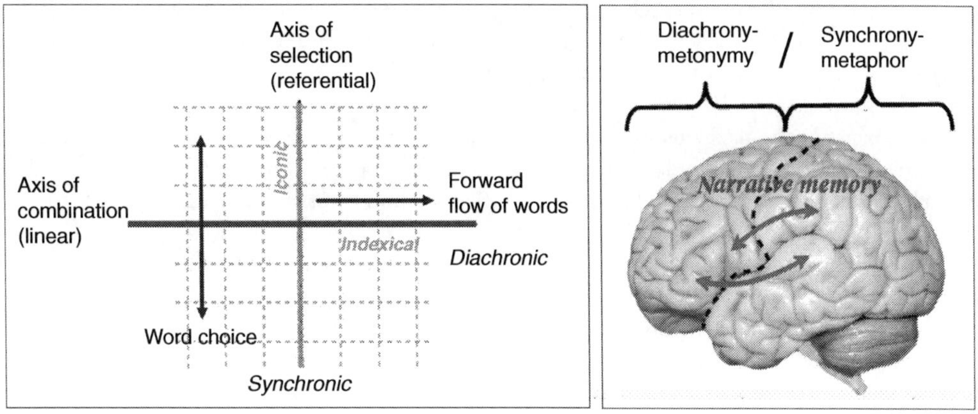

Figure 2.4 Two-dimensional view of neurolinguistic processes

Roman Jakobson's two-dimensional analysis of language processes (left panel) and his hypothesis concerning how they are segregated between frontal and posterior regions of the cerebral cortex (right panel). I have linked Jakobson's synchronic-metaphoric dimension with iconic interpretive processes in general and his diachronic-metonymic dimension with indexical interpretive processes in general. As discussed in the text, I also argue that the two orthogonal modes of mnemonic consolidation (described as procedural and episodic memory processes, respectively, and which are supported by distinct neural substrates) are brought into synergistic relation to one another by symbolic language, giving rise to a human-unique mnemonic capacity: narrative memory.

simultaneous choice options drawn from within a hierarchically nested set of similar sentential units, such as metaphoric associations (e.g., lion–cat). Notice that syntagmatic-metonymic relations involve indexical interpretive processes and paradigmatic-metaphoric relations involve iconic interpretive processes. In his brief essay on aphasia (found in Jakobson, 2018: Chapter 5), he suggests that posterior cortical regions are critical for the paradigmatic functions, such as the choice of the appropriate word in a given sentential position; while frontal cortical regions are critical for the syntagmatic functions, such as shifting from one word to another different complementarily functioning word. This can be interpreted to suggest that frontal processes enable shifts from one posterior iconic state to another, and that word sounds should be spatially-cortically correlated with the sensorimotor features that serves as mnemonic cues to their referents.

Putting these insights together provides a view of symbolic interpretive processes that effectively involves most of the cerebral cortex, not merely a few "language specialized" cortical areas, as the classic Broca-Wernicke theory would suggest. Indeed, recent functional magnetic resonance imaging research suggests that support for word meaning is distributed throughout the cerebral cortex in both hemispheres (Huth et al., 2016). This suggests that we should begin to think of the generation and interpretation of sentences as a differentiation process (Deacon, 2016a) – not as a word-and-phrase combination process – which therefore takes advantage of the same iconic-indexical differentiation logic as other forms of perception and action. It should not be surprising, then, that imagistic processes are common correlates of the conception and interpretation of sentences.

Mnemonic implications

This further provides insight into a unique mnemonic innovation that symbolic processes have provided to human cognition, and that is unavailable to other species (Deacon, 2016b). This can be described as narrative memory. In all mammal (and probably most vertebrate) brains, mnemonic functions are divided into two quite distinct neurological systems supporting two quite distinct and to some extent functionally incompatible means of storage and recovery (for an overview, see Baars & Gage 2007).

The acquisition of a motor skill is accomplished by repetition of an activity, which progressively improves precision and efficiency of the activity. Repetition progressively increases its automaticity and reduces the need for consciously monitoring its production. It is generally assumed that repetition strengthens some complex synaptic pathways and weakens others. Thus, retention and recall of this information are facilitated by the way the signaling has become canalized by redundant synaptic strengthening. This mnemonic strategy is often called *procedural* memory for these reasons. It exemplifies the general principle that mnemonic strength and accessibility is a function of statistical redundancy.

In contrast, it is also critical to be able to store and retrieve experiential information in contexts where repetition is not possible. What has been called *episodic* or declarative memory is memory (I find this latter term misleading because of its linguistic framing) for events or episodes that occurred once, uniquely, are not repeated, or involve little in the way of repeatable actions. This requires the generation of redundancy of a different sort: redundancy of associations. This creates memory traces for singular experiences by correlations between features. Thus, when we try to recall a specific experience from our past, it is generally necessary to triangulate to it using correlated associations, involving dates, places, typical social frames, and so forth. This form of mnemonic redundancy is formally orthogonal to the redundancy characteristic of procedural memory.

Because of this mutually incompatible difference in the role played by redundancy, procedural memory formation and episodic memory formation are supported by quite distinct neural substrates. Therefore, procedural memory is dependent on cerebral cortical (especially frontal) interaction with basal ganglia and cerebellar structures, whereas episodic memory is dependent on cerebral cortical (especially sensory) interaction with the hippocampus and adjacent structures.

Because of this functional segregation of these mnemonic systems, language has come to play an interesting and unique mediating role. It has become the foundation upon which an unprecedented new form of memory has emerged in human evolution. Early in the process of language acquisition, articulatory and syntactical combinatorial skills are acquired procedurally, via the many thousands of repetitions of similar word sounds and syntactic habits. In contrast, the symbolic references that constitute word meanings and their penumbra of semantic and experiential associations are necessarily acquired episodically in a growing web of associations. Because of this synergistic use of mnemonic systems, language enables each mnemonic system to reciprocally cue the other. In Jakobsonian terms, procedurally acquired syntagmatic associations can cue episodically acquired paradigmatic associations, which in turn can cue new syntagmatic associations and so on. This metonymic-metaphoric and indexical-iconic alternation is facilitated by the fact that the sign vehicles (e.g., words and phrases) of language are unencumbered by the need to share intrinsic properties with what they refer to.

Narrative memory is the result. It forms the basis for promising, reasoning, and theorizing, as well as creating our identities, histories, politics, and art. Essentially, every form of socially maintained pragmatic knowledge, from religious belief to technology, is built from a growing matrix of shared narratives of diverse forms. Hence, although the neural substrates supporting these distinct mnemonic systems have not fundamentally been altered in human evolution from the ancestral primate condition, human cognition has been restructured radically by this novel mnemonic affordance made possible by the evolution of our unprecedented symbolic interpretive competence.

Summary and conclusions

This has been a highly speculative effort to find common ground between the neurosciences and a "science" of semiosis. To accomplish this at even a superficial level of detail has required rethinking assumptions that are currently taken for granted in each field.

In the neurosciences, this has required abandoning both the computational metaphor and the view that the basic functional unit of recognition and memory can be identified with neuronal response properties. Instead, it suggests that the basic neurosemiotic unit is a dynamical attractor that likely involves the collective activity of thousands of neurons, forming a vastly distributed network within a local cortical area, modulated by its distinctive patterns of input and output relations.

For semiotic theory, this has required abandoning a categorical structuralist conception of the sign relation, adopting a process perspective in which iconic, indexical, and symbolic relations are understood as phases in a multistep interpretive process rather than as sign vehicle properties. This further requires that semiosis is understood as hierarchically constructive, with iconic interpretation as the most basic interpretive process, indexical interpretation as dependent on prior iconic interpretation processes, and symbolic interpretation as dependent on prior indexical interpretation processes.

The result is a reframing of neurological processes as semiological processes and vice versa. From this synthetic perspective, the basic neurosemiotic function is understood to be iconic interpretation, whether perceptual, mnemonic, or behavioral. Higher order indexical and symbolic forms of cognitive inference or communication are understood in terms of recursive complexifications of iconic processes. Although this is not sufficient to provide a theory of subjective experience, it does provide the necessary semiotic foundation without which contemporary theories of consciousness will remain cryptically dualistic.

Reflecting on where things currently stand, this is at least a beginning. To date, the cognitive neurosciences have been almost completely oblivious to the potential relevance of semiotic theory. On the one hand, this is the result of reluctance within the cognitive sciences to address the presumed philosophical challenges posed by the problem of mental representation and instead to frame research in a purely mechanistic paradigm. On the other hand, it is the result of the failure of semiotic theory to grapple with its physical implementation, and instead to mostly address problems within the humanities where the concept of mental representation can simply be taken for granted.

As a result, for the most part people working in each of these fields know little or nothing about current theorizing in the other. This has impeded advances in both fields and has made the problem of explaining conscious experience and agency intractable. It has also led to a resurgence of scholarly interest in the extremes of eliminative materialism and panpsychism. This is not inevitable, but it cannot be overcome without finding a common neurosemiotic methodology.

I have argued that to achieve this, it will be necessary to challenge many common assumptions in each field and to embrace Peirce's core insight: that both cognition and communication involve the production of signs – that what goes on in brains is also just the generation of signs to interpret signs, no more and no less. To provide an example of how this might be approached, I have described how the hierarchic interpretive dependence of symbols on indices and indices on icons can be understood in terms of neural processes taking place in the cerebral cortex and related brain structures. Of course, only when we are able to trace a specific empirical example of this process in some detail from process to process and structure to structure in the brain will this achieve the status of a semiotic theory of brain function. This may still be a long way off, but we cannot achieve this unless researchers in these currently isolated fields develop some common conceptual tools. I hope to have provided some hints as to how this might be accomplished.

In conclusion, this has necessarily been a highly schematic and abstract account, which will require considerable empirical study to elaborate, clarify, and test. But it offers a basis from which to begin to formulate a new synthesis: a semiotic cognitive neuroscience.

Notes

1 Standard volume and paragraph reference for the *Collected Papers of C. S. Peirce* (1931–1958).

2 The idea that the generic function of cerebral cortical circuits is iconic is similar to the theory that cortical circuits have evolved for memory storage, recall, and recognition that is presented in the 2005 book *On Intelligence* by Jeff Hawkins (the inventor of the PalmPilot) with co-author Sarah Blakeslee (Hawkins & Blakeslee, 2005).

3 Indeed, the 2014 Nobel Prize in Medicine was awarded for single neuron recording studies that demonstrated correlations with spatial location.

References

Baars, B. J. & Gage, N. M. (2007). *Cognition, Brain, and Consciousness: Introduction to Cognitive Neuroscience*. London: Elsevier.

Breakspear, M. (2017). Dynamic models of large-scale brain activity. *Nature Neuroscience, 20*, 340–352. doi: 10.1038/nn.4497

Brette, R. (2019). Is coding a relevant metaphor for the brain? *Behavioral and Brain Sciences, 42*, 1–44. doi: 10.1017/S0140525X19000049

Copeland, B. J. (2020). The Church-Turing thesis. In E. Zalta (Ed.), *The Stanford Encyclopedia of Philosophy*. Stanford. CA: Stanford University Press. https://plato.stanford.edu/archives/sum2020/entries/church-turing

Cossert, R., Aronov, D. & Yuste, R. (2003). Attractor dynamics of network UP states in the neocortex. *Nature 423*(6937), 283–288.

Deacon, T. (1989). Holism and associationism in neuropsychology: An anatomical synthesis. In E. Perecman (Ed.), *Integrating Theory and Practice in Clinical Neuropsychology* (pp. 1–47). London: Routledge.

Deacon, T. (2016a). The emergent process of thinking as reflected in language processing. In D. Schoeller, & V. Saller (Eds.), *Thinking Thinking: Practicing Radical Reflection* (pp. 135–158). Freiburg: Verlag Karl Alber.

Deacon, T. (2016b). On human (symbolic) nature: How the word became flesh. In T. Fuchs. & C. Tewes (Eds.). *Embodiment in Evolution and Culture* (pp. 129–150). Tübingen: Mohr Siebeck.

Deacon, T. (2018). Beneath symbols: Convention as a semiotic phenomenon. In S. C. Hayes, & D. S. Wilson (Eds.). *Evolution & Contextual Behavioral Science: A Reunification*. (pp. 67–84). Oakland, CA: New Harbinger.

Freeman, W. J., & Skarda, C. A. (1990). Representations: Who needs them? In J. L. McGaugh, N. M. Weinberger, & G. Lynch (Eds.). *Brain Organization and Memory* (pp. 375–380). New York: Oxford University Press.

Gibson, J. J. (1966). *The Senses Considered as Perceptual Systems*. Boston: Houghton Mifflin.

Halley, A., Baldwin, M., Cooke, D., Englund, M. & Krubitzer, L. (2020). Distributed motor control of limb movements in rat motor and somatosensory cortex: The sensorimotor amalgam revisited. *Cerebral Cortex, 30*, 6296–6312.

Harnad, S. (1990). The symbol grounding problem. *Physica D: Nonlinear Phenomena, 42*(1–3), 335–346. doi: 10.1016/0167-2789(90)90087-6

Hawkins, J., & Blakeslee, S. (2005). *On Intelligence: How a New Understanding of the Brain will Lead to the Creation of Truly Intelligent Machines*. New York: St. Martin's Press.

Huth, A., de Heer, W., Griffiths, T., Theunissen, F., & Gallant, J. (2016). Natural speech reveals the semantic maps that tile human cerebral cortex. *Nature, 532*, 453–458. doi: 10.1038/nature17637

Jakobson, R. (2018). Two aspects of language and two types of aphasic disturbances. In *Studies on Child Language and Aphasia* (pp. 49–74). Berlin: De Gruyter Mouton.

Newell, S. W., & Simon, H. A. (1972). *Human Problem Solving*. Englewood Cliffs, NJ: Pearson Prentice-Hall.

Newell, S. W., and Simon, H. A. (1976). Computer science as empirical inquiry: Symbols and search. *Communications of the ACM, 19*(3), 113–126. doi: 10.1145/360018.360022

Peirce, C. S. (1931–1958). *Collected Papers of Charles Sanders Peirce*. Vol. 1–6, C. Hartshorne &, P. Weiss (Eds.); vols. 7–8, A. W. Burks (Ed.). Cambridge, MA: Harvard University Press.

Penfield, W. (1958). *The Excitable Cortex in Conscious Man* (The Sherrington Lectures). Liverpool: Liverpool University Press.

Penfield, W., & Rasmussen, T. B. (1950). *The Cerebral Cortex of Man*. New York: Macmillan.

Raczaszek-Leonardi, J., Nomikou, I., Rohlfing, K., & Deacon T. (2018). Language development from an ecological perspective: Ecologically valid ways to abstract symbols. *Ecological Psychology, 30*(1), 39–73. doi: 10.1080/10407413.2017.1410387

Schoonover, C., Ohashi, S., Axel, R., & Fink, A. (2021). Representational drift in primary olfactory cortex. *Nature, 594*, 541–546. doi: 10.1038/s41586-021-03628-7

Vezoli, J, Magrou, L, Goebel, R, Wang, X., Knoblauch, K., Vinck, M., & Kennedy, H. (2021) Cortical hierarchy, dual counterstream architecture and the importance of top-down generative networks. *NeuroImage, 225*, 117479. doi: 10.1016/j.neuroimage.2020.117479

Vilarroya, O. (2017) Neural representation. A survey-based analysis of the notion. *Frontiers in Psychology, 8*, 1458. doi: 10.3389/fpsyg.2017.01458

Ward, L. (2001). *Dynamical Cognitive Science*. Cambridge, MA: MIT Press.

Yuste, R. (2015). From the neuron doctrine to neural networks. *Nature Reviews Neuroscience, 16*, 487–497. doi: 10.1038/nrn3962

3

AN ACTIVE INFERENCE APPROACH TO SEMIOTICS

A variational theory of signs

Antoine Milette-Gagnon, Samuel P. L. Veissière, Karl J. Friston, and Maxwell J. D. Ramstead

Introduction

Recent decades have borne witness to the emergence of new frameworks in psychology (Chemero, 2009; Gibson, 1979), neuroscience (Eliasmith, 2005; Varela, 1996; Varela et al., 1991), anthropology (Deacon, 2011a), and philosophy (Thompson, 2010), each more committed than the last to explaining the cognitive feats of organisms from their own point of view.

New mechanistic theories, drawing on dynamical systems theory and information theory, evince a growing interest in the study of the workings of meaning and signification. Previous theories had tended to approach living systems either from a detached, reductionist stance that disregarded conscious experience (Fodor, 1975; 1983; Watson, 1913) or – in contrast – from a purely subjective perspective, without much concern for the physical processes that underwrite our experience of a meaningful world (Ingold, 2000). The dual reality of living systems – as mechanistic, but also perspectival and capable of signification – increasingly drives research on sentient systems. It would be a mistake to think that adopting a mechanistic approach commits one to reductionism and to mindless conceptions of the living (Ramstead et al., 2018; Thompson, 2010).

The terms "signification" and "meaning" are polysemic. Sometimes their referents seem elusive because the phenomena at play in attributions of significance are multilayered. We use the terms "signification" and "meaning" to refer to a specific kind of interpretive ability and its output, whereby an agent can make use of signs to convey specific meanings – or to interpret signs provided to them as meaning this or that. As emphasized by many philosophical traditions (notably, stoicism), humans do not interact with the world in an unmediated way (as a naïve realist or phenomenological account might hold), but rather apprehend it via the meaning that they assign to their experience.

We argue that active inference can provide some mechanistic insights about signification and meaning-making abilities in humans. Active inference is the newest creature-centered framework to come out of information theory (Friston, 2020), and it represents a promising new avenue for the study of mind in cultural context (Ramstead et al., 2016; Veissière et al., 2020). Active inference explains how organisms are able to generate rolling cycles of belief-guided, adaptive action and perception (Clark, 2015; Ramstead et al., 2019a). The framework casts perception, learning, and action as forms of inference – and provides a formal model for the study of hierarchically

DOI: 10.4324/9781003051817-5

nested systems (Badcock et al., 2019a; Kirchhoff et al., 2018). The active inference framework has been applied to explain varied phenomena, such as the generation of adaptative behavior by living creatures (Friston et al., 2017), the hierarchical and nested structure of biological systems (Ramstead et al., 2019b), the construction by creatures of their ecological niche (Constant et al., 2018), and the coevolution of human genes and culture (Veissière et al., 2020), cooperative communication systems (Vasil et al., 2019), linguistic capacity (Friston et al., 2020), and hermeneutics (Friston & Frith, 2015a). We believe many of the questions addressed by active inference echo those addressed in the field of neurosemiotics, which intends to study – among other things – the processes that underwrite the general capacity of organisms to behave meaningfully, or to generate meaning, within their environment (Bouissac, 1985; Jorna, 2006).

The main claim of this chapter is that a theory of signs akin to classical, Peircean semiotics can be (partially) formulated using active inference, in light of the conceptual analogies between the two frameworks, notably the shared commitment to the notion of abductive inference in living (and cognitive) systems. Furthermore, we argue that Peirce's construct of semiotic interpretant – the interpreter's understanding of the relation between a signifier and what it signifies – can be given a formal interpretation under active inference by associating it with the construct of generative model in active inference. Generative models are probabilistic mappings, from a set of unobserved or latent causes to their observed sensory consequences. Under active inference, such models underlie the generation of adaptive action. We argue that active inference allows us to model signification and meaning-making as inference in a hierarchical generative model, where inferential processes at superordinate layers of the hierarchical model arise from – and constrain – those unfolding at subordinate levels (Friston, 2008). Based on this argument, we reinterpret Peirce's typology of signs (as icons, indices, and symbols) via active inference. We place special emphasis on the notion of abductive inference (going beyond the sensory data at hand) in resolving the ill-posed problem of inferring what our sensations connote (Seth, 2015).

The remainder of this chapter will be divided in two parts. In the next section, we introduce the active inference framework. We then detail the conceptual analogies between active inference and classical (Peircean) semiotics, before offering a partial but formal mapping of key semiotic notions, notably the icon/index/symbol triad, onto central constructs of active inference. We close with proposals for future work.

Active inference

An introduction to the active inference framework

Active inference is a theory that explains how living systems preserve their nonequilibrium steady state (Friston, 2020). According to the fluctuation theorems that generalize the second law of thermodynamics, the entropy of any system tends to increase – and living systems must counter its dispersive effects to remain alive (Parr et al., 2020; Seifert, 2012). In this context, entropy is a measure of disorder: it quantifies the total number of configurations in which the system being examined can find itself. Most inanimate systems in nature self-organize to equilibrium, which means that they consume the gradients around which they self-organize. For instance, the lightning bolt, in striking, self-organizes around – and dissolves – a charge gradient, thereby increasing the entropy and disorder of the surrounding air molecules. Living systems, in contrast, tend to resist this tendency towards entropic disorder and maintain their internal organization. By definition, this means they exist far from thermodynamic equilibrium – which is death (Schrödinger, 1944). For example, the body temperature of mammals is far from the room temperature (and for most animals, to find their body at the ambient temperature of the environment entails death). How is this feat accomplished by living organisms?

This question has been tackled by an emerging field of work centered around the free-energy principle, a variational principle of least action that underwrites active inference (Friston, 2010, 2020).

The central claim is that for a self-organizing system to exist at nonequilibrium steady state means that it looks as if it minimizes its variational free energy (Ramstead et al., 2019a). In a nutshell, this free energy quantifies the discrepancy between the current sensory state and the expected sensory state. At its simplest, this means everything that lives this must show some form of homoeostasis (Bernard, 1974) – that is, a minimization of the discrepancy between sensed states of being and homoeostatic (or allostatic) setpoints (Ramsay & Woods, 2014; Seth & Friston, 2016; Stephan et al., 2016; Sterling & Eyer, 1988). In information theoretic terms, this discrepancy is measured by free energy, which provides a measurable proxy for self-information or surprisal. The average self-information is entropy, so any minimizing free energy counters an increase in entropy (Friston, 2010). One could then reformulate the problem in the following way: "How do organisms resist entropic decay? By minimizing free energy." This is, in essence, the free-energy principle.[1] Of course, stating this without further investigation would be begging the question "How do organisms minimize their free energy?" This question can be answered by appealing to Markov blankets and generative models.

Markov blankets and generative models

We can associate a system of interest with the states in which it can find itself, which we call internal states. The rationale for this is intuitive. For a system to be considered as a system, it must evince a minimal form of independence from its surrounding environment (external states), lest it simply dissolve into that environment when perturbed – or indeed measured. This is not to say that the system of interest is completely separated from its environment (i.e., isolated or closed in a thermodynamic sense), but rather that its influence on the system is mediated, such that the embedding environment can change without the system being entrained without question.

In the active inference framework, this form of conditional independence is underwritten by the presence of a Markov blanket (Friston, 2013), a statistical construct originally developed in the context of statistical inference over random variables (Pearl, 1988). For our purposes, it operationalizes the intuitive notion of a mediated coupling to the environment (Kirchhoff et al., 2018; Ramstead et al., 2018). A Markov blanket mediates between internal and external states, and the blanket itself is composed of sensory states, which influence but are not influenced by internal states, and active states, which influence but are not influenced by external states (see Figure 3.1).

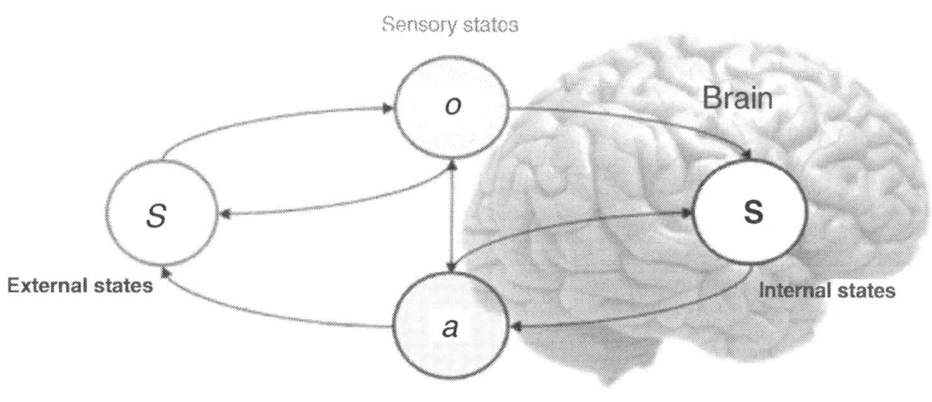

Figure 3.1 Markov blanket and its variables

This figure depicts a Markov blanket, illustrating the influences between the variables that constitute the blanket. Here, internal states – denoted s – are influenced by (but do not influence) sensory states or observations (o); while external states – denoted s – are influenced by (but do not influence) active states (a). From Ramstead, Kirchhoff, and Friston (2019). See e-book for a fullcolor version of this figure.

From this vantage point, every living creature is enshrouded by a Markov blanket, which mediates its access to the world in which it is embedded. Yet what lies behind the shroud is of critical significance to the creature because everything of relevance to it – be it potential predators, food items, or mates – lies there. This is reminiscent of the concept of the *Umwelt* developed by Jakob von Uexküll. The *Umwelt* can be understood as the embodied perspective (i.e., the viewpoint) that biological beings take on their world, and this perspective is the union of the *effector world* and the *perceptor world* (von Uexküll, 1982). This means the subjective world of organisms is not composed of a series of objects with "objective" properties, but rather is better understood as a set of objects that are made meaningful in the organism's perceptual field by its action capacities: for foxes, given their specific set of hunting capacities, a field of grass is a support for walking towards their prey; but for worm-eating birds, given their action capacities, the field grass is the "pantry" itself, so to speak.

The existence of a Markov blanket implies a form of inference, implicit in the minimization of free energy that scores the likelihood of sensations, given an *Umwelt* associated to the internal states. This means that to exist – in the sense of being separable from the environment – is to *infer* the external causes of sensory impressions that are hidden behind the Markov blanket. These hidden causes are the external states. In active inference, inference about the most probable hidden cause of sensory data is accomplished thanks to what is known as a generative model, a statistical formulation of the *Umwelt* as a model of the process that generates sensations. In other words, it is a model of how sensory impressions are generated – including, crucially, the actions of the organism. Technically, a generative model is a joint probability distribution or density over sensory outcomes and their hidden causes (Friston, 2010; Friston et al., 2018).

The idea is that organisms entertain and evaluate competing models or hypotheses (*Umwelten*) and select the one for which there is the most evidence (i.e., the hypothesis that renders the sensations the most likely or least surprising). Crucially, this evidence is the complement of the free energy above. In other words, minimizing free energy minimizes the discrepancy between sensory states and those expected under a generative model. This is mathematically the same as maximizing the evidence for the generative model. Heuristically, variational free energy therefore provides a measure of the evidence for a creature's generative model. To select the model that minimizes the discrepancy between what is predicted and what is sensed (i.e., variational free energy) is the same as selecting the model that is supported by the most evidence (Friston, 2020) – that is, a form of self-evidencing (Hohwy, 2016). The links between this self-evidencing and Peircean abductive inference will be fleshed out below.

We emphasize the inferential and perspectival nature of active inference. Generative models scaffold the probabilistic beliefs of an organism. These Bayesian beliefs[2] reflect the existence of the organism itself. They have been shaped by evolutionary history: the preferred states of the organism, encoded in its model, can be cast as a "best guess" about the causal structure of the econiche as experienced by the phenotype in question (Badcock et al., 2019b; Campbell, 2016). In other words, organisms are constantly trying to infer states of affairs in the external world, given current evidence provided by sensory states and its prior beliefs – and, indeed, given the kind of creature that it is. For instance, for a human to find oneself suddenly submerged in water would be quite surprising, whereas such a situation would be expected for a fish. What is important to note is that the generative model is not an objective map of the world; it is formed as a function of the needs and concerns of the creature (Ramstead et al., 2019a; Tschantz et al., 2019). Thus, generative models harness these species-specific expectations about the lived world (just like in the *Umwelt*).

A simple generative model: Likelihood mappings and prior beliefs

Given sensory data, the system is trying to infer what external states have caused these outcomes. The relation between hidden causes and sensory outcomes is formalized in a generative model through a likelihood mapping (Figure 3.2), which in discrete-state space generative models, like

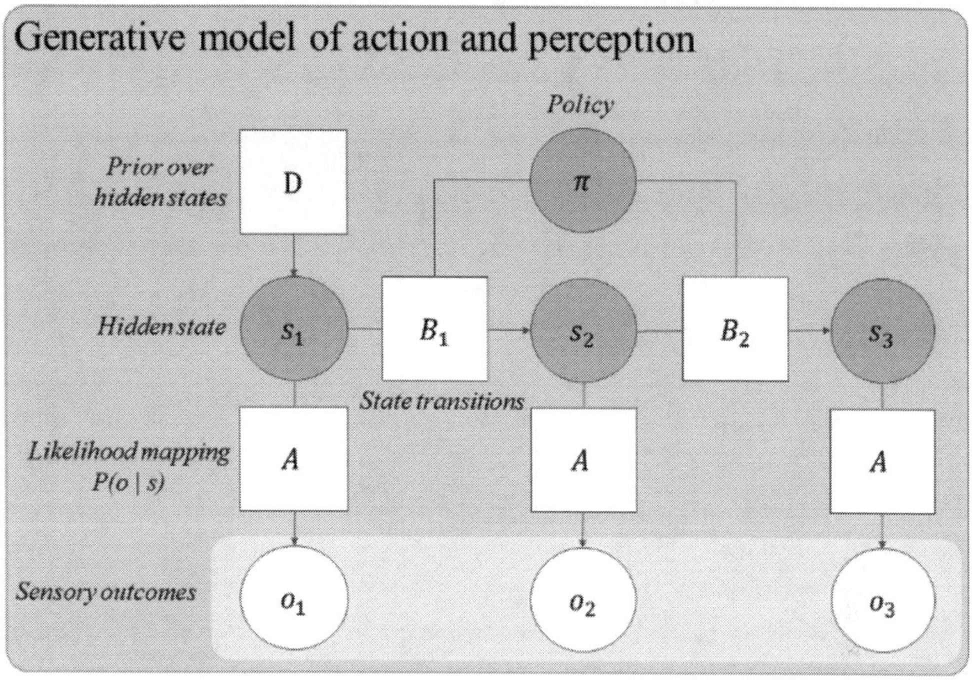

Figure 3.2 Generative model of action perception

In active inference, perception amounts to the (Bayesian) inversion of a generative model. This inversion corresponds to inference or abduction. The organism has access to its sensory observations (o), its beliefs about how its observations map onto states in the world (A), and its prior beliefs about the state of the world before seeing observations (D). More sophisticated generative models include beliefs about state transitions (B) that depend upon plans or policies. The policies (π) that are selected are those that minimize expected free energy that depends upon prior beliefs about final states (C). Please see Parr and Friston (2018) for a technical explanation of the equations that describe the implicit belief updating, given sensory outcomes. See e-book for a full-color version of this figure.

finite state machines or partially observed Markov decision processes is usually denoted by a matrix A. Technically, this mapping tells us the probability of some observation, given that some state of the world is the case – which is denoted *P* (o | s). This likelihood is supplemented with some prior Bayesian beliefs about how states change over time, usually encoded by a probability transition matrix called B. These state transitions depend upon action or plans. Prior beliefs about final and initial hidden states are usually encoded in vectors called C and D. It may seem strange to reduce a generative model, or *Umwelt*, of the world in this way; however, the functional form of this generative model is universal and very expressive (see below). Crucially, committing to a particular functional form allows one to simulate the minimization of free energy and accompanying self-organization. In this setting, the minimization of free energy corresponds to Bayesian belief updating and, with the above form, looks very much like message passing in neuronal circuits (for further details, see Parr and Friston, 2018).

Starting from prior beliefs and its sensory states, the organism must solve the inverse inference problem that of determining which state of the world is most probable, given its observations and prior beliefs – denoted *P* (s | o). Thus, we say that perception "inverts" the generative model that maps from unobservable (external) causes to observable (sensory) consequences to obtain the inverse mapping – namely, the most probable cause of current sensory states. This inverse mapping from consequences to causes is the essence of inference and self-evidencing, which can also be viewed as an act of abduction.

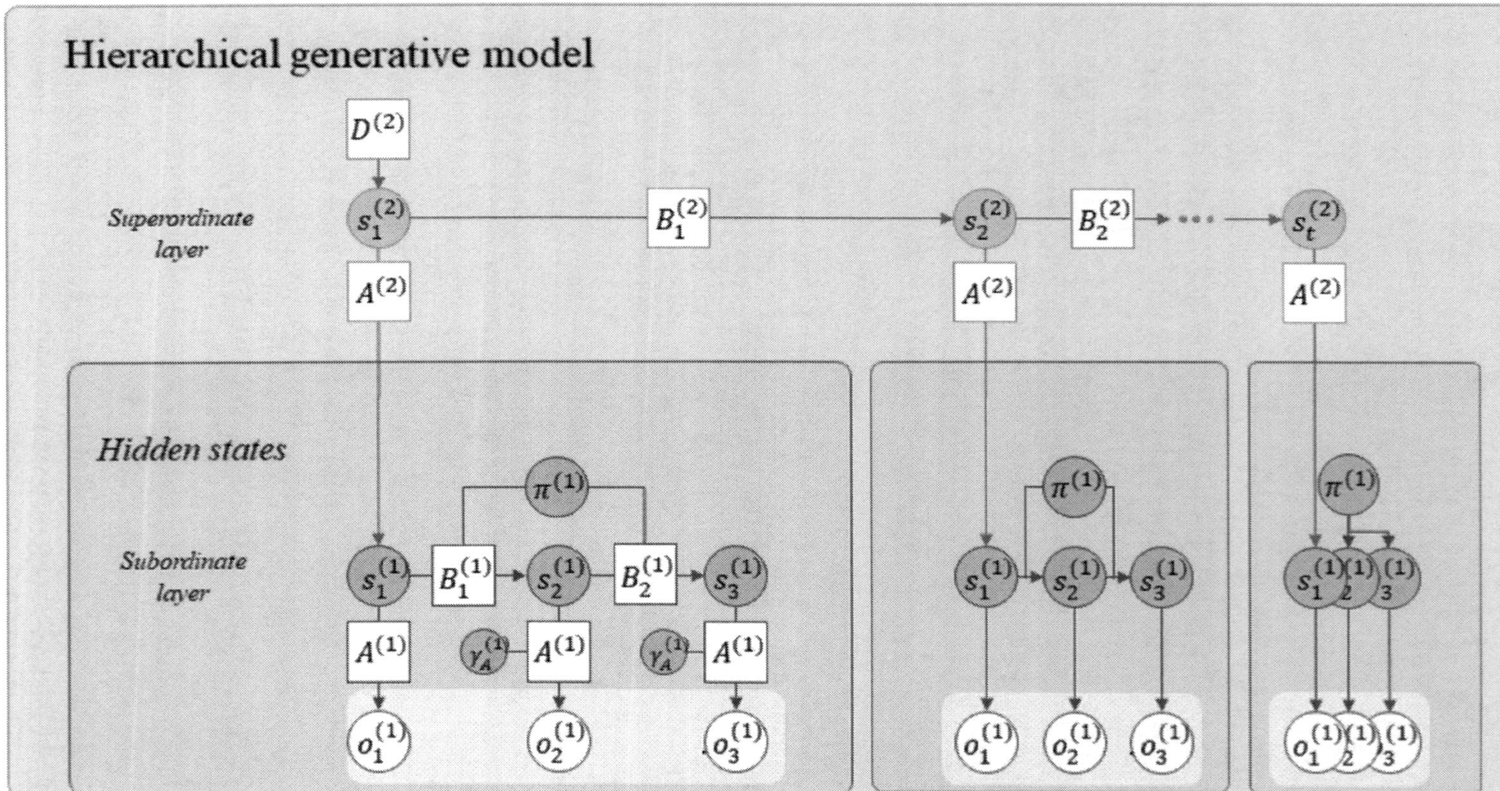

Figure 3.3 Hierarchical generative model

The generative models presented here can be hierarchically extended. In such hierarchical models, state estimation at the subordinate level is used as sensory evidence (i.e., observations) for state inference at the superordinate level. Please see Parr and Friston (2018) for a discussion of the implicit belief updating dynamics. See e-book for a full-color version of this figure.

Crucially, to be endowed with beliefs about state transitions opens the door to action on the world. After all, the ability to act depends on the ability to anticipate the (sensory) consequences of action, which in turn implies the ability to plan into the future. Under active inference, beliefs about possible courses of action are called policies. The selection of policies is implemented as the selection of specific beliefs about state transitions – namely, beliefs informed by the foreseen consequences of action and prior beliefs about final outcomes. Action is cast as a self-fulfilling prophecy: creatures fulfill their expectations through policy selection (Friston et al., 2017). Policy selection, in turn, is driven by expected free energy – namely, the free energy expected under a given policy. Differences in expected free energy over competing policies drive policy selection, as creatures enact the policy associated with the lowest expected free energy, thereby working towards predictable outcomes that constitute the free energy minimizing, evidence maximizing, nonequilibrium steady-state dynamics that characterize the creature in question.

Crucially, for our purposes, the generative models used in active inference can be endowed with a hierarchical structure. Such a scheme is depicted in Figure 3.3, in which state estimation at the subordinate level is used as sensory data (as observations) for state inference at the superordinate level. Note the higher-order likelihood matrix A(2), which links lower-level states (1) – now taken as sensed outcomes – to higher-level state inference (2). This setup effectively equips the agent with higher-order beliefs, e.g., higher-order beliefs about state transitions, which would be denoted by B(2), that contextualize beliefs and inferences at the subordinate layers of the model. In short, a hierarchical generative model of this sort equips the creature with a sense of the future (i.e., temporal depth) at different temporal scales, which finesses planning and policy selection – based upon the future consequences of action.

Toward a variational semiotics

We are now in a position to establish a preliminary mapping between semiotic constructs and structures within the active inference framework. We first expand the general theme of our variational rendition of semiotics by showcasing the conceptual similarities between the two frameworks. More precisely, we claim that Peircean interpretants can be associated formally with generative models in active inference. We then describe how Peirce's most famous typology of signs into icons, indices, and symbols can be recast in the active inference framework.

As foreshadowed in our brief presentation of active inference, we note that the theoretical structure of active inference is strikingly similar to that of Peircean semiotics, allowing us to map some of the constructs of active inference (at least partially) onto those of Peirce's semiotics, namely abductive inference and the sign triad of icons, indices, and symbols. Does that mean we can *reduce* semiotics to active inference? Our aim is rather to show that active inference is semiotic in its logic. In some sense, our attempt to explain some of the semiotic concepts by appealing to the resources of the active inference framework is not far from the intent of Peirce himself. As Short argues, "a central thrust of Peirce's mature semeiotic is that intentionality may be explained naturalistically" (Short, 2007: 8).

Active inference and deflationary semantics

Before touching on the semiotic structure of active inference, we have to address one major concern about generative models, which is their capacity to address the very notion of "meaning" that is at stake within neurosemiotics. Indeed, some critics have pointed out that information-theoretic constructs should not be conflated with the phenomenon of "meaning" (Brier, 2008). Thus, it is fair to ask whether active inference and generative models are up to the task. Our goal here is not to demonstrate that a global reduction of the phenomenon of meaning is within the purview of active inference, but rather to point toward how active inference can deal with certain specific aspects of meaning. As stated before, the term "meaning" itself is polysemic; one could follow Morris and distinguish between multiple dimensions of meaning, namely *semantics* (or the "reference" or "aboutness" of signs), *syntactics* (the reference to other signs or symbols) and *pragmatics* (the concrete use of signs in real-life situations).[3] This leaves out the *phenomenal* or *experienced* aspect of meaning, arguably infusing all other dimensions to different degrees. While we do not pretend to directly solve the issue of *naturalizing* phenomenality as the complexity of the issue as generated more than 100 years of active philosophical and scientific debate (see Ramstead, 2015 for a discussion), this chapter still aims to convince the reader that active inference can at least provide some partial account of the "meaningful" drive of organisms that can be also described as dynamical systems.

The *semantic* aspect of meaning within active inference has been studied by Ramstead et al. (2020). In the active inference conceptual context, *semantics* is used to describe the relation between internal states of the system and external states – that is, an *aboutness* of internal states (and not meaning as a subjective feeling or experience). The authors, following Egan (2019), propose to cast, in a deflationary fashion, the aboutness of internal states in terms of the mathematical function that these states accomplish within physical systems, rather than by some "gloss" of cognitive content. The key to understanding how this (mathematical) aboutness is at play is that we can describe a given system with the tools of systems theory, as a dynamical flow within over some state space, or using information theoretic tools, providing a statistical description of this flow. In brief, under the free-energy principle, we can describe the internal states of a system as containing a *statistical manifold*, a space in which the coordinates are *sufficient statistics* of beliefs over external states (e.g., the mean and variance of a Bayesian belief).

Under the free energy principle, given the Markovian partition of internal and external states (which are conditionally independent), it follows that internal states act as (the *sufficient statistics* of) beliefs about external states – that is, given the internal state, a consumer of the state can find the probability distribution of external states (just like any normal distribution can be reproduced given its mean and variance, which are its *sufficient statistics*). In short, the *aboutness* of internal states is formalized under the free-energy principle as a relationship between internal and external states, with internal states *parametrizing* probability densities over external states – a technical treatment of the mathematical foundations of this observation can be found in Friston (2020) and Friston et al. (2020). Philosophically, the important point to understand is that, in this context, the emphasis is placed on the *relations of meaning* rather than on the *content of meaning*. Furthermore, in active inference, the relations of meaning are always enacted: the internal states also encode the *consequences* of action on external states (via active states).

The limitation of this account is that we have to accept a "deflationary" account of semantic content (Egan, 2019), in which semantic content is only an intentional gloss that can serve heuristic purposes to guide scientific research about cognitive activities (Ramstead, 2019c). That is, the association of internal states with external states and the role of this association for the description of the behavior of a far-from-equilibrium steady states system can be explained mathematically, but not the complete integrated experience of meaning. Nevertheless, we still maintain that active inference displays some basic aspects of a semiotic structure. With these deflationary caveats in place, we now attempt to connect systematically active inference and Peirce's semiotics.

A basic semiotic structure

Signs are first and foremost things that stand for other things. This is in line with the commitments of active inference, which states that creatures do not have access to things in an unmediated way (as we have presented in comparison with Uexküll's *Umwelt*). This is why we believe that, at its core, active inference is compatible with many aspects of (Peircean) semiotics. Indeed, the abductive nature of the inferential processes under the free-energy principle has recently been compared with Peircean abduction (or abductive inference) (Pietarinen & Beni, 2021). Briefly, they describe self-evidencing processes in the following fashion:

1. Y (a sensory datum) is surprising (in the information-theoretical sense described above);
2. if X (a prior or a fact about the world) were to be the case, then Y would be less surprising;
3. therefore, let us see to it that/there is reason to suspect that X (to "believe-X" about external states) is to be part of the generative model. (Adapted from Pietarinen & Beni, 2021; see also Parr and Friston, 2018, for a technical explanation of the equations that describe the implicit belief updating, given sensory outcomes.)

The inferential nature of semiosis has also been described within the field of biosemiotics. For instance, Kull et al. (2011) argue that conditional forms of logic (i.e., if → then) are embodied in the forms and habits of organisms and are in this sense a "bio-logic." As they explicitly state,

> semiosis facilitates the development of an organism's capacity to behave in a way that is both consistent with its environment and implicitly inferential. "Logic" as we are using it here is not something to be considered as a product of abstract cognition in humans, but rather we simply intend to highlight the inference-like architecture of biological function, which we take to also be the basis of semiosis in general.
>
> *(Kull et al., 2011: 33)*

This "inference-like" architecture is precisely what is at play within active inference under the free-energy principle, following the fact that internal states of organisms are conditionally independent of external states, given the Markov blanket partition.

In this line of thought, we propose that the Peircean concept of *interpretant* can be mapped to the concept of generative models, an idea that has already been sketched, but not developed enough, in Campbell (2012). The interpretant, for Peirce, is the "understanding" (at least implicit) that a semiotic agent has of the signifier–signified relationship – or, as Peirce puts it, the effect of the sign on the interpreter (Peirce, 1902). This construct reflects the idea that a signifier must be taken as standing for something. That an agent can relate a signified to its signifier assumes that they have acquired the relevant skill, or evolved the disposition, to interpret the sign as a sign. At bottom, a Peircean interpretant is a way to sample, and organize our perception of, the world around us.

Generative models accomplish the same thing as interpretants – namely, organizing perception of (and action in) the world. Indeed, generative models are joint probability distributions of sensory states and what caused them, including the action of the organism itself. In other words, the inferential process at the core of life – the *bio-logic* as described by Kull and colleagues – takes the form of a generative model within active inference. This affinity between semiotic and variational frameworks makes us believe in the possibility of a (partial) formalization of semiotics as a *naturalized* theory of signification. The aim here is not to replace the field of semiotics, but rather to suggest that semiotic processes can be explained rigorously by appeal to active inference framework. Moreover, this correspondence can facilitate the work of understanding semiotic constructs at different temporal scales because active inference provides a principled (and possibly unified) account of life processes, including signification and semiosis.

Variational icons ("looks like")

We now turn to a partial breakdown of the Peircean typology in variational terms, starting with the simplest signs: icons. Icons signify by virtue of a shared quality (often an apparent physical similarity) between the sign-vehicle (signifier) and the object (signified) (Peirce, 1902). An illustrative example of an iconic sign is a photograph of a friend. Unless affected by prosopagnosia or placed under undue strain, persons can leverage the palpable similarity between the photograph and their friend and recognize the image as being a photograph *of* this friend.

Iconic signs underlie the most elementary forms of perception, since members of a given perceptual category bear iconic resemblance to each other, for the interpreter. Perceptual categorization is thus dependent on iconicity – in the general sense of shared quality or similarity – because a category is simply a set of members sharing certain features, which means that they signify each other iconically (for the interpreter who uses the category).

From the variational point of view, we argue that a sign signifies iconically when its action on the interpreter is mediated by a likelihood mapping (or matrix A). Thus, two different icons refer to the same thing (object, event, etc.) if they trigger the same inferences. If a given signifier is similar enough to what it signifies, it will cause the creature to infer the same hidden cause as when it observes the thing signified by the icon. In short, iconic signifiers trigger the same state inferences as the direct, firsthand perception of their signified "in the flesh": both the signifier and the signified itself map onto the same underlying latent state. Our proposal here is similar to Deacon's description of icons: the most basic sense of iconicity is that of "non-distinction" – that is, that the same interpretative processes are in play for two things, making them "iconic" of each other (Deacon, 1997: 76–77). The neuroanatomical correlates of this matrix A function will be explored in the next section, linking icons (A matrices) and indices (B matrices).

Variational indices ("points to")

Indices can also be formalized via active inference, through the correspondence between the process of indexical inference and beliefs about state transitions (i.e., B matrices). The capacity of indices to signify is based upon causal or correlative relationships between them and their signified. For example, because of the causal relation between them, symptoms can be indices of a disease. Here, we follow Deacon's hierarchical model of semiotics, in the sense that simpler types of signification are embedded within more complex types – that is, there is a nested structure of signs at play in the constitution of more complex semiotic relations. To recognize a sign as the index of some signified, the creature needs to recognize (iconically) the two elements composing the indexical relation (e.g., symptom and disease) and relate them using a superordinate sign. We argue that this structural (and hierarchical) characteristic is similar to the way that, in active inference, moment-to-moment state inference (based on likelihood mappings and prior beliefs) is contextualized by beliefs about state transitions.

Recall that state transition (B) matrices embody – in neuronal or chemical connections such as the brain connections or a cell's intracellular kinetic pathways – a creature's beliefs about how states transition into others, and about what sensory outcomes these future hidden states typically cause. Moreover, when one is talking about a causal relationship between things (one of the hallmarks of indexical signification), one is really talking about transitions between one state and the next, at least insofar as this relation of co-occurrence is believed to hold by the interpreter. What we mean is that causality is not necessary "objective" – for example, a lab mouse can have a model of the transition between a red light and an electric shock, whether or not the red light really *causes* the electric shock. Therefore, we argue that the transition probabilities (the B matrices) function, in semiotic terms, indexically, since they imply a succession of moment-to-moment state inferences based on likelihood mappings and priors, just as indices imply an association of icons. This is particularly so for generative models based upon discrete state spaces, where the only thing that distinguishes one state from another is its index – and the only operational meaning of these indices are the transition (or likelihood) mappings to the indices of other states (or sensory outcomes) – see Friston and Buzsaki (2016) for treatment of indexing time in this setting.

Interestingly, the general structure of these (perceptual) inferences can be related to neuroanatomical architecture (Hipólito et al., 2021; Parr & Friston, 2018). This is in line with the good regulator theorem (Conant & Ashby, 1970), stating that a good regulator must be a model of what it regulates. For active inference, this means that generative models and brain anatomy are mutually constraining – that is, that the space of plausible brain architectures is constrained by the free energy principle (Parr & Friston, 2018).

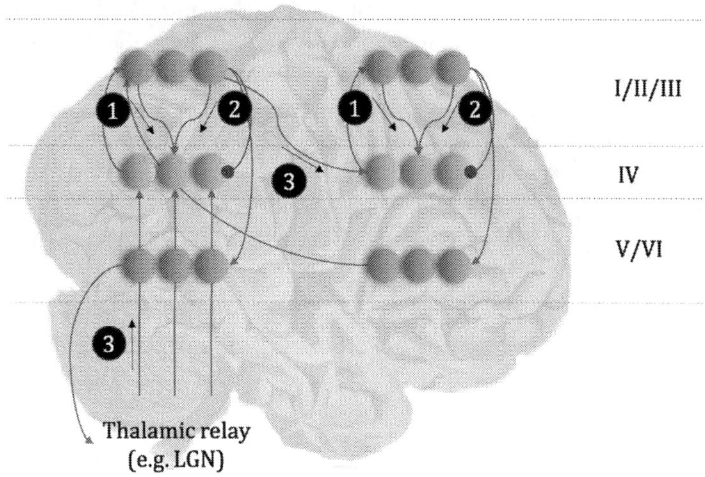

Figure 3.4 Active inference model mapped onto a brain diagram

Neurons in cortical layer IV represent the spiny stellate cells that receive input from relay nuclei of the thalamus, and from lower cortical areas. The appropriate thalamic relay depends upon the system in question. In the context of the visual system, it is the lateral geniculate nucleus (LGN). In the somatosensory or auditory systems, it is the ventral posterior nucleus or the medial geniculate nucleus, respectively. Layer IV cells in this network signal prediction errors (a measure of surprisal), computed by comparing the optimal estimate (obtained by combining the messages from its Markov blanket) with the current belief, represented in superficial cortical layers (adapted from Parr and Friston, 2018). See e-book for a full-color version of this figure.

Active inference models have been mapped onto known neuroanatomy. Consider the simplified model of the brain presented in Figure 3.4, adapted from Parr and Friston (2018). In this representation, the superficial layers of the brain encode an agent's expectations: the units in superficial layers encode beliefs about states at three time-points (immediate past, current time, and immediate future). In this neuronal representation, the likelihood mapping is encoded by specific neural populations (which implement the A-matrix that as we have seen encodes the probability of an observation given a discrete hidden state) and passed on via the thalamic relay (by the lateral geniculate nucleus for the visual system or the medial geniculate nucleus for the auditory system). Conversely, the neural messages carrying signals encoded by B matrices (state transitions) are passed on and processed by populations encoding past states and future states, which are thought to be implemented by the connections between superficial layers and layer IV spiny stellate cells. In turn, these neurons are thought to represent prediction errors, which as they arise and are quashed drive the system towards better predictions. This forms a biologically plausible neural architecture that can implement icons and indexes as discussed above.

Let us use an example to see the possible implications of such framework. Imagine a creature walking in a forest – this example is inspired by Deacon (1997: 77–78). Suddenly, a new sensory outcome is made available – one that updates its current belief about the state of affairs in the world. After correcting for prediction error, the creature infers (that is, *believes that*) what it is seeing is smoke. This first (predictive) inference allows the agent to attribute the changes in its sensory states to a cause – namely, to a black column rising from the trees. Armed with the likelihood mappings already formed within the organism's generative model, the animal infers that smoke is the most probable hidden cause of the current sensory outcomes. Here, as Deacon suggests, smoke is perceived iconically, in the sense that the current appearance of the black column bears an iconic resemblance to past occurrences of smoke. As we saw in the previous section, active inference formalizes this kind of relationship with likelihood mappings. The organism can make this inference because it has a good generative model of an econiche that features things that "smoke."

With the presence of the smoke inferred, other beliefs get to work. Through its previous experiences with its niche (made of combustible trees), the organism has become endowed with beliefs about state transitions (B matrices). Now that smoke has been identified as the probable cause of the current sensory outcome, uncertainty can be reduced further by leveraging these beliefs. Our creature has learned that *the most probable cause* of smoke is fire. It is thus able to perform a nested indexical inference (namely, that the state "smoke" often transitions into the state "fire"), so to perceive smoke motivates the inference that there is probably a fire nearby, with (action) related sensory outcomes associated with the hidden state "fire" (e.g., heat, light, burning, pain), thus motivating policy selection to ensure movement away from the source of smoke (even if there is not a *real* fire).

Variational symbols ("refers to, within a convention")

We now turn to symbols, the most complex case in the semiotic theory of signs. A symbol signifies by virtue of a convention (Peirce, 1902). Although this definition is generally agreed upon, it leaves much to the imagination. This definition is vague enough to lead to multiple usages of the term. Thankfully, the construct was taken up by Deacon (2011b), who characterized two major usages of the word "symbol" in the literature:

1. *Non-linguistic symbols.* In the social sciences, the word "symbol" refers to meanings that are conventionally invested in or projected onto artifacts that are culturally determined. The meaning is typically learned and culturally specific. For example, crowns are symbols of monarchy and its related political institutions, as when we refer to a monarchy as "The Crown."
2. *Linguistic, code-like symbols.* In mathematics and logic, the word "symbol" refers to written traces that are conventionally mapped to other such traces, and that can be combined to form other, distinct written traces according to explicit rules.

We argue that (1) the conventional aspect of symbols can be understood as an effect of collective patterns of inference based on the same, shared generative model; and (2) the syntactical aspect of symbols (symbol to symbol transitions, as are commonplace in language) can be recast as superordinate beliefs about (semiotic) state transitions.

Deontic cues and the conventionalization of signs

We believe that studying the *conventional* aspect of symbols is akin to studying cultural patterns inside a given group or society – that is, studying a multi-agent phenomenon. How can the active inference framework explain these phenomena? The trick is to reformulate the question: How can multiple agents arrive at a shared understanding of the meaning of some cues in their (shared) environment? We believe we can recast the conventional aspect of symbols as *deontic cues under a shared generative model.*

Indeed, what we call "culture" – that is, the inheritable behavioral differences among conspecifics that are acquired through learning – can be understood as underwritten by shared generative models. Thus, to share a culture is to share a set of expectations about "how creatures like myself behave in specific contexts," a model of the "generic other" reminiscent of Mead (1934). This notion of a shared generative model, in turn, has motivated work on shared manners of attending to the world – what we have called regimes of attention and expectation (Constant et al., 2019). These comprise shared manners of sampling of the world and shared patterns of attributing salience to things in the world.

In a very minimalist sense, a cultural practice can be described as a shared, socially patterned way of acting and perceiving the world (Veissière et al., 2020). In other words, people sharing the same culture will share the same (or similar enough) generative models, which means they share the same expectations about how the world is and how agents can act within it. Shared regimes of attention manifest themselves to the organisms through shared behavioral repertoires underwritten by shared expectations about the value of policies; these are *cultural* affordances because they are not innate, but instead learned through immersive practice and imitation.

How can a generative model become "shared" among multiple agents? For simple agents, like songbirds, the *attunement* of two (or more) generative models can be described as "neural hermeneutics," which describes the process by which two interpreters can come to understand one another – a process that rests on sharing a generative model. In short, two coupled interlocutors attune themselves to each other until they converge on the same beliefs about each other's internal states (Friston & Frith, 2015a, 2015b; see also Veissière et al., 2020). For humans (and any other potential *cultural* species), the story is, of course, more complicated.

A key notion when it comes to understanding these phenomena is that of *niche construction under the free energy principle* – that is, the modification of the environment by the organism to better fit its own expectations, as formalized within the active inference framework (Constant et al., 2018). Indeed, active inference is not a process situated solely in the brain, but rather is embodied and embedded in the environment. The modifications of the environment by the organism are targeted towards elements that can be modified to better fit its own phenotype, and thus minimize its free energy in that environment. These modifications are "traces" of the action of the organism; the environment embodies the preferences of the organisms that shape it. Reciprocally, that means the organism can later rely on environmental features to guide its behavior (or policy selection), a concept known in the philosophy of biology as the *scaffolding* of cognitive processes (Sterelny, 2010). Under the active inference framework, policy selection – involving environmental features – can have an *epistemic value* or a *pragmatic value* (Constant et al., 2019). *Epistemic value* is a function of the reduction of uncertainty, while *pragmatic value* is a function of the potential fulfillment of preferred sensory outcomes (innate or prior preferences over phenotypic states of being).

The more organisms that act on its environment in a certain way, the more the environment becomes *robust* to change (like a path in a field whose groves grow deeper and cleaner at each passage, and thus comes to "embody" the preferred path of the individuals who take it). In this context, generic "cues" (i.e., iconic/indexical signs) that have an epistemic and/or pragmatic value (e.g., like the link between smoke and fire) will consolidate into *deontic cues* (i.e., conventional signs) as a function of the action of the organisms within the environment (Constant et al., 2019). A *deontic* cue informs the organism about what ought to be done given the current context and situation, and is socially determined. This is because the more organisms act on their environment, the more their actions are carved into their niche – and the more the niche will reliably inform other members about the expectations of a *generic like me other* in this (now socio-cultural) niche. Hence the opportunity for deontic policy selection, where denizens scaffold their inference through the environment in a reciprocal causation loop. Thus, the environmental niche itself becomes a model of its inhabitants, in the sense that this reciprocal loop performs a "caching" of beliefs about actions in this environment. In other words, *generic cues consolidate into deontic cues through agential actions on the environment.*

Conventions – that is, shared ways of acting and perceiving the world – are thus generated through the actions and the recognition of the action of the others, eventually amounting to a local "social-cultural world" where mutually recognized utterances and environmental cues have a specific "meaning," or a certain epistemic and pragmatic affordance (or value) (Veissière et al., 2020). This is also reminiscent of the Morris *pragmatics* dimension of meaning as described earlier. The deontic cues that make up the niche encode the preferences of the "generic other" and can take the form of indexical artifacts that acquire a deontic value through the repeated actions of multiple agents and *point to* broader symbolic conventions for navigating the world. Roads, for example, point to the expected presence of other humans – who also know how to operate cars – to be utilized in certain explicit ways (via traffic signs as additional guides) and many more implicit ways encoded in cultural conventions. We believe that these deontic cues – as characterized within active inference – capture the conventional aspect of symbols – that is, environmental and cultural cues that have a shared value and will influence and be interpreted by different members of a community in roughly the same way. Technically, in Peircean nomenclature, this conventional feature is characteristic of *legisigns* – that is, sign-vehicles that are generated and used conventionally, whereas symbols are a specific kind of legisigns (see Short, 2007 for a more detailed account of the Peircean typology of signs.

The syntactic aspect of symbols

The second aspect of *symbols* is more akin to the linguistic notion – that is, signs that can indicate other signs or, in the hierarchical model of Deacon, *indices of indices* (Deacon, 1997). Based on generative models with deep temporal structure (e.g. Friston et al., 2020), we suggest that the best way to implement syntactic constraints in a generative model is to use a hierarchical model that has a superordinate B matrix. It has already been argued that statistical notions could yield a working paradigm for understanding language processing, acquisition and evolution, which could provide an alternative to the innateness of language structures (Christiansen & Chater, 2016). Indeed, what is a syntax if not a set of rules ascribing the correct and incorrect transition from one symbol to the next, and which symbols can indicate which other symbols. An important feature of (linguistic) symbols is the fact that they can refer to other symbols. This can be described as a syntax (Deacon, 1997; Luuk & Luuk, 2012). Interestingly, it is precisely this kind of hierarchical and relational indexing that underlies most of modern computational linguistics (Khani et al., 2018; Kleinschmidt & Jaeger, 2015; MacKay & Peto, 1995; Roy, 2005; Teh et al., 2006), sometimes with an explicit nod to semiotics.

With a generative model of two systems able to play the 20 questions game, Friston et al. (2020) suggest that transition between words in a sentence is analogous to policy selection – namely, selecting the best symbol given precedent symbols, future symbols, and the general context of the conversation. Symbols can be recast as state transitions, beliefs about state transitions beliefs, or B matrices at a superordinate level of the generative model, which contextualize subordinate B matrices. This is the variational version of indices of indices. This refers to transitions between symbols (e.g., selecting which word will come next in a sentence). This rendition is, of course, not a finished model of all linguistic processes that, in itself, could count as a dynamical explanation of syntax, but rather functions to illustrate the potential of active inference to construct such a model.

Conclusion

We hope we have demonstrated the possible fruitful connections that can be made between the field of semiotics, which provides tools to understand signification, and the active inference framework, which provides tools to understand living systems from a formalized and principled statistical perspective. The work presented here is a first sketch of what could be called variational semiotics. We hope this discussion will motivate interdisciplinary investigations at the intersection of semiotics and the sciences of life and mind, progressing towards the establishment of neurosemiotics to understand the unyielding drive to construe meaning in humans (and possibly other species).

Acknowledgments

We are grateful to Casper Hesp, Pierre Poirier, and Simon Tardif for helpful comments and discussions that contributed to our work on this chapter. We are also grateful to Lars Sandved Smith for permission to use his figure template for Figures 3.2 and 3.3 and Thomas Parr for permission to use Figure 3.4. Researchers on this article were supported by the Fond de recherche du Québec – Société et Culture (AMG), Social Sciences and Humanities Research Council of Canada (MJDR) and by a Wellcome Trust Principal Research Fellowship (Ref: 088130/Z/09/Z) (KJF).

Notes

1 Technically, the free energy principle turns this on its head to show that systems that resist entropic decay (i.e., possess a nonequilibrium steady state) look as if they are minimizing free energy, thereby furnishing a teleological normative account of self-organization.
2 Probabilistic or Bayesian beliefs are simply conditional or posterior probability distributions over external states that are parameterized by internal states. They do not connote personal or propositional beliefs. For example, a virus can encode Bayesian beliefs about its external milieu in its internal molecular states.
3 This characterization of Morris has been described as non-Peircean (Pietarinen, 2012); nevertheless, it proves useful in our situation to relate certain aspects of meaning with certain aspects of active inference.

References

Badcock, P. B., Friston, K. J., & Ramstead, M. J. D. (2019a). The hierarchically mechanistic mind: A free-energy formulation of the human psyche. *Physics of Life Reviews*, *31*, 104–121. doi: 10.1016/j.plrev.2018.10.002

Badcock, P. B., Friston, K. J., Ramstead, M. J., Ploeger, A., & Hohwy, J. (2019b). The hierarchically mechanistic mind: An evolutionary systems theory of the brain, mind and behavior. *Cognitive, Affective, and Behavioral Neuroscience*, *19*, 1319–1351. doi: 10.3758/s13415-019-00721-3

Bernard, C. (1974). *Lectures on the Phenomena Common to Animals and Plants* (H. Hoff, R. Guillemin, & L. Guillemin, Trans.). Springfield, IL: Charles C. Thomas.

Bouissac, P. (1985). Neurosemiotics: A definition. *Recherches sémiotiques/Semiotics Inquiry*, *5*(3), 323–325.

Brier, S. (2008). *Cybersemiotics: Why Information is Not Enough!* Toronto: University of Toronto Press.

Campbell, J. O. (2012). Bayesian inference and the world mind. https://arxiv.org/pdf/1210.8031.pdf

Campbell, J. O. (2016). Universal Darwinism as a process of Bayesian inference. *Frontiers in Systems Neuroscience*, *10*. doi: 10.3389/fnsys.2016.00049

Chemero, A. (2009). *Radical Embodied Cognition*. Cambridge, MA: MIT Press.

Christiansen, M. H. & Chater, N. (2016). *Creating Language: Integrating Evolution, Acquisition, and Processing*. Cambridge, MA: MIT Press.

Clark, A. (2015). *Surfing Uncertainty: Prediction, Action, and the Embodied Mind*. Oxford: Oxford University Press.

Conant, R. C., & Ross Ashby, W. (1970). Every good regulator of a system must be a model of that system. *International Journal of Systems Science*, *1*(2), 89–97. doi: 10.1080/00207727008920220

Constant, A., Ramstead, M. J., Veissiere, S. P., Campbell, J. O., & Friston, K. J. (2018). A variational approach to niche construction. *Journal of the Royal Society Interface*, *15*(141), 20170685. doi: 10.1098/rsif.2017.0685

Constant, A., Ramstead, M. J., Veissière, S. P., & Friston, K. J. (2019). Regimes of expectations: An active inference model of social conformity and human decision making. *Frontiers in Psychology*, *10*, 679. doi: 10.3389/fpsyg.2019.00679

Deacon, T. (1997). *The Symbolic Species: The Co-evolution of Language and the Brain*. New York: W.W. Norton.

Deacon, T. (2011a). *Incomplete Nature: How Mind Emerged from Matter*. New York: W.W. Norton.

Deacon, T. (2011b). The symbol concept. In K. R. Gibson & M. Tallerman (Eds.), *The Oxford Handbook of Language Evolution* (pp. 393–405). Berkeley, CA: University of California Press.

Egan, F. (2019). The nature and function of content in computational models. In M. Sprevak & M. Colombo (Eds.), *The Routledge Handbook of the Computational Mind* (pp. 247–258). London: Routledge.

Eliasmith, C. (2005). A new perspective on representational problems. *Journal of Cognitive Science*, *6*, 97–123.

Fodor, J. A. (1975). *The Language of Thought, Vol. 5*. Cambridge, MA: Harvard University Press.

Fodor, J. A. (1983). *The Modularity of Mind: An Essay on Faculty Psychology*. Cambridge, MA: MIT Press.

Friston, K. (2008). Hierarchical models in the brain. *PLoS Computational Biology*, *4*(11), e1000211. doi: 10.1371/journal.pcbi.1000211

Friston, K. & Buzsaki, G. (2016). The functional anatomy of time: What and when in the brain. *Trends in Cognitive Sciences*, *20*(7), 500–511. doi: 10.1016/j.tics.2016.05.001

Friston, K., Parr, T., Yufik, Y., Sajid, N., Price, C. J., & Holmes, E. (2020). Generative models, language and active inference. *PsyArXiv Preprints*. doi: 10.31234/osf.io/4j2k6

Friston, K. J. (2010). The free-energy principle: a unified brain theory? *Nature Reviews Neuroscience*, *11*(2), 127–138. doi: 10.1038/nrn2787

Friston, K. J. (2013). Life as we know it. *Journal of the Royal Society Interface*, *10*(86). doi: 10.1098/rsif.2013.0475

Friston, K. J. (2020). A free energy principle for a particular physics. ArXiv. 1906.10184v1

Friston, K. J., FitzGerald, T., Rigoli, F., Schwartenbeck, P., & Pezzulo, G. (2017). Active inference: A process theory. *Neural Computation*, *29*(1), 1–49. doi: 10.1162/NECO_a_00912

Friston, K. J., & Frith, C. D. (2015a). Active inference, communication and hermeneutics. *Cortex*, *68*, 129–143. doi: 10.1016/j.cortex.2015.03.025

Friston, K. J., & Frith, C. (2015b). A duet for one. *Consciousness and Cognition, 36*, 390–405. doi: 10.1016/j.concog.2014.12.003

Friston, K. J., Rosch, R., Parr, T., Price, C., & Bowman, H. (2018). Deep temporal models and active inference. *Neuroscience & Biobehavioral Reviews, 90*, 486–501. doi: 10.1016/j.neubiorev.2017.04.009

Friston, K. J., Wiese, W., & Hobson, J. A. (2020). Sentience and the origins of consciousness: From Cartesian duality to Markovian monism. *Entropy, 22*(5), 516. doi: 10.3390/e22050516

Gibson, J. J. (1979). *The Ecological Approach to Visual Perception*. Hove: Psychology Press.

Hipólito, I., Ramstead, M. J., Convertino, L., Bhat, A., Friston, K., & Parr, T. (2021). Markov blankets in the brain. *Neuroscience & Biobehavioral Reviews, 125*, 88–97. doi: 10.1016/j.neubiorev.2021.02.003

Hohwy, J. (2016). The self-evidencing brain. *Noûs, 50*(2), 259–285. doi: 10.1111/nous.12062

Ingold, T. (2000). *The Perception of the Environment: Essays on Livelihood, Dwelling and Skill.* New York: Routledge.

Jorna, R. J. J. M. (2006). Neurosemiotics. In M.D. Binder, N. Hirokawa, & U. Windhorst (Eds.), *Encyclopedic Reference of Neuroscience*. Berlin: Springer.

Khani, F., Goodman, N. D., & Liang, P. (2018). Planning, inference and pragmatics in sequential language games. *Transactions of the Association for Computational Linguistics, 6*, 543–555. doi: 10.1162/tacl_a_00037

Kirchhoff, M., Parr, T., Palacios, E., Friston, K., & Kiverstein, J. (2018). The Markov blankets of life: Autonomy, active inference and the free energy principle. *Journal of the Royal Society Interface, 15*(138). doi: 10.1098/rsif.2017.0792

Kleinschmidt, D. F. & Jaeger, T. F. (2015). Robust speech perception: Recognize the familiar, generalize to the similar, and adapt to the novel. *Psychological Review, 122*(2), 148–203. doi: 10.1037/a0038695

Kull, K., Deacon, T., Emmeche, C., Hoffmeyer, J., & Stjernfelt, F. (2011). Theses on biosemiotics: Prolegomena to a theoretical biology. In C. Emmeche & K. Kull (Eds.), *Towards a Semiotic Biology: Life is the Action of Signs* (pp. 25–41). Singapore: Imperial College Press.

Luuk, E. & Luuk, H. (2012). Natural language – no infinity and probably no recursion. *Proceedings of the Annual Meeting of the Cognitive Science Society, 34.*

MacKay, D. J. C. & Peto, L. C. B. (1995). A hierarchical Dirichlet language model. *Natural Language Engineering, 1*(3), 289–308. doi: 10.1017/S1351324900000218

Mead, G. H. (1934). *Mind, Self and Society*. Chicago: University of Chicago Press.

Parr, T., Da Costa, L., & Friston, K. (2020). Markov blankets, information geometry and stochastic thermodynamics. *Philosophical Transactions of the Royal Society A, 378*(2164), 20190159. doi: 10.1098/rsta.2019.0159

Parr, T., & Friston, K. J. (2018). The anatomy of inference: Generative models and brain structure. *Frontiers in Computational Neuroscience, 12*(90). doi: 10.3389/fncom.2018.00090

Pearl, J. (1988). *Probabilistic Reasoning in Intelligent Systems: Networks of Plausible Inference*. San Francisco, CA: Morgan Kaufmann.

Peirce, C. S. (1902). Logic as semiotic: The theory of signs. *Philosophical writings of Peirce*. Mineola, NY: Dover.

Pietarinen, A. V. J. (2012). Peirce and Deacon on the meaning and evolution of language. In T. Schilhab, F. Stjernfelt, & T. Deacon, *The Symbolic Species Evolved* (pp. 65–80). Dordrecht: Springer.

Pietarinen, A. V. & Beni, M. D. (2021). Active inference and abduction. *Biosemiotics, 14*, 499–517. doi: 10.1007/s12304-021-09432-0

Ramsay, D. S. & Woods, S. C. (2014). Clarifying the roles of homeostasis and allostasis in physiological regulation. *Psychological Review, 121*(2), 225–247. doi: 10.1037/a0035942

Ramstead, M. J. (2015). Naturalizing what? Varieties of naturalism and transcendental phenomenology. *Phenomenology and the Cognitive Sciences, 14*(4), 929–971. doi: 10.1007/s11097-014-9385-8

Ramstead, M. J., Badcock, P. B., & Friston, K. J. (2018). Answering Schrödinger's question: A free-energy formulation. *Physics of Life Reviews, 24*, 1–16. doi: 10.1007/s11097-014-9385-8

Ramstead, M. J., Constant, A., Badcock, P. B., & Friston, K. J. (2019b). Variational ecology and the physics of sentient systems. *Physics of Life Reviews, 31*, 188–205. doi: 10.1016/j.plrev.2018.12.002

Ramstead, M. J., Kirchhoff, M. D., Constant, A., & Friston, K. J. (2019c). Multiscale integration: Beyond internalism and externalism. *Synthese, 198*, 41–70. doi: 10.1007/s11229-019-02115-x

Ramstead, M. J., Kirchhoff, M. D., & Friston, K. J. (2019a). A tale of two densities: Active inference is enactive inference. *Adaptive Behavior, 28*(4), 225–239. doi: 10.1177/1059712319862774

Ramstead, M. J., Friston, K. J. & Hipólito, I. (2020). Is the free-energy principle a formal theory of semantics? From variational density dynamics to neural and phenotypic representations. *Entropy*, 22(8), 889, doi: 10.3390/e22080889

Ramstead, M. J., Veissière, S. P., & Kirmayer, L. J. (2016). Cultural affordances: Scaffolding local worlds through shared intentionality and regimes of attention. *Frontiers in Psychology*, 7. doi: 10.3389/fpsyg.2016.01090

Roy, D. (2005). Semiotic schemas: A framework for grounding language in action and perception. *Artificial Intelligence, 167*(1–2), 170–205. doi: 10.1016/j.artint.2005.04.007

Sterelny, K. (2010). Minds: extended or scaffolded? *Phenomenology and the Cognitive Sciences, 9*(4), 465–481. doi: 10.1007/s11097-010-9174-y

Schrödinger, E. (1944). *What is Life?* Cambridge: Cambridge University Press.

Seifert, U. (2012). Stochastic thermodynamics, fluctuation theorems and molecular machines. *Reports on Progress in Physics*, *75*(12). doi: 10.1088/0034-4885/75/12/126001

Seth, A. K. (2015). Inference to the best prediction. In T. K. Metzinger & J. M. Windt (Eds.), *Open MIND*. Frankfurt am Main: MIND Group.

Seth, A. K. & Friston, K. J. (2016). Active interoceptive inference and the emotional brain. *Philosophical Transactions of the Royal Society B: Biological Sciences*, *371*(1708). doi: 10.1098/rstb.2016.0007

Short, T. L. (2007). *Peirce's Theory of Signs*. Cambridge: Cambridge University Press.

Stephan, K. E., Manjaly, Z. M., Mathys, C. D., Weber, L. A. E., Paliwal, S., Gard, T., Tittgemeyer, M., Fleming, S. M., Haker, H., Seth, A. K., Petzschner, F. H. (2016). Allostatic self-efficacy: A metacognitive theory of dyshomeostasis-induced fatigue and depression. *Frontiers in Human Neuroscience*, *10*, 550. doi: 10.3389/fnhum.2016.00550

Sterling, P. & Eyer, J. (1988). Allostasis: A new paradigm to explain arousal pathology. In S. Fisher & J. Reason (Eds.), *Handbook of Life Stress, Cognition and Health* (pp. 629–649). New York: John Wiley & Sons.

Teh, Y. W., Jordan, M. I., Beal, M. J., & Blei, D. M. (2006). Hierarchical Dirichlet processes. *Journal of the American Statistical Association*, *101*(476), 1566–1581. doi: 10.1198/016214506000000302

Thompson, E. (2010). *Mind in Life: Biology, Phenomenology, and the Sciences of Mind*. Cambridge, MA: Harvard University Press.

Tschantz, A., Seth, A. K., & Buckley, C. L. (2019). Learning action-oriented models through active inference. bioRxiv. doi: 10.1101/764969

Varela, F. J. (1996). *Neurophenomenology: A Methodological Remedy for the Hard Problem*. Exeter: Imprint Academic.

Varela, F. J., Thompson, E., & Rosch, E. (1991). *The Embodied Mind: Cognitive Science and Human Experience*. Cambridge, MA: MIT Press.

Vasil, J., Badcock, P. B., Constant, A., Friston, K., & Ramstead, M. J. (2019). A world unto itself: Human communication as active inference. arXiv, arXiv: 1906.10538

Veissière, S. P., Constant, A., Ramstead, M. J., Friston, K. J., & Kirmayer, L. J. (2020). Thinking through other minds: A variational approach to cognition and culture. *Behavioral and Brain Sciences*, *43*, e90. doi: 10.1017/S0140525X19001213

von Uexküll, J. (1982). The theory of meaning. *Semiotica*, *42*(1), 25–79. doi: 10.1515/semi.1982.42.1.25

Watson, J. B. (1913). Psychology as the behaviorist views it. *Psychological Review*, *20*(2), 158–177. doi: 10.1037/h0074428

4

EXPERIMENTAL SEMIOTICS

Past, present, and future

Jonas Nölle and Bruno Galantucci

Introduction

We humans are distinct from other animals in that our life is permeated by constant creation and manipulation of semiotic systems such as languages, writing systems, and the pictograms we exchange through our phones (Cassirer, 1953; Deacon, 1997). How do such semiotic systems come about? Over the last two decades, research performed in experimental semiotics (ES) has addressed this question empirically by studying in the lab how people develop novel semiotic systems.

In this chapter, we first situate ES within its historical context. We then describe a sample of the key scientific contributions ES has offered since its inception. These have a broad scope, ranging from insights into the fundamentals of human semiosis to findings concerning its cognitive and social underpinnings. In other words, despite its recent origins, ES has already demonstrated great potential as an engine of discovery in the cognitive, language, and social sciences. We conclude by discussing current challenges faced by ES and how these can be approached in the future with novel technology and a tighter integration with neuroscientific methods, to the mutual benefit of both disciplines and in the best spirit of the neurosemiotic framework.

Historical context of experimental semiotics

ES has both ancient and modern precursors. The question of how humans can create a novel communication system has sparked interest since at least around 600 BCE, when Pharao Psamtik I conducted an isolation experiment with two human infants to investigate whether language is innate. Such unethical experiments (usually resulting in severe damage to the infants) were repeated several times in history and can to some extent be considered precursors to ES as well as precursors to isolation studies into the innateness of bird song (e.g., Fehér et al., 2009: 564–568; Thorpe, 1958: 535–570). More modern precursors to laboratory experiments on communication can be traced back to psychologists such as Bartlett (1932) and Bavelas (1952: 1–44), who studied in the lab how information transmission leads to the creation of "stereotypical" memory patterns or the emergence of leadership. Although these scholars were interested in different questions, their paradigms resemble ES insofar they involve senders, receivers, and pressures concerning the processes through which people exchange information. Similarly, there were early attempts to use artificial miniature languages to study language change (e.g., Esper, 1925; Wolfle, 1933: 313–315), which in many ways resemble some

DOI: 10.4324/9781003051817-6

of the modern ES paradigms. Finally, recent precursors include strands of related research (Galantucci, 2017), such as experimental pragmatics (Noveck & Sperber, 2004), in which participants use pre-existing forms of communication – that is, their native language – to solve communicative problems. Such studies usually address how interlocutors design utterances to express their intention in a given context. Phenomena of interest are usually pragmatic aspects of communication such as relevance, degree of specificity, and efficient utterance formation for successful communication (Gibson et al., 2019: 389–407; Grice, 1975: 183–198; Rubio-Fernandez & Jara-Ettinger, 2020: 13399–13404), often in the context of contemporary theoretical frameworks such as the *rational speech-act model* (Goodman & Frank, 2016: 818–829). To study actual communication in the lab, these studies typically rely on communication tasks, in which participants can succeed only if they communicate accurately about the entities of a specific experimental context (Clark & Wilkes-Gibbs, 1986: 1–39; Horton & Keysar, 1996: 91–117; Krauss & Weinheimer, 1964: 113–114). For instance, Garrod and colleagues used the Maze Game – where dyads have to communicate locations of gate-opening switches in two-dimensional mazes – to show that such problem-solving leads to routinization of communicative conventions (Garrod & Anderson, 1987: 181–218). In a follow-up study, it was found that these conventions would diffuse in a community of interacting partners (Garrod & Doherty, 1994: 181–215). The cooperative Maze Game has since been used in a number of studies addressing interactional phenomena, such as alignment (Garrod & Pickering, 2009: 292–304), repair (Healey, 2008: 13–39), and how linguistic conventions are shaped by environmental factors such as different maze configurations (Nölle, et al., 2020: 1–10).

The main difference between ES and experimental pragmatic studies is that ES focuses on the emergence of *de novo* communication systems in the lab. In other words, rather than allowing participants to communicate through their shared language, ES forces them to establish a novel semiotic system to solve the task at hand. For instance, in Galantucci's (2005: 737–767) experiment, participants had to communicate locations in a similar vein to the Maze Game, but could only communicate by drawing on a device that systematically distorted the drawings. In this respect, ES also resembles earlier attempts to simulate the emergence of linguistic structure or communication systems using formal mathematical models or populations of agents. Such models have been used to simulate cultural transmission of novel communicative signals as well as situations where such signals have to be established in interaction to achieve successful communication (e.g., Brighton et al., 2005: 177–226; Griffiths & Kalish, 2007: 441–480; Steels, 2011: 339–356; Kirby & Hurford, 2002: 121–147). One of the main achievements of ES studies has been to demonstrate that such research can also be conducted with humans to investigate how their own natural constraints shape the fundamental structures of communication (see also Box 4.1 later in the chapter). While rigorously controlled, these experiments offer higher levels of ecological validity than computational models because they do not rely on *ad hoc* assumptions concerning human nature (Galantucci & Roberts, 2012: 1–13).[1]

Over the two decades that have elapsed since its inception, ES has offered a number of scientific contributions, from insights into the fundamentals of human semiosis to discoveries concerning its cognitive and social underpinnings. In this chapter, we will present and discuss a sample of these contributions, with no claims of exhaustiveness. ES began thriving after it was spontaneously developed in a few different scientific communities. Reviewing the full body of research generated through this methodology is beyond the scope of this article; instead, we opted to present a sample of contributions that, in our opinion, best highlight the potential of ES as an engine of scientific discovery.

The fundamentals of human semiosis

Some of the early ES studies focused on fundamental aspects of human semiosis, such as how humans ground symbols and how these symbols organize themselves in highly functional semiotic systems, such as signed and spoken languages.

Symbol grounding

The origins of symbolic language have sometimes been referred to as the "hardest problem in science" (Christiansen & Kirby, 2003: 1–15), requiring interdisciplinary efforts and a wide variety of empirical methods to be addressed (Fitch, 2017: 3–33; Nölle, Hartmann, et al., 2020: 3–26). Besides the biological, cognitive, and sociocultural prerequisites for human language (see, e.g., Fitch, 2010; Kirby, 2017: 118–137; Tomasello, 2008, 2014), a central question concerns the "symbol grounding problem" (Harnad, 1990: 335–346): How does a population of agents with no symbolic communication system ground such a system with non-symbolic means?

Early ES studies by Galantucci (2005: 737–767) and Garrod et al. (2007: 961–987) provide two significant contributions to answer this question. First, they show that in the context of joint actions with clear goals, humans can readily solve the symbol grounding problem. The second is that the problem itself provides a fertile experimental framework to study human semiotic behavior under controlled laboratory conditions. In particular, these studies showed that when participants who could not use their native language were asked to solve communication problems in a graphical communication medium, they would usually try to bootstrap signs based on motivated icons or indexical signals. Typically, these motivated forms were directly related to properties of the task participants were performing or the environment in which they were immersed. Over time, these initial forms would then gradually evolve into symbols. For instance, in Garrod et al.'s (2007: 961–987) 'Pictionary' drawing task, initially participants tried to communicate referents by using very descriptive drawings such as a smoking cowboy to express "Clint Eastwood." These drawings tended to gradually evolve into simplified symbols (e.g., a circle and arrow indicating "East"), which were more efficient to produce but less transparent to outsiders (see also Box 4.1 and Figure 2). This process of "symbolification" illustrates how ES studies offer an opportunity to observe the emergence of fundamental hallmarks of human symbolic systems such as arbitrariness and conventionality (de Saussure, 1916).

Design features

At first glance, one could question whether the highly abstract and simplified communication games in ES studies, which usually feature a single well-defined communicative objective and very restricted degrees of behavioral freedom, can provide a fertile terrain to grow something akin to a full-blown language in the lab. After all, the communication systems that emerge in such settings usually consist of very small inventories of signs that are just about sufficient to solve the task at hand (see Galantucci, Garrod, et al., 2012: 477–493 for detailed examples). However, to the contrary, this restrictedness is one of the main strengths of ES because its experimental settings can be tailored to zoom in on a specific property of communication and isolate the variables that influence its emergence. In this way, ES studies have been able to investigate most of the "design features" proposed by Hockett (1960) to capture the essence of human language as a semiotic system distinct from animal communication.

These include *duality of patterning* – the fact that languages rely on both *combinatorial* and *compositional* structure. Combinatoriality is the ability to integrate discrete, meaningless forms into an indefinite number of meaningful combinations. In this way, spoken or signed languages use small inventories to make up words from combinations of phonemes or discrete features of manual gestures. Galantucci, Kroos, and Rhodes (2010: 100–111) showed that one pressure leading to the emergence of combinatoriality is another design feature, namely *rapidity of fading* – the fact that signed or spoken languages are evanescent (in contrast to, say, writing). They observed that participants dealing with more rapidly fading signals were more likely to reuse and combine simple elements to achieve communicative success. Further studies (Little et al., 2017: 1–15; Roberts et al., 2015: 52–66) have shown that arbitrariness likewise fosters combinatoriality because, when the meaning space (*what* is communicated) does not easily map onto the form space (*how* it is communicated), the pressure for efficient message transmission prevails over other communicative pressures. Since combinatorial signs greatly enhance efficient message transmission, people tend to prefer them over other sign types.

In addition to combinatoriality, human communication systems are also *compositional* and *systematic* (Dingemanse et al., 2015: 603–615). They allow systematically recombining a finite set of existing meanings to express an open-ended set of possible meanings in the form of new words and sentences. Early computer simulations suggested that compositional structures could be the outcome of pressures from learning and communication acting upon communication systems as they are used and transmitted over generations (rather than derived from innate biology; see Brighton, 2002: 25–54; Christiansen & Chater, 2008: 489–509). However, it was ES that allowed researchers to demonstrate for the first time that this emergence of structure could be observed in humans in the lab. In various studies, participants were given unstructured input – for example, objects with random labels in an artificial language – or were asked to communicate a set of meanings with recurring dimensions (such as shape, color, and texture) in a novel communication medium (Kirby et al., 2014: 108–114). A recurring finding has been that, over time, emerging communication systems become increasingly compositional in response to various pressures. For example, studies by Kirby and colleagues (2008: 10681–10686; 2015: 87–102) showed that initially holistic signals, where a random character string like *tupim* encodes a meaning like "red triangle," could evolve into compositional labels in which, for example, the first syllable encodes the shape and the second syllable encodes the color. This compositionality allows the expression of many possible shape–color combinations with a finite set of meanings, similar to how the English utterances *green triangle*, and *blue triangle* reuse a shared element. Systematic structure of this kind has been observed to emerge in different settings in studies by Theisen et al. (2010: 14–32) and Motamedi et al. (2019: 1–21), who had their participants communicate concepts belonging to specific semantic categories (e.g., writing, school, teacher, cooking, chef, restaurant) through either drawing or gestures. In these experiments, certain elements of the drawings or single gestures people used to communicate would be reused so that, for instance, a "cooking" gesture could be combined with a systematic gesture marking "building" or "person" to express *restaurant* or *chef*. A related gesture study by Nölle et al. (2018: 93–104) showed that this tendency to evolve markers for systematic categories was amplified in an open-ended environment where new meanings were constantly introduced (see also Carr et al., 2017: 892–923; Selten & Warglien, 2007: 7361–7366). The study further found that another design feature, *displacement*, had an impact on the degree of systematicity: dyads communicating about absent entities were more likely to introduce systematic gestures, presumably because categorizing referents made it easier to reason about the task and set of target referents in working memory.

Together, these findings suggest that ES does not just allow studying design features of communication systems such as combinatoriality, rapidity of fading, systematicity, or displacement, but also offers insights to be gained into their interrelations. Furthermore, ES has proven to be an excellent tool to study other aspects of human semiosis. For instance, some studies have tested how communication systems developed in the lab adapt to the communicative situation in which they are used and found that different contexts determine the extent to which signals become holistic, underspecified, or systematic (Nölle et al., 2018: 93–104; Silvey et al., 2015: 212–226; Winters et al., 2015: 415–449).

The cognitive and social underpinnings of human semiosis

Thanks to ES methods, researchers have performed a host of studies aimed at uncovering, through experimental manipulations, the cognitive and social underpinnings of human semiosis. We describe a sample of these studies, focusing on sets of them that have emerged as more or less coherent lines of research in the literature.

Cognitive underpinnings: Impact of modality

Graphical media like drawing or gesture provide a strong affordance for iconicity, since they allow representing concepts via forms that resemble their referents. Some authors have therefore argued that gesture is better suited for bootstrapping communication systems (Fay et al., 2013: 1356–1367, 2014: 1–12). However, how effectively a meaning can be represented iconically in a specific medium also depends on its semantics. While manual gestures can easily depict actions or objects – for example, emotions can easily be expressed by facial expressions or vocalizations (Perlman et al., 2015: 1–16; Perlman & Lupyan, 2018: 1–14) – in the language sciences, it is becoming increasingly accepted that human communication is multimodal and relies on large variety of integrated communication channels such as speech, gesture, and facial expressions (Holler & Levinson, 2019: 639–652; Perniss, 2018: 1–5). ES can help tease apart the contributions of these channels and how they became integrated in the first place (e.g., Zlatev et al., 2017: 465–488). Paradigms affording iconicity further lend themselves to the study of more specific aspects of language in detail, since the medium allows participants to quickly and reliably ground communication systems in the lab. Thus, silent gesture experiments have recently become a popular tool for studying the origins of specific grammatical structures, such as cross-linguistic word order preferences that seem to reflect cognitive processes, which can be observed in the lab (Culbertson et al., 2020: 696–717; Goldin-Meadow et al., 2008: 9163–9168; Ortega & Özyürek, 2020: 51–67; Schouwstra & de Swart, 2014: 431–436). The manual modality is of special interest, since recently emerged natural sign-languages show similar evolutionary stages as gesture systems that emerge in the lab, such as high degrees of iconicity in early generations of users and the gradual development of discrete combinatorial elements that become organized in a system (Fusellier-Souza, 2006: 30–56; Motamedi et al., 2019: 1–21; Senghas, 2004: 1779–1782). Here, lab experiments offer not just a parallel to naturalistic data, but can help shed light on the underlying mechanisms that lead to the emergence of structure. This includes the lab observations that prevalent iconicity can impede combinatoriality (Little et al., 2017: 1–15; Roberts & Galantucci, 2012: 297–318; Roberts et al., 2015: 52–66), which are reflected in the real-world case of Al Sayyid Bedouin Sign Language, which developed in an isolated village community (Sandler et al., 2011: 503–543), or the finding that spatial modulation to differentiate event arguments across discourse requires several generations of signers to develop, which has been attested both in the lab (Motamedi et al., 2018) and in Nicaraguan Sign Language (Kocab et al., 2015: 1–13).

Other communicative modalities frequently used in ES include written miniature languages comprising small lexicons of artificial words (e.g., Kirby et al., 2008: 10681–10686, 2015: 87–102; Smith et al., 2017: 1–13; Tinits et al., 2017: 148–159; Winters et al., 2015: 415–449), sequences of symbols such as letters or pictograms (e.g., Ruiter et al., 2010: 51–77; Selten & Warglien, 2007: 7361–7366; Winters & Morin, 2019: 1–17) or different types of trackpads, touchscreens, and motion control (e.g., Eryilmaz & Little, 2017: 1748–1768; Galantucci, 2005: 737–767; Morin et al., 2018: 91–93). To evoke complex structures, like duality of patterning, experiments need to include both a meaning space that affords compositional reference (e.g., recurring meaning dimensions such as color, shape, etc.), and a continuous signaling space that affords creating both holistic and combinatoric messages. This has, for instance, been achieved with a slide whistle (Verhoef, 2012: 357–380; Verhoef et al., 2014: 57–68) or the Leap Motion device (Eryilmaz & Little, 2017: 1748–1768), which allow for discrete patterns to emerge from an initially continuous and unstructured signal.

Social underpinnings: Horizontal and vertical transmission

Over the years, ES researchers have developed a wide range of experimental paradigms to address different questions in the field (see also Tamariz & Kirby, 2016: 39). Early ES studies mainly relied on one of two basic designs. The first is dyadic interaction, where two participants solve a coordination problem (e.g., Galantucci, 2005: 737–767; Scott-Phillips et al., 2009: 226–233) or perform a referential communication task (Garrod et al., 2007: 961–987). As we described above, such studies have provided insights into how humans could bootstrap symbolic communication in the first place. The second design is the so-called 'iterated learning' paradigm, where an initial "generation" *n* of participants are trained on an artificial language and have to reproduce it. Next, their output becomes the input for the subsequent generation *n* + 1 and so forth, hence allowing to observe how the system evolves over time in reaction to learning biases present in the learners (see Kirby et al., 2014: 108–114 for a review).

These different approaches led to the realization that different types of interaction and population dynamics affect communication systems in different ways (Fay et al., 2010: 351–386; Smith et al., 2013: 1348–1353), which resulted in refinement of these design and further paradigms (Figure 4.1).

Generally, interaction puts communicative pressures on signaling systems. Signals need to be expressive and informative so interlocutors can readily interpret what their partner is signaling to solve the task at hand, while also being simple and efficient to reduce production costs and facilitate communication. Pairs in dyadic-only studies therefore often settle on very efficient symbolic solutions, which rarely involve systematic structures or redundant elements that are not crucial for solving the task (e.g., see Fay et al., 2013: 1–9; Galantucci, 2005: 737–767; cf. Nölle et al., 2018: 93–104; Raviv

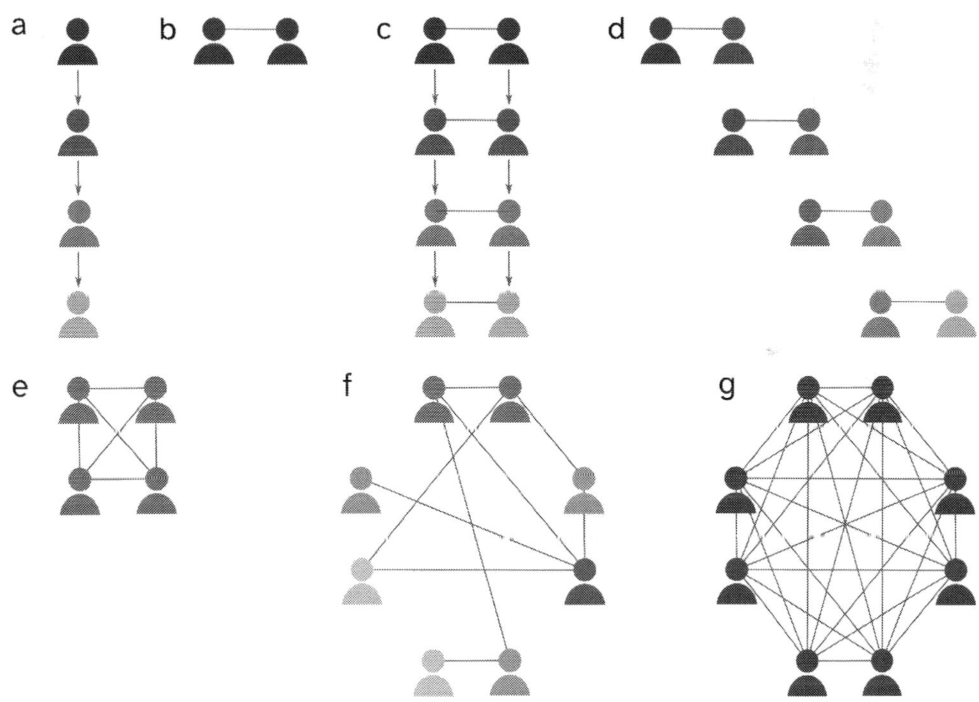

Figure 4.1 Common experimental designs used in experimental semiotics studies

Arrows indicate vertical transmission; solid lines indicate horizontal interaction. (a) Transmission only: An iterated learning chain modelling cultural transmission of a communication system over four generations). (b) Dyadic interaction only: pairs of participants solve a communication game in each experimental session). (c) Transmission and interaction: Dyads interact within an iterated chain, where the output of a dyad becomes the input for the next generation. (d) Replacement method: Dyads interact, and after some time one dyad member is replaced with a new participant, simulating population turnover (in this case, five participants in total). (e–f) Micro-societies: Participants interact with several members of an artificial 'community' to simulate the spread of variants in a population. Different population sizes (e.g., e vs f) and social network topologies (e.g., fully connected networks in e and g vs a sparse network in f) allow studying how population dynamics affect the evolution of the communication systems that emerge in these settings. See e-book for a full-color version of this figure.

et al., 2019: 151–164). By contrast, transmission creates biases for simplicity and learnability. Variants are more likely to get passed on if they are easier to remember. Participants in iterated learning studies therefore favor compressible analytic structures that are easier to learn over simple holistic signals, which creates a bottleneck for compositional structure to pass through (Kirby et al., 2008: 10681–10686). However, the most learnable systems are not necessarily very expressive and useful for communication (e.g., a single label that applies to all available meanings). Newer studies have therefore begun to combine interaction and transmission paradigms by using chains of dyads and consistently shown that this results in languages that are both easy to learn and transmit, and expressive and efficient for communication (Kirby et al., 2015: 87–102; Motamedi et al., 2019: 1–21).

Other paradigms have been added, such as replacement and community paradigms that allow studying how symbol variants evolve as they diffuse in a population, and how local usage events and changes can lead to the emergence of global conventionalized patterns (Fay et al., 2010: 351–386; Fay & Ellison, 2013: 1–9; Galantucci, Theisen, et al., 2012: 583–590). In this context, ES can be used to study the relationship between language and its wider environment: Raviv and colleagues (2019: 151–164) tested a correlation that has been found between grammatical complexity and population size in spoken (Lupyan & Dale, 2010) and signed languages (Meir et al., 2012: 247–291). They had participants interacting in micro-societies with four or eight members in fully connected networks (see Figure 4.1, for example) and found that larger communities developed more systematic languages and did so faster, which corroborates the patterns among natural languages.

Box 4.1 Summary of the experimental semiotics approach

To illustrate how ES studies give rise to a novel communication system in the lab, Figure 4.2 provides an overview of common components of ES experiments.

Each sign system ultimately derives from form-meaning mappings. The signaling space (Figure 2a top) determines the form – that is, which communication channel is chosen. The modality of the channel (e.g., gesture, vocalization, drawing) provides affordances for iconicity and determines how signals can be motivated. For example, in Fay et al.'s (2007) drawing study, participants improvised iconic drawings of concepts such as *computer screen* (bottom). This allows grounding communicative signals and enables a process of conventionalization whereby, due to the interactive nature of the game, gradual symbolification turns icons into arbitrary symbols. The meaning space (Figure 2b) determines the semantic content the signals are mapped onto – that is, *what* is talked about. This could, for example, be the location of four rooms with corresponding symbols, such as in Galantucci's (2005) original coordination game (left), or a set of cartoon pictures with systematic elements, such as in Nölle et al.'s (2018) silent gesture study (right). In most cases, the sign inventory (or lexicon of an artificial language) will come to reflect the referential targets that have to be communicated. The wider task environment (Figure 2c) can exert further pressures by highlighting salient properties or making aspects of the referential environment (ir-)relevant. This can include aspects of where the experiment is situated, like different layouts in the Maze Game (top) that make specific ways of describing locations particularly salient (Garrod & Anderson, 1987; Nölle, Fusaroli, et al., 2020), or the presence of features in the referential context itself. If referential targets include different shapes (center left), each signal is likely to be mapped onto a shape; however, if both shape and color are relevant meaning dimensions (center right), then the communication system will likely encode both (Silvey et al., 2015; Winters et al., 2015). Furthermore, aspects of the communicative environment itself can shape sign systems (bottom left). Referring to visible objects on a table is vastly different from communicating things that are displaced from the communicative context (e.g., shown briefly on a screen before communication takes place), since strategies such as pointing are disabled. Lastly, the social environment, such as community size or network structure,

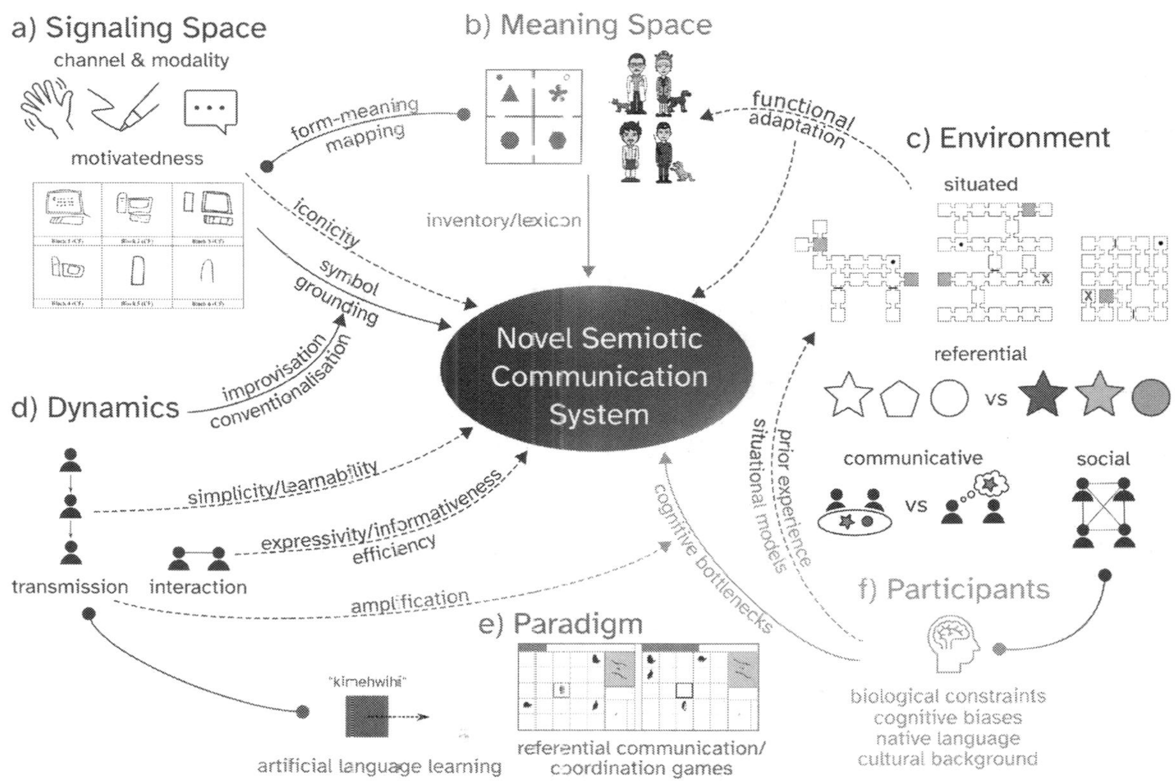

Figure 4.2 Components of experimental semiotics studies that give rise to a novel semiotic communication system

Solid lines indicate processes and mechanisms in the evolution of a sign system, dashed lines indicate pressures shaping its core properties. See e-book for a full-color version of this figure.

can shape aspects such as complexity of the sign system or the diffusion of variants (Fay & Ellison, 2013; Raviv et al., 2019, 2020). The paradigm that is chosen for an ES experiment is tightly linked to task dynamics. For example, artificial language learning is usually used when studying vertical transmission (Figure 2e, left), like in iterated learning designs (Kirby et al., 2014). By contrast, communication studies use referential tasks or coordination games to study horizontal interaction. For example, Roberts and Galantucci (2012) had dyads communicate targets from a set of referents placed on a grid via a track pad for graphical communication (Figure 2e, right). The task dynamics (Figure 2d), in turn, then shape the characteristics of the communication system in different ways: Transmission puts pressure on systems to become simpler, more compressible and easier to learn, whereas interaction puts pressure on signals to become more efficient over time, and makes them informative and expressive in the given context (i.e., satisfy the meaning space and be functionally adaptive to the environment). These pressures are necessary to give rise to design features such as systematicity or duality of patterning (see section 3.2). For more details on variations of task dynamics, see also Figure 4.1 above. A final set of constraints comes from participants' biological and cognitive biases (Figure 2f). This involves, for example, innate learning biases that are amplified over transmission and lead to regularity (Kirby et al., 2007). Additionally, linguistic background should be controlled for depending on the phenomena of interest – for example, when studying the emergence of noun phrase word order with English speakers, it makes sense to use a post-nominal language to preclude native biases, and silent gesture experiments should not be conducted with fluent signers who are more experienced in the manual modality. Lastly, the cultural background and cognitive style might affect the pre-established grammatical or conceptual categories (e.g., color, space) that participants will impose on the task, which can lead to different outcomes. ES studies therefore try to control for such variables and/or study samples from different populations for a cross-cultural perspective that provides insights into universals and variation of human semiotic behavior.

Open challenges and future directions

Limitations

Although ES has delivered many of its promises and proven to be a powerful engine of discovery for the cognitive, language, and social sciences, it does not come without limitations. While ES has successfully modelled mechanisms underlying the basic building blocks of communication, we are still far from observing the emergence of full-fledged "languages," in the sense of fully productive, flexible, and open-ended communication systems. This is in part because artificial communication systems are often miniature versions of languages consisting of small inventories of form-meaning mappings that can only be applied in the restricted context of the task itself. Additionally, ES has focused on isolating the core properties of language and has only more recently been integrated with research into more concrete phenomena – for example, after the success of ES paradigms in uncovering cognitive biases and mechanisms shaping communication systems, artificial language learning experiments are now used more routinely to investigate the origins of typological patterns such as word order universals (Culbertson et al., 2020: 696–717), animacy markers (Vihman et al., 2018: 552–565), or person systems (Maldonado & Culbertson, 2020: 1–42). Furthermore, the general forces that shape communication systems in ES experiments, such as pressures for expressivity/informativeness and simplicity/learnability, have – beyond lab experiments – been confirmed to shape features of natural languages, such as semantic category system – for example, to express kinship (Kemp & Regier, 2012: 1049–1054) or colors (Gibson et al., 2019: 389–407). ES has also been applied to subfields such as sociolinguistics, simulating the formation of dialects (Sneller & Roberts, 2018: 298–311), phonology (Roberts & Clark, 2020: 121–139), and experimental pragmatics (Tinits et al., 2017: 128–159;

Rubio-Fernandez & Jara-Ettinger, 2020: 13399–13404). Roberts and Sneller (2020: 188–229) therefore view ES as part of a newly "integrated science of language evolution" that allows studying both the emergence of structure and its ongoing change and variation (see also Roberts, 2017: 1–13, as well as Hartmann, 2020: 15–39 on the distinction between language evolution and language change). For the near future, the challenge for ES is to demonstrate that it cannot only serve as a tool for simulating the emergence of simple task-oriented communication systems but also help explain the full richness and complexity of natural language.

Tamariz (2017: 402) identified several "future issues" for the field. Some of these have been advanced in recent years, such as integrating ES more with other disciplines as described above, or the manipulation of population size and structure in experiments, which have since been conducted (see previous section). However, other challenges remain: the differential contribution of children and adults to the emergence of language is still poorly understood, and only few studies have begun to address this question (Kempe et al., 2015: 247–254, 2019; Raviv & Arnon, 2018: 160–173).

Another challenge lies in the use of more "naturalistic games" (Tamariz, 2017: 403), which pertains to the ecological validity of ES experiments. To get humans who already speak or sign a language to create novel forms of communication in the lab, researchers have conceived elegant, but ultimately highly artificial, settings that hardly resemble real communicative interactions. This in turn makes it unclear whether the results are representative of and generalizable to real-world phenomena. For a long time, it has virtually been agreed upon that ecological validity is something that needs to be sacrificed to gain experimental control (e.g., to isolate the causal effect of a variable). However, as Peeters (2019) points out, these two aspects of experimental design are actually orthogonal properties rather than the ends of a continuum. This becomes clear when considering recent advances in technology, such as immersive virtual reality (VR). Using VR, it is possible to design immersive and realistic communication tasks that still allow for full experimental control of all variables. This has, for instance, been used to study how spatial language adapts to the environment (Nölle, Kirby, et al., 2020: 321–323) and could easily be extended to other multimodal communication tasks. Similarly, smartphone apps now offer a novel opportunity for studying the emergence and diffusion of communication systems in large populations for which computational models were previously required (Morin et al., 2018: 91–93, 2020). We thus believe that several limitations of ES can be overcome, as novel technologies and the integration of ES paradigms into other disciplines will greatly expand what the approach is capable of.

Integration of ES and neuroscience in a neurosemiotic framework

While ES has been applied successfully in the language and psychological sciences, other fields still bear a lot of potential for cross-fertilization and a tighter integration of ES methods. In neuroscience, recent years have seen calls for a tighter integration with the social sciences and application of neuroscientific findings (Ibáñez et al., 2017) – for instance, to better understand how social processes such as value-based decision-making, influence and persuasion (Falk & Scholz, 2018: 329–356), or social cognitive abilities like mentalizing and theory of mind (Frith & Frith, 2012: 287–313), are actually embedded in situated social interactions.

As we have seen, ES allows studying human meaning-making in *situated* and *social settings* (see Box 4.1, Figure 2c), in which interlocutors must rely on exactly these social processes embedded in joint actions to create shared symbols and coordinate successfully (e.g., Clark, 1996). Building common ground and establishing form-meaning mappings based on feedback from the interlocutor and environment requires joint attention, perspective-taking and mentalizing abilities, and even so, some individual participants still fail at solving ES tasks successfully (Galantucci, 2005: 737–767). This offers the perfect opportunity to study the underlying social and affective neural processes under "extreme" conditions and, with advances in paradigms and technology (such as VR), in naturalistic but controlled settings.

In the past, neuroscience has focused mostly on studying cognitive processes in individual brains. One way to study social phenomena with neuroscientific methods is the social observation approach, whereby participants in the brain scanner passively encounter social stimuli. More recently, some studies have looked explicitly at symbolic behavior. For instance, Rocca et al. (2020: 1–16) used contextualized dialogical narratives in the fMRI scanner to show that spatial demonstratives ("this," "that"), which are used to establish joint attention in interaction, rely on neural resources for perception, attention, and extra-linguistic cognition. Tylén et al. (2016: 105–112) combined a behavioral task with a brain scan to show how symbolic artefacts engage social brain areas. Participants had to collective build symbolic representations of abstract concepts using LEGO bricks. Viewing photographs of the models was associated with social areas in the brain, and more interestingly contrasting activation for viewing one's own models or those created by other groups, suggesting that neural activity can capture a perceiver's attitude towards a cultural symbol.

A new "second-person" neuroscience tries to go even further by directly studying brain-to-brain couplings with a "dual-brain approach" (Hasson et al., 2012: 114–121) or "hyperscanning" (Montague, 2002: 1159–1164), where two participants in separate fMRI scanners interact directly with each other (Redcay & Schilbach, 2019: 495–505). Such an approach allows measuring coupling (synchronous activity in the same regions of both brains) as well as inter-brain connectivity (brain activity in one participant that correlates with brain activity in a distinct area in another participant) in direct social interaction, and has demonstrated how the brains of two interlocutors are coupled/misaligned during successful/failed communication using speech (Stephens et al., 2010: 14425–14430) or gesture (Schippers et al., 2010: 9388–9393). This dual-brain approach allows studying social cognitive processes such as mentalizing, joint attention, reciprocal interaction, and group dynamics (see Redcay & Schilbach, 2019: 495–505 for a review).

Combining ES with this second-person neuroscience approach will allow investigating the brain-to-brain coupling processes involved in symbol grounding, how this neural coupling emerges gradually as common ground is established between participants, and the extent to which it is required for successful communication. Some initial studies in this direction have already been conducted: Stolk et al. (2014: 25–34) used transcranial magnetic stimulation during an ES-style communication task to show which areas are necessary for action understanding when establishing communication. In this vein, the combination of ES and modern neuroscience techniques allows deriving both a behavioral and neural picture of how people establish conceptual alignment (Pickering & Garrod, 2004: 169–225; Stolk et al., 2016: 180–191) and resolve ambiguity, uncertainty, and asymmetries to successfully communicate (Stolk et al., 2020; see also Chapter 17 in this volume).

As part of an integrated neurosemiotic framework that views human meaning-making as both socially and biologically grounded (see Deacon, 1997; Plebe & Cruz, 2016 and other chapters in this volume), ES can not only inspire neuroscience to integrate more socially focused interaction paradigms, but likewise benefit from the use of neuroscientific methods. Behavioral data can provide only a sketchy picture of the cognitive, emotional, and social processes involved in ES experiments, and people are notoriously unreliable in describing them at a subjective level. Neural data (fMRI, MEG, EEG), as well as biological markers and physiological measures (heart rate, skin conductance), can provide insights into the neurobiological underpinnings of embodied synchronizations and interpersonal synergies that are necessary to achieve meaning-making but have mostly been studied on a behavioral level (Fusaroli & Tylén, 2016: 145–171; Louwerse et al., 2012: 1404–1426).

Conclusions

Taken together, the first decade of ES research established it as a serious approach for studying human semiosis and the evolution of communication systems in the lab using direct interaction under controlled conditions (Galantucci, Garrod, et al., 2012: 477–493). During its second decade, ES has proven to be a reliable tool that can be applied in various disciplines and fields to study the full range of human semiosis. It is our hope that, in its third decade, ES will improve upon some of its limitations. This includes more naturalistic tasks and a tighter integration of neurological and biological perspectives, to understand not only how humans are able to create sign systems at the behavioral level but also which neurobiological processes are underlying meaning-making in these contexts. ES can thus serve as an important set of methods in a modern neurosemiotic framework that approaches human semiosis in its natural ecology, namely goal-oriented face-to-face interaction between embodied agents situated in an environment.

Note

1 Computational models, in turn, allow execution of experiments that would be unethical or unpractical to perform with humans.

References

Bartlett, F. C. (1932). *Remembering. A Study in Experimental and Social Psychology*. Cambridge: Cambridge University Press.

Bavelas, A. (1952). Communication patterns in problem-solving groups. In H. von Foerster (Ed.), *Cybernetics. Circular, Causal and Feedback Mechanisms in Biological and Social Systems. Transactions of the Ninth Conference* (pp. 1–44). New York: Josiah Macy Jr. Foundation.

Brighton, H. (2002). Compositional syntax from cultural transmission. *Artificial Life*, *8*(1), 25–54. doi: 10.1162/106454602753694756

Brighton, H., Smith, K., & Kirby, S. (2005). Language as an evolutionary system. *Physics of Life Reviews*, *2*(3), 177–226. doi: 10.1016/j.plrev.2005.06.001

Carr, J. W., Smith, K., Cornish, H., & Kirby, S. (2017). The cultural evolution of structured languages in an open-ended, continuous world. *Cognitive Science*, *41*(4), 892–923. doi: 10.1111/cogs.12371

Cassirer, E. (1953). *The Philosophy of Symbolic Forms. Vol. I: Language* (pp. xiv, 328). New Haven, CT: Yale University Press.

Christiansen, M. H., & Chater, N. (2008). Language as shaped by the brain. *Behavioral and Brain Sciences*, *31*(5), 489–509. doi: 10.1017/S0140525X08004998

Christiansen, M. H., & Kirby, S. (2003). Language evolution: The hardest problem in science. In M. H. Christiansen & S. Kirby (Eds.), *Language Evolution* (pp. 1–15). Oxford: Oxford University Press.

Clark, H. H. (1996). *Using Language*. Cambridge: Cambridge University Press.

Clark, H. H., & Wilkes-Gibbs, D. (1986). Referring as a collaborative process. *Cognition*, *22*(1), 1–39. doi: 10.1016/0010-0277(86)90010-7

Culbertson, J., Schouwstra, M., & Kirby, S. (2020). From the world to word order: Deriving biases in noun phrase order from statistical properties of the world. *Language*, *96*(3), 696–717. doi: 10.1353/lan.2020.0045

de Saussure, F. (1916). *Cours de linguistique générale*. Paris: Payot.

Deacon, T. W. (1997). *The Symbolic Species: The Co-evolution of Language and the Brain*. New York: W.W. Norton.

Dingemanse, M., Blasi, D. E., Lupyan, G., Christiansen, M. H., & Monaghan, P. (2015). Arbitrariness, iconicity, and systematicity in language. *Trends in Cognitive Sciences*, *19*(10), 603–615. doi: 10.1016/j.tics.2015.07.013

Eryilmaz, K., & Little, H. (2017). Using leap motion to investigate the emergence of structure in speech and language. *Behavior Research Methods*, *49*(5), 1748–1768. doi: 10.3758/s13428-016-0818-x

Esper, E. A. (1925). *A Technique for the Experimental Investigation of Associative Interference in Artificial Linguistic Material*. Washington, DC: Linguistic Society of America.

Falk, E., & Scholz, C. (2018). Persuasion, influence, and value: Perspectives from communication and social neuroscience. *Annual Review of Psychology*, *69*(1), 329–356. doi: 10.1146/annurev-psych-122216-011821

Fay, N., Arbib, M., & Garrod, S. (2013). How to bootstrap a human communication system. *Cognitive Science*, *37*(7), 1356–1367. doi: 10.1111/cogs.12048

Fay, N., & Ellison, T. M. (2013). The cultural evolution of human communication systems in different sized populations: Usability trumps learnability. *PLoS ONE*, *8*(8), e71781. doi: 10.1371/journal.pone.0071781

Fay, N., Garrod, S., Roberts, L., & Swoboda, N. (2010). The interactive evolution of human communication systems. *Cognitive Science*, *34*(3), 351–386. doi: 10.1111/j.1551-6709.2009.01090.x

Fay, N., Lister, C. J., Mark Ellison, T., & Goldin-Meadow, S. (2014). Creating a communication system from scratch: Gesture beats vocalization hands down. *Frontiers in Psychology*, *5*, 1–12. doi: 10.3389/fpsyg.2014.00354

Fehér, O., Wang, H., Saar, S., Mitra, P. P., & Tchernichovski, O. (2009). De novo establishment of wild-type song culture in the zebra finch. *Nature*, *459*(7246), 564–568. doi: 10.1038/nature07994

Fitch, W. T. (2010). *The Evolution of Language*. Cambridge: Cambridge University Press.

Fitch, W. T. (2017). Empirical approaches to the study of language evolution. *Psychonomic Bulletin & Review, 24*(1), 3–33. doi: 10.3758/s13423-017-1236-5

Frith, C. D., & Frith, U. (2012). Mechanisms of social cognition. *Annual Review of Psychology, 63*, 287–313. doi: 10.1146/annurev-psych-120710-100449

Fusaroli, R., & Tylén, K. (2016). Investigating conversational dynamics: Interactive alignment, interpersonal synergy, and collective task performance. *Cognitive Science, 40*(1), 145–171. doi: 10.1111/cogs.12251

Fusellier-Souza, I. (2006). Emergence and development of signed languages. *Sign Language Studies*, 7(1), 30–56. doi: 10.1353/sls.2006.0030

Galantucci, B. (2005). An experimental study of the emergence of human communication systems. *Cognitive Science, 29*(5), 737–767. doi: 10.1207/s15516709cog0000_34

Galantucci, B. (2017). Experimental semiotics. In B. Galantucci (Ed.), *Oxford Research Encyclopedia of Linguistics*. Oxford: Oxford University Press. doi: 10.1093/acrefore/9780199384655.013.210

Galantucci, B., Garrod, S., & Roberts, G. (2012). Experimental semiotics. *Language and Linguistics Compass, 6*(8), 477–493. doi: 10.1002/lnc3.351

Galantucci, B., Kroos, C., & Rhodes, T. (2010). The effects of rapidity of fading on communication systems. *Interaction Studies, 11*(1), 100–111. doi: 10.1075/is.11.1.03gal

Galantucci, B., & Roberts, G. (2012). Experimental semiotics: An engine of discovery for understanding human communication. *Advances in Complex Systems, 15*(3–4), 1150026. doi: 10.1142/S0219525911500263

Galantucci, B., Theisen, C., Gutierrez, E. D., Kroos, C., & Rhodes, T. (2012). The diffusion of novel signs beyond the dyad. *Language Sciences, 34*(5), 583–590. doi: 10.1016/j.langsci.2012.03.013

Garrod, S., & Anderson, A. (1987). Saying what you mean in dialogue: A study in conceptual and semantic co-ordination. *Cognition, 27*(2), 181–218. doi: 10.1016/0010-0277(87)90018-7

Garrod, S., & Doherty, G. (1994). Conversation, co-ordination, and convention: An empirical investigation of how groups establish linguistic conventions. *Cognition, 53*(3), 181–215. doi: 10.1016/0010-0277(94)90048-5

Garrod, S., Fay, N., Lee, J., Oberlander, J., & MacLeod, T. (2007). Foundations of representation: Where might graphical symbol systems come from? *Cognitive Science, 31*(6), 961–987. doi: 10.1080/03640210701703659

Garrod, S., & Pickering, M. J. (2009). Joint action, interactive alignment, and dialog. *Topics in Cognitive Science, 1*(2), 292–304. doi: 10.1111/j.1756-8765.2009.01020.x

Gibson, E., Futrell, R., Piantadosi, S. P., Dautriche, I., Mahowald, K., Bergen, L., & Levy, R. (2019). How efficiency shapes human language. *Trends in Cognitive Sciences, 23*(5), 389–407. doi: 10.1016/j.tics.2019.02.003

Goldin-Meadow, S., So, W. C., Özyürek, A., & Mylander, C. (2008). The natural order of events: How speakers of different languages represent events nonverbally. *Proceedings of the National Academy of Sciences, 105*(27), 9163–9168. doi: 10.1073/pnas.0710060105

Goodman, N. D., & Frank, M. C. (2016). Pragmatic language interpretation as probabilistic inference. *Trends in Cognitive Sciences, 20*(11), 818–829. doi: 10.1016/j.tics.2016.08.005

Grice, H. P. (1975). Logic and conversation. In P. Cole & J. L. Morgan (Eds.), *Syntax and Semantics*, Vol. III (pp. 183–198). Cambridge, MA: Academic Press.

Griffiths, T. L., & Kalish, M. L. (2007). Language evolution by iterated learning with Bayesian agents. *Cognitive Science, 31*(3), 441–480. doi: 10.1080/15326900701326576

Harnad, S. (1990). The symbol grounding problem. *Physica D: Nonlinear Phenomena, 42*(1), 335–346. doi: 10.1016/0167-2789(90)90087-6

Hartmann, S. (2020). Language change and language evolution: Cousins, siblings, twins? *Glottotheory, 11*(1), 15–39. doi: 10.1515/glot-2020-2003

Hasson, U., Ghazanfar, A. A., Galantucci, B., Garrod, S., & Keysers, C. (2012). Brain-to-brain coupling: A mechanism for creating and sharing a social world. *Trends in Cognitive Sciences, 16*(2), 114–121. doi: 10.1016/j.tics.2011.12.007

Healey, P. G. T. (2008). Interactive misalignment: The role of repair in the development of group sub-languages. In R. Cooper & R. Kempson (Eds.), *Language in Flux* (pp. 13–39). New York: Palgrave Macmillan.

Hockett, C. F. (1960). The origin of speech. *Scientific American, 203*(3), 88–97. doi: 10.2307/24940617

Holler, J., & Levinson, S. C. (2019). Multimodal language processing in human communication. *Trends in Cognitive Sciences, 23*(8), 639–652. doi: 10.1016/j.tics.2019.05.006

Horton, W. S., & Keysar, B. (1996). When do speakers take into account common ground? *Cognition, 59*(1), 91–117. doi: 10.1016/0010-0277(96)81418-1

Ibáñez, A., Sedeño, L., & García, A. M. (2017). *Neuroscience and Social Science: The Missing Link*. New York: Springer.

Kemp, C., & Regier, T. (2012). Kinship categories across languages reflect general communicative principles. *Science, 336*(6084), 1049–1054. doi: 10.1126/science.1218811

Kempe, V., Gauvrit, N., & Forsyth, D. (2015). Structure emerges faster during cultural transmission in children than in adults. *Cognition, 136*, 247–254. doi: 10.1016/j.cognition.2014.11.038

Kempe, V., Gauvrit, N., Gibson, A., & Jamieson, M. (2019). Adults are more efficient in creating and transmitting novel signaling systems than children. *Journal of Language Evolution, 4*(1), 44–70. doi: 10.1093/jole/lzy012

Kirby, S. (2017). Culture and biology in the origins of linguistic structure. *Psychonomic Bulletin & Review, 24*(1), 118–137. doi: 10.3758/s13423-016-1166-7

Kirby, S., Cornish, H., & Smith, K. (2008). Cumulative cultural evolution in the laboratory: An experimental approach to the origins of structure in human language. *Proceedings of the National Academy of Sciences, 105*(31), 10681–10686. doi: 10.1073/pnas.0707835105

Kirby, S., Dowman, M., & Griffiths, T. L. (2007). Innateness and culture in the evolution of language. *Proceedings of the National Academy of Sciences, 104*(12), 5241–5245. doi: 10.1073/pnas.0608222104

Kirby, S., Griffiths, T., & Smith, K. (2014). Iterated learning and the evolution of language. *Current Opinion in Neurobiology, 28*, 108–114. doi: 10.1016/j.conb.2014.07.014

Kirby, S., & Hurford, J. R. (2002). The emergence of linguistic structure: An overview of the iterated learning model. In A. Cangelosi & D. Parisi (Eds.), *Simulating the Evolution of Language* (pp. 121–147). New York: Springer.

Kirby, S., Tamariz, M., Cornish, H., & Smith, K. (2015). Compression and communication in the cultural evolution of linguistic structure. *Cognition, 141*, 87–102. doi: 10.1016/j.cognition.2015.03.016

Kocab, A., Pyers, J., & Senghas, A. (2015). Referential shift in Nicaraguan Sign Language: A transition from lexical to spatial devices. *Frontiers in Psychology, 5*. doi: 10.3389/fpsyg.2014.01540

Krauss, R. M., & Weinheimer, S. (1964). Changes in reference phrases as a function of frequency of usage in social interaction: A preliminary study. *Psychonomic Science, 1*(1), 113–114. doi: 10.3758/BF03342817

Little, H., Eryılmaz, K., & de Boer, B. (2017). Signal dimensionality and the emergence of combinatorial structure. *Cognition, 168*, 1–15. doi: 10.1016/j.cognition.2017.06.011

Louwerse, M. M., Dale, R., Bard, E. G., & Jeuniaux, P. (2012). Behavior matching in multimodal communication is synchronized. *Cognitive Science, 36*(8), 1404–1426. doi: 10.1111/j.1551-6709.2012.01269.x

Lupyan, G., & Dale, R. (2010). Language structure is partly determined by social structure. *PloS one*, 5(1), e8559.

Maldonado, M., & Culbertson, J. (2020). Person of interest: Experimental investigations into the learnability of person systems. *Linguistic Inquiry*, 1–42. doi: 10.1162/ling_a_00406

Meir, I., Israel, A., Sandler, W., Padden, C. A., & Aronoff, M. (2012). The influence of community on language structure: Evidence from two young sign languages. *Linguistic Variation, 12*(2), 247–291. doi: 10.1075/lv.12.2.04mei

Montague, P. (2002). Hyperscanning: Simultaneous fMRI during linked social interactions. *NeuroImage, 16*(4), 1159–1164. doi: 10.1006/nimg.2002.1150

Morin, O., Winters, J., Müller, T., & Morisseau, T. (2020). An overview of the "Color Game" app project. *SocArXiv Papers*. doi: 10.31235/osf.io/cjaxw

Morin, O., Winters, J., Müller, T. F., Morisseau, T., Etter, C., & Greenhill, S. J. (2018). What smartphone apps may contribute to language evolution research. *Journal of Language Evolution, 3*(2), 91–93. doi: 10.1093/jole/lzy005

Motamedi, Y., Schouwstra, M., Smith, K., Culbertson, J., & Kirby, S. (2019). Evolving artificial sign languages in the lab: From improvised gesture to systematic sign. *Cognition, 192*, 103964. doi: 10.1016/j.cognition.2019.05.001

Motamedi, Y., Smith, K., Schouwstra, M., Culbertson, J., & Kirby, S. (2018). The emergence of systematic argument distinctions in artificial sign languages. *PsyArXiv*. doi: 10.31234/osf.io/p6zy4

Nölle, J., Fusaroli, R., Mills, G. J., & Tylén, K. (2020). Language as shaped by the environment: Linguistic construal in a collaborative spatial task. *Palgrave Communications, 6*(1), 1–10. doi: 10.1057/s41599-020-0404-9

Nölle, J., Hartmann, S., & Tinits, P. (2020). Language evolution research in the year 2020: A survey of new directions. *Language Dynamics and Change, 10*(1), 3–26. doi: 10.1163/22105832-bja10005

Nölle, J., Kirby, S., Culbertson, J., & Smith, K. (2020). Does environment shape spatial language? A virtual reality approach. In A. Ravignani, C. Barbieri, M. Martins, M. Flaherty, Y. Jadoul, E. Lattenkamp, H. Little, K. Mudd, & T. Verhoef (Eds.), *The Evolution of Language: Proceedings of the 13th International Conference (EvoLang13)* (321–323). doi: 10.17617/2.3190925

Nölle, J., Staib, M., Fusaroli, R., & Tylén, K. (2018). The emergence of systematicity: How environmental and communicative factors shape a novel communication system. *Cognition, 181*, 93–104. doi: 10.1016/j.cognition.2018.08.014

Noveck, I. A., & Sperber, D. (Eds.). (2004). *Experimental Pragmatics*. London: Palgrave Macmillan.

Ortega, G., & Özyürek, A. (2020). Systematic mappings between semantic categories and types of iconic representations in the manual modality: A normed database of silent gesture. *Behavior Research Methods, 52*(1), 51–67. doi: 10.3758/s13428-019-01204-6

Peeters, D. (2019). Virtual reality: A game-changing method for the language sciences. *Psychonomic Bulletin & Review*, 26(3), 894–900. doi: 10.3758/s13423-019-01571-3

Perlman, M., Dale, R., & Lupyan, G. (2015). Iconicity can ground the creation of vocal symbols. *Royal Society Open Science*, *2*(8), 150152. doi: 10.1098/rsos.150152

Perlman, M., & Lupyan, G. (2018). People can create iconic vocalizations to communicate various meanings to naïve listeners. *Scientific Reports*, *8*(1), 2634. doi: 10.1038/s41598-018-20961-6

Perniss, P. (2018). Why we should study multimodal language. *Frontiers in Psychology*, *9*. doi: 10.3389/fpsyg.2018.01109

Pickering, M. J., & Garrod, S. (2004). Toward a mechanistic psychology of dialogue. *Behavioral and Brain Sciences*, *27*(2). doi: 10.1017/S0140525X04000056

Plebe, A., & Cruz, V. M. D. L. (2016). *Neurosemantics: Neural Processes and the Construction of Linguistic Meaning*. New York: Springer.

Raviv, L., & Arnon, I. (2018). Systematicity, but not compositionality: Examining the emergence of linguistic structure in children and adults using iterated learning. *Cognition*, *181*, 160–173. doi: 10.1016/j.cognition.2018.08.011

Raviv, L., Meyer, A., & Lev-Ari, S. (2019). Compositional structure can emerge without generational transmission. *Cognition*, *182*, 151–164. doi: 10.1016/j.cognition.2018.09.010

Raviv, L., Meyer, A., & Lev-Ari, S. (2020). The role of social network structure in the emergence of linguistic structure. *Cognitive Science*, *44*(8), e12876. doi: 10.1111/cogs.12876

Redcay, E., & Schilbach, L. (2019). Using second-person neuroscience to elucidate the mechanisms of social interaction. *Nature Reviews Neuroscience*, *20*(8), 495–505. doi: 10.1038/s41583-019-0179-4

Roberts, G. (2017). The linguist's Drosophila: Experiments in language change. *Linguistics Vanguard*, *3*(1). doi: 10.1515/lingvan-2016-0086

Roberts, G., & Clark, R. (2020). Dispersion, communication, and alignment: An experimental study of the emergence of structure in combinatorial phonology. *Journal of Language Evolution*, *5*(2), 121–139. doi: 10.1093/jole/lzaa004

Roberts, G., & Galantucci, B. (2012). The emergence of duality of patterning: Insights from the laboratory. *Language and Cognition*, *4*(04), 297–318. doi: 10.1515/langcog-2012-0017

Roberts, G., Lewandowski, J., & Galantucci, B. (2015). How communication changes when we cannot mime the world: Experimental evidence for the effect of iconicity on combinatoriality. *Cognition*, *141*, 52–66. doi: 10.1016/j.cognition.2015.04.001

Roberts, G., & Sneller, B. (2020). Empirical foundations for an integrated study of language evolution. *Language Dynamics and Change*, *10*(2), 188–229. doi: 10.1163/22105832-bja10001

Rocca, R., Coventry, K. R., Tylén, K., Staib, M., Lund, T. E., & Wallentin, M. (2020). Language beyond the language system: Dorsal visuospatial pathways support processing of demonstratives and spatial language during naturalistic fast fMRI. *NeuroImage*, *216*, 116128. doi: 10.1016/j.neuroimage.2019.116128

Rubio-Fernandez, P., & Jara-Ettinger, J. (2020). Incrementality and efficiency shape pragmatics across languages. *Proceedings of the National Academy of Sciences*, *117*(24), 13399–13404. doi: 10.1073/pnas.1922067117

Ruiter, J. P. de, Noordzij, M. L., Newman-Norlund, S., Newman-Norlund, R., Hagoort, P., Levinson, S. C., & Toni, I. (2010). Exploring the cognitive infrastructure of communication. *Interaction Studies*, *11*(1), 51–77. doi: 10.1075/is.11.1.05rui

Sandler, W., Aronoff, M., Meir, I., & Padden, C. (2011). The gradual emergence of phonological form in a new language. *Natural Language & Linguistic Theory*, *29*(2), 503–543. doi: 10.1007/s11049-011-9128-2

Schippers, M. B., Roebroeck, A., Renken, R., Nanetti, L., & Keysers, C. (2010). Mapping the information flow from one brain to another during gestural communication. *Proceedings of the National Academy of Sciences*, *107*(20), 9388–9393. doi: 10.1073/pnas.1001791107

Schouwstra, M., & de Swart, H. (2014). The semantic origins of word order. *Cognition*, *131*(3), 431–436. doi: 10.1016/j.cognition.2014.03.004

Scott-Phillips, T. C., Kirby, S., & Ritchie, G. R. S. (2009). Signalling signalhood and the emergence of communication. *Cognition*, *113*(2), 226–233. doi: 10.1016/j.cognition.2009.08.009

Selten, R., & Warglien, M. (2007). The emergence of simple languages in an experimental coordination game. *Proceedings of the National Academy of Sciences*, *104*(18), 7361–7366. doi: 10.1073/pnas.0702077104

Senghas, A. (2004). Children creating core properties of language: Evidence from an emerging sign language in Nicaragua. *Science*, *305*(5691), 1779–1782. doi: 10.1126/science.1100199

Silvey, C., Kirby, S., & Smith, K. (2015). Word meanings evolve to selectively preserve distinctions on salient dimensions. *Cognitive Science*, *39*(1), 212–226. doi: 10.1111/cogs.12150

Smith, K., Perfors, A., Fehér, O., Samara, A., Swoboda, K., & Wonnacott, E. (2017). Language learning, language use and the evolution of linguistic variation. *Philosophical Transactions of the Royal Society B: Biological Sciences*, *372*(1711), 20160051. doi: 10.1098/rstb.2016.0051

Smith, K., Tamariz, M., & Kirby, S. (2013). Linguistic structure is an evolutionary trade-off between simplicity and expressivity. In M. Knauff, M. Pauen, N. Sebanz, & I. Wachsmuth (Eds.), *Cooperative Minds: Social Interaction and Group Dynamics* (pp. 1348–1353). Seattle, WA: Cognitive Science Society.

Sneller, B., & Roberts, G. (2018). Why some behaviors spread while others don't: A laboratory simulation of dialect contact. *Cognition*, *170*, 298–311. doi: 10.1016/j.cognition.2017.10.014

Steels, L. (2011). Modeling the cultural evolution of language. *Physics of Life Reviews*, *8*(4), 339–356. doi: 10.1016/j.plrev.2011.10.014

Stephens, G. J., Silbert, L. J., & Hasson, U. (2010). Speaker-listener neural coupling underlies successful communication. *Proceedings of the National Academy of Sciences*, *107*(32), 14425–14430. doi: 10.1073/pnas.1008662107

Stolk, A., Bašnáková, J., & Toni, I. (2020). Joint epistemic engineering: The neglected process of context construction in human communication. *PsyArXiv*. doi: 10.31234/osf.io/rwfe6

Stolk, A., Noordzij, M. L., Volman, I., Verhagen, L., Overeem, S., van Elswijk, G., Bloem, B., Hagoort, P., & Toni, I. (2014). Understanding communicative actions: A repetitive TMS study. *Cortex*, *51*, 25–34. doi: 10.1016/j.cortex.2013.10.005

Stolk, A., Verhagen, L., & Toni, I. (2016). Conceptual alignment: How brains achieve mutual understanding. *Trends in Cognitive Sciences*, *20*(3), 180–191. doi: 10.1016/j.tics.2015.11.007

Tamariz, M. (2017). Experimental studies on the cultural evolution of language. *Annual Review of Linguistics*, *3*(1), 389–407. doi: 10.1146/annurev-linguistics-011516-033807

Tamariz, M., & Kirby, S. (2016). The cultural evolution of language. *Current Opinion in Psychology*, *8*, 37–43. doi: 10.1016/j.copsyc.2015.09.003

Theisen, C. A., Oberlander, J., & Kirby, S. (2010). Systematicity and arbitrariness in novel communication systems. *Interaction Studies*, *11*(1), 14–32. doi: 10.1075/is.11.1.08the

Thorpe, W. H. (1958). The learning of song patterns by birds, with especial reference to the song of the chaffinch Fringilla coelebs. *Ibis*, *100*(4), 535–570. doi: 10.1111/j.1474-919X.1958.tb07960.x

Tinits, P., Nölle, J., & Hartmann, S. (2017). Usage context influences the evolution of overspecification in iterated learning. *Journal of Language Evolution*, *2*(2), 148–159. doi: 10.1093/jole/lzx011

Tomasello, M. (2008). *Origins of Human Communication*. Cambridge, MA: MIT Press.

Tomasello, M. (2014). *A Natural History of Human Thinking*. Cambridge, MA: Harvard University Press.

Tylén, K., Philipsen, J. S., Roepstorff, A., & Fusaroli, R. (2016). Trails of meaning construction: Symbolic artifacts engage the social brain. *NeuroImage*, *134*, 105–112. doi: 10.1016/j.neuroimage.2016.03.056

Verhoef, T. (2012). The origins of duality of patterning in artificial whistled languages. *Language and Cognition*, *4*(4), 357–380. doi: 10.1515/langcog-2012-0019

Verhoef, T., Kirby, S., & De Boer, B. (2014). Emergence of combinatorial structure and economy through iterated learning with continuous acoustic signals. *Journal of Phonetics*, *43*, 57–68. doi: 10.1016/j.wocn.2014.02.005

Vihman, V.-A., Nelson, D., & Kirby, S. (2018). Animacy distinctions arise from iterated learning. *Open Linguistics*, *4*(1), 552–565. doi: 10.1515/opli-2018-0027

Winters, J., Kirby, S., & Smith, K. (2015). Languages adapt to their contextual niche. *Language and Cognition*, 7(3), 415–449. doi: 10.1017/langcog.2014.35

Winters, J., & Morin, O. (2019). From context to code: Information transfer constrains the emergence of graphic codes. *Cognitive Science*, *43*(3), e12722. doi: 10.1111/cogs.12722

Wolfle, D. L. (1933). The relative stability of first and second syllables in an artificial language. *Language*, *9*(4), 313–315. doi: 10.2307/409418

Zlatev, J., Wacewicz, S., Żywiczyński, P., & van de Weijer, J. (2017). Multimodal-first or pantomime-first? Communicating events through pantomime with and without vocalization. *Interaction Studies*, *18*(3), 465–488. doi: 10.1075/is.18.3.08zla

5

BEYOND THE HUMAN ANIMAL

Towards a cross-species neurosemiotics

Morten Tønnessen

Introduction

This chapter takes a biosemiotic perspective on neurobiology as its starting point in assessing neurosemiotics across species. A semiotic understanding of comparative neurobiology can shed light on questions such as: how different are humans from non-humans? What do we have in common with (some) other animals? And what is uniquely human?

I build mainly on the neurosemiotics that is implicit in the *Umwelt* theory of the Baltic-German biologist Jakob von Uexküll (1864–1944) and contemporary interpretations of this theory. This angle has been chosen because Uexküll's pioneering thinking on neurosemiotics has influenced classical ethology as well as contemporary biosemiotics, code biology, and cognitive semiotics. Uexküll's work, which includes a number of interrelated neurosemiotic constructs, is thus seen as relevant for semioticians and biologists alike. It furthermore shares some perspectives with prominent contemporary approaches to cognition across species, including cognitive ethology and comparative psychology.

Biosemiotician Jesper Hoffmeyer (2002: 32) conjectured that "the evolutionary origin of consciousness" might be found in primitive organisms that had acquired "a sensitivity, or a susceptibility to impressions." With reference to an article by Maxine Sheets-Johnstone (1998), he outlines the deep connection between consciousness and movement as follows:

> Plants do not have to move, thus they do not have the problem that forced primitive animals a long time ago to evolve the nervous system. Movement demands that muscle cells at one corner of the organism instantaneously, that is, in microseconds, coordinate their activity with muscle cells at the other end. To achieve this coordination – from the perspective of a single cell – long-distance communication became the very art of nerve cells.
>
> *(Hoffmeyer, 2002: 32)*

A precondition for movement is that "the body constantly registers its own change" (2002: 32). This is achieved via "proprioception," the collection of inner sensations through which we sense our own movement. In the words of Sheets-Johnstone (1998: 275), this "astoundingly varied and intricately detailed biological faculty that allows knowing one's own body and body movement … in the most basic sense allows knowing the world," and should be recognized as "a dimension of consciousness,"

 DOI: 10.4324/9781003051817-7

which she suggests to name "corporeal consciousness." Alexei Sharov (2017: 172) relatedly describes proprioception as an "important sensorial scaffold," which enables the body "to facilitate neural-based learning."

Uexküll's *Umwelt* theory is of foundational importance to biosemiotics (Brentari, 2015) and incorporates neurosemiotic ideas. Uexküll operates with a pluralistic approach to neurobiology and behavior. In terms of *Umwelt* theory, neurosemiotic traits across species should be considered in a case-specific manner rather than in gradualistic terms (taking human neurobiology as the measure) or exceptionalistic terms (denying the relevance of any comparison). From Uexküll's perspective, the measure of an organism's biology is its specific needs, which follow from its physiological constitution and its range of related behaviors. While some neurosemiotic traits are in this view uniquely human, their particular character is regarded within a worldview in which the human organism is not the only organism that has unique neurosemiotic traits.

More recently, zoologist Donald Griffin (1915–2003) advanced *cognitive ethology*, an approach to ethology that emphasizes animal consciousness (Allen & Bekoff, 1999; Griffin, 2001). As he observed, a "truly comparative neuroscience of consciousness has begun to develop" (Griffin & Speck, 2004: 15). This is also reflected in the emergence within cognitive science of embodied perspectives focused on "situated living bodies" and "their enacted activity, history and social world," which, according to Ezekiel A. di Paulo (2020: 252), "owe much to Uexküllian thinking." In a parallel development, *comparative psychology* has been reaffirmed as a multidisciplinary field devoted to study "the similarities and differences in the behavior of organisms with special emphases on the development and evolution of the behaviors" (Hill, Guarino, & Dietrich, 2017: 1).

In semiotics, issues related to cognitive science have been addressed particularly by biosemiotics and related subfields (zoosemiotics, ecosemiotics), code biology, and cognitive semiotics, all of which engage systematically with natural science. Identifying both as a biosemiotician and as a cognitive semiotician, Frederik Stjernfelt (2013: 2) emphasizes the need to accomplish a semiotic understanding of cognitive phenomena and pinpoints the need to reject "untenable dreams of the complete reduction of things semiotic to psychology," which the emergence and growth of cognitive science has actualized.

From the perspective of more contemporary biosemiotics, acts of interpretation are involved in the functioning of the nervous system, but also in other biological processes, including simpler processes that are also found in non-sentient organisms. Here, however, opinions differ. For example, biosemioticians working within a Peircean framework tend to believe that acts of interpretation occur even at low levels of biological organization, whereas code biologists such as Marcello Barbieri believe that lower-level biological processes are generally code-based. As we will see, such conceptual disagreements are reflected in contrasting views on neural codes and the functioning of the nervous system.

A key term that will serve as a central reference point in our comparisons of neurosemiotic capabilities across species is *neurosemiotic agency*. In a biosemiotic outlook, all sentient organisms are endowed with neurosemiotic agency – that is, an agentive capability to relate to sign-related aspects of neural-based phenomena. The exact character of this agency, however, varies from species to species. By extension, sentient organisms also differ in how, and maybe also whether, they relate to objects, understood as discernable, unified wholes. This concerns *objecthood* as an issue within semiotics and studies of cognition and perception across species.

In the remainder of this chapter, I start out by discussing whether the neural code can be understood as a semiotic concept and if so, how – given the perspectives of biosemiotics and code biology. I then present the basic features of the neurosemiotics of Jakob von Uexküll before discussing how the neural code can be understood in light of the *Umwelt* theory. Next, I discuss objecthood in perception and the capacity of different organisms to relate to objects. This discussion is informative in terms of diverging views on the different forms of subjectivity among sentient organisms. At the end of the chapter, a biosemiotic perspective on species-related methodological issues in neurobiology is presented, with focus on anthropocentrism, the relation between the observer and the observed, and the general shortfall within neurobiology of qualitative studies of subjectivity and individuality.

The "neural code": A semiotic concept?

In this section, I discuss the conception of a neural code – or codes – in light of different biosemiotic frameworks, including that of code biology. This discussion is central to neurosemiotics at large because it concerns the nature of the operation of the nervous system across species and the mechanisms at work in this context.

The neural code can be characterized as something that triggers "a signal that carries an abstract representation of some signal or process of interest," with "neural coding" being conducted in neurons that "act as information-processing channels that take incoming information, integrate it, and produce a signal that contains information encoded in the neuronal ... electrical activity pattern" (Richmond, 2014: 1).

Discussions about the neural code intersect with those on the role of representations in the workings of the nervous system and consciousness. There are heated debates in neuroscience about whether or not such representations exist. The theoretical construct of a "mental representation" is central to the computational theory of mind, which holds that "cognitive states and processes are constituted by the occurrence, transformation and storage (in the mind/brain) of information-bearing structures (representations)" (Pitt, 2020: para. 1). In a wider sense, a mental representation can be understood as "a mental object with semantic properties" (Pitt, 2020: para. 2). Most biosemioticians maintain representationalism in some form, but oppose computational theories. Gładziejewski (2016: 560) points to the general problem that many "theories which are heralded as representation-invoking turn out to be representational in name only" because they "often use the term 'representation' in such a liberal and unconstrained way that it no longer denotes structures that could be regarded as representational in any recognizable or explanatorily useful manner."

Given the prominence of the notion of a "neural *code*" (my emphasis) within neurobiology, one would perhaps assume that the relevance of semiotics for neurobiology was obvious. However, despite the almost ubiquitous use of the term, the utility of the code metaphor in this context has been questioned. In a recent target article in *Behavioral and Brain Sciences*, which has triggered a lively debate, neuroscientist Romain Brette (2019: 2) argues that neural codes are "unstructured and therefore unable to represent relations." According to his view, "the neural coding metaphor cannot provide a valid basis for theories of brain function, because it is incompatible with both the causal structure of the brain and the representational requirements of cognition." Of note, Brette refers to Uexküll's work (specifically to Uexküll, 1909), as well as to the theoretical biology of Robert Rosen (1985), in acknowledging a form of intrinsic information that may be related to the notion of the *Umwelt* or to other conceptions of organisms' internal models of the world.

Neurobiologist and anthropologist Terrence Deacon and cognitive psychologist and linguist Joanna Rączaszek-Leonardi – both biosemioticians – agree with Brette that the coding metaphor entails more problems than solutions for neurocognitive theories (Deacon & Rączaszek-Leonardi, 2019). They argue that cognitive functioning should, nevertheless, be framed in semiotic terms. As the two point out, the assumption that some form of coding must be involved in neural processes has been reinforced by methods enabling measurement of spike trains in individual neurons following stimulus presentation (Deacon & Rączaszek-Leonardi, 2019). More specifically, observation of correlations between stimulus features and fast neuronal spikes has been understood to support the view that such features are somehow encoded by the neuronal activity (Deacon & Rączaszek-Leonardi, 2019). However, the conceptual framework of coding has led researchers to surmise that mapping such correlations or covariant dynamics amounts to *explaining* neural processes, when in fact it only implies *describing* them.

Deacon and Rączaszek-Leonardi (2019) reject a standard response to criticism of the coding metaphor, which entails abandoning the concept of representation and instead using terminology related to covarying coupled dynamics. This kind of response emerges from various versions of the so-called "dynamical approach" to cognition, which holds that "cognitive systems should be studied as brain processes in continuous dynamical interaction with the body and the immediate environment" (Haselager, de Groot, & van Rappard, 2003: 6) without any need to refer to internal representations. This, Deacon and Rączaszek-Leonardi argue, merely replaces one mapping relation with another, without reconceptualizing and improving our understanding of the involved dynamics.

As an alternative, they propose a synthesis between the reductionist encoding paradigm and those approaches that speak exclusively about neural dynamics (Deacon & Rączaszek-Leonardi, 2019) established by drawing on insights from the dynamical systems perspective and the semiotic framework of Charles S. Peirce. With reference to the work in theoretical biology of Pattee (1973) and Polanyi (1968), Deacon and Rączaszek-Leonardi (2019) emphasize the importance of studying the relationship between constraints and dynamics to gain insights on the very logic of living processes. According to Polanyi (1968: 1312), "recognition of the impossibility of understanding living things in terms of physics and chemistry [only], far from setting limits to our understanding of life, will guide it in the right direction." In the interpretation of Deacon and Rączaszek-Leonardi, this is the context in which semiotics, informed by a systems dynamics approach, can contribute crucially. Specifically, a biosemiotic perspective can explain how living things work *in relation to* their physical and chemical organization but governed by laws and constraints *that cannot be derived* from the dynamics of mere matter.

What the systems dynamics perspective adds to the Peircean framework is an understanding that signs constrain ongoing dynamics, and that, of necessity, semiotic constraints must be different from the dynamics on which they operate (Deacon & Rączaszek-Leonardi, 2019). This distinction is ignored by the coding framework and by other accounts that conceive of cognition exclusively as correlated dynamics (Deacon & Rączaszek-Leonardi, 2019). In this dynamical semiotic approach, constraints on neural activity constitute sign vehicles that should be treated as information structures, which regulate the dynamics underlying the generation of other sign vehicles (Deacon & Rączaszek-Leonardi, 2019). In this perspective, it does make sense to refer to *neural representations*, but these representations must be understood to be dynamical – and, given a conventional understanding of codes as fixed rules, this rejects any conception of a neural code.[1]

Code biologist and biosemiotician Marcello Barbieri (2003, 2015) takes a different approach to neural codes, arguing that code biology provides the coding framework in neuroscience with a suitable theoretical foundation. The main idea of code biology is that various organic or biological codes, starting with the genetic code, are fundamental for the functioning of organisms. In this perspective, neural codes represent one class of organic codes among other types of codes at work in the living realm, and an important advancement in evolutionary history that made the emergence of conscious life-forms possible. Barbieri (2013: 278) stresses that at "the origin of mind, the key event was the appearance of feelings." His hypothesis is that the neural code was "as instrumental to the production of feelings as the genetic code was to the production of proteins."

In Barbieri's words, the concept of a neural code "stands for the unknown mechanism by which the signals from sense organs are transformed into feelings and sensations." An important question is whether there is really something akin to a universal neural code, rather than different neural codes for different animals.

Barbieri (2014: 245) characterizes neural codes as "sets of rules" that mediate between sensory signals and "mental images, or high-level neural states." In his reading (Barbieri, 2014: 245, my emphasis), "neurobiology has made it abundantly clear that there are no *necessary* connections between sensory inputs and mental, or neural, images." However, there may be arbitrary, conventional connections. This would fit with the general idea of codes in code biology, where codes are conceived as fixed rules that mediate between entities or phenomena in two independent realms (cf. Barbieri, 2003: 5; Barbieri, 2014: 245).

With reference to Nicolelis and Ribeiro (2006), Barbieri (2013: 278) proposes that the evidence for the existence of a nearly universal neural code can be found in "the physiological processes that transform the mechanical stimuli into tactile sensations," which "are the same in all animals," a finding that "does suggest that there is a universal mechanism at work." A key point is that the sense organs that produce electrical signals, thus transforming and transmitting sensory input, "arise from the basic histological tissues of the body" (Barbieri, 2013: 279). The four fundamental types of animal tissue are epithelial (i.e., inner and outer surface tissue), connective, muscular, and nervous tissues, and these "are the same in all triploblastic animals" (Barbieri, 2013: 279).[2]

Barbieri (2013: 279) concludes that all sensory signals "come from organs produced by a limited number of universal tissues, and that does make it plausible that they represent a limited number of universal inputs." The next question is whether there are also a limited number of universal outputs. Barbieri thinks this is the case, since feelings and perceptions are associated with certain corresponding actions that largely derive from basic instincts – for example, related to hunger, survival, and reproduction. Barbieri (2013: 279) states: "The neural correlates of the basic histological tissues are associated with the basic animal instincts and these appear to be virtually the same in all triploblastic animals."

Summing up, Barbieri observes that there is

> a universal set of basic histological tissues on one side, a universal set of basic animal instincts on the other side, and a set of neural transformation processes in between. The most parsimonious explanation is that the neural processes in between are also a universal set of operations. And since there is no necessary physical link between sense organs and feelings, we can conclude that the bridge between them can only be the result of a virtually universal *neural code*.
>
> *Barbieri (2013: 279)*

It is worth noting that the neural code is sometimes referred to in the singular form, and other times in the plural form. One finds the singular form in Barbieri (2013), but the plural form in Barbieri (2014). In the latter, he addresses "the appearance of different neural codes in the evolution of the brain" (Barbieri 2014: 245). Barbieri (2014: 245) goes on to suggest: "The increase in the number of neural codes would explain the increase in complexity that took place in brain evolution" over time. However, the outcome of an increasing number of neural codes, understood as various fixed rules for transforming sensory input into neural images, would be limited to a greater diversity of animals "whose behavior is almost entirely pre-programmed, or hardwired" (Barbieri, 2014: 245). It cannot explain the emergence of behavior that is more flexible. While some animals "do have virtually hardwired reactions" – which, according to Barbieri (2014: 245) makes it possible to account for their behavior in large measure by reference to neural codes, "it is a fact that some animals evolved the ability to interpret what goes on in the world around them, and this skill is a true evolutionary novelty, something that is not reducible to coding." Such more adaptable – and perhaps more advanced – subjective experience is, in Barbieri's outlook, within the realm of Peircean semiosis, in which "interpretation" is a relevant concept. In this view, complex neural representations occurring in multicellular animals are interpretation-based, just as much as they are code-based, but they still depend on the operation of a nearly universal neural code, and several more specific neural codes.

In relation to the biosemiotic perspectives of Deacon and Rączaszek-Leonardi (2019) and that of Barbieri (2013, 2014), a middle path may be possible in which the terminology of codes is maintained but reconceptualized, along with an understanding that gives interpretation ample space. This presupposes that a distinction is made between fixed codes and flexible codes. Within this framework, neural codes exemplify fixed codes, but in cognitively complex animals neural representations also rely on ecological codes, which are flexible codes and not fixed rules. As Timo Maran (2012: 149) details, "It is plausible to assume that codes on the ecological level are not strict regulations, but rather ambiguous and fuzzy linkages based on analogies and correspondences." In the interpretation of Tønnessen (2018: 142), "we can assume that neural codes and ecological codes coalesce in the functioning of the search image," which plays an important role in Uexküll's *Umwelt* theory by linking sensation, perception, and action by way of anticipation – on Uexküll's notion of search images, see also Chien (2006).

To recapitulate, we have learned that a Peircean version of biosemiotics and code biology have contrasting views on the utility of conceptualizing neurosemiotic mechanisms in terms of neural codes. Embarking on a middle path by emphasizing the ecological context of sentient organisms makes it possible to maintain a role for neural codes in interplay with ecological (inter-individual) codes that are more flexible and open to interpretation.

Neurosemiotics in Jakob von Uexküll's *Umwelt* theory

The centrality of neurobiology in the biological approach of Jakob von Uexküll is demonstrated already in one of the first pages of his scientific monograph on theoretical biology. The introduction to *Theoretische biologie*, translated here by M. Tønnessen, makes clear not only how *Umwelt* theory builds on philosopher Immanuel Kant's outlook on subject-dependent aspects of reality, but also how it differs from it:

> The task of biology consists in expanding the lessons of Kant's research in two directions: 1. to take into account the role of our bodies, particularly our sense organs and our central nervous system, and 2. to study other subjects' (the animal's) relations to objects.
>
> *(Uexküll 1928: 9)*

In light of this programmatic statement, we can observe that what *Umwelt* theory treats as its subject-matter consists of subject-dependent aspects of reality that are related to the functioning of human and animal bodies and particularly the functioning of the sense organs and central nervous systems of humans and animals.[3] It is also worth noting that Uexküll identifies objecthood, which we will discuss later on, as a core research interest of *Umwelt* theory.

In his first monograph on *Umwelt* theory, *Umwelt und Innenwelt der Tiere* (Uexküll 1909 [first edition], 1921 [second edition]; see also Mildenberger & Herrman, 2014), Uexküll focused on the ways in which the subjective experiential world of humans and animals is of a dual nature, by involving not only an *Umwelt* (outer subjective world) but also an *Innenwelt* (inner subjective world), with the boundary of the body distinguishing the one from the other. In this conception, the *Umwelt* is composed of *Umwelt* objects (or carriers of traits, as Uexküll might have preferred to say) that a human being or animal typically experiences as being present to it somewhere in its proximity, *outside* itself. In contrast, the neurosemiotic construct of the *Innenwelt* is concerned with capturing the experience a human being or animal has of itself, including its own body (this partly corresponds to what is in contemporary literature called "interoception" – that is, the perception of sensations from inside the body). As characterized by Thomas Sebeok (1986: 23), the *Umwelt* in this sense of incorporating an internal and an external environment involves "a qualitative and meaningful model of a species' significant surrounding" (the *Umwelt*) as well as "the individual's actualized version of that surround orchestrated by its nervous system" (the *Innenwelt*).

In terms of semiotic conceptualization, *Umwelt* theory finds its most developed form in *Bedeutungslehre* (Uexküll, 1940; reprinted in Uexküll, 1956 [1934/1940] and most recently published in English translation in Uexküll, 2010 [1934/1940]), Uexküll's final major work. Here the neurosemiotic constructs *Merkwelt* (perceptual world) and *Wirkwelt* (operational world), which together constitute the *Umwelt*, are at a lower level of biological organization explained in terms of the functioning of *Merkzeichen* (perceptual signs) and *Wirkzeichen* (operational signs). According to Uexküll, such signs operate at a cellular level and represent the biosemiosis that is the underlying foundation of consciously experienced phenomena. This sheds light on one of Uexküll's chief insights: that the physiological "machinery" of organisms is always run by cellular or corporeal "machine operators" (*Maschinisten*) and involves sign exchange and what we can call semiotic agency (Uexküll 1956 [1934/1940]: 24). The mechanisms of living organisms are operated by way of agentive biosemiosis (cf., 1956 [1934/1940]: 84). As Roepstorff (1999: 762–763) underlines,

> the *Innenwelt* is not in the trivial sense determined by the *Bauplan* [the organism's physiological and functional organization]; rather the actual connection between *Merkwelt* and *Wirkwelt* is to some extent mediated via experience and communication, that is, via earlier *Umwelt* interactions.

At the time of *Bedeutungslehre* (Uexküll, 1940), Uexküll's position was that being endowed with an *Umwelt* composed of a *Merkwelt* and a *Wirkwelt* was the prerogative of animals with a nervous system. Since they have no sense organs and no nerves, he notes, plants' entire existence appears to play out in a *Wirkwelt* (Uexküll, 1956 [1940]: 123). In the first version of *Umwelt und Innenwelt der Tiere* (Uexküll, 1909), the *Umwelt* notion was attributed more widely, and this was to some extent the case even in *Streifzüge durch die Umwelten von Tieren und Menschen: Ein Bilderbuch unsichtbarer Welten* (Uexküll, 1934; see particularly Uexküll, 1956 [1934]: 48–53), where he refers to the *Umwelt* of unicellular organisms. Throughout his work, Uexküll explicates that the *Umwelt* is a biological version of what Kant refers to as the *Erscheinungswelt* (phenomenal world), with the main difference being that Uexküll applies the term to animals as well as human beings.

Uexküll wrote a number of scientific journal articles on neurobiology, especially early on in his career as a biologist, in 1894–1899, but also quite frequently over a longer period, in 1892–1915, followed by further contributions in the 1920s and 1930s (cf. Uexküll, 1956 [1934/1940]: 172).[4] It was the findings from Uexküll's studies in neurobiology that convinced him he could contribute beyond making observations on selected species of animals by developing theoretical concepts of relevance to biology at large (Mildenberger & Herrman, 2014: 252), as he started doing in Uexküll (1909). In Uexküll (1929), he discusses neuro-muscular feedback and "reaches an important conclusion" (Kull, 2001: 28–29):

> The task of the stimuli is not to convey knowledge about the external world to the animal, but rather to show it the 'right way' through a world that is entirely unknown to it. That is also why the *Merkwelt* is [...] so meager and [...] the *Wirkungswelt* so certain and planned for.
> *(Uexküll, 1929: 762 – German quote translated by M. Tønnessen)*[5]

Only a selection of the physical "effects" of the environment are treated as sensory stimuli by the organism (Uexküll, 1956 [1934/1940]: 111). In *Umwelt und Innenwelt der Tiere*, Uexküll (1921: 166) notes that different kinds of external stimuli can give rise to the same sign, on the condition that a certain lower threshold of stimuli intensity has been passed. Once formed, the perceptual sign, as Uexküll would later call it, only varies in its intensity, which is covariant with the intensity of the stimuli – for a more detailed presentation of Uexküll's views, see Brentari (2013: 11–12). This line of thinking is consistent with Uexküll's thoughts (1928) in *Theoretische Biologie* about the ways in which the *Umwelten* of different species are differently configured with regard to the range of sensory stimuli to which they are sensitive – see also Feiten, Holland, & Chemero (2020: 5). The parameters for lower and upper thresholds for this sensitivity are in effect decided by the physiological features of the organism.

Even though the current biosemiotic understanding of *Umwelten* draws on the works of Uexküll, as Tønnessen et al. (2016: 143) point out, contemporary biosemiotic interpretations of Uexküll have "brought along some transformations of the initial meaning of the concept." This includes a greater emphasis on phenomena and qualia, a development that reflects the change in focus in related disciplines. Köchy (2020: 61) thus notes that "recent developments in neuroscience and behavioral research have led to the repealing of previous restrictions and now the investigation of internal representations of mental events is regarded as the main concern of cognitive neuroscience."

As noted previously, however, the existence and explanatory role of internal cognitive representations are debated. Enactivism is among the schools of thought that explain "cognition as non-representational processes of embodied dynamic interaction" (Heras-Escribano & de Jesus, 2018: 250). "Biosemiotic enactivism," first introduced by Paulo de Jesus (2016), seeks to "develop an account of cognition as creative processes of sign-use among and between species of living organisms," with a conception of signs that does not rely on internal mental representations (Heras-Escribano & de Jesus, 2018: 250). This builds on an enactive reinterpretation of Uexküll's *Umwelt* theory and Peirce's theory of signs (2018: 252–253).

To recapitulate, in this section we have learned that neurobiology played a central role in Uexküll's work from the outset, and that his neurosemiotic outlook convinced him that *Umwelt* theory could be of wider interest. On some points his views matured over time, resulting in a sharper distinction between sentient and other organisms in his last major work. The understanding of neurosemiotic aspects of *Umwelt* theory has kept developing after Uexküll as well, with new syntheses being proposed up until contemporary times.

The neural code across species in light of *Umwelt* theory

In this section, I consider how the neural code or codes can be understood in light of *Umwelt* theory. This is pertinent since the notion of neural codes was not introduced until after Uexküll's death.

In his discussion on proprioception, Hoffmeyer (2002: 33) observes that the movement of an animal "is guided by an internal model, that is being constantly updated," fueled by the organism's ongoing interpretation of external stimuli. It "seems likely," he notes (Hoffmeyer, 2002: 34), that the "internal model" underlying proprioception "constitutes the very primordial basis of consciousness." Hoffmeyer suggests that we "should imagine that when animals in the course of evolution developed the conglomerates of nerve cells we call brains, there emerged, little by little, the capacity for making … internal models" (Hoffmeyer, 2002: 34). In Uexküllian terminology, such models constitute the *Innenwelt* (insofar as they model occurrences within the organism) and the *Umwelt* (insofar as they model occurrences outside the organism) of an organism. In most biosemiotic interpretations, these involve cognitive representations of some kind. In Sebeok's (1996: 107–108) view, the neural codes that trigger such representations constitute an important part of the endosemiosis (i.e., internal, bodily semiosis) of sentient organisms, alongside genetic, immune, and metabolic codes.

This may be compatible with so-called "predictive coding theory" in contemporary cognitive science, according to which cognitive systems control action by inferring "the most likely worldly causes of incoming sensory signals" (Gładziejewski, 2016: 561). A key feature of cognitive systems is, in this view, that they attempt to minimize prediction errors. One way to achieve this is by making "perceptual inferences" and "active inferences" (directly related to action) in a dynamic manner, so "perceiving the world (perceptual inference) and acting on it (active inference) turn out to be two sides of … the same process of minimizing prediction error" (Gładziejewski, 2016: 562). In this view, "Our cognitive engagement with the environment rests on a constant oscillation between perceptual and active inference" (Gładziejewski, 2016: 562–563).

Revisiting Barbieri's discussion of the neural code, we can now reevaluate his hypothesis that "a virtually universal *neural code*" mediates between "a universal set of basic histological tissues" and "a universal set of basic animal instincts" by way of "a set of neural transformation processes" (Barbieri, 2013: 279). As it stands, Barbieri's hypothesis does not explain the wide variety of animal behavior we can observe, which varies from species to species and in some cases even from individual to individual. Barbieri's hypothesis will be strengthened if supplemented by Uexküll's (1921, 1928) view on how the *Umwelten* of different species are differently configured depending on each organism's specific physiology, particularly with regard to sensory and motor capacities. By setting the parameters for the organism's sensitivity to sensory stimuli, the organism's specific physiology defines the possible scope of the subjective experience of an animal. Furthermore, for animals capable of learning, each organism's life experience further configures the animal's sensory sensitivity and contextualizes its experience. The neural code (or codes) is thereby utilized in ways that make sense for the animal, and that lead to diverse and context-dependent behaviors.

As Alexei Sharov (2017: 172) points out, "the studies of the body and meaningful neural processes that roughly correspond to mind are poorly connected." For example, embryology and cognitive science are rarely seen in relation to each other. With "its emphasis on studying agency and specifically composite agency," biosemiotics "offers a new way of bridging this gap" by considering "body and mind as two subagents connected via reciprocal guiding interactions" and exploring "how internal senses, such as pain, serve as a guiding scaffold for the developing mind, and how mental functions affect the development and evolution of the body" (Sharov, 2017: 172).

To recapitulate, in this section we have learned that our understanding of neural codes can be improved by drawing on *Umwelt* theory because the *Innenwelt* notion can substantiate and provide a framework for the internal models and modelling that the operation of neural codes presupposes. This also goes for Barbieri's view on the existence of a universal neural code, which cannot in itself explain the wide variety in animal behavior. But combined with Uexküll's approach to species-specific physiologies and subjective worlds, it can.

Neurosemiotic agency and objecthood across species

We have seen that there are substantial disagreements about how neurosemiotic mechanisms, and neural codes – if any – should be understood, even among those who apply semiotic perspectives in biology. In this section I proceed to discuss neurosemiotics across species with a focus that brings us one step closer to sentient organisms as individuals endowed with subjectivity. The subjectivity of organisms, however, cannot be addressed without investigating how they relate to objects, which also requires some reflections on their agency.

A key question in this context is: What kind of *neurosemiotic agency* – agentive capability to relate to sign-related aspects of neural-based phenomena – do different organisms have? Answering that question will make clear what sort of things or phenomena they are able to relate to and act on. Another key question concerns *whether* and *how* different sentient organisms are capable of relating to objects, understood as discernable, unified wholes. Arguably, only organisms that are capable of relating to objects in this sense are *subjective* in the sense of being able to engage in subject–object relations. This, in turn, warrants a distinction between *proper subjects* (i.e., organisms capable of having coherent experience) and *quasi-subjects* (i.e., organisms with some sort of experience that is, however, disorganized or scattered):

> Proper subjects stand out because their lives have another dimension – namely, unified, cohesive experience of their surroundings – which quasi-subjects lack. Quasi-subjects such as plants, fungi and animals with decentralized bodies also have semiotic agency and quasi-experience, but only proper subjects have cohesive, integrated experience.
>
> *(Tønnessen, 2016: 81)*

By having semiotic agency – that is, by being an agent that engages purposefully in semiosis) – even a quasi-subject has something resembling subjective experience, but *proper* subjective experience should be distinguished from what only resembles it. In a biosemiotic perspective, subjectivity (and by extension individuality) is in this sense a graded phenomenon, as Hoffmeyer (1996) has stressed. What distinguishes what I call proper subjects in terms of biosemiotic theory is that they are either conscious and therefore capable of immediate muscular coordination coupled with their (partly) conscious interpretative experience of signs (see Hoffmeyer, 2002: 32; Uexküll, 1921, 1928, 1934) or unicellular and therefore capable of immediate full body coordination based on their cellular semiosis (Uexküll, 1921). Quasi-subjects, in contrast, rely on intercellular semiosis which does not result in any similarly coherent experience or in any immediate coordination or action.

Taking one step back from sentient organisms to organisms in general, the question concerning objecthood can be rephrased like this: of all the Earth's organisms, which ones are capable of relating to objects, and in what ways?

Sharov and Vehkavaara (2015) introduce a distinction between "protosemiosis" and "eusemiosis," with the latter being associated with a capacity for relating to objects. In the terminology used in this chapter, quasi-subjects only engage in protosemiosis, whereas proper subjects are also engaged in eusemiosis. Within this framework, semiotic agents that are merely capable of engaging in protosemiosis (e.g., bacteria) "associate signs directly with actions … whereas in eusemiosis, agents associate signs with objects and only then possibly with actions" (Sharov & Vehkavaara, 2015: 103). While protosemiosis is mostly at work at a molecular level within cells, "eusemiosis supports higher-level cellular functions and cell interactions in various organs, especially in the neural system" (2015: 108). In this outlook, it is primarily animals with a nervous system that are capable of relating to objects.

The line between organisms that have cohesive experience of their surroundings and those that do not can be drawn in different places. Some opt for drawing this line somewhere *within* the class of animals that have a central nervous system.[6] Hoffmeyer (2004) discusses snakes as a border case:

> The snake may well go on searching for the prey at the spot where it disappeared, but it will not calculate the eventual path the prey may have taken. […] This lack of true intermodality in the snake makes it "hard to imagine that the snake can harbor some form of a concept of a mouse in its brain" (Sjölander, 1995: 5). The snake apparently cannot integrate its sense modalities to form a central construct.
>
> *(Hoffmeyer, 2004: 90)*

While undoubtedly a semiotic agent, in Hoffmeyer's perspective the snake is an example of an animal with a central nervous system that operates with "a direct coupling of stimulus and behavior" Hoffmeyer, 2004: 91) and does not relate to objects. This "does not necessarily mean that snakes are totally deprived of an experienced world, but if indeed they have experiences, these must be lacking in inner coherence" (Hoffmeyer, 2004: 91). In the snake's *Umwelt*, in this view, there are only "things to be searched for, things to be stroked, and things for swallowing" (Hoffmeyer, 2004: 91), but no dynamic objects corresponding to moving objects in the snake's actual surroundings. With respect to the definition of objects presented earlier, we could say that snakes experience some things as discernible but not as unified wholes.

As for human beings, at a quite early stage in human ontogeny, we become proper subjects capable of eusemiosis and relating to objects, after developing a "sense-saturated *Umwelt*" at the fetal stage (Tønnessen, 2014: 293). Objects then emerge gradually, with different kinds of objects emerging at various developmental stages, first in the womb and then, after birth, in increasing numbers and with increasing complexity. Human ontogeny, however, also includes an embryonic stage in which the human *Umwelt* is much simpler. We start out as quasi-subjects (Tønnessen, 2014: 289–290). Only gradually do we become genuinely human, with our potentially advanced ways of relating to objects.

To recapitulate, while all sentient organisms are endowed with neurosemiotic agency, and thus actively relate to signs in the context of neural-based phenomena, they differ in their exact capabilities. An important line can be drawn between those organisms that are able to relate to objects understood as unified, discernable wholes, and those that are not. Biosemioticians disagree on where this line should be drawn.

A biosemiotic perspective on anthropocentrism in behavioral neuroscience

More than a century ago, Lloyd Morgan suggested that we ought to err on the side of caution when interpreting the psychological capacities of non-humans, by formulating what is known as "Morgan's canon" (Morgan, 1903: 59): "In no case is an animal activity to be interpreted in terms of higher psychological processes if it can be fairly interpreted in terms of processes which stand lower in the scale of psychological evolution and development."

Zoosemiotician Dario Martinelli (2007: 276) has suggested turning Morgan's canon upside-down by asserting that "in no case should actions or behaviors be interpreted as the result of an inferior psychic faculty, when it is possible to interpret them as a result of a superior faculty" (see also Martinelli & Bankov, 2008). This too would involve erring on the side of caution, albeit from another angle, operating with an anti-anthropocentric stance as default rather than having an anthropocentric point of view as the default position. These two opposing programmatic statements appear to be equally justifiable in terms of both logics and scientific merit.[7]

Several species-related methodological issues derive from the difference between the role of the observer and the role of the observed in neurobiology. The fact that only humans can serve as scientific observers has profound implications. Operating with an Uexküllian perspective on neuroscience, Gomez-Marin (2019: 29) notes that to

> be an organism is to have a point of view ... What is meaningful for an organism – or even what is possibly apprehensible – need not be meaningful for the scientist studying it, and *vice versa* ... A clash of *Umwelts* [*Umwelten*, in proper German] is going on in our laboratories.

The methodological challenge for mainstream contemporary biology derives from the fact that "an observer-independent reality is erected" despite the fact that biologists "are subjects whose objects of study are subjects too" (Gomez-Marin, 2019: 29). In behavioral neuroscience, this results in a gap between observer and observed. Gomez-Marin (2019: 29) posits that "computational neuroscience can benefit from insights of theoretical ethology to transform its anthropomorphic bias."

As Deacon and Rączaszek-Leonardi (2019) remark, the "aboutness" in the neural processes underlying perceptual experience is designated by the experimenter and not necessarily any intrinsic property of the neural processes themselves. In the big scheme of things, this concerns the mind–body problem, one of the core problems of modern philosophy and science. Polanyi (1968) addresses the issue of the observer's position in cognitive studies by distinguishing between *at*-knowledge, which originates from an external (i.e., third person) perspective, and *from*-knowledge, which originates from an internal (i.e., first person) perspective:

> The mind-body problem arises from the disparity between the experience of a person observing an external object – for example, a cat and a neurophysiologist observing the bodily mechanism by means of which the person sees the cat. The difference arises from the fact that the person observing the cat has a *from*-knowledge of the bodily responses evoked by the light in his sensory organs and this *from*-knowledge integrates the joint meaning of these responses to form the sight of the cat, whereas the neurophysiologist, looking at these responses from outside, has only an *at*-knowledge of them, which, as such, is not integrated to form the sight of the cat.
>
> *(Polanyi, 1968: 1312)*

As central as a subjective, first-person perspective is in ordinary experience, it has nevertheless largely been anathema in science. "Natural science," as Hoffmeyer (2002: 32) would have it, "is about phenomena that can be described in the third person singular," whereas "consciousness is a phenomenon that can only be known from within" (Hoffmeyer, 2002: 31). In Hoffmeyer's view, while natural science "cannot deal with consciousness as such, it is possible by way of science to try to understand what is needed in order for a system to have consciousness."

The methodological tradition within natural science of studying naturally occurring phenomena *objectively* is so strong that it has also shaped the theoretical and methodological outlook of ethology, the study of animal behavior. This is evident in Nikolaas Tinbergen's (1963) programmatic statements concerning the four aims of ethology: to explain animal behavior by studying mechanism; adaptive value; ontogeny; and phylogeny. In this classical approach to ethology, the animal's subjective perspective is systematically left out, or at any rate sidelined. However, not so long ago, Gordon M. Burghardt (1997), drawing on *Umwelt* theory, suggested supplementing Tinbergen's four aims of ethology with a fifth: "private experience."

Owing to some peculiarities in German biology in the period 1900–1930, Uexküll himself did not want people to associate *Umwelt* theory with the *Tierpsychologie* (animal psychology) of his time. This should not be taken to imply that Uexküll denied that *Umwelt* theory involves a genuine subjective aspect. As Mildenberger and Herrman (2014: 298) remark, Uexküll's rejection of animal psychology must be understood in light of what passed as animal psychology among his contemporaries. This included suggestions that horses could solve mathematical problems and communicate the results to humans in coded form. The implication of Uexküll's rejection of contemporary "animal psychology," therefore, is not at all that Uexküll thought that scientific studies of subjective animal experience were unfeasible – indeed, the entire *Umwelt* theory is testament to the opposite. Instead, the message of this historical incident is that Uexküll stressed that any "*Umwelt* research" (*Umweltforschung*) worthy of the name must be based on empirical studies carried out within a sound methodological and theoretical framework in which anthropomorphic biases are avoided.

The unavoidable human bias, or perspective, entrenched in the study of neurobiology has, along with a more normatively loaden anthropocentric bias in ethics, politics, and science, had consequences for how researchers have approached issues of individuality in animals. A common assumption is that whereas both quantitative and qualitative methods are applicable to human subjects, qualitative methods are applicable only to human subjects, meaning in effect that animals can only be studied in quantitative terms. That might work quite well for the stereotypical animal, but not necessarily for individual animals. This methodological understanding has led to an unfortunate neglect of scientific studies of animal individuality. There is a considerable gap between the typical descriptions of animal behavior offered by animal keepers (small-scale farmers, zookeepers, pet owners, etc.) and most objective scientific descriptions of animal behavior, in that animal keepers acknowledge that animals have individual traits and personalities to a much greater extent than researchers currently do. In theoretical as well as methodological terms, the field of biosemiotics is equipped to facilitate qualitative studies of animals, supplementary to and in combination with more quantitative studies of animal cognition and behavior. Inspiration for new directions for research on animals is also to be found in Dominique Lestel's (2011) call for a more interactive ethology, which rests on the assumption that active interaction with animals often provides the best setting for the display and study of animal behavior.

To recapitulate, several methodological issues in behavioral neuroscience derive from a lack of attentivity to the difference between the role of the observer and the role of the observed. The fact that we can experience and engage with the subjectivity involved in the human observer role first hand, while having no similar access to animal subjectivity, should not lead us to think that animals do not have a similarly subjective experiential perspective. Animal subjectivity has been neglected in biology, and is still seriously understudied. *Umwelt* theory informed by contemporary biosemiotics can contribute to the theoretical foundation for the new approaches to animal subjectivity that are needed.

Concluding remarks

In the discussion of whether the neural code is a semiotic concept, and if so how it should be understood within a semiotic framework for biology, I favor an approach that incorporates the wider ecological context of sentient organisms and makes it possible to maintain a notion of neural codes in interplay with ecological, more flexible codes that operate inter-individually. The basic neurosemiotic features of Jakob von Uexküll's *Umwelt* theory integrates semiotics and biology, with ideas about neurosemiotics across species playing a central role. I have argued that code biology's conception of neural codes is most viable if supplemented with Uexküll's neurosemiotic ideas, and underlined the connections between the subjectivity and agency of different sentient organisms and how they relate to and interact with objects understood as discernible, unified wholes. The biosemiotic understanding of subjectivity and agentive capabilities amounts to acknowledging that these are graded phenomena, with some organisms having more complex capabilities than others. I have also addressed species-related methodological issues in behavioral neuroscience, focused on the anthropocentrism that is to some extent unavoidable given our human perspective in neurosemiotic studies.

While some historically important and overtly anthropocentric biases in neurobiological research have been abandoned in favor of a genuinely comparative neuroscience, implicit anthropocentric biases still abound and continue to distort our understanding of sentient organisms. This is first of all due to the long-standing neglect of subjectivity and individuality in animals. Where they occur, these biases weaken the credibility of findings in comparative neurobiological studies, and also shut us out of research avenues that we might otherwise have pursued. The best way to avoid such biases is to study the neurosemiotics of various species on their own terms.[8]

Notes

1 Deacon and Rączaszek-Leonardi (2019) remark that within a coding framework, the neural activity of any of a potentially large number of neurons located along the path that links the first registration of a stimulus to a specific neuron that is thus caused to become active could similarly be understood as encoding the same stimulus. This suggests that simple encoding/decoding models of neural processes may be a poor match with empirical reality, and that encoding/decoding models that are either more complex or more dynamic potentially have a higher degree of credibility.

2 Triploblastic animals are animals with body tissues that are derived from three germ layers. Most multicellular animals are triploblastic.

3 See also Uexküll (1956 [1934/1940]: 14, 111, and 168), where the central role of the central nervous system for the constitution of the *Umwelt* is reiterated.

4 The appendix of Uexküll 1956 [1934/1940] lists more than 100 texts by Uexküll. Those referred to here from the period 1892–1915 are categorized as being "Aus dem Gebiet der Nerven- und Muskelphysiologie" – that is, from the field of nerve and muscle physiology.

5 The original quote reads like this: "Die Aufgabe [der Reize] ist es nicht, dem Tier die Kenntnis der Aussenwelt zu vermitteln, sondern den 'richtigen Weg' durch eine ihm völlig unbekannte Welt zu weisen. Deshalb ist auch die Merkwelt … so dürftig und … Wirkungswelt so sicher und planmässig." Here Uexküll refers to the "*Wirkungswelt*" (literally, the "world of effects") rather than the "*Wirkwelt*" (the operational world).

6 This might reasonably include Barbieri (2014), given his characterization of animals whose behavior is mostly or entirely hardwired. If so, interpretative skills are in this view a precondition for having cohesive experience, whereas quasi-subjective animals that rely predominantly on neural codes alone are bound to lack cohesion in their experience.

7 Martinelli defends a methodological application of anthropomorphism in some cases. The attribution of traits found in humans to animals should according to Martinelli (2007: 288) "not be avoided, [but] in fact encouraged, when, through empathy, it helps comprehend the given phenomenon."

8 The author acknowledges his involvement, in the context of this chapter, in the program area for research at University of Stavanger (UIS) "Philosophy and subjectivity" (IN-11746), and in the Cognitive and Behavioral Neuroscience Lab (UIS).

References

Allen, C., & Bekoff, M. (1999). *Species of Mind: The Philosophy and Biology of Cognitive Ethology*. Cambridge, MA: MIT Press.

Barbieri, M. (2003). *The Organic Codes: An Introduction to Semantic Biology*. Cambridge: Cambridge University Press.

Barbieri, M. (2013). Organic semiosis and Peircean semiosis. *Biosemiotics*, *6*(2), 273–289. doi: 10.1007/s12304-012-9161-5
Barbieri, M. (2014). From biosemiotics to code biology. *Biological Theory*, *9*, 239–249. doi: 10.1007/s13752-013-0155-6
Barbieri, M. (2015). *Code Biology: A New Science of Life*. Cham: Springer.
Brentari, C. (2013). How to make worlds with signs. Some remarks on Jakob von Uexküll's *Umwelt* theory. *Rivista Italiana di Filosofia del Linguaggio (RIFL)*, 7(2), 8–21. doi: 10.4396/20130701
Brentari, C. (2015). *Jakob von Uexküll. The Discovery of the Umwelt Between Biosemiotics and Theoretical Biology*. Dordrecht: Springer.
Brette, R. (2019). Is coding a relevant metaphor for the brain? *Behavioral and Brain Sciences*, *42*, E215. doi: 10.1017/S0140525X19000049
Burghardt, G. M. (1997). Amending Tinbergen: A fifth aim for ethology. In R. W. Mitchell, N. S. Thompson, & H. Ly Miles (Eds.), *Anthropomorphism, Anecdotes and Animals* (pp. 254–276). New York: State University of New York Press.
Chien, J.-P. (2006). From animals to humans: Uexküll's *Umwelt* as read by Lacan and Canguilhem. *Concentric: Literary and Cultural Studies*, *32*(2), 45–69.
de Jesus, P. (2016). From enactive phenomenology to biosemiotic enactivism. *Adaptive Behavior*, *24*(2), 130–146. doi: 10.1177/1059712316636437
Deacon, T. W., & Rączaszek-Leonardi, J. (2019). Abandoning the code metaphor is compatible with semiotic process. *Behavioral and Brain Sciences*, *42*, E224. doi: 10.1017/S0140525X19001419
Di Paulo, E. A. (2020). Afterword: A future for Jakob von Uexküll. In F. Michelini, & K. Köchy (Eds.), *Jakob von Uexküll: Life, Environments, Anthropology* (pp. 252–256). London: Routledge.
Feiten, T. E., Holland, K., & Chemero, A. (2020). Worlds apart? Reassessing von Uexküll's *Umwelt* in embodied cognition with Canguilhem, Merleau-Ponty, and Deleuze. *Journal of French and Francophone Philosophy*, *28*(1), 1–26. doi: 10.5195/jffp.2020.929
Gładziejewski, P. (2016). Predictive coding and representationalism. *Synthese*, *193*, 559–582. doi: 10.1007/s11229-015-0762-9
Gomez-Marin, A. (2019). A clash of *Umwelts*: Anthropomorphism in behavioral neuroscience. *Behavioral and Brain Sciences*, *42*, E229. doi: 10.1017/S0140525X19001237
Griffin, D. R. (2001). *Animal Minds: Beyond Cognition to Consciousness*. Chicago: University of Chicago Press.
Griffin, D. R., & Speck, G. B. (2004). New evidence of animal consciousness. *Animal Cognition*, 7, 5–18. doi: 10.1007/s10071-003-0203-x
Haselager, P., de Groot, A., & van Rappard, H. (2003). Representationalism vs. anti-representationalism: A debate for the sake of appearance. *Philosophical Psychology*, *16*(1), 5–24. doi: 10.1080/0951508032000067761
Heras-Escribano, M., & de Jesus, P. (2018). Biosemiotics, the extended synthesis, and ecological information: Making sense of the organism-environment relation at the cognitive level. *Biosemiotics*, *11*(2), 245–262.
Hill, H. M., Guarino, S., & Dietrich, S. (2017). The field of comparative psychology. In T. K. Shackelford, & V. A. Weekes-Shackelford (Eds.), *Encyclopedia of Evolutionary Psychological Science*. Cham: Springer. https://link.springer.com/referenceworkentry/10.1007/978-3-319-19650-3_2637
Hoffmeyer, J. (1996). *Signs of Meaning in the Universe*. Bloomington, IN: Indiana University Press.
Hoffmeyer, J. (2002). Proprioception. In C. Emmeche, K. Kull, & F. Stjernfelt (Eds.), *Reading Hoffmeyer, Rethinking Biology* (pp. 31–34) (C. Emmeche & M. Sheets-Johnstone, Trans.). Tartu: Tartu University Press.
Hoffmeyer, J. (2004). Uexküllian Planmässigkeit. *Sign Systems Studies*, *32*(1–2), 73–97.
Köchy, K. (2020). Uexküll's legacy: Biological reception and biophilosophical impact. In F. Michelini, & K. Köchy (Eds.), *Jakob von Uexküll: Life, Environments, Anthropology* (pp. 52–69). London: Routledge.
Kull, K. (2001). Jakob von Uexküll: An introduction. *Semiotica*, *134*(1–4), 1–59. doi: 10.1515/semi.2001.013
Lestel, D. (2011). What capabilities for the animal? *Biosemiotics* *4*(1), 83–102.
Maran, T. (2012). Are ecological codes archetypal structures? In T. Maran, K. Lindström, R. Magnus, & M. Tønnessen (Eds.), *Semiotics in the Wild: Essays in Honour of Kalevi Kull on the Occasion of his 60th Birthday* (pp. 147–156). Tartu: Tartu University Press.
Martinelli, D. (2007). *Zoosemiotics: Proposals for a Handbook (Acta semiotica Fennica 26)*. Imatra: Finnish Network University of Semiotics.
Martinelli, D., & Bankov, K. (2008). Bankov's razor versus Martinelli's canon. A confrontation around Biosemiotics. *Biosemiotics*, *1*(3), 397–418. doi: 10.1007/s12304-008-9022-4
Mildenberger, F., & Herrman, B. (2014). *Uexküll: Umwelt and Innenwelt der Tiere* (reprint of Uexküll 1921, with commentary). Berlin: Springer Spektrum.
Morgan, C. L. (1903). *An Introduction to Comparative Psychology* (2nd ed.). Newcastle: Walter Scott.
Nicolelis, M., & Ribeiro, S. (2006). Seeking the neural code. *Scientific American*, *295*, 70–77. doi: 10.1038/scientificamerican1206-70

Pattee, H. H. (1973). The physical basis and origin of hierarchical control. In H. H. Pattee (Ed.), *Hierarchy Theory. The Challenge of Complex Systems* (pp. 73–108). New York: G. Braziller.

Pitt, D. (2020). Mental representation. In E. N. Zalta (Ed.), *The Stanford Encyclopedia of Philosophy*. Stanford, CA: Stanford University Press. https://plato.stanford.edu/entries/mental-representation

Polanyi, M. (1968). Life's irreducible structure. *Science, 160*(3834), 1308–1312. doi: 10.1126/science.160.3834.1308

Richmond, B. (2014) Neural coding. In D. Jaeger, & R. Jung (Eds.), *Encyclopedia of Computational Neuroscience*. New York: Springer. doi: 10.1007/978-1-4614-7320-6_398-1

Roepstorff, A. (1999). Brains in scanners: An Umwelt of cognitive neuroscience. *Semiotica 134*(1–4), 747–765. doi: 10.1515/semi.2001.051

Rosen, R. (1985). *Anticipatory Systems: Philosophical, Mathematical and Methodological Foundations*. Oxford: Pergamon Press.

Sebeok, T. A. (1986). *I Think I am a Verb: More Contributions to the Doctrine of Signs*. New York: Springer.

Sebeok, T. A. (1996). Signs, bridges, origins. In J. Trabant (Ed.)., *Origins of Language* (pp. 89–115). Budapest: Collegium Budapest.

Sharov, A. (2017). Composite agency: Semiotics of modularity and guiding interactions. *Biosemiotics, 10*(2), 157–178. doi: 10.1007/s12304-017-9301-z

Sharov, A. A., & Vehkavaara, T. (2015). Protosemiosis: Agency with reduced representation capacity. *Biosemiotics, 8*(1), 103–123. doi: 10.1007/s12304-014-9219-7

Sheets-Johnstone, M. (1998). Consciousness: A natural history. *Journal of Consciousness Studies, 5*(2), 260–294.

Sjölander, S. (1995). Some cognitive breakthroughs in the evolution of cognition and consciousness and their impact on the biology of language. *Evolution and Cognition, 1*(1), 3–11.

Stjernfelt, F. (2013). The generality of signs: The actual relevance of anti-psychologism. *Semiotica, 2013*(194), 1–33. doi: 10.1515/sem-2013-0023

Tinbergen, N. (1963). On aims and methods of Ethology. *Zeitschrift für Tierpsychologie, 20*(4), 410–433. doi: 10.1111/j.1439-0310.1963.tb01161.x

Tønnessen, M. (2014). The ontogeny of the embryonic, foetal and infant human umwelt. *Sign Systems Studies, 42*(2), 281–307. doi: 10.12697/SSS.2014.42.2-3.06

Tønnessen, M. (2016). Agency in biosemiotics and enactivism. In J. Zlatev, G. Sonesson, & P. Konderak (Eds.), *Meaning, Mind and Communication: Explorations in Cognitive Semiotics* (pp. 69–82). Frankfurt: Peter Lang.

Tønnessen, M. (2018). The search image as a link between sensation, perception and action. *BioSystems, 164*, 138–146. doi: 10.1016/j.biosystems.2017.10.016

Tønnessen, M., Magnus, R., & Brentari, C. (2016). The biosemiotic glossary project: *Umwelt*. With appendix (supplementary material available online). *Biosemiotics, 9*(1), 129–149. doi: 10.1007/s12304-016-9255-6

Uexküll, J. von (1909). *Umwelt und Innenwelt der Tiere* (1st edn). Berlin: Verlag von Julius Springer.

Uexküll, J. von (1921). *Umwelt und Innenwelt der Tiere* (2nd edn). Berlin: Verlag von Julius Springer.

Uexküll, J. von (1928). *Theoretische Biologie* (2nd edn). Berlin: Verlag von Julius Springer.

Uexküll, J. von (1929). Reflexumkehr: Starker und schwacher Reflex. In A. Bethe, G. von Bergmann, G. Embden, & A. Ellinger (Eds.), *Handbuch der normalen und pathologischen Physiologie: Mit Berücksichtigung der experimentellen Pharmakologie, Vol. 9*, pp. 755–762). Berlin: Verlag von Julius Springer.

Uexküll, J. von (1934). *Streifzüge durch die Umwelten von Tieren und Menschen: Ein Bilderbuch unsichtbarer Welten*. Berlin: Verlag von Julius Springer.

Uexküll, J. von (1940). *Bedeutungslehre*. Leipzig: Verlag von J. A. Barth.

Uexküll, J. von (1956 [1934/1940]). *Streifzüge durch die Umwelten von Tieren und Menschen: Ein Bilderbuch unsichtbarer Welten. Bedeutungslehre*. Leipzig: Rowohlt.

Uexküll, J. von (2010 [1934/1940]). *A Foray into the Worlds of Animals and Humans with a Theory of Meaning* (J. D. O'Neil, Trans.). Minneapolis MN: University of Minneapolis Press.

PART II

Language and its pathways to meaning

6

NEURAL BASES OF MULTIMODAL SEMANTICS

Maya Visser

Introduction

Our capacity to construe meaning is an important aspect of human social behavior. Over the centuries, it has been investigated in multiple disciplines, including semiotics, philosophy, neuropsychology, and neuroscience. Come the twenty-first century, the field of neurosemiotics tries to integrate insights from all these fields to grapple with the issue of concept formation (Jorna, 2008). To inform this agenda, this chapter focuses on the neural basis of multimodal semantics, a research field within semiotics (Føllesdal, 1997)

Semantics involves, among other processes, the understanding of objects and concepts. If we see a cat, we can easily retrieve related information: it is a relatively small pet, it says "meow," it is furry, and so on. This type of information lies at the core of semantic memory, a system dealing with the meaning of words, pictures, sounds, and general information about the world. As you might expect, losing the ability to process semantic information will affect both mundane and professional activities. This is demonstrated in patients with semantic dementia, who are unable to recognize objects, such as a cat, and all related information (i.e., the fact that it is a pet that meows and is furry). Interestingly, their impairment is restricted to affect solely semantic processing, at least in the early stages of this progressive disease. For example, these patients speak fluently and retain the ability to recall day-to-day events (episodic memory). As such, they are aware of their condition and how it affects them on an everyday basis, especially during the early stages of the disease. A more detailed explanation of the problems that these patients face is described in Murre et al. (2001) and Witoonpanich et al. (2015). Understanding the neural basis of semantic memory aids in understanding the core deficits seen in these patients. Such are the goals of this chapter.

First, I will introduce the concept of semantic memory, followed by a short history of semantic research and an overview of relevant models. Emphasis will be placed on the hub-and-spoke model (Lambon Ralph et al., 2016), which proposes that a hub system regulates the interaction between modality-specific (e.g., visual and verbal) regions to allow for generalization, among other faculties. In a neurosemiotic spirit, details of this specific model will be delineated based on behavioral and neuroimaging data from healthy individuals and clinical populations, alongside insights from computational modeling.

DOI: 10.4324/9781003051817-9

Semantic memory

Semiotics tends to focus on determining the meaning of signs and messages (Spapé et al., 2019). Signs are the basis that enable us to make generalizations and abstractions about the world (Oakley, 2007). They can be verbal (words, phrases) or non-verbal (gestures, pictures, paintings) (Oakley, 2007; Spapé et al., 2019). That is to say, signs depend on different modalities and contextual aspects, and therefore must rely on an interactive neural network that underlies these different cognitive functions (Spapé et al., 2019). The hub-and-spoke model describes such a network.

To understand this hub-and-spoke model, it is important to grasp a correct definition of semantic memory. Together with episodic memory, semantic memory is integral to declarative (or explicit) memory systems – for further details, see Carlson & Birkett (2017). Semantic memory differs from episodic memory in that it does not deal with information about when and how we interacted with a certain concept (Eichenbaum, 2017; Tulving, 1972; Vatansever, Smallwood, & Jefferies, 2021). For example, if we think about a dog, our semantic memory will guide the understanding that it is a pet that barks and needs to be taken care of. In contrast, episodic memory refers to an event in which you came in contact with a certain dog. In other words, you can remember the exact time and place of this "episodic" event. Classic embodied theories suggest that semantic concepts are formed over time by the accumulated knowledge from episodic verbal and non-verbal experiences (Eggert, 1977). In other words, the repetitive episodic encounters with a certain concept (e.g., a dog you saw on a certain day) will shape the semantic knowledge of that concept. The focus in this chapter will fall primarily on semantic memory – on the relationship between semantic and episodic memory, see Greenberg & Verfaellie (2010) as well as Duff et al. (2020).

The history of semantic research

Semantic memory is involved in many cognitive processes, such as producing and comprehending speech and making non-verbal associations. The first attempts to investigate these processes date back to the nineteenth century, spearheaded by neurologists Pierre Paul Broca and Carl Wernicke (Carlson & Birkett, 2017; Eggert, 1977). They suggested that speech comprehension relies heavily on the posterior temporal lobe (Wernicke's area), whereas expression relies heavily on the inferior frontal lobe (Broca's area) (Figure 6.1).

Classical language models constructed in the following years added several neural regions that had a contributing and specifically defined role in concept processing (Carlson & Birkett, 2017; Eggert, 1977). For example, the semantic network included visual regions that process form and color as well as temporal regions involved in auditory sensory input. Classical language models suggest that a semantic concept arises due to the direct interaction between these modality-specific regions (Eggert, 1977; Lambon Ralph et al., 2016). Subsequently, many semantic memory models emerged that focused on category and/or modality-specific regions – for a review, see Capitani et al. (2003). These models aim to establish the exact neural underpinnings of each category or modality and their interaction. These embodied (modality-specific) systems are discussed in Chapter 7.

One of the latest developments in this tradition is the hub-and-spoke model, which proposes the bilateral anterior temporal lobes (bATLs) as a core system regulating the interaction between these modality-specific regions (Lambon Ralph et al., 2016) (Figure 6.1). Although this new model has been mostly construed and refined by professor Lambon Ralph and colleagues (for review, see Lambon Ralph et al., 2016), some of the earlier category or modality-specific models already mentioned the possibility of an additional supramodal convergence zone integrating information from sensorimotor areas (Caramazza et al., 1994; Hoenig et al., 2008; Simmons & Barsalou, 2003). Similarly, Lambon Ralph et al. (2016) suggest that their model is in line with these category- and/or modality-specific models, with the additional focus on this supramodal hub.

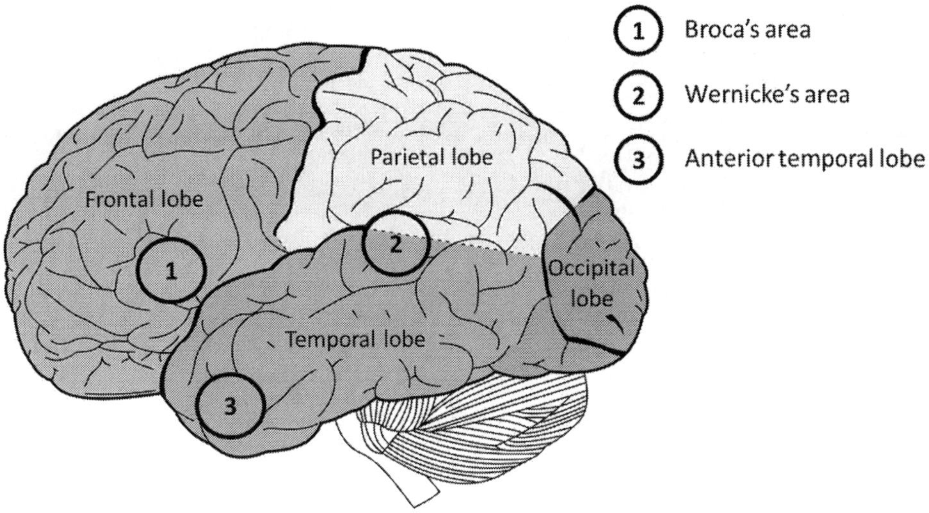

Figure 6.1 Brain regions associated with language and semantic processing

(1) Broca's area is involved in language production. (2) Wernicke's area is involved in language comprehension. (3) The bilateral anterior temporal lobe is thought to have a pivotal role within the semantic system by guiding the formation of a semantic concept through connections with modality specific regions situated throughout the neocortex. The image is taken and adapted from a publicly available source (Wikimedia). See e-book for a full-color version of this figure.

Some of the key assumptions of the hub-and-spoke model are, in fact, based on previously developed ideas. Over the last decades, several famous language models have been constructed that highlight (1) the reuse of modality-specific regions for concept processing (Martin & Chao, 2001; Pulvermüller, 1999, 2018); (2) the importance of hub regions or convergence zones (Binder, 2016; Damasio, 1989; Simmons & Barsalou, 2003); and (3) the role of the ATL in conceptual processing (Hickok & Poeppel, 2007; Poeppel et al., 2012). It is beyond the scope of this chapter to discuss and compare all these models, but for the interested reader it is certainly advisable to read this related literature.

The neural basis of semantic memory

As explained above, classical models of the neural basis of semantic memory suggest that conceptual knowledge arises directly from networks of modality-specific brain regions distributed throughout the cortex – for reviews, see Capitani et al. (2003), Humphreys & Forde (2001), and Martin (2007). In other words, specific brain regions have been acknowledged to process visual, auditory, and verbal information streams, the interactions of which give rise to semantic concepts. Specifically, if we think about the concept of a cat, visual regions will provide information about its form and color; auditory regions would contribute information about the possible sounds associated with the animal; and verbal regions would be involved in expressing this information. All these regions are simultaneously activated and interact directly to form the semantic concept we have of cats (Figure 6.2a).

However, early computational models have shown that the addition of an intermediate hidden layer is required to support generalizations across related concepts that can have different property profiles (Plaut, 2002; Rogers et al., 2004). In Figure 6.2b, we can see a graphical example of such a hidden layer, which is represented as a circle named "hub." This hub (or intermediate hidden layer in computational models) guides the information of the modality-specific regions (the spokes) to form semantic concepts. The idea is that this is pivotal for everyday generalization of semantic concepts. For

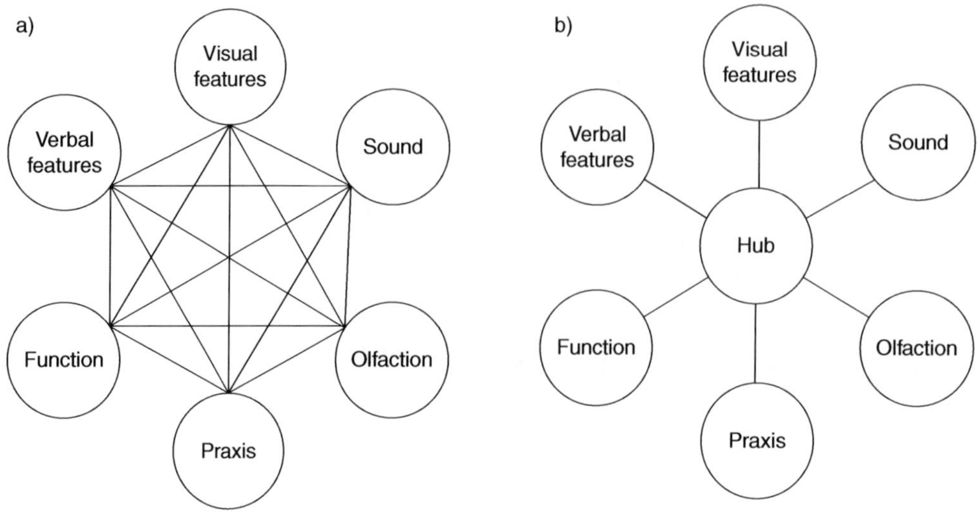

Figure 6.2 Models of communication between modality-specific areas

(a) The "classical" distributed semantic model proposes that modality specific regions communicate directly to form semantic concepts. (b) The hub-and-spoke theory incorporates a "hub," guiding transmission of information between modality-specific systems, while at the same time diminishing the number of required functional connections. These figures are based on the hub-and-spoke theory described in Lambon Ralph et al. (2016, 2010) and in Rogers et al. (2004).

example, dogs and parrots look and behave very differently, yet they share many conceptual relations that humans can easily use to support categorical generalizations (e.g., they are animals, they breathe air, they are pets). In addition, the use of a hub may decrease the number of connections required for communication among modality-specific regions, making it a more efficient system to glean information from different modality-specific systems as illustrated in Figure 6.2b (Lambon Ralph et al., 2010, 2016).

This model's "hub" integrates all necessary information to form coherent transmodal concepts through connections with perceptual and modality-specific regions (Lambon Ralph et al., 2010, 2016). This is an adjustment of the classical proposal by Meynert and Wernicke (Lambon Ralph et al., 2016). Both models assume that multimodal experiences are essential to learn semantic concepts. In addition, both models suggest that multimodal information is encoded in modality-specific regions throughout the brain. However, the main difference is that the hub-and-spoke theory attributes a vital funcion to the "hub" region, located in the bATLs. The reminder of this chapter will outline the existing evidence for such a hub, including behavioral patient studies, transcranial magnetic stimulation (TMS), computational modelling, and functional magnetic resonance imaging (fMRI).

Semantic dementia

Let us first consider patient data. If such a hub exists, then damage to the bATLs should lead to a loss of semantic knowledge in all domains, including verbal and non-verbal semantic information. This is exactly the pattern observed in persons with semantic dementia (SD), whose damage is mostly restricted to the bATLs (Galton et al., 2001; Kopelman, 2002; Mummery et al., 2000; Nestor et al., 2006). The disorder is also known as primary progressive fluent aphasia and it was first described about two decades ago (Hodges et al., 1992; Mummery et al., 2000; Snowden et al., 1996). The unique aspect of this dementia is that, as the disease progresses, the semantic knowledge of these patients diminishes whereas other cognitive functions (e.g., episodic memory, sensory, and grammar skills) remain relatively intact (Hodges et al., 1992; Snowden, 2002). Semantic memory is affected in all modalities, including verbal (written and spoken language), non-verbal (e.g., sounds and visual objects), and tactile stimuli. Moreover, if knowledge of a semantic concept is lost, it is lost in all these modalities at the same time (Bozeat et al., 2000; Jefferies & Lambon Ralph, 2006). In other words, if a patient loses the concept "parrot," they cannot recognize the sound it makes, ascertain its visual aspects, or describe any information about the animal (e.g., it is a pet, often depicted with pirates, and so on). Based on these patient studies, the bATLs have been proposed as a core region for semantic memory, or a semantic hub (Lambon Ralph et al., 2010, 2016). Furthermore, the level of comprehension difficulties in these patients reflects both the degree of ATL atrophy and the extent of functional connectivity reduction within the hub-and-spoke network (Guo et al., 2013), building a strong case for the bATLs as a semantic hub region. Similarly, damage to the bATLs leads to impaired semantic performance in other diseases such as Alzheimer's disease, temporal lobe epilepsy (TLE), and herpes simplex encephalitis (Rice et al., 2018; Rogers et al., 2004; Visser et al., 2018). As a final note, it seems counterintuitive that this important semantic region has never been suggested in the classical language models by Broca and Wernicke and others; however, these models were based on patients with middle cerebral artery stroke, which is unlikely to damage the middle to ventral ATL due to its neuroanatomical position (Lambon Ralph et al., 2016; Phan et al., 2005).

Overall, findings from SD demonstrate that semantic memory is a selective cognitive process that can be damaged independently. These patients are restricted in their everyday activities and professional lives. Research on this patient group has not only led to improved clinical profiling and therapies; it has also furthered basic science. Based on this patient group, the bATLs have been revealed to be a core region of semantic processing, which subsequently led to the hub-and-spoke model as described above. This has been an important step in the field of semantics and, consequently, neurosemiotics.

Semantic problems in temporal lobe epilepsy patients

Temporal lobe epilepsy (TLE) is a chronic form of epilepsy that causes recurrent seizures originating in the temporal lobe. Seizures can affect consciousness (the patient is unaware of their surroundings), but this is not always the case. In some cases, the seizure evolves from focal to generalized, so it spreads to regions outside the temporal lobe, leading to convulsions. If medical treatment with anticonvulsants is ineffective, a unilateral resection of the ATL is sometimes undertaken to control severe epilepsy.

Surprisingly, the literature very rarely describes semantic problems in these patients, casting doubts on the semantic role of the bATLs. Clinical neuropsychological assessment typically focuses on episodic memory and naming problems, known to be impaired in TLE patients, but omits semantic memory. However, over a decade ago, some researchers suggested that anomia (i.e., naming problems) is actually a sign of an underlying mild semantic disorder (Bell & Giovagnoli, 2007; Lambon Ralph et al., 2012). Indeed, recent research has shown that TLE patients with unilateral resection show mild semantic problems; however, this deficit is only apparent when looking at the patients' reaction times or when probing more demanding (e.g., level-specific, low-frequency, or abstract) concepts (Lambon Ralph et al., 2012; Rice et al., 2018; Visser et al., 2018).

Knowing that the bATLs have a prominent role in semantic memory, it is surprising that the removal of the whole left or right ATL results in such a small semantic impairment. This means that the semantic system must be flexible and have the ability to re-organize after unilateral damage. Recent combined TMS-fMRI studies showed that (temporal) damage to the unilateral ATL indeed leads to an upregulation in the contralateral ATL (Binney & Lambon Ralph, 2015; Jung & Lambon Ralph, 2016). Specifically, induced damage (by TMS) to the left ATL led to an upregulation of semantic function in the right ATL and improved connectivity between the two ATLs. The authors interpreted these results as evidence that the semantic system consists of a flexible adaptive bilateral system that is able to support functional recovery after unilateral ATL damage in patients (Jung & Lambon Ralph, 2016). Similarly, the usefulness of such a resilient bilateral system has been imitated through a computational model by Schapiro et al. (2013). This computational model confirms that a bilateral semantic system would be very resilient to unilateral damage, as it was able to mimic the same pattern of impairments as TLE patients after unilateral damage (i.e., semantic concepts are relatively preserved except for low-frequency concepts). In contrast, when the same degree of damage was divided over the left and right semantic hub (similar to SD patients), semantic impairments were much worse (Schapiro et al., 2013).

In summary, investigating the semantic problems of TLE patients has proven important to fully describing their clinical profile, all while improving basic neurosemantic science. Although both the left and right ATL have a slightly different function (with respect to verbal and non-verbal information, respectively), both regions are highly interactive and damage to either side leads to an upregulation on the remaining ATL. In other words, these studies suggest that the semantic hub entails a highly interconnected left and right ATL, with overlapping, although slightly differing, functions with respect to verbal and non-verbal concepts. Therefore, these studies have made an important contribution for the development of the hub-and-spoke model. Consequently, this is an important step forward in the field of semantics and neurosemiotics.

Neuroimaging

Patient data can be difficult to interpret for various reasons. First, it can be hard to ascertain the relation between damaged area and behavioral impairment, given that surrounding or even peripheral tissue can take over functions. In addition, many patients at least attempt to adopt strategies to overcome their impairments (Wise, 2003). Accordingly, it is important to use other methods to derive convergent evidence. As such, for over two decades, the bATLs have been connected with semantic memory by studies using repetitive TMS (Lambon Ralph et al., 2009; Pobric et al., 2007); transcranial direct current stimulation (Díez et al., 2017); intracortical recordings in neurosurgical patients (Halgren et al., 1994); and functional neuroimaging studies of comprehension using positron emission tomography (PET) (Devlin et al., 2000; Perani et al., 1999; Vandenberghe et al., 1996) and magnetoencephalography (MEG) (Marinkovic et al., 2003).[1] However, fMRI studies have long overlooked the role of the bATLs in semantic memory, mainly because (1) the blood-oxigen-level-dependent (BOLD) signal is affected by geometrical distortions in the inferior ATL; and (2) limited brain coverage during data acquisition usually led to exclusion of the inferior ATL (Devlin et al., 2000; Halai et al., 2014; Visser et al., 2010a; Visser et al., 2010b) – Figure 6.3. As fMRI has dominated the neuroimaging literature over the last 20 years, older models of semantic memory tend to exclude the ATL (Catani & Ffytche, 2005; Martin, 2007). However, newer techniques allow modern fMRI studies to capture signals from the ATL (Halai et al., 2015), confirming its key role in semantic memory (Binney et al., 2010; Halai et al., 2015; Rice et al., 2015a; Visser et al., 2012; Visser et al., 2010a; Visser & Lambon Ralph, 2011).

In line with studies on SD patients, neuroimaging data have shown that the bATLs are engaged in semantic processing of all input modalities and conceptual categories (Binney et al., 2010; Vandenberghe et al., 1996; Visser & Lambon Ralph, 2011). Also, both the left and right ATL have been implicated in processing verbal and non-verbal semantic information (Pobric, Jefferies, & Lambon Ralph, 2010; Visser et al., 2012). This is in line with the interactive bilateral ATL system described in the previous section on TLE patients and is an exception (one of several) to the normally heavily left lateralization for verbal processing. Moreover, although patient data originally associated the bATLs with semantic processing, exact localization based on patient data is difficult as neural damage usually covers extended areas. In particular, accruing evidence points to the ventrolateral portion of the ATL as the core region underlying this multimodal hub (for review, see Lambon Ralph et al., 2016). Overall, novel neuroimaging techniques have revealed the semantic role of the bATLs. Nonetheless,

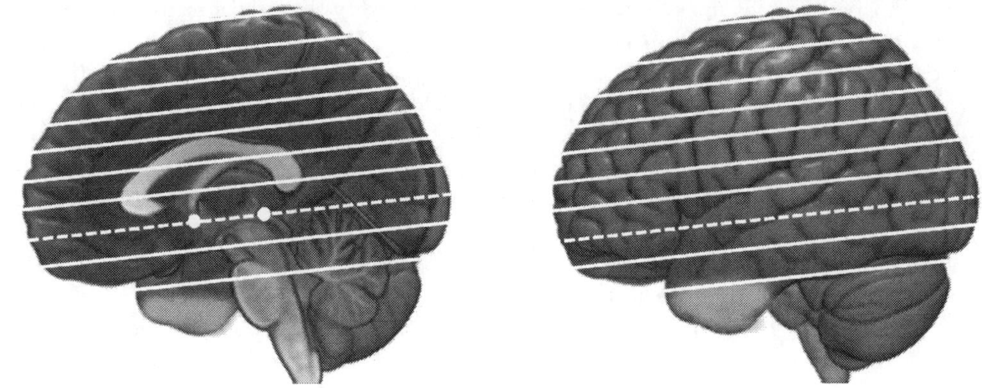

Figure 6.3 Exclusion of the bilateral anterior temporal lobe during fMRI data acquisition

Most fMRI studies use axial data acquisition. The BOLD signal is obtained slice by slice from top to bottom (usually in an interleaved fashion). The slice inclination follows the striped line which is positioned to cross both the anterior and posterior commissure (white circles). The number of slices is limited due to time restrictions. As such, the inferior ATL (depicted in light gray) is often excluded from data acquisition due to its anatomical position (Visser, Jefferies, et al., 2010). Figure created using MRIcroGL (www.nitrc.org/projects/mricrogl).

note that if an fMRI study does not actively seek to extract signal from the ATL, this region might still often be excluded from data aquisition and analysis. Knowing the limitations and strengths of neuroimaging techniques such as fMRI enables us to advance better-informed semantic memory models.

The frequency effect

The objective of most theoretical models is to be able to explain the peculiarities of the respective cognitive process. One of the peculiarities of semantics is the frequency effect, whereby words or items that are encountered more frequently are processed faster. For example, in natural language the word *dog* is encountered more frequently than *chihuahua* or *poodle*. As a consequence, people find it easier to use the word *dog* compared with *poodle*, which is reflected in reaction times (i.e., it takes them longer to produce the word *poodle* compared with the word *dog*).

Early neurally based computational models explained the word frequency effect in terms of differences in the weights of distributed connections within the semantic network (e.g., Plaut et al., 1996; Rogers et al., 2004; Seidenberg & McClelland, 1989). In line with classical semantic models, as well as the hub-and-spoke theory, these computational accounts assume that semantic items are represented across different modality-specific neural regions (i.e., network units). A semantic item arises from connections between these different network units, and the strength of these connections depends on the frequency of exposure to a semantic concept. Consequently, a high-frequency item (e.g., *dog*) comprises strong connections, meaning that associated semantic information can be recovered rapidly. As such, we can easily recognize a dog and retrieve all semantic knowledge of this concept, but this will be a slower and less accurate process for a low-frequency concept like *poodle*. If the ATL is a core region for semantic memory, then it should be associated with the semantic frequency effect. Neuroimaging and patient data suggest that this is indeed the case.

First, the retrieval of low-frequency information requires more effort, which is reflected in higher neural activation for low- than high-frequency item (Hoffman et al., 2015). Note that many studies on the frequency effect still omit the ATL, as this region often remains excluded from data adquisition and analyses. Instead, they tend to associate the frequency effect dominantly with frontal regions – but see Hoffman et al. (2011, 2013) for an alternative explanation. However, the hub-and-spoke model suggests that both regions should show a frequency effect as they are esential regions for semantic memory (Jefferies, 2013; Lambon Ralph et al., 2016).

Second, damage to the ATL in SD patients results in a gradual loss of semantic memory (Jefferies & Lambon Ralph, 2006). Patients first lose the knowledge of low-frequency items, whereas high-frequency semantic concepts are relatively well preserved. As the disease progresses, higher-frequency items also become more difficult to retrieve (Jefferies & Lambon Ralph, 2006). This is in line with the idea that high-frequency items are supported by well-established connections within the network and are therefore relatively resilient againts neural damage. As such, the hub-and-spoke theory is able to explain the frequency effect. The ATL hub is the center of all connections and, as such, its gradual deterioration will first affect low-frequency concepts and can subsequently be noticed with higher-frequency concepts. Similarly, this explains the observation described in the section on TLE that these patients only struggle with low-frequency objects as these are represented by fewer and weaker connections within the semantic representational system, and are therefore more prone to be lost after unilateral damage.

Overall, the frequency effect is a well-known and heavily investigated phenomenon that can be explained by the hub-and-spoke theory. This theory does not just provide a neural foundation for this effect, but also explains the clinical characteristics that occur when the semantic system is damaged, thereby advancing both basic and clinical neuroscience. Finally, it shows how the architecture of a natural language is reflected in the neural forming of concepts.

Lateralization within the semantic network

So far, we have discussed the semantic hub a bilateral system, without differentiation between the left and right ATL. However, over a century of research has shown that each hemisphere subserves different functions during language processing. In more detail, most (but not all) language functions are left-lateralized, whereas the right hemisphere is involved in non-verbal processes like recognizing geometric forms and establishing spatial patterns, as well as in the verbalization of these concepts (Carlson & Birkett, 2017; Eggert, 1977). Based on this hemispheric division, it seems logical that the left and right ATL have at least a somewhat different role within the semantic network. Indeed, neuropsychological studies on SD patients associate left ATL damage with increased anomia (i.e., problems expressing thoughts, usually measured with a picture naming task), whereas right ATL damage results in greater prosopagnosia (i.e., inability to recognise faces) (Chan et al., 2009; Graham et al, 1995; Josephs et al., 2008; Lambon Ralph et al., 2001; Woollams & Patterson, 2018). More generally, it seems that the left ATL is relatively more involved in verbal processing, whereas non-verbal semantic items rely more strongly on the right ATL (Mion et al., 2010; Woollams & Patterson, 2018).

However, the hub-and-spoke theory suggests that this hemispheric difference is graded and not absolute (Lambon Ralph et al., 2010, 2016; Rice et al., 2015a). That is to say that both verbal processing and non-verbal processing require the ATL of each hemisphere, even though there is an asymmetry reflected by a relative left and right hemispheric difference, respectively. This is in line with the results of a large-scale fMRI meta-analysis, which indicated that semantic processing takes place in the bilateral ATL hub, but with a predilection of the left ATL for verbal stimuli (Rice et al., 2015b). Furthermore, computational modelling suggests that this interactive, bilateral semantic hub system with left–right graded differences correctly reflects the semantic impairments seen in SD patients with asymmetric ATL damage (Lambon Ralph aet al., 2001), while also explaining the relatively strong resilience to semantic impairments associated with unilateral damage in TLE patients (Schapiro et al., 2013).

Overall, the lateralization within the bATLs is present but more graded compared to other neural regions. This knowledge aids in the understanding of the semantic system and how it forms concepts from multimodal information, including both verbal and non-verbal resources. It thus shows how the brain captures and organizes input from a multimodal environment.

Semantic control system

Conceptual processing also hinges on semantic control, the ability to focus on semantic aspects that are relevant for the task or circumstances at hand (Jackson, 2021; Jefferies, 2013; Lambon Ralph et al., 2016; Noonan et al., 2013; Thompson-Schill et al., 1999). Essential tasks of the semantic control system are task switching, inhibiting task-irrelevant features, accessing lower-frequency concepts, and resolving ambiguity or incongruent meanings (Jefferies, 2013). The semantic control system is thought to be amodal, based on the impairment pattern seen in semantic aphasia (SA) patients. Similar to SD patients, SA patients exhibit multimodal semantic impairments. However, the impairments are caused by damage to the left fronto-parietal executive system. As opposed to the bATLs, this "control" system is dominantly, but not solely, left-organized (Jefferies, 2013).

The impairment pattern seen in SA patients clearly differs from that of SD patients, aligning with the idea that both are caused by damage to distinct cognitive systems. For example, the performance of SA patients can be influenced by cueing or varying task demands. This demonstrates that SA patients have preserved semantic representations but problems accessing the semantic item (Jefferies & Lambon Ralph, 2006; Sylvester & Shimamura, 2002). In contrast, cueing does not affect performance in SD patients because the underlying concepts are degraded and cannot be reinstituted (Jefferies & Lambon Ralph, 2006; Sylvester & Shimamura, 2002). These results prompted the Controlled Semantic Cognitive Framework, which frames the semantic system as an interactive neural network comprising (1) the representation system subserved by the bATLs and (2) fronto-parietal executive circuitry (Jackson, 2021; Jefferies, 2013; Lambon Ralph et al., 2016). Two extensive meta-analyses of fMRI data contrasting semantic tasks with either high or low semantic control demands (Jackson, 2021; Noonan et al., 2013) provided aligning evidence for this executive semantic control network, although the role of the parietal lobe is questioned by Jackson (2021). Although the details of this interaction still remain to be fully fleshed out, the integration of semantic and executive mechanisms in this model incarnates the non-compartmentalist ethos of neurosemiotics.

Conclusion

To summarize, semantic memory refers to our general knowledge about the world, including the meaning of words, pictures, objects, sounds, and faces. Damage to the bATLs leads to impaired semantic performance in Alzheimer's disease, SD, TLE, and herpes simplex encephalitis, suggesting that the bATLs are a core region for semantic representation (Lambon Ralph et al., 2016; Rogers et al., 2004). Specifically, through connections with perceptual and modality-specific regions, the bATLs integrate all necessary information to form coherent transmodal concepts (Lambon Ralph et al., 2010, 2016). The more *frequent* a concept, the stronger the connections are, making them more readily available and more robust to damage (Lambon Ralph et al., 2016; Rogers et al., 2004). These factors are reflected in the performance of SD patients, who demonstrate degraded knowledge in all semantic tasks and across different modalities, alongside better performance on high-frequency/ familiar items (Jefferies & Lambon Ralph, 2006). Similarly, unilateral ATL damage in TLE patients only affects low-frequency concepts, but high-frequency concepts remain intact (Rice et al., 2018; Visser et al., 2018).

Apart from patient studies, neuroimaging data has reliably corroborated the ATL as an amodal semantic hub region, aligning with the hub-and-spoke theory (Rice et al., 2015b). The large set of neuroimaging and patient data depicts a bilateral amodal semantic hub that shows a graded lateralization for verbal and non-verbal semantic processing. This means that, although both ATLs are involved in verbal and non-verbal semantic processing, an asymmetry exists in which the left and right ATL are relatively more engaged in verbal and non-verbal concept processing, respectively (Rice et al., 2015b).

Finally, the bATLs interact closely with the fronto-parietal executive system. Whereas the former supports semantic representations, the latter underlies semantic "control," which is required to manipulate/select specific semantic information needed to perform a task in an appropriate manner (Jackson, 2021; Noonan et al., 2013; Thompson-Schill et al., 1999). Damage to these regions leads to SA, in which patients have preserved semantic representations but present problems using and selecting semantic information in a task-appropriate manner (Jefferies & Lambon Ralph, 2006; Sylvester & Shimamura, 2002). Their performance can be improved significantly by cueing, whereas cueing does not affect performance in SD patients because the underlying concepts are degraded and cannot be reinstituted (Jefferies & Lambon Ralph, 2006; Sylvester & Shimamura, 2002). This means the semantic system is an interactive neural network comprising the bATLs representation system and fronto-parietal executive circuitry (Jackson, 2021; Jefferies, 2013).

As explained at the outset, signs can be verbal (words and phrases) or non-verbal (gestures, pictures, and paintings). The hub-and-spoke model captures this multimodal fact, thus aligning with core assumptions of neurosemiotics. Importantly, with its clinical implications, this account extends the translational possibilities of future neurosemiotic research.

Still, this scholarly space is not without limitations. First, our conceptual skills allow us to build complex social relations and create novel ideas that shape major advances of humankind (e.g., spirituality, money, nations). Beyond concept-formation, future work could concentrate on placing this semantic system in a broader perspective that maps continuities between individual and social semantic phenomena. Similarly, Hoffman et al. (2020) point out that most language research focuses on isolated signs and forms (words, pictures) and how these are paired with their related meaning. However, real-world speech uses different levels of grammatical descriptions, from words to phrases to larger pieces of discourse. According to Hoffman et al. (2020), all these different levels of grammatical description can be seen as form-meaning pairs (also referred to as constructs). Future research on the hub-and-spoke theory should delve into these larger semantic elements, expanding the intersections between the model and neurosemiotics at large.

Note

1 The objective of this paragraph is to demonstrate that several neuroimaging techniques have independently associated the bATLs with semantic memory. It goes beyond the scope of this chapter to explain each technique, but the interested reader can read Siebner et al. (2009) for further information.

References

Bell, B. D., & Giovagnoli, A. R. (2007). Recent innovative studies of memory in temporal lobe epilepsy. *Neuropsychology Review* 17(4), 455–476.

Binder, J. R. (2016). In defense of abstract conceptual representations. *Psychonomic Bulletin & Review, 23*(4), 1096–1108.

Binney, R. J., Embleton, K. V., Jefferies, E., Parker, G. J. M., & Lambon Ralph, M. A. (2010). The ventral and inferolateral aspects of the anterior temporal lobe are crucial in semantic memory: Evidence from a novel direct comparison of distortion-corrected fMRI, rTMS, and semantic dementia. *Cerebral Cortex, 20*(11), 2728–2738.

Binney, R. J., & Lambon Ralph, M. A. (2015). Using a combination of fMRI and anterior temporal lobe rTMS to measure intrinsic and induced activation changes across the semantic cognition network. *Neuropsychologia, 76*, 170–181.

Bozeat, S., Lambon Ralph, M. A., Patterson, K., Garrard, P., & Hodges, J. R. (2000). Non-verbal semantic impairment in semantic dementia. *Neuropsychologia, 38*(9), 1207–1215.

Capitani, E., Laiacona, M., Mahon, B., & Caramazza, A. (2003). What are the facts of semantic category-specific deficits? A critical review of the clinical evidence. *Cognitive Neuropsychology, 20*(3–6), 213–261.

Caramazza, A., Hillis, A., Leek, E. C., & Miozzo, M. (1994). The organization of lexical knowledge in the brain: Evidence from category- and modality-specific deficits. *Mapping the Mind*, 68–84.

Carlson, N. R., & Birkett, M. A. (2017). *Physiology of Behavior* (12th edn). London: Pearson Education .

Catani, M., & Ffytche, D. H. (2005). The rises and falls of disconnection syndromes. *Brain, 128*(Pt 10), 2224–2239.

Chan, D., Anderson, V., Pijnenburg, Y., Whitwell, J., Barnes, J., Scahill, R., Stevens, J. M., Barkhof, F., Scheltens, P., Rossor, M. N., & Fox, N. C. (2009). The clinical profile of right temporal lobe atrophy. *Brain, 132*(5), 1287–1298.

Damasio, A. R. (1989). Time-locked multiregional retroactivation: A systems-level proposal for the neural substrates of recall and recognition. *Cognition, 33*(1–2), 25–62.

Devlin, J. T., Russell, R. P., Davis, M. H., Price, C. J., Wilson, J., Moss, H. E., Matthews, P. M., & Tyler, L. K. (2000). Susceptibility-induced loss of signal: Comparing PET and fMRI on a semantic task. *NeuroImage, 11*(6I), 589–600. doi: 10.1006/nimg.2000.0595

Díez, E., Gómez-Ariza, C. J., Díez-Álamo, A. M., Alonso, M. A., & Fernandez, A. (2017). The processing of semantic relatedness in the brain: Evidence from associative and categorical false recognition effects following transcranial direct current stimulation of the left anterior temporal lobe. *Cortex, 93*, 133–145.

Duff, M. C., Covington, N. V., Hilverman, C., & Cohen, N. J. (2020). Semantic memory and the hippocampus: Revisiting, reaffirming, and extending the reach of their critical relationship. *Frontiers in Human Neuroscience, 13*, 471.

Eggert, G. H. (1977). *Wernicke's Works on Aphasia: A Sourcebook and Review*. Paris: Mouton.

Eichenbaum, H. (2017). Memory: Organization and control. *Annual Review of Psychology, 68*, 19–45.

Føllesdal, D. (1997). Semantics and semiotics. In M. L. Chiara, K. Doets, D. Mundici, & J. Van Benthem (Eds.), *Structures and Norms in Science* (pp. 449–457). Dordrecht: Springer.

Galton, C. J., Patterson, K., Graham, K., Lambon-Ralph, M. A., Williams, G., Antoun, N., Sahakian, B. J., & Hodges, J. R. (2001). Differing patterns of temporal atrophy in Alzheimer's disease and semantic dementia. *Neurology, 57*(2), 216–225.

Graham, K., Patterson, K., & Hodges, J. R. (1995). Progressive pure anomia: Insufficient activation of phonology by meaning. *Neurocase, 1*(1), 25–38.

Greenberg, D. L., & Verfaellie, M. (2010). Interdependence of episodic and semantic memory: Evidence from neuropsychology. *Journal of the International Neuropsychological Society, 16*(5), 748–753.

Guo, C. C., Gorno-Tempini, M. L., Gesierich, B., Henry, M., Trujillo, A., Shany-Ur, T., Jovicich, J., Robinson, S. D., Kramer, J. H., Rankin, K. P., Miller, B. L., & Seeley, W. W. (2013). Anterior temporal lobe degeneration produces widespread network-driven dysfunction. *Brain, 136*(10), 2979–2991.

Halai, A. D., Parkes, L. M., & Welbourne, S. R. (2015). Dual-echo fMRI can detect activations in inferior temporal lobe during intelligible speech comprehension. *NeuroImage, 122*, 214–221. doi: 10.1016/j.neuroimage.2015.05.067

Halai, A. D., Welbourne, S. R., Embleton, K., & Parkes, L. M. (2014). A comparison of dual gradient-echo and spin-echo fMRI of the inferior temporal lobe. *Human Brain Mapping, 35*(8), 4118–4128. doi: 10.1002/hbm.22463

Halgren, E., Baudena, P., Heit, G., Clarke, M., & Marinkovic, K. (1994). Spatio-temporal stages in face and word processing. 1. Depth recorded potentials in the human occipital and parietal lobes. *Journal of Physiology – Paris, 88*(1), 1–50. doi: 10.1016/0928-4257(94)90092-2

Hickok, G., & Poeppel, D. (2007). The cortical organization of speech processing. *Nature Reviews Neuroscience, 8*(5), 393–402. doi: 10.1038/nrn2113

Hodges, J. R., Patterson, K., Oxbury, S., & Funnell, E. (1992). Semantic dementia: Progressive fluent aphasia with temporal lobe atrophy. *Brain, 115*(6), 1783–1806. doi: 10.1093/brain/115.6.1783

Hoenig, K., Sim, E. J., Bochev, V., Herrnberger, B., & Kiefer, M. (2008). Conceptual flexibility in the human brain: Dynamic recruitment of semantic maps from visual, motor, and motion-related areas. *Journal of Cognitive Neuroscience, 20*(10), 1799–1814. doi: 10.1162/jocn.2008.20123

Hoffman, P., Cogdell-Brooke, L., & Thompson, H. E. (2020). Going off the rails: Impaired coherence in the speech of patients with semantic control deficits. Neuropsychologia, 146, Article 107516. doi: 10.1016/j.neuropsychologia.2020.107516

Hoffman, P., Lambon Ralph, M. A., & Rogers, T. T. (2013). Semantic diversity: A measure of semantic ambiguity based on variability in the contextual usage of words. *Behavior Research Methods, 45*(3), 718–730. doi: 10.3758/S13428-012-0278-X

Hoffman, P., Lambon Ralph, M. A., & Woollams, A. M. (2015). Triangulation of the neurocomputational architecture underpinning reading aloud. *Proceedings of the National Academy of Sciences of the United States of America, 112*(28), 3719–3728. doi: 10.1073/pnas.1502032112

Hoffman, P., Rogers, T. T., & Ralph, M. A. L. (2011). Semantic diversity accounts for the "missing" word frequency effect in stroke aphasia: Insights using a novel method to quantify contextual variability in meaning. *Journal of Cognitive Neuroscience, 23*(9), 2432–2446. doi: 10.1162/JOCN.2011.21614

Humphreys, G. W., & Forde, E. M. (2001). Hierarchies, similarity, and interactivity in object recognition: "category-specific" neuropsychological deficits. *The Behavioral and Brain Sciences, 24*(3), 453–509. https://pubmed.ncbi.nlm.nih.gov/11682799

Jackson, R. L. (2021). The neural correlates of semantic control revisited. *NeuroImage, 224*. doi: 10.1016/j.neuroimage.2020.117444

Jefferies, E. (2013). The neural basis of semantic cognition: Converging evidence from neuropsychology, neuroimaging and TMS. *Cortex, 49*(3), 611–625. doi: 10.1016/j.cortex.2012.10.008

Jefferies, E., & Lambon Ralph, M. A. (2006). Semantic impairment in stroke aphasia versus semantic dementia: A case-series comparison. *Brain, 129*(8), 2132–2147. doi: 10.1093/brain/awl153

Jorna, R. J. (2008). Neurosemiotics. In *Encyclopedia of Neuroscience* (pp. 2830–2833). Springer Berlin Heidelberg. doi: 10.1007/978-3-540-29678-2_3946

Josephs, K. A., Whitwell, J. L., Vemuri, P., Senjem, M. L., Boeve, B. F., Knopman, D. S., Smith, G. E., Ivnik, R. J., Petersen, R. C., & Jack, C. R. (2008). The anatomic correlate of prosopagnosia in semantic dementia. *Neurology, 71*(20), 1628–1633.

Jung, J. Y., & Lambon Ralph, M. A. (2016). Mapping the dynamic network interactions underpinning cognition: A cTBS-fMRI study of the flexible adaptive neural system for semantics. *Cerebral Cortex, 26*(8), 3580–3590.

Kopelman, M. D. (2002). Disorders of memory. *Brain, 125*(10), 2152–2190.

Lambon Ralph, M. A., Ehsan, S., Baker, G. A., & Rogers, T. T. (2012). Semantic memory is impaired in patients with unilateral anterior temporal lobe resection for temporal lobe epilepsy. *Brain, 135*(1), 242–258. doi: 10.1093/brain/awr325

Lambon Ralph, M. A., Jefferies, E., Patterson, K., & Rogers, T. T. (2016). The neural and computational bases of semantic cognition. *Nature Reviews Neuroscience, 18*(1), 42–55.

Lambon Ralph, M. A., McClelland, J. L., Patterson, K., Galton, C. J., & Hodges, J. R. (2001). No right to speak? The relationship between object naming and semantic impairment: Neuropsychological evidence and a computational model. *Journal of Cognitive Neuroscience, 13*(3), 341–356. doi: 10.1162/08989290151137395

Lambon Ralph, M. A., Pobric, G., & Jefferies, E. (2009). Conceptual knowledge is underpinned by the temporal pole bilaterally: Convergent evidence from rTMS. *Cerebral Cortex, 19*(4), 832–838. doi: 10.1093/cercor/bhn131

Lambon Ralph, M. A., Sage, K., Jones, R. W., & Mayberry, E. J. (2010). Coherent concepts are computed in the anterior temporal lobes. *Proceedings of the National Academy of Sciences of the United States of America, 107*(6), 2717–2722.

Marinkovic, K., Dhond, R. P., Dale, A. M., Glessner, M., Carr, V., & Halgren, E. (2003). Spatiotemporal dynamics of modality-specific and supramodal word processing. *Neuron, 38*(3), 487–497. doi: 10.1016/S0896-6273(03)00197-1

Martin, A. (2007). The representation of object concepts in the brain. *Annual Review of Psychology, 58*(1), 25–45. doi: 10.1146/annurev.psych.57.102904.190143

Martin, A, & Chao, L. (2001). Semantic memory and the brain: structure and processes. *Current Opinion in Neurobiology, 11*(2), 194–201. doi: 10.1016/s0959-4388(00)00196-3

Mion, M., Patterson, K., Acosta-Cabronero, J., Pengas, G., Izquierdo-Garcia, D., Hong, Y. T., Fryer, T. D., Williams, G. B., Hodges, J. R., & Nestor, P. J. (2010). What the left and right anterior fusiform gyri tell us about semantic memory. *Brain, 133*(11), 3256–3268.

Mummery, C. J., Patterson, K., Price, C. J., Ashburner, J., Frackowiak, R. S. J., & Hodges, J. R. (2000). A voxel-based morphometry study of semantic dementia: Relationship between temporal lobe atrophy and semantic memory. *Annals of Neurology, 47*(1), 36–45.

Murre, J. M. J., Graham, K. S., & Hodges, J. R. (2001). Semantic dementia: Relevance to connectionist models of long-term memory. *Brain, 124*(4), 647–675. doi: 10.1093/brain/124.4.647

Nestor, P. J., Fryer, T. D., & Hodges, J. R. (2006). Declarative memory impairments in Alzheimer's disease and semantic dementia. *NeuroImage, 30*(3), 1010–1020. doi: 10.1016/j.neuroimage.2005.10.008

Noonan, K. A. K. A., Jefferies, E., Visser, M., & Lambon Ralph, M. A. M. A. (2013). Going beyond inferior prefrontal involvement in semantic control: Evidence for the additional contribution of dorsal angular gyrus and posterior middle temporal cortex. *Journal of Cognitive Neuroscience, 25*(11), 1824–1850. doi: 10.1162/jocn_a_00442

Oakley, T. (2007). Attention and semiotics. *Cognitive Semiotics, 1*, 25–45. doi: 1515/COGSEM.2007.1.FALL2007.25

Perani, D., Schnur, T., Tettamanti, M., Gorno-Tempini, M., Cappa, S. F., & Fazio, F. (1999). Word and picture matching: A PET study of semantic category effects. *Neuropsychologia, 37*(3), 293–306. doi: 10.1016/s0028-3932(98)00073-6

Phan, T. G., Donnan, G. A., Wright, P. M., & Reutens, D. C. (2005). A digital map of middle cerebral artery infarcts associated with middle cerebral artery trunk and branch occlusion. *Stroke, 36*(5), 986–991. doi: 10.1161/01.STR.0000163087.66828.e9

Plaut, D. C. (2002). Graded modality-specific specialisation in semantics: A computational account of optic aphasia. *Cognitive Neuropsychology, 19*(7), 603–639. doi: 10.1080/02643290244000112

Plaut, D. C., McClelland, J. L., Seidenberg, M. S., & Patterson, K. (1996). Understanding normal and impaired word reading: Computational principles in quasi-regular domains. *Psychological Review*, *103*(1), 56–115. doi: 10.1037/0033-295X.103.1.56

Pobric, G., Jefferies, E., & Lambon Ralph, M. A. (2010). Amodal semantic representations depend on both anterior temporal lobes: Evidence from repetitive transcranial magnetic stimulation. *Neuropsychologia*, *48*(5), 1336–1342. doi: 10.1016/j.neuropsychologia.2009.12.036

Pobric, G., Jefferies, E., & Ralph, M. A. L. (2007). Anterior temporal lobes mediate semantic representation: Mimicking semantic dementia by using rTMS in normal participants. *Proceedings of the National Academy of Sciences of the United States of America*, *104*(50), 20137–20141. doi: 10.1073/pnas.0707383104

Poeppel, D., Emmorey, K., Hickok, G., & Pylkkänen, L. (2012). Towards a new neurobiology of language. *Journal of Neuroscience*, *32*(41), 14125–14131. doi: 10.1523/JNEUROSCI.3244-12.2012

Pulvermülller, F. (1999). Words in the brain's language. *Behavioral and Brain Sciences*, *22*(2), 253–279. doi: 10.1017/S0140525X9900182X

Pulvermüller, F. (2018). Neural reuse of action perception circuits for language, concepts and communication. *Progress in Neurobiology*, *160*, 1–44. doi: 10.1016/j.pneurobio.2017.07.001

Rice, G. E., Caswell, H., Moore, P., Hoffman, P., & Lambon Ralph, M. A. (2018). The roles of left versus right anterior temporal lobes in semantic memory: A neuropsychological comparison of postsurgical temporal lobe epilepsy patients. *Cerebral Cortex*, *28*(4), 1487–1501. doi: 10.1093/cercor/bhx362

Rice, G. E., Hoffman, P., & Lambon Ralph, M. A. (2015a). Graded specialization within and between the anterior temporal lobes. *Annals of the New York Academy of Sciences*, *1359*(1), 84–97. doi: 10.1111/nyas.12951

Rice, G. E., Ralph, M. A. L., & Hoffman, P. (2015b). The roles of left versus right anterior temporal lobes in conceptual knowledge: An ALE meta-analysis of 97 functional neuroimaging studies. *Cerebral Cortex*, *25*(11), 4374–4391. doi: 10.1093/cercor/bhv024

Rogers, T. T., Lambon Ralph, M. A., Garrard, P., Bozeat, S., McClelland, J. L., Hodges, J. R., & Patterson, K. (2004). Structure and deterioration of semantic memory: A neuropsychological and computational investigation. *Psychological Review*, *111*(1), 205–235. doi: 10.1037/0033-295X.111.1.205

Schapiro, A. C., McClelland, J. L., Welbourne, S. R., Rogers, T. T., & Ralph, M. A. L. (2013). Why bilateral damage is worse than unilateral damage to the brain. *Journal of Cognitive Neuroscience*, *25*(12), 2107–2123. doi: 10.1162/jocn_a_00441

Seidenberg, M. S., & McClelland, J. L. (1989). A distributed, developmental model of word recognition and naming. *Psychological Review*, *96*(4), 523–568. doi: 10.1037/0033-295X.96.4.523

Siebner, H. R., Bergmann, T. O., Bestmann, S., [illegible] Rossini, P. M. (2009). Consensus paper: Combining transcranial stimulation with neuroimaging. *Brain Stimulation*, *2*(2), 58–80. doi: 10.1016/j.brs.2008.11.002

Simmons, W. K., & Barsalou, L. W. (2003). The similarity-in-topography principle: Reconciling theories of conceptual deficits. *Cognitive Neuropsychology*, *20*(3–6), 451–486. doi: 10.1080/02643290342000032

Snowden, J. (2002). Disorders of semantic memory. In A. Baddeley, B. Wilson, & M. Kopelman (Eds.), *Handbook of Memory Disorders* (pp. 293–314). Chichester: John Wiley.

Snowden, J., Griffiths, H. L., & Neary, D. (1996). Semantic-episodic memory interactions in semantic dementia: Implications for retrograde memory function. *Cognitive Neuropsychology*, *13*(8), 1101–1139. doi: 10.1080/026432996381674

Spapé, M., Harjunen, V., Ahmed, I., Jacucci, G., & Ravaja, N. (2019). The semiotics of the message and the messenger: How nonverbal communication affects fairness perception. *Cognitive, Affective and Behavioral Neuroscience*, *19*(5), 1259–1272. doi: 10.3758/s13415-019-00738-8

Sylvester, C.Y. C., & Shimamura, A. P. (2002). Evidence for intact semantic representations in patients with frontal lobe lesions. *Neuropsychology*, *16*(2), 197–207. Doi: 10.1037//0894-4105.16.2.197

Thompson-Schill, S. L., D'Esposito, M., & Kan, I. P. (1999). Effects of repetition and competition on activity in left prefrontal cortex during word generation. *Neuron*, *23*(3), 513–522. doi: 10.1016/s0896-6273(00)80804-1

Tulving, E. (1972). Episodic and semantic memory. In E. Tulving & W. Donaldson (Eds.), *Organization of Memory* (pp. 381–402). New York: Academic Press.

Vandenberghe, R., Price, C., Wise, R., Josephs, O., & Frackowiak, R. S. J. (1996). Functional anatomy of a common semantic system for words and pictures. *Nature*, *383*(6597), 254–256. doi: 10.1038/383254a0

Vatansever, D., Smallwood, J., & Jefferies, E. (2021). Varying demands for cognitive control reveals shared neural processes supporting semantic and episodic memory retrieval. *Nature Communications*, *12*(1), 2134. doi: 10.1038/s41467-021-22443-2

Visser, M., Embleton, K.V., Jefferies, E., Parker, G. J., & Ralph, M. A. L. (2010a). The inferior, anterior temporal lobes and semantic memory clarified: Novel evidence from distortion-corrected fMRI. *Neuropsychologia*, *48*(6). doi: 10.1016/j.neuropsychologia.2010.02.016

Visser, M., Forn, C., Lambon Ralph, M. A. A., Hoffman, P., Gómez Ibáñez, A., Sunajuán, A., Rosell Negre, P., Villanueva, V., & Ávila, C. (2018). Evidence for degraded low frequency verbal concepts in left resected temporal lobe epilepsy patients. doi: 10.1162/jocn.2009.21309

Visser, M., Jefferies, E., Embleton, K.V., & Ralph, M. A. L. (2012). Both the middle temporal gyrus and the ventral anterior temporal area are crucial for multimodal semantic processing: Distortion-corrected fMRI evidence for a double gradient of information convergence in the temporal lobes. *Journal of Cognitive Neuroscience, 24*(8). 1766–1778. doi: 10.1162/jocn_a_00244

Visser, M., Jefferies, E., & Lambon Ralph, M. A. (2010b). Semantic processing in the anterior temporal lobes: A meta-analysis of the functional neuroimaging literature. *Journal of Cognitive Neuroscience, 22*(6). doi: 10.1162/jocn.2009.21309

Visser, M., & Lambon Ralph, M. A. (2011). Differential contributions of bilateral ventral anterior temporal lobe and left anterior superior temporal gyrus to semantic processes. *Journal of Cognitive Neuroscience, 23*(10), 3121–3131. doi: 10.1162/jocn_a_00007

Wise, R. J. S. (2003). Language systems in normal and aphasic human subjects: functional imaging studies and inferences from animal studies. *British Medical Bulletin*, 65(1), 95–119. doi: 10.1093/bmb/65.1.95

Witoonpanich, P., Crutch, S. J., Warren, J. D., & Rossor, M. N. (2015). The undiscovered syndrome: Macdonald Critchley's case of semantic dementia. *Neurocase, 21*(4), 408–412. doi: 10.1080/13554794.2014.910307

Woollams, A. M., & Patterson, K. (2018). Cognitive consequences of the left–right asymmetry of atrophy in semantic dementia. *Cortex, 107*, 64–77. doi: 10.1016/j.cortex.2017.11.014

7

EMBODIED MECHANISMS AND THE SHAPING OF SEMANTICS

Giovanni Buccino

Introduction

Neurosemiotics is an emergent field that aims to provide a holistic understanding of human communicative behavior by integrating social and biological sciences (Ibáñez et al., 2017). In particular, a neurosemiotic approach to language and communication targets the neurobiological mechanisms underlying our capacity to engage in symbolic interactions, with special reference to the construal and transmission of meaning in everyday interactive contexts (García et al., 2020). This chapter reviews the main empirical findings concerning the way the brain conveys meaning to words, the most common symbols humans use to communicate. Empirical results will be discussed in light of the so-called *embodied approach* to cognition, according to which individuals understand words expressing specific contents by recruiting the neural substrates used to experience those contents in motor, sensory, and even emotional domains.

Both embodied and neurosemiotic approaches emphasize the importance of conceptualizing linguistic communication as fundamentally grounded in human experience, also considering the role of emotions, empathy, theory of mind, and non verbal cues from the multimodal context in which language is learned and processed, contrasting with a more classical approach according to which language is amodal – that is, disentangled from the neural structures involved in experiencing the content of words (e.g., Chatterjee, 2010; Fodor, 1975; Mahon & Caramazza, 2005; Pylyshyn, 1984).

In the Western philosophical tradition, at least two milestones anticipate the current neuroscientific approach to explain the capacity of human individuals to give meaning to words. According to the Aristotelian standpoint, ideas or essences are not separate entities, but exist as embedded in material and concrete objects. Thus, human beings can grasp concepts as they can "abstract" (extrapolate) them from physical instantiations. Note that abstraction, in this context, refers to a general process through which any concept is formed. The Aristotelian point of view underwent developments that are interesting for what follows in the next sections, especially as far as the British empiricist tradition is concerned. John Locke, for instance, claimed that human beings could gain their ideas from experience. In Locke's view, ideas can be divided into two broad classes: simple ideas and complex ones. Simple ideas correspond with elementary aspects of external reality as grasped by our senses, such as the coldness or hardness of ice, the whiteness of a lily, or the sweetness of sugar. Complex ideas – such as beauty, gratitude, humanity, army, and universe – derive from the sum of many different simple ideas already acquired from experience. Therefore, in Locke's view, complex ideas have the same

DOI: 10.4324/9781003051817-10

origin as the simple ones – that is, experience. Complex ideas are so because of the complexity of the experiences to which they refer.

In recent times, the way the brain codes and interprets concepts and symbols in communicative and social contexts has become a debated matter in neuroscience, especially in light of the embodied approach to cognitive processes and functions. As anticipated, when focusing on language, according to such approach, the meaning of all linguistic expressions derives from actual, real-life experiences grounded in the neural substrates underpinning those experiences. For example, to understand the verb "to grasp," individuals recruit the same neural structures actually involved in performing grasping actions (Gallese, 2003; Gallese & Lakoff, 2005; Glenberg, 1997; Jirak et al., 2010; Lakoff, 1987; Pulvermüller, 2002; Zwaan & Taylor, 2006). While the embodied approach to language has achieved significant empirical results, it provided less straightforward results in the domain of abstract words, by definition far from single actual experiences (see Buccino et al., 2019 for a review).

The present chapter is structured as follows. First, we will review the literature concerning how the brain processes verbs expressing a specific motor content, embedded or not in a sentence. Second, we will consider literature on nouns referring to concrete objects, again embedded or not in a sentence. Third, the processing of words expressing emotional contents will be discussed. The choice of these three main topics is justified by the fact that verbs and nouns are the most common lexical categories used in linguistic communication. Furthermore, there is well-established empirical evidence, collected over the last 20 years, about the neural substrates involved in the processing of these lexical categories. As for words expressing emotional content, for many authors (e.g., Barsalou, 2008; Vigliocco et al., 2013) they represent a bridge between concrete words and those expressing abstract concepts. Accordingly, the study of these words would open the possibility to extend the embodied approach into the processing of words expressing abstract concepts. Finally, a fourth, integrative section is proposed in which we highlight epistemological continuities and opportunities for cross-fertilization between neurosemiotics and embodied approaches to language.

Processing verbs

Actions are at the basis of our experience of the world. By means of actions, we can interact with objects in the environment and with other individuals. It is not by chance that some authors, such as Piaget (1963) and Montessori (1914), consider the sensorimotor system and motor experiences fundamental for cognitive development. Words referring to actions are verbs, which for this reason play a central role in language as actions in everyday life. Within the embodiment theoretical framework, several empirical studies have focused on verbs expressing a typical motor content, an action that can be executed by a biological effector like a hand, a foot, or the mouth – for example, "to grasp" or "to bite."

Neural structures of verbs processing

By means of functional magnetic resonance imaging (fMRI), some early and pivotal studies have shown a clear involvement of the neural structures responsible for action execution during the processing of verbs expressing a specific action content (Hauk et al., 2004; Tettamanti et al., 2005). In these studies, reading or listening to verbs expressing hand, foot, or mouth actions led to the activation of distinct sectors of the motor and premotor areas, where motor representations of hand, foot, and mouth actions, respectively, have been described (Buccino et al., 2001; Dalla Volta et al., 2015; Sakreida et al., 2005; Wheaton et al., 2004). As a whole, these studies support the notion that overlapping sectors within the motor system are similarly recruited during the observation/execution of hand, foot, and mouth actions as well as the processing of verbs expressing those same actions

(Aziz-Zadeh et al., 2006; Baumgaertner et al., 2007). In keeping with this, it has been shown that the application of repetitive transcranial magnetic stimulation – rTMS, which allows for a reversible inactivation of a specific area – on the premotor cortex resulted in impaired comprehension of sentences describing manual actions (Tremblay et al., 2012). Similarly, recent evidence shows that that non-invasive stimulation of the primary motor cortex can also selectively reduce comprehension of action meanings even in naturalistic narratives (Birba et al., 2020).

Behavioral evidence

Some behavioral studies have demonstrated that the execution of a motor response is facilitated when participants have to process sentences that describe actions taking place in the same direction as the motor response (e.g., Glenberg & Kaschak, 2002; Kaschak & Borreggine, 2008; Zwaan & Taylor, 2006). This modulation of motor responses is known as action-sentence compatibility effect (ACE). That said, it is worth stressing that in a recent multicentric study (Morey et al., 2021), the e ACE has not been replicated. Insights into a crucial (and possibly causal) role of the recruitment of the motor system in language processing were obtained in several behavioral studies by asking participants an early (within 200 ms from stimulus presentation) motor response to action verbs stimuli (Boulenger et al., 2006; Buccino et al., 2005; Dalla Volta et al., 2009; de Vega et al., 2013 Sato et al., 2008). For example, when participants were asked to make a semantic decision on listened verbs (expressing either hand- or foot-related actions), they gave slower hand motor responses when they had to judge language material concerning hand actions as compared to foot actions. In a similar manner, they gave slower foot motor responses when they had to judge foot action related language material, compared with hand verbs (Buccino et al., 2005). This evidence has been interpreted as an interference effect. Since the same neural resources (namely, the same sectors of the motor system) were involved in giving motor responses and judging the presented language material, participants paid a cost showing a slowing down of their motor responses. Indeed, an interference effect seems more causally related to a direct involvement of the motor system in verb comprehension.

In general terms, the modulation of motor responses during the understanding of words embedded or not in sentences seems to be rather complex, depending on the task and the time at which the response is given (for a review, see García & Ibáñez, 2016).

Time-course of verb understanding

Empirical evidence showing a crucial role of motor system recruitment in processing action verbs has been collected by means of neurophysiological techniques such as electroencephalography (EEG), magnetoencephalography (MEG), and TMS.

In this respect, studies carried out by means of these techniques allow researchers to gain insights on the precise time course of cognitive events such as language processing and understanding because of their temporal resolution (Pulvermüller et al., 2001; for a review, see Pulvermüller et al., 2009). As in the brain imaging studies reviewed above, when using these techniques it has been demonstrated that passive reading or listening to verbs expressing hand and/or foot actions recruit specific sectors of the motor and premotor cortex corresponding to those active during the actual execution of hand and/or foot actions. Interestingly, this recruitment occurs within 150–170 ms from the stimulus presentation, thus ruling out the possibility that the recruitment of the motor system during the processing of verbs could be due to motor imagery or motor preparation. Complementary to these results, using the same task reported earlier (see Buccino et al., 2005) in a TMS experiment, it has been shown that when TMS stimuli were delivered within 200 ms from language material presentation, motor evoked potentials (MEPs) recorded from hand muscles decreased in amplitude when participants were listening to hand vs. foot action-related sentences. Opposite results have been obtained when MEPs were recorded from foot/leg muscles. The decrease of MEPs amplitude is in line with the interference effect seen in behavioral tasks.

It is worth stressing that the results of these experiments showing an interference effect on motor responses while processing language material do not contrast with EEG and MEG studies (Pulvermüller et al., 2009) documenting an early recruitment of the motor system during language comprehension. Instead, they seem to further support this evidence, indicating that the motor system is not only involved early during language processing, but also that this involvement is potentially crucial to language understanding since it specifically affects the cognitive performance of healthy individuals. A MEG study (Klepp et al., 2015) has shed light on the neurophysiological mechanisms responsible for this interference effect. During the execution of actions, a suppression of β rhythm, normally recorded in motor/premotor areas, occurs. If a motor response is requested while processing language material, this suppression is weaker, indicating that the system is less prompt to actually execute an action. Furthermore, this effect correlates with the "imageability" of the processed verbs: the stronger the imageability, the weaker the suppression of β rhythm. Similarly, EEG studies showed the modulation of fronto-central mu rhythm during action sentences processing (Moreno, de Vega, & León, 2013; Moreno et al., 2015; van Elk et al., 2010). Both mu and beta rhythms are equally considered neural signatures of motor processes.

Taken together, the behavioral studies reviewed in the previous paragraph, as well as the neurophysiological findings reviewed here, allow one to conclude that the modulation of the motor system during language processing changes over time, going from an early interference, operating between 100–200 ms after stimulus onset, to a subsequent facilitation, operating later than 200 ms after stimulus presentation (García & Ibáñez, 2016). It is worth noting that the late recruitment of the motor system, possibly leading to a facilitation of motor responses, has been interpreted by some authors as a side-effect, at the motor level, of distinct, causal, and upstream cognitive processes underlying language processing. According to these authors, at most it may represent a way to enrich conceptual processing and provide it with a relational context (Mahon & Caramazza, 2005; Tomasino et al., 2007). However, this interpretation appears less plausible when considering an early recruitment of the motor system (150–170 ms after stimulus presentation). Although in this case one cannot completely rule out that the recruitment of the motor system occurs because of upstream cognitive processes, it may reasonably be excluded that it follows as a side-effect due, for example, to motor preparation or motor imagery of the verb content or just to provide it with a relational context. Indeed, these should be slower processes, occurring after semantic processing has been completed.

Embodiment in movements disorders

Increasing evidence of a causal role of the recruitment of the motor system in language processing comes from lesion studies. By using six different tasks aimed at probing knowledge of action concepts in a large group of brain-damaged patients, it has been shown that lesion sites included brain regions within the fronto-parietal sensorimotor systems (Kemmerer et al., 2012). In another study (Desai et al., 2015) the authors tested manual and semantic abilities in chronic stroke patients. They found that the degree of impairment for action word processing showed correlation with the impairment in manual performance. In keeping with this, another work showed that reversible inactivation of hand pre-motor cortex (obtained with rTMS) in healthy individuals may hinder the comprehension of sentences expressing hand actions (Tremblay et al., 2012). In the clinical domain, several studies (Bak et al., 2001, 2006; Cardona et al., 2013; Cotelli et al., 2007; Fernandino et al., 2013; García et al., 2018; García & Ibáñez, 2018; for a review, see also Birba et al., 2017) have shown that lesions affecting the motor system, even at the subcortical level, may lead to impairment in action word processing, thus supporting the notion of a close and causal relationship between sensorimotor and conceptual systems of the brain. Overall, these results show that the brain motor system is critically, and possibly causally, involved in processing action verbs.

Mirror neurons and their potential role in language processing

The involvement of the motor system in different cognitive functions, ranging from action observation/recognition to motor imagery, including language, finds its cornerstone in the discovery of mirror neurons (Rizzolatti et al., 1996a, 1996b), originally described in a sector of the monkey premotor cortex (the so-called area F5). Later on, mirror neurons where also found in the monkey parietal lobe, indicating that they are combined in fronto-parietal circuits (for reviews, see Borra & Luppino, 2019; Sakreida et al., 2016). These neurons are endowed with a mirror mechanism – that is, the capacity to match an observed action with its motor counterpart. In the monkey, mirror neurons are active both when an animal performs an action upon an object (e.g., grasping a cup) and when it observes the same action executed by another individual (Fabbri-Destro & Rizzolatti, 2008; Rizzolatti & Craighero, 2004). Additionally, some mirror neurons also respond to the typical sound of some actions (e.g., nut-cracking), suggesting that they may be engaged by multi-modal inputs – that is, by visual as well as auditory information (Kohler et al., 2002). This is a key observation as the linguistic signal is usually mediated by auditory inputs (as well as by visual inputs in the cases of sign languages and reading). It is worth underlining that the monkey premotor sector where mirror neurons were described (area F5) largely coincide with the human inferior frontal gyrus where Broca's region is located (Petrides et al., 2005). In humans, this region is classically considered to be devoted to the control of speech and communicative acts.

So far, there is no electrophysiological evidence, at the single neuron level, of the existence of mirror neurons in areas homologue to those where mirror neurons were found in the monkey. However, brain imaging studies have shown that the observation of actions carried out with different biological effectors (i.e., a hand or a foot) leads to the activation of different sectors of fronto-parietal regions (Buccino et al., 2001; Dalla Volta et al., 2015; Sakreida et al., 2005; Wheaton et al., 2004), largely overlapping with those active during the execution and imagination of those same actions (for a review, see Hardwick et al, 2018). The brain areas that are recruited during both the execution and the observation of actions are more properly defined as the mirror neuron system (Fabbri-Destro & Rizzolatti, 2008; Rizzolatti & Craighero, 2004). Some authors have proposed that the mirror neuron system may subserve complex tasks such as understanding others' actions and social interactions (Hari & Kujala, 2009). Moreover, the mirror neuron system displays a somatotopical organization: executed and observed actions for different biological effectors are segregated in distinct parieto-frontal regions. Areas within the mirror neuron system overlap with those active during the processing of verbs expressing actions performed with the mouth, a hand, and a foot, respectively. Therefore, the mirror neuron system seems to be able to discriminate action domains in relation to the involved biological effector; discrimination of action domains may also help discriminating semantic domains (e.g., "kick" vs. "grasp"). Taken together, these considerations make it reasonable to hypothesize that understanding the meaning of action verbs may rely on the mirror neuron system in the human brain, thus supporting the view that linguistic meaning is rooted in the brain circuits engaged in actual sensorimotor experiences.

The role of the mirror neuron system in processing verbs has been also highlighted in a paper (Kemmerer & Castillo, 2010) aimed at reviewing empirical data supporting the so-called two-level theory of verb meaning (Levin & Rappaport Hovav, 2005; Pinker, 2007). According to this theory, verbs have two distinct levels of meaning. One level reflects the uniqueness of every verb and is called the "root-level." The other one is a common representation shared by all verbs belonging to a specific "action-structure" class (e.g., the verbs "to spray," "to splash," and "to squirt" all have the same action-structure as in "Carol sprayed/splashed/squirted the flowers with water"). This common structure is captured by the "template-level." In their article, Kemmerer & Castillo (2010) propose that the root level (essentially the one we discuss in this chapter) may have its neural counterpart in mirror neurons somatotopically organized in different sectors of the premotor cortex. The template-level may be processed in Broca's region in the inferior frontal gyrus, where a few studies have found a common representation for verbs describing actions actually performed by different body parts (Baumgaertner et al., 2007; Tettamanti et al., 2005), or presented through different modalities (either verbally or acoustically).

For the sake of completeness, it should be mentioned that the role of the mirror neuron system in language processing has been disputed (Hickok, 2009, 2013). These criticisms mainly point to some weaknesses of the current research on mirror neurons. While these criticisms may help better define the role of mirror neurons and mirror mechanisms in language processing, definitively they should not be considered a reason to abandon this line of research.

Processing concrete nouns

Most actions performed by human individuals are directed to objects. Several empirical findings in neuroscience have shown that specific circuits in the brain are involved in coding the sensorimotor features of objects (e.g., their shape, size, and so on) to act upon them in the most proper manner (Borra & Luppino, 2019; Jeannerod et al., 1995; Sakreida et al. 2016). The verbal counterpart of objects is nouns. Hence, within the embodiment approach, the representation of nouns should overlap with those of their corresponding objects.

As we have seen in the previous section, there is broad evidence for a role of the motor cortex (motor/premotor sectors and the parietal sectors to which they are connected) in action verbs understanding, embedded, or not in sentences. In contrast, there has been much less focus on the neural structures responsible for conveying meaning to nouns. According to linguistic theory, all languages have different lexical categories, and all languages distinguish between nouns and verbs (albeit in different ways). This, in turn, has been considered as an index of a different representation of these lexical categories in the brain. Indeed, clinical, brain imaging, and neurophysiological studies (see Vigliocco et al., 2011 for a review) support the notion that distinct neural structures are recruited during processing of nouns and verbs.

However, since nouns refer to objects, and objects are known to be represented in the motor/premotor cortex, in the embodied perspective it is be expected that nouns (at least those referring to concrete graspable objects), like verbs, are represented in the motor system.

Neural representation of objects

The manipulation of actual objects recruits a fronto-parietal circuit in the brain both of monkeys and humans (Binkofski et al., 1999; Jeannerod et al., 1995; Rizzolatti et al., 2004), reflecting sensorimotor transformations – that is, the transformation of specific object features in appropriate motor plans to interact upon them. Furthermore, both in non-human primates and humans, the mere observation of objects alone also modulates the activity of the motor system. For monkeys in particular, a set of neurons, now referred to as "canonical neurons," have been shown to respond during the perception of manipulable objects (Murata et al., 1997; Raos et al., 2006; Rizzolatti et al., 1988). Similar findings have been demonstrated in the human brain using brain imaging techniques (Grèzes et al., 2003a, 2003b). In sum, the perception of objects that have the potential for being manipulated activates the very system responsible for actual manipulation. In other words, the brain responds to the affordances (Gibson, 1977, 1979) of an object. A TMS study has highlighted the relationships between motor activity and the properties/affordances of manipulable objects by showing that changing the physical (affording) properties of an object changes the motor response to it (Buccino et al., 2009), as revealed by MEPs. For example, when participants observe an object with a whole handle and MEPs are recorded from their hand muscles, MEPs are modulated as if participants had to actually grasp the observed object. On the other hand, when they observe a broken object, MEPs recorded from hand muscles are modulated as if the observed object could be not grasped. It seems likely that, in the same way that mirror neurons could underlie verb processing, canonical neurons could underlie noun processing and enable the recruitment of the motor system.

Neural representation of concrete nouns

Differently from verbs, only few studies have addressed the issue of the activation of the motor cortex during language tasks with nouns as stimuli. A TMS study using nouns presented as single words found an involvement of the ventral premotor cortex (PMv) for the processing of tool-related items (Cattaneo et al., 2010). A few brain imaging studies reported the activation of different systems during the processing of nouns denoting natural objects and artifacts, including acoustic, visual, and sensorimotor systems, depending on the attribute accompanying the noun (Hoenig et al., 2008; Kiefer et al, 2008). At the behavioral level, there is some evidence that the presentation of graspable nouns can interact with motor activity. For instance, a kinematic study by Glover et al. (2004) showed that reading nouns referring to small and large objects (e.g., "grape" or "apple"), requiring respectively a precision grip or a power grip, interfered with the planning of grasping movements directed to targets of different size. Similar findings were reported by Tucker and Ellis (2004), who used a categorization task in which nouns referring to different size objects were used as stimuli and responses were given by manipulating a mechanical device requiring a precision grip or a power grip. The authors found faster motor responses when there was a compatibility between the grip implied by the noun and the grip required to respond. A consistency effect between action preparation and noun processing was subsequently observed by Lindemann et al. (2006), who stressed that planning grasping-to-use movements directed toward everyday objects (e.g., a glass) facilitates the semantic activation of nouns that are related to the action goals of the object use (e.g., mouth). Moreover, Myung et al. (2006) showed that words denoting human-made objects that share elements of manipulation knowledge (e.g., "piano" and "typewriter") prime one another in a lexical decision task. It has been shown, more specifically, that the manipulation knowledge evoked by words of human-made objects includes details of specific hand movements associated with both the overall volumetric properties of objects and their conventional use (Bub et al., 2008). When comparing these results with those obtained with verbs, one could argue that a "priming" effect, similar to ACE, is also operating when considering nouns expressing concrete, graspable objects. Processing these nouns facilitates, as a whole, hand motor responses. Although the interaction between noun processing and motor activity has already been addressed in behavioral studies, the issue of timing remains. As for verbs, it is of great relevance to distinguish between an early recruitment of the motor system (within 150–200 ms), which in turn might be considered crucial to language processing and understanding, and later phenomena that could represent an interaction between language and the motor system, not necessarily relevant to language *per se*. To our knowledge, only Boulenger et al. (2006, 2008) has assessed the time course of linguistic-motor activation using nouns. However, since these nouns referred to non-graspable objects, no definitive conclusions can be drawn on the matter.

Time-course of concrete nouns processing

To assess the time course of the modulation of the motor system during noun processing, Marino et al. (2013) have investigated the involvement of the motor system in noun processing, following a similar paradigm used for verbs. Right-handed participants were presented with foot-related nouns, hand-related nouns, and abstract nouns. They were required to indicate by hand responses (left or right) when a word was concrete. Effects were tested at an early (150 ms) and a late (1150 ms) go-signal delivery. The time points were chosen to coincide with those of a previous behavioral experiment on verbs, which showed a clear interference effect early in word processing, an effect that disappeared when the motor response was given by the late time point (Sato et al., 2008).

Furthermore, the authors tested the involvement of left and right hemisphere primary motor areas (right or left hand). At the early go-signal, the results showed slower right-hand responses for hand-related nouns compared with foot related nouns; the opposite pattern was found for the left hand. These findings demonstrate an early, lateralized modulation of the motor system during noun processing, most likely crucial for noun comprehension. Moreover, a TMS study was carried out to compare modulation of the motor system when subjects read nouns referring to artificial vs. natural and graspable vs. ungraspable objects (Gough et al., 2012). TMS was applied to the primary motor cortex representation of the first dorsal interosseous (FDI) muscle of the right hand at 150 ms after noun presentation.

Analyses of MEPs revealed that, across the duration of the task, nouns referring to graspable artifacts (tools) were associated with significantly greater MEP areas. Analyses of the initial presentation of items revealed a main effect of graspability. The findings are in line with an embodied view of nouns, with MEPs measures modulated according to whether nouns denoted natural objects or artifacts (tools). These findings confirm tools as a special class of items in motor terms. In this context, it is worth underlining that there is evidence of tool-specific activity in the human parietal cortex (Valyear et al., 2007), an area that appears to be phylogenetically specific of human primates (Peeters et al., 2009). Of interest is the fact that, as for verb processing as well as for nouns, it seems that the motor system is modulated according to a specific time course: within the first 200 ms from stimulus presentation, an interference effect occurs, so that the biological effector normally used to interact with processed nouns (i.e., a hand) is slower in giving motor responses. Late processing leads to a facilitation of motor responses.

This evidence has been confirmed in a behavioral study where participants had to judge whether objects presented through pictures or nouns were sensitive or not (Marino et al., 2013). Objects could be graspable or non-graspable. Participants had to respond at an early (150 ms) and late time point (1150 ms) from stimulus presentation. The results have shown that early hand motor responses were slower for graspable vs. non-graspable objects, whatever the type of stimulus (picture or noun). This interference effect disappeared in late responses. Interestingly, a similar modulation pattern has been also demonstrated in a study where participants had to judge the same kind of stimuli with nouns expressed in a second language – L2 (Buccino et al., 2017). In this study, hand motor responses were slower for graspable objects (either pictures or nouns) compared with non-graspable objects. These findings seem to reinforce the notion that, as for verbs, there is a motor experience at the basis of noun processing, and motor responses are similarly affected when a specific graspable object is expressed in L1 or L2.

Finally, in parallel with verbs, patients with motor impairment, such as Parkinson's disease patients, fail to process nouns as well as pictures denoting graspable objects (Buccino et al., 2018). Relevant to the perspective taken in this chapter, the modulation of the motor system during the processing of words denoting motor properties has been also shown while presenting adjectives expressing either negative or positive pragmatic features (Gough et al., 2013). Using TMS, MEPs were recorded from two antagonistic muscles, the FDI of a hand and the extensor communis digitorum (EC) of the forearm. The FDI is involved in grasping actions and the EC in releasing. TMS pulses were delivered while participants were reading adjectives expressing either negative or positive pragmatic properties (e.g., thorny or soft, respectively), at 150 ms after presentation of language material. Overall, findings showed an interaction of adjective type (positive, negative) and muscle (FDI, EC), the effect being driven by a significant difference for negative adjectives. Further analysis aimed at investigating the effectiveness of positive adjectives showed a similar, but opposite, pattern of effects for the positive words in the two initial blocks. These results indicate that, as for verbs and nouns, adjectives recruit the sensorimotor system, and their processing is best explained by an embodied rather than an amodal approach to language.

Summing up, the findings of several neuroscientific studies strongly support a crucial role of the sensorimotor systems in the capacity to process and understand words such as verbs, nouns, and even adjectives, at least when these lexical categories refer to and express concrete situations and entities. It has been proposed (Buccino et al., 2016) that what is crucial for the comprehension of words is the re-enactment of specific experiences related to words. We know "by experience" what a cup is for, how we can use it, its physical and pragmatic features, and so on. Indeed, these experiences are sensorimotor by nature and are coded in the brain's sensorimotor systems. Whenever we read or listen to a specific word, we re-enact our experience concerning a specific object (a noun) or a specific action (a verb), and in this manner we can convey meaning to nouns, verbs, or even words that describe specific features of an object (adjectives). Figure 7.1 shows the common representation in the brain for hand actions and hand-related verbs, and hand objects and their nouns, respectively, as revealed by neurophysiological and brain imaging studies.

At the very end, communicating with words means sharing experiences related to those words. This is relevant for at least two reasons. First, it may account for the fact that the recruitment of brain systems devoted to coding the underlying experiences is crucial for processing words expressing those experiences. This also suggests that the distinction between word categories may be rooted in the motor and sensory experience, rather than in a priori defined parts of speech (Vigliocco et al., 2011). In other words, there are no areas in the brain devoted to understand nouns different or distinct from those coding for verbs, but rather areas coding for specific motor or sensory content (semantic fields) conveyed by different word categories. Second, it provides with a theoretical framework empirical evidence showing common neural substrates for words expressed in different languages (e.g., Abutalebi, 2008; Buchweitz et al., 2012; Van de Putte et al., 2018). Since the meaning of a word – whatever the language used – expresses a similar experience, the neural basis for processing will be shared across languages.

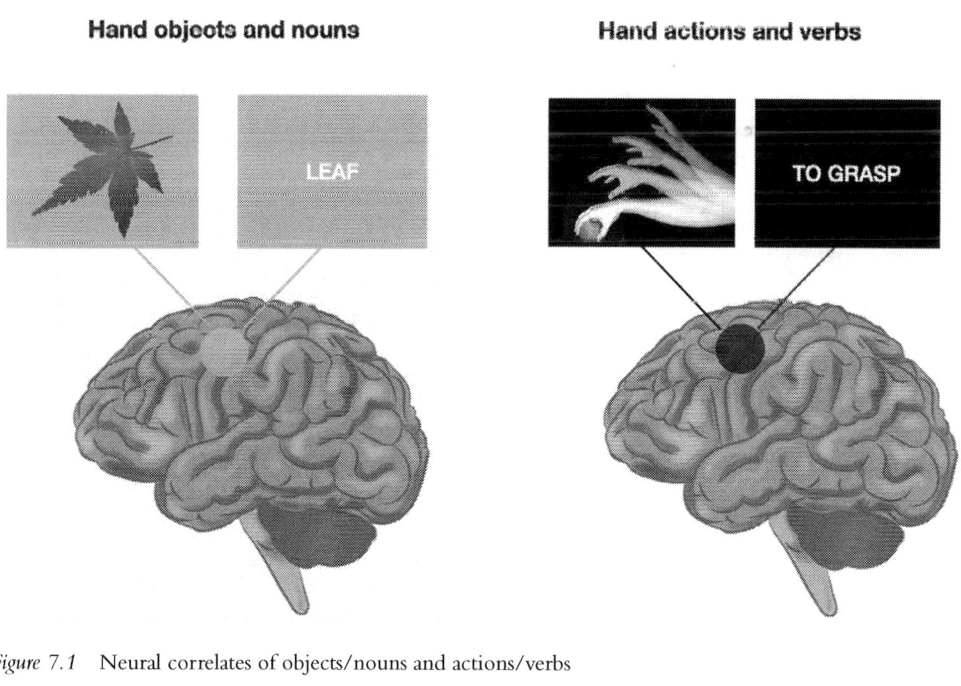

Figure 7.1 Neural correlates of objects/nouns and actions/verbs

Experimental evidence supports the view of a common representation in the cerebral cortex of visually presented hand objects and nouns in the same category, and hand related actions and verbs in the same category. Orange and black dots indicate the motor cortex endowed with hand motor representation. See e-book for a full-color version of this figure.

The language of emotions

So far, we have reviewed papers strongly supporting the notion that verb and noun processing is mediated by the same neural structures actually involved in coding the actions expressed by verbs or in coding the objects expressed by nouns. However, all experiments reported assessed the modulation of the motor system due to language material referring to concrete objects or to specific actions. What about emotions? Are words related to emotions embodied like words referring to concrete objects or actions? Before considering how language of emotions may be processed in the brain, it is worth considering how we can recognize and understand whether another individual is angry, happy, or sad. It has recently been suggested that the neural mechanisms devoted to the comprehension of emotional states are no different from those responsible for the comprehension of actions. As described above, the comprehension of an observed action is possibly mediated by a mirror mechanism matching the observed action on the same neural structures that are active when the action is performed. Following this approach, the comprehension of emotions could be based on a mechanism that allows individuals to "feel" the emotions of other people by recruiting the same neural structures through which they feel those same emotions. This view has been supported by several studies.

An fMRI study showed that the observation and the imitation of facial expressions related to emotions (e.g., fear, anger, happiness, disgust, sadness) recruits the same neural structures (i.e., insula, amygdala, and PMv) that are active during the actual production of those same facial expressions (Carr et al., 2003). It may be argued that these neural structures are endowed with a mirror mechanism devoted to the recognition and understanding of emotions similar to the one encoded by mirror neurons and devoted to the understanding of actions.

In the same vein, Wicker et al. (2003) used fMRI to assess what cortical areas are active during the personal experience of disgust, obtained by inhalation of disgusting substances and during the observation of other individuals inhaling the same substances and feeling the same emotion. The results of this study have demonstrated that the anterior part of the left insula is active both during the actual experience of disgust and during the observation and recognition of the same emotion in other people's faces. It is most likely, therefore, that in this part of the brain there are neurons endowed with a mirror mechanism specifically devoted to disgust. Along similar lines, during immersive reading of literary extracts with a strong emotional content, it has been reported an activation of the mid-cingulate cortex, classically involved in coding emotion (Hsu et al., 2014; Hsu et al., 2015). Further evidence in this direction comes from clinical practice: a patient with a lesion centered in the anterior insula was unable to feel disgust but, most importantly for the aim of our reasoning, he was not able to recognize this emotion on the face of other individuals.

Summing up, from the empirical data reviewed above it may be argued that the comprehension of emotions recruits, at least to some extent, the same neural structures involved in the subjective and actual experience of those emotions. Interestingly, even in the case of pain there might be a mirror mechanism subserving our capacity to perceive and recognize the pain felt by other individuals. Despite the fact that pain is not an emotion in the strict sense of the word, there is no doubt that it is accompanied by several emotional states. By recording the activity in the neurons of the anterior cingulate cortex in one patient, it has been shown that there are neurons in this area involved both during the subjective perception of pain and when painful stimuli were applied to the bodies of other individuals (Hutchison et al., 1999). Complementary to this, the presentation of fearful or threatening stimuli presented in various modalities, including written words, modulated the activity of the amygdala as revealed by brain potentials recorded with intracranial electrodes (Naccache et al., 2005). In a similar manner, in an interesting fMRI study, the anterior insula and anterior cingulate cortex were recruited during the delivery of painful stimuli to the participants, but also during the painful stimulation of other people. This recruitment was modulated by the kind of personal relationship with the person who underwent painful stimulation (Singer et al., 2004). Obviously, this is not to say that this first-person, experiential manner of recognizing and interpreting emotions is the only way we have to interpret other people's emotions. There might be situations where other strategies come into play.

Within an embodied view of language processing, it may be assumed that processing words expressing or related to emotions will engage the same neural systems involved in the actual experience of those same emotions (Niedenthal, 2007), similarly to what happens with the motor systems. For the study of words expressing emotions, there are of course several difficulties due to the intrinsic multimodal nature of emotions – which implies, for example, facial expressions, viscero-motor aspects, emotional states so that language can impact emotion, even when there is no direct reference to emotion states (Havas & Matheson, 2013). Think of the sentence "The water park is refreshing on the hot summer day": even if there is no specific emotional content, there is no doubt that it will induce positive feelings, or even smiling – especially for someone experiencing a hot summer. Despite these complications, there is increasing evidence that the processing of words expressing emotions recruits cortical and subcortical neural structures (including the anterior cingulate cortex, insula, PMv, and amygdala) like the corresponding emotional states do (for a review, see Citron, 2012). For instance, Ponz et al. (2014) (see also Gu et al., 2021) showed that during the processing of words expressing disgust, there is a recruitment of the insula in the same manner as when individuals feel disgust or observe other people experiencing this emotion (Wicker et al., 2003). The fact that emotional language is most likely embodied, like language material referring to actions and objects, may be at the basis of what Adam Smith (1759: 11) noted when he wrote:

> Our joy for the deliverance of those heroes of tragedy who interest us, is as sincere as our grief for their distress, and our fellow-feeling with their misery is not more real than that with their happiness. We enter into their gratitude towards those faithful friends who did not desert them in their difficulties; and we heartily go along with their resentment against those perfidious traitors who injured, abandoned, or deceived them

Even the charm of literature, to some extent, may reside in a mirror mechanism that allows us to internally re-enact the experiences and emotions of our heroes.

Embodied communication in a neurosemiotic framework

Recent years have seen calls for a tighter integration of (neuro)biological and social sciences to better understand human meaning-making in concrete communicative contexts (Ibáñez et al., 2017).

A step in this direction has been taken by the emergent field of neurosemiotics, which aims to track the convergences of the neurocognitive, perceptual, sensorimotor, and visceral processes that jointly shape our individual and social semiotic experiences (e.g., Brier, 2015). We propose that the experimental evidence reviewed in this chapter can provide a more general framework for neurosemiotics, by anchoring the emergence and transmission of meaning to the re-enactment of neural structures that allow individuals engaged in communication to share real-world experiences. Consider, for instance, the word "halt." The message implies that people have to stop their running or driving. If you use a red triangle to indicate the same command, the same neural structures are possibly involved, since the consequence of this command, at the behavioral level, is exactly the same. Since the use of a red light in the traffic light provides the same content, again the neural structures coding for that content will come into play. In this respect, our tenet is that whatever the shared symbols or signs we use, the brain codes this symbol re-enacting the neural substrates where the meaning of that symbol or sign is experienced. That is, sharing the meaning of words and symbols equals to share the underlying experiences. The integration of neuroscience and semiotic theory in light of embodiment has promoted, for instance, a better understanding of the emergence of new communication systems among human and artificial agents (Galantucci & Garrod, 2010; Galantucci & Steels, 2008), and opened up new opportunities for studying meaning transmission in situated social interactions (e.g., Hasson et al., 2012). It has been suggested in this respect that the body is the fundamental basis for constructing meaningful communicative exchanges, not only because it allows for the coding, perception, and reproduction of shared symbols, but also because it can be used to set up frames of joint attention (e.g., by pointing or eye gaze) and coordinated action (e.g., conversational turn-taking) in face-to-face contexts. These data suggest that an embodied approach to meaning may provide neurosemiotics with new tools to integrate the social and biological components of communication. Of note, technological advancements will arguably help neuroscience to design more immersive and ecological communication tasks in order to investigate human semiosis in more realistic settings than traditional in-lab conditions.

Conclusion

The experimental findings reviewed in this chapter support an embodied approach to semantic processing. First, these data support the notion that individuals can process and understand a specific word, denoting an action, an object, or even a feeling, by recruiting the brain areas and systems that are active during the actual experience of the content of those same words. Second, the data overall suggest that different lexical categories such as verbs, nouns, and adjectives are not coded in specific and distinct neural substrates, but rather in those areas where the content of the word is represented. The different word classes therefore seem coded in terms of semantic fields: verbs expressing concrete actions may be intermingled with nouns expressing concrete objects. Verbs and nouns are assembled in the brain like actions and objects are combined in everyday life. Third, we forward that this experimental evidence will provide a more general framework for neurosemiotics, in which coding symbols and signs implies the re-enactment of neural structures that allow individuals to make experience of that specific content.

References

Abutalebi, J. (2008). Neural aspects of second language representation and language control. *Acta Psychologica, 128*(3), 466–478. doi: 10.1016/j.actpsy.2008.03.014

Aziz-Zadeh, L., Wilson, S. M., Rizzolatti, G., & Iacoboni, M. (2006). Congruent embodied representations for visually presented actions and linguistic phrases describing actions. *Current Biology, 16*(18), 1818–1823. doi: 10.1016/j.cub.2006.07.060

Bak, T.H., O'Donovan, D.G., Xuereb, J.H., Boniface, S., & Hodges, J.R. (2001). Selective impairment of verb processing associated with pathological changes in Brodmann areas 44 and 45 in the motor neurone disease-dementia-aphasia syndrome. *Brain* 124, 103–120. doi: 10.1093/brain/124.1.103

Bak, T.H., Yancopoulou, D., Nestor, P.J., Xuereb, J.H., Spillantini, M.G., Pulvermüller, F., & Hodges, J.R., (2006). Clinical, imaging and pathological correlates of a hereditary deficit in verb and action processing. *Brain*, 129, 321–332. doi: 10.1093/brain/awh701

Baumgaertner, A., Buccino, G., Lange, R., McNamara, A., & Binkofski, F. (2007). Polymodal conceptual processing of human biological actions in the left inferior frontal lobe. *European Journal of Neuroscience, 25*(3), 881–889. doi: 10.1111/j.1460-9568.2007.05346.x

Binkofski, F., Buccino, G., Posse, S., Seitz, R. J., Rizzolatti, G., & Freund, H. (1999). A fronto-parietal circuit for object manipulation in man: Evidence from an fMRI-study. *European Journal of Neuroscience, 11*(9), 3276–3286. doi: 10.1046/j.1460-9568.1999.00753.x

Birba, A., García-Cordero, I., Kozono, G., Legaz, A., Ibáñez, A., Sedeño, L., & García, A. M. (2017). Losing ground: Frontostriatal atrophy disrupts language embodiment in Parkinson's and Huntington's disease. *Neuroscience & Biobehavioral Reviews, 80*, 673–687. doi: 10.1016/j.neubiorev.2017.07.011

Birba, A., Vitale, F., Padrón, I., Dottori, M., de Vega, M., Zimerman, M., … García, A. M. (2020). Electrifying discourse: Anodal tDCS of the primary motor cortex selectively reduces action appraisal in naturalistic narratives. *Cortex, 132*, 460–472. doi: 10.1016/j.cortex.2020.08.005

Borra, E., & Luppino, G. (2019). Large-scale temporo-parieto-frontal networks for motor and cognitive motor functions in the primate brain. *Cortex, 118*, 19–37. doi: 10.1016/j.cortex.2018.09.024

Boulenger, V., Roy, A. C., Paulignan, Y., Deprez, V., Jeannerod, M., & Nazir, T. A. (2006). Cross-talk between language processes and overt motor behavior in the first 200 msec of processing. *Journal of Cognitive Neuroscience, 18*(10), 1607–1615. doi: 10.1162/jocn.2006.18.10.1607

Boulanger, V., Mechtouff, L., Thobois, S., Broussolle, E., Jeannerod, M., & Nazir, T. A. (2008). Word processing in Parkinson's disease is impaired for action verbs but not for concrete nouns. *Neuropsychologia, 46*(2), 743–756. doi: 10.1016/j.neuropsychologia.2007.10.007

Brier, S. (2015). Can biosemiotics be a "science" if its purpose is to be a bridge between the natural, social and human sciences? *Progress in Biophysics and Molecular Biology, 119*(3), 576–587. doi: 10.1016/j.pbiomolbio.2015.08.001

Bub, D. N., Masson, M. E. J., & Cree, G. S. (2008). Evocation of functional and volumetric gestural knowledge by objects and words. *Cognition, 106*(1), 27–58. doi: 10.1016/j.cognition.2006.12.010

Buccino, G., Binkofski, F., Fink, G. R., Fadiga, L., Fogassi, L., Gallese, V., ... Freund, H. J. (2001). Action observation activates premotor and parietal areas in a somatotopic manner: An fMRI study. *European Journal of Neuroscience, 13*(2), 400–404. doi: 10.1111/j.1460-9568.2001.01385.x

Buccino, G., Colagè, I., Gobbi, N., & Bonaccorso, G. (2016). Grounding meaning in experience: A broad perspective on embodied language. *Neuroscience and Biobehavioral Reviews, 69*, 69–78. doi: 10.1016/j.neubiorev.2016.07.033

Buccino, G., Colagè, I., Silipo, F., & D'Ambrosio, P. (2019). The concreteness of abstract language: An ancient issue and a new perspective. *Brain Structure and Function, 224*(4), 1385–1401. doi: 10.1007/s00429-019-01851-7

Buccino, G., Dalla Volta, R., Arabia, G., Morelli, M., Chiriaco, C., Lupo, A., ... Quattrone, A. (2018). Processing graspable object images and their nouns is impaired in Parkinson's disease patients. *Cortex, 100*, 32–39. doi: 10.1016/j.cortex.2017.03.009

Buccino, G., Marino, B. F., Bulgarelli, C., & Mezzadri, M. (2017). Fluent speakers of a second language process graspable nouns expressed in L2 like in their native language. *Frontiers in Psychology, 8*, 1306. doi: 10.3389/fpsyg.2017.01306

Buccino, G., Riggio, L., Melli, G., Binkofski, F., Gallese, V., & Rizzolatti, G. (2005). Listening to action-related sentences modulates the activity of the motor system: A combined TMS and behavioral study. *Cognitive Brain Research, 24*(3), 355–363. doi: 10.1016/j.cogbrainres.2005.02.020

Buccino, G., Sato, M., Cattaneo, L., Rodà, F., & Riggio, L. (2009). Broken affordances, broken objects: A TMS study. *Neuropsychologia, 47*(14), 3074–3078. doi: 10.1016/j.neuropsychologia.2009.07.003

Buchweitz, A., Shinkareva, S. V., Mason, R. A., Mitchell, T. M., & Just, M. A. (2012). Identifying bilingual semantic neural representations across languages. *Brain and Language, 120*(3), 282–289. doi: 10.1016/j.bandl.2011.09.003

Cardona, J. F., Gershanik, O., Gelormini-Lezama, C., Houck, A. L., Cardona, S., Kargieman, L., ... Ibáñez, A. (2013). Action-verb processing in Parkinson's disease: New pathways for motor-language coupling. *Brain Structure and Function*, 218(6), 1355–1373. doi 10.1007/s00429-013-0510-1.

Carr, L., Iacoboni, M., Dubeau, M. C., Mazziotta, J. C., & Lenzi, G. L. (2003). Neural mechanisms of empathy in humans: A relay from neural systems for imitation to limbic areas. *Proceedings of the National Academy of Sciences of the United States of America, 100*(9), 5497–5502. doi: 10.1073/pnas.0935845100

Cattaneo, Z., Devlin, J. T., Salvini, F., Vecchi, T., & Silvanto, J. (2010). The causal role of category-specific neuronal representations in the left ventral premotor cortex (PMv) in semantic processing. *NeuroImage, 49*(3), 2728–2734. doi: 10.1016/j.neuroimage.2009.10.048

Chatterjee, A. (2010). Disembodying cognition. *Language and Cognition, 2*(1), 79–116. doi: 10.1515/langcog.2010.004

Citron, F. M. (2012). Neural correlates of written emotion word processing: A review of recent electrophysiological and hemodynamic neuroimaging studies. *Brain and Language, 122*(3), 211–226. doi: 10.1016/j.bandl.2011.12.007

Cotelli, M., Borroni, B., Manenti, R., Zanetti, M., Arévalo, A., Cappa, S. F., & Padovani, A. (2007). Action and object naming in Parkinson's disease without dementia. *European Journal of Neurology, 14*(6), 632–637. doi: 10.1111/j.1468-1331.2007.01797.x

Dalla Volta, R., Fasano, F., Cerasa, A., Mangone, G., Quattrone, A., & Buccino, G. (2015). Walking indoors, walking outdoors: An fMRI study. *Frontiers in Psychology, 6*, 1502. doi: 10.3389/fpsyg.2015.01502

Dalla Volta, R., Gianelli, C., Campione, G. C., & Gentilucci, M. (2009). Action word understanding and overt motor behavior. *Experimental Brain Research, 196*(3), 403–412. doi: 10.1007/s00221-009-1864-8

de Vega, M., Moreno, V., & Castillo, D. (2013). The comprehension of action-related sentences may cause interference rather than facilitation on matching actions. *Psychological Research*, 77(1), 20–30. doi: 10.1007/s00426-011-0356-1

Desai, R. H., Herter, T., Riccardi, N., Rorden, C., & Fridriksson, J. (2015). Concepts within reach: Action performance predicts action language processing in stroke. *Neuropsychologia*, 71, 217–224. doi: 10.1016/j.neuropsychologia.2015.04.006

Fabbri-Destro, M., & Rizzolatti, G. (2008). Mirror neurons and mirror systems in monkeys and humans. *Physiology, 23*(3), 171–179. doi: 10.1152/physiol.00004.2008

Fernandino, L., Conant, L. L., Binder, J. R., Blindauer, K., Hiner, B., Spangler, K., & Desai, R. H. (2013). Parkinson's disease disrupts both automatic and controlled processing of action verbs. *Brain and Language*, 127(1), 65–74. doi: 10.1016/j.bandl.2012.07.008. S0093-934X(12)00140-X

Fodor, J. A. (1975). *The Language of Thought*. Cambridge, MA: Harvard University Press.

Galantucci, B., & Garrod, S. (2010). Experimental semiotics: A new approach for studying the emergence and the evolution of human communication. *Interaction Studies: Social Behaviour and Communication in Biological and Artificial Systems*, *11*(1), 1–13. doi: 10.1075/is.11.1.01gal

Galantucci, B., & Steels, L. (2008). The emergence of embodied communication in artificial agents and humans. In I. Wachsmuth, M. Lenzen, & G. Knoblich (Eds.), *Embodied Communication in Humans and Machines* (pp. 229–256). Oxford: Oxford University Press.

Gallese, V. (2003). A neuroscientific grasp of concepts: From control to representation. *Philosophical Transactions of the Royal Society B: Biological Sciences*, *358*(1435), 1231–1240. doi: 10.1098/rstb.2003.1315

Gallese, V., & Lakoff, G. (2005). The brain's concepts: The role of the sensory-motor system in conceptual structure. *Cognitive Neuropsychology*, *22*(3–4), 455–479. doi: 10.1080/02643290442000310

García, A. M., Bocanegra, Y., Herrera, E., Moreno, L., Carmona, J., Baena, A., … Ibáñez, A. (2018). Parkinson's disease compromises the appraisal of action meanings evoked by naturalistic texts. *Cortex*, *100*, 111–126. doi: 10.1016/j.cortex.2017.07.003

García, A. M., Franco-O'Byrne, D., & Ibáñez, A. (2020). Neurosemiotics: Blurbing a field beyond the "two cultures divide." In L. Lacková, C. Rodríguez, & K. Kull (eds.), *Gatherings in Biosemiotics XX* (pp. 92–97). Tartu: University of Tartu Press.

García, A. M., & Ibáñez, A. (2016). A touch with words: Dynamic synergies between manual actions and language. *Neuroscience and Biobehavioral Reviews*, *68*, 59–95. doi: 10.1016/j.neubiorev.2016.04.022

García, A. M., & Ibáñez, A. (2018). When embodiment breaks down: Language deficits as novel avenues into movement disorders. *Cortex*, *100*, 1–7. doi: 10.1016/j.cortex.2017.12.022

Gibson, J. J. (1977). The theory of affordances. In R. Shaw, & J. Bransford (Eds.), *Perceiving, Acting and Knowing: Toward an Ecological Psychology* (pp. 67–82). London: Routledge.

Gibson, J. J. (1979). *The Ecological Approach to Visual Perception*. Boston: Houghton Mifflin.

Glenberg, A. M. (1997). What memory is for. *Behavioral and Brain Sciences*, *20*(1), 1–19. doi: 10.1017/S0140525X97000010

Glenberg, A. M., & Kaschak, M. P. (2002). Grounding language in action. *Psychonomic Bulletin & Review*, *9*(3), 558–565. doi: 10.3758/BF03196313

Glover, S., Rosenbaum, D. A., Graham, J., & Dixon, P. (2004). Grasping the meaning of words. *Experimental Brain Research*, *154*, 103–108. doi: 10.1007/s00221-003-1659-2

Gough, P. M., Campione, G. C., & Buccino, G. (2013). Fine tuned modulation of the motor system by adjectives expressing positive and negative properties. *Brain and Language*, *125*(1), 54–59. doi: 10.1016/j.bandl.2013.01.012

Gough, P. M., Riggio, L., Chersi, F., Sato, M., Fogassi, L., & Buccino, G. (2012). Nouns referring to tools and natural objects differentially modulate the motor system. *Neuropsychologia*, *50*(1), 19–25. doi: 10.1016/j.neuropsychologia.2011.10.017

Grèzes, J., Armony, J. L., Rowe, J., & Passingham, R. E. (2003a). Activations related to "mirror" and "canonical" neurones in the human brain: An fMRI study. *NeuroImage*, *18*(4), 928–937. doi: 10.1016/S1053-8119(03)00042-9

Grèzes, J., Tucker, M., Armony, J., Ellis, R., & Passingham, R. E. (2003b). Objects automatically potentiate action: an fMRI study of implicit processing. *European Journal of Neuroscience*, *17*(12), 2735–2740. doi: 10.1046/j.1460-9568.2003.02695.x

Gu, B., Wang, H., Beltrán, D., Liu, B., Liang, T., Wang, X., & de Vega, M. (2021). Embodied processing of disgust in Mandarin words: An ERP study. *Journal of Neurolinguistics*, *58*, 100981. doi: 10.1016/j.jneuroling.2020.100981

Hardwick, R. M., Caspers, S., Eickhoff, S. B., & Swinnen, S. P. (2018). Neural correlates of action: Comparing meta-analyses of imagery, observation, and execution. *Neuroscience & Biobehavioral Reviews*, *94*, 41–44. doi: 10.1016/j.neubiorev.2018.08.003

Hari, R., & Kujala, M. V. (2009). Brain basis of human social interaction: From concepts to brain imaging. *Physiological Reviews*, *89*(2), 453–479. doi: 10.1152/physrev.00041.2007

Hasson, U., Ghazanfar, A. A., Galantucci, B., Garrod, S., & Keysers, C. (2012). Brain-to-brain coupling: A mechanism for creating and sharing a social world. *Trends in Cognitive Sciences*, *16*(2), 114–121. doi: 10.1016/j.tics.2011.12.007

Hauk, O., Johnsrude, I., & Pulvermüller, F. (2004). Somatotopic representation of action words in human motor and premotor cortex. *Neuron*, *41*(2), 301–307. doi: 10.1016/S0896-6273(03)00838-9

Havas, D. A., & Matheson, J. (2013). The functional role of the periphery in emotional language comprehension. *Frontiers in Psychology*, *4*, 294. doi: 10.3389/fpsyg.2013.00294

Hickok, G. (2009). Eight problems for the mirror neuron theory of action understanding in monkeys and humans. *Journal of Cognitive Neuroscience*, *21*(7), 1229–1243. doi: 10.1162/jocn.2009.21189

Hickok, G. (2013). Do mirror neurons subserve action understanding? *Neuroscience Letters*, *540*, 56–58. doi: 10.1016/j.neulet.2012.11.001

Hoenig, K., Sim, E. J., Bochev, V., Herrnberger, B., & Kiefer, M. (2008). Conceptual flexibility in the human brain: Dynamic recruitment of semantic maps from visual, motor, and motion-related areas. *Journal of Cognitive Neuroscience*, *20*(10), 1799–1814. doi: 10.1162/jocn.2008.20123

Hsu, C. T., Conrad, M., & Jacobs, A. M. (2014). Fiction feelings in Harry Potter: Haemodynamic response in the mid-cingulate cortex correlates with immersive reading experience. *NeuroReport*, *25*(17), 1356–1361. doi: 10.1097/WNR.0000000000000272

Hsu, C. T., Jacobs, A. M., & Conrad, M. (2015). Can Harry Potter still put a spell on us in a second language? An fMRI study on reading emotion-laden literature in late bilinguals. *Cortex*, *63*, 282–295. doi: 10.1016/j.cortex.2014.09.002

Hutchison, W. D., Davis, K. D., Lozano, A. M., Tasker, R. R., & Dostrovsky, J. O. (1999). Pain-related neurons in the human cingulate cortex. *Nature Neuroscience*, *2*(5), 403–405. doi: 10.1038/8065

Ibáñez, A., Sedeño, L., & García, A. M. (2017). *Neuroscience and Social Science: The Missing Link*. New York: Springer.

Jeannerod, M., Arbib, M. A., Rizzolatti, G., & Sakata, H. (1995). Grasping objects: The cortical mechanisms of visuomotor transformation. *Trends in Neurosciences*, *18*(7), 314–320. doi: 10.1016/0166-2236(95)93921-J

Jirak, D., Menz, M. M., Buccino, G., Borghi, A. M., & Binkofski, F. (2010). Grasping language: A short story on embodiment. *Consciousness and Cognition*, *19*(3), 711–720. doi: 10.1016/j.concog.2010.06.020

Kaschak, M. P., & Borreggine, K. L. (2008). Temporal dynamics of the action–sentence compatibility effect. *Quarterly Journal of Experimental Psychology*, *61*(6), 883–895. doi: 10.1080/17470210701623852

Kiefer, M., Sim, E. J., Herrnberger, B., Grothe, J., & Hoenig, K. (2008). The sound of concepts: Four markers for a link between auditory and conceptual brain systems. *Journal of Neuroscience*, *28*(47), 12224–12230. doi: 10.1523/JNEUROSCI.3579-08.2008

Kohler, E., Keysers, C., Umiltà, M. A., Fogassi, L., Gallese, V., Rizzolatti, G., Umilta, M. A., Fogassi, L., Gallese, V., & Rizzolatti, G. (2002). Hearing sounds, understanding actions: Action representation in mirror neurons. *Science*, *297*(5582), 846–848. doi: 10.1126/science.1070311

Lakoff, G. (1987). *Women, Fire, and Dangerous Things: What Categories Reveal About the Mind*. Chicago: University of Chicago Press.

Levin, B., & Rappaport Hovav, M. (2005). *Argument Realization*. Cambridge. Cambridge University Press.

Lindemann, O., Stenneken, P., & van Schie, H. T. (2006) Semantic activation in action planning. *Journal of Experimental Psychology*, 32(3), 633–643. doi: 10.1037/0096-1523.32.3.633

Kemmerer, D., & Gonzalez-Castillo, J. (2010). The two-level theory of verb meaning: An approach to integrating the semantics of action with the mirror neuron system. *Brain and Language*, *112*(1), 54–76. doi: 10.1016/j.bandl.2008.09.010

Kemmerer, D., Rudrauf, D., Manzel, K., & Tranel, D. (2012). Behavioral patterns and lesion site associated with impaired processing of lexical and conceptual knowledge of actions. *Cortex*, *48*, 826–848. doi: 10.1016/j.cortex.2010.11.001

Klepp, A., Niccolai, V., Buccino, G., Schnitzler, A., & Biermann-Ruben, K. (2015). Language–motor interference reflected in MEG beta oscillations. *NeuroImage*, *109*, 438–448. doi: 10.1016/j.neuroimage.2014.12.077

Mahon, B. Z., & Caramazza, A. (2005). The orchestration of the sensory-motor systems: Clues from neuropsychology. *Cognitive Neuropsychology*, *22*(3–4), 480–494. doi: 10.1080/02643290442000446

Marino, B. F., Gough, P. M., Gallese, V., Riggio, L., & Buccino, G. (2013). How the motor system handles nouns: A behavioral study. *Psychological Research*, 77(1), 64–73. doi: 10.1007/s00426-011-0371-2

Montessori, M. (1914). *Dr. Montessori's Own Handbook*. New York: Frederick A. Stokes.

Moreno, I., de Vega, M., & León, I. (2013). Understanding action language modulates oscillatory mu and beta rhythms in the same way as observing actions. *Brain and Cognition*, *82*(3), 236–242. doi: 10.1016/j.bandc.2013.04.010

Moreno, I., De Vega, M., León, I., Bastiaansen, M., Lewis, A. G., & Magyari, L. (2015). Brain dynamics in the comprehension of action-related language: A time-frequency analysis of mu rhythms. *NeuroImage*, *109*, 50–62. doi: 10.1016/j.neuroimage.2015.01.018

Morey, R. D., Kaschak, M. P., Díez-Álamo, A. M., Glenberg, A. M., Zwaan, R. A., … Ziv-Crispel, N. (2021). A pre-registered, multi-lab non-replication of the action-sentence compatibility effect (ACE). *Psychonomic Bulletin & Review*, *29*, 613–626. doi: 10.3758/s13423-021-01927-8

Myung J, Blumstein SE, Sedivy JC. (2006). Playing on the typewriter, typing on the piano: Manipulation knowledge of objects. *Cognition*, *98*, 223–43. doi: 10.1016/j.cognition.2004.11.010

Murata, A., Fadiga, L., Fogassi, L., Gallese, V., Raos, V., & Rizzolatti, G. (1997). Object representation in the ventral premotor cortex (area F5) of the monkey. *Journal of Neurophysiology, 78*(4), 2226–2230. doi: 10.1152/jn.1997.78.4.2226

Naccache, L., Gaillard, R., Adam, C., Hasboun, D., Clémenceau, S., Baulac, M., … Cohen, L. (2005). A direct intracranial record of emotions evoked by subliminal words. *Proceedings of the National Academy of Sciences of the United States of America, 102*(21), 7713–7717. doi: 10.1073/pnas.0500542102

Niedenthal, P. M. (2007). Embodying emotion. *Science, 316*(5827), 1002–1005. doi: 10.1126/science.1136930

Peeters, R., Simone, L., Nelissen, K., Fabbri-Destro, M., Vanduffel, W., Rizzolatti, G., & Orban, G. A. (2009). The representation of tool use in humans and monkeys: Common and uniquely human features. *Journal of Neuroscience, 29*(37), 11523–11539. doi: 10.1523/JNEUROSCI.2040-09.2009

Petrides, M., Cadoret, G., & Mackey, S. (2005). Orofacial somatomotor responses in the macaque monkey homologue of Broca's area. *Nature, 435*(7046), 1235–1238. doi: 10.1038/nature03628

Piaget, J. (1963). Intellectual operations and their development. In H. E. Gruber & J. J. Vonéche (eds.), *The Essential Piaget: An Interpretive Reference and Guide* (pp. 342–358). New York: Basic Books.

Pinker, S. (2007). *The Stuff of Thought: Language as a Window onto Human Nature.* New York: Viking.

Ponz, A., Montant, M., Liegeois-Chauvel, C., Silva, C., Braun, M., Jacobs, A. M., & Ziegler, J. C. (2014). Emotion processing in words: A test of the neural re-use hypothesis using surface and intracranial EEG. *Social Cognitive and Affective Neuroscience, 9*(5), 619–627. doi: 10.1093/scan/nst034

Pulvermüller, F. (2002). *The Neuroscience of Language.* Cambridge: Cambridge University Press.

Pulvermüller, F., Härle, M., & Hummel, F. (2001). Walking or talking? Behavioral and neurophysiological correlates of action verb processing. *Brain and Language, 78*(2), 143–168. doi: 10.1006/brln.2000.2390

Pulvermüller, F., Shtyrov, Y., & Hauk, O. (2009). Understanding in an instant: Neurophysiological evidence for mechanistic language circuits in the brain. *Brain and Language, 110*(2), 81–94. doi: 10.1016/j.bandl.2008.12.001

Pylyshyn, Z. (1984). *Computation and Cognition: Toward a Foundation for Cognitive Science.* Cambridge, MA: MIT Press.

Raos, V., Umiltá, M. A., Murata, A., Fogassi, L., & Gallese, V. (2006). Functional properties of grasping-related neurons in the ventral premotor area F5 of the macaque monkey. *Journal of Neurophysiology, 95*(2), 709–729. doi: 10.1152/jn.00463.2005

Rizzolatti, G., Camarda, R., Fogassi, L., Gentilucci, M., Luppino, G., & Matelli, M. (1988). Functional organization of inferior area 6 in the macaque monkey. *Experimental Brain Research, 71*(3), 491–507. doi: 10.1007/BF00248742

Rizzolatti, G., & Craighero, L. (2004). the Mirror-Neuron System. *Annual Review of Neuroscience, 27*(1), 169–192. doi: 10.1146/annurev.neuro.27.070203.144230

Rizzolatti, G., Fadiga, L., Gallese, V., & Fogassi, L. (1996a). Premotor cortex and the recognition of motor actions. *Cognitive Brain Research,* 3(2), 131–141. doi: 10.1016/0926-6410(95)00038-0

Rizzolatti, G., Fadiga, L., Matelli, M., Bettinardi, V., Paulesu, E., Perani, D., & Fazio, F. (1996b). Localization of grasp representations in humans by PET: 1. Observation versus execution. *Experimental Brain Research, 111*(2), 246–252. doi: 10.1007/BF00227301

Rizzolatti, G., Fogassi, L., & Gallese, V. (2004). Cortical mechanisms subserving object grasping, action understanding and imitation. In M. S. Gazzaniga (Ed.), *The New Cognitive Neurosciences* (3rd edn). Cambridge: MIT Press.

Sakreida, K., Effnert, I., Thill, S., Menz, M. M., Jirak, D., Eickhoff, C. R., … & Binkofski, F. (2016). Affordance processing in segregated parieto-frontal dorsal stream sub-pathways. *Neuroscience & Biobehavioral Reviews, 69,* 89–112. doi: 10.1016/j.neubiorev.2016.07.032

Sakreida, K., Schubotz, R. I., Wolfensteller, U., & von Cramon, D. Y. (2005). Motion class dependency in observers' motor areas revealed by functional magnetic resonance imaging. *Journal of Neuroscience, 25*(6), 1335–1342. doi: 10.1523/JNEUROSCI.4170-04.2005

Sato, M., Mengarelli, M., Riggio, L., Gallese, V., & Buccino, G. (2008). Task related modulation of the motor system during language processing. *Brain and Language, 105*(2), 83–90. doi: 10.1016/j.bandl.2007.10.001

Singer, T., Seymour, B., O'Doherty, J., Kaube, H., Dolan, R. J., & Frith, C. D. (2004). Empathy for pain involves the affective but not sensory components of pain. *Science, 303*(5661), 1157–1162. doi: 10.1126/science.1093535

Smith, A. (1976) *The Theory of Moral Sentiments.* Edited by D. D. Raphael and A. L. Macfie. Oxford: Oxford University Press.

Tettamanti, M., Buccino, G., Saccuman, M. C., Gallese, V., Danna, M., Scifo, P., … Perani, D. (2005). Listening to action-related sentences activates fronto-parietal motor circuits. *Journal of Cognitive Neuroscience, 17*(2), 273–281. doi: 10.1162/0898929053124965

Tomasino, B., Werner, C. J., Weiss, P. H., & Fink, G. R. (2007). Stimulus properties matter more than perspective: An fMRI study of mental imagery and silent reading of action phrases. *NeuroImage, 36,* T128-T141. doi: 10.1016/j.neuroimage.2007.03.035

Tremblay, P., Sato, M., & Small, S. L. (2012). TMS-induced modulation of action sentence priming in the ventral premotor cortex. *Neuropsychologia, 50*(2), 319–326. doi: 10.1016/j.neuropsychologia.2011.12.002

Tucker, M., & Ellis, R. (2004). Action priming by briefly presented objects. *Acta Psychologica, 116*(2), 185–203. doi: 10.1016/j.actpsy.2004.01.004

Valyear, K. F., Cavina-Pratesi, C., Stiglick, A. J., & Culham, J. C. (2007). Does tool-related fMRI activity within the intraparietal sulcus reflect the plan to grasp? *NeuroImage, 36*, T94–T108. doi: 10.1016/j.neuroimage.2007.03.031

Van de Putte, E., De Baene, W., Price, C. J., & Duyck, W. (2018). Neural overlap of L1 and L2 semantic representations across visual and auditory modalities: A decoding approach. *Neuropsychologia, 113*, 68–77. doi: 10.1016/j.neuropsychologia.2018.03.037

van Elk, M., van Schie, H. T., Zwaan, R. A., & Bekkering, H. (2010). The functional role of motor activation in language processing: Motor cortical oscillations support lexical-semantic retrieval. *NeuroImage, 50*(2), 665–677. doi: 10.1016/j.neuroimage.2009.12.123

Vigliocco, G., Kousta, S., Vinson, D., Andrew, M., & Del Campo, E. (2013). The representation of abstract words: What matters? Reply to Paivio's (2013) comment on Kousta et al. (2011). *Journal of Experimental Psychology: General*, 142(1), 288–291. doi: 10.1037/a0028749

Vigliocco, G., Vinson, D. P., Druks, J., Barber, H., & Cappa, S. F. (2011). Nouns and verbs in the brain: A review of behavioural, electrophysiological, neuropsychological and imaging studies. *Neuroscience & Biobehavioral Reviews, 35*(3), 407–426. doi: 10.1016/j.neubiorev.2010.04.007

Wheaton, K. J., Thompson, J. C., Syngeniotis, A., Abbott, D. F., & Puce, A. (2004). Viewing the motion of human body parts activates different regions of premotor, temporal, and parietal cortex. *NeuroImage, 22*(1), 277–288. doi: 10.1016/j.neuroimage.2003.12.043

Wicker, B., Keysers, C., Plailly, J., Royet, J.P., Gallese, V., Rizzolatti, G., (2003). Both of us disgusted in my insula. *Neuron* 40, 655–664, doi: 10.1016/ S0896-6273(03)00679-2.

Zwaan, R. A., & Taylor, L. J. (2006). Seeing, acting, understanding: Motor resonance in language comprehension. *Journal of Experimental Psychology: General, 135*(1), 1–11. doi: 10.1037/0096-3445.135.1.1

8
THE FIGURATIVE BRAIN

Valentina Cuccio

Introduction

As an integral part of everyday communication, figurative language is a core topic in the agenda of neurosemiotics. Figurative uses of language imply something by saying something else. For example, in the metaphor "This surgeon is a butcher," we describe a surgeon (and their professional qualities) by referring to a butcher (and their professional qualities). The sentence is literally false, but the violation of the assumption that we usually say what we believe to be true (Grice, 1957) is functional to convey a specific meaning about the surgeon's ability. The violation is therefore only illusory, since the truth-assumption is restored thanks to the inferential processes that allow us to make sense of the sentence and to understand what the speaker is implying beyond what is explicitly said. Metaphors, irony, and indirect speech are different forms of figurative language. This chapter will be devoted to describing their biological bases, focusing on metaphors from a pragmatic, context-sensitive approach.

Pragmatics explores the role of context in the semiotic processes that lead to the construction of linguistic meaning. Without understanding the speaker's intentions, which are considered as an integral part of the context of utterance of a sentence, and without understanding the situation in which the sentence is uttered, we could not make sense of the butcher metaphor above. Pragmatics is always relevant in the process of linguistic meaning construction, but its role is especially compelling in the case of figurative meaning. For this reason, a basic knowledge of the pragmatic of language is propaedeutic to the study of the biological bases of figurative language.

At the same time, the study of figurative language is crucially relevant for the field of neurosemiotics, since figurative uses of language, as a cogent exemplification of how language production/comprehension exceeds coding/decoding operations, offer us a privileged perspective to investigate the mechanisms underlying the construction of meaning and their neural correlates. On the other hand, a neurosemiotic perspective on figurative language can illuminate the understanding of this phenomenon at large, since the process of construction of figurative meaning can be contextualized and understood in the framework of the more general human ability to communicate through signs and meanings, which are not limited to linguistic ones.

Since this chapter is devoted to the understanding of the biological bases of figurative meaning construction, and considering that the pragmatic dimension is fundamental in this process, the next section provides a basic description of the core aspects of a pragmatic account of language. This will serve as a guide to the experiments that will be discussed in subsequent paragraphs. The following

DOI: 10.4324/9781003051817-11

section will then be devoted to the discussion of the neural correlates of figurative language, including the role of embodied simulation in the processing of metaphors. A description will be provided of the neural time course of metaphor processing, which will be discussed in the framework of a semiotic account of language understanding. To conclude, final remarks will be made on the relevance of these findings in the context of neurosemiotics.

Pragmatic insights for a neurosemiotics of figurative language

Today, pragmatics is the subject of a lively internal debate that concerns fundamental aspects of this paradigm. Although different currents of thought can be identified in this debate, different aspects can be identified as the core of any pragmatic approach to the study of language.

A starting point for the identification of these defining features is the distinction between *what is literally said* and *what is intended* through an utterance (Gibbs, 1999; Grice, 1989). This distinction suggests that the semantic level only, with compositionality rules, is not sufficient to understand our linguistic activity. In other words, we cannot grasp the meaning of a sentence only on the basis of the meaning of its constituent parts plus a set of rules on how to combine them. This is so because meaning is much more than a combination of fixed lexical entries. In fact, sentences are largely underdetermined with respect to the meaning they communicate. The gap between *what is said* (the literal expression or sentential meaning) and *what is intended* through an utterance (its implicit meaning or speaker meaning) is thus filled thanks to (pragmatic) processes, which are deeply grounded in the context of use of the sentence. Without any context, we could hardly make sense of language: decades of research in the pragmatics of language have widely shown that our linguistic expressions need to be contextually enriched and disambiguated in order to be understood – for a discussion, see Recanati (2004). It is worth noting that the notion of context is used here in its broadest sense: it is the physical context where a linguistic exchange takes place; it is the co-text (i.e., the other sentences that surround a linguistic expression); it is the background (encyclopaedic) knowledge of the speakers and their mental states (Carapezza & Cuccio, 2018). The notion of context is clearly of paramount importance in any pragmatic account of the semiotic process underlying meaning construction. How context contributes to different levels of this process is still under debate. The object of investigation, from a neuroscientific perspective, are the neural mechanisms that underpin the integration of contextual information in the process of semiosis.

We can now turn to another point: *Linguistic meaning is the product of a mutual identification of communicative intentions*. This theoretical assumption dates back to Grice's program (e.g., Grice, 1957) to analyze linguistic meaning in terms of communicative intentions and to its legacy in the current debate (e.g., the relevance-theoretic approach). In this perspective, without the possibility of understanding other people's mental states (including their beliefs, opinions, hopes, and attitudes), and in particular their communicative intentions (what other people want to communicate to us by means of the words they are uttering), language would be a mere code, thus making figurative language merely impossible. Consider this example. You are finally allowed to go to the beach after several weeks of lockdown because of a pandemic and it suddenly starts to rain exactly when you are leaving your apartment. Looking out the window, you say: "How lucky am I, that I get to stay home and do all the work I have postponed in the last weeks?" This ironic statement is a clear example of figurative meaning. In this case, you might want to express something (namely, your disappointment) by referring to something else (namely, a mood which actually is different from what you are really experiencing). The listener, to understand the irony in your sentence, needs to understand your attitude towards your own sentence and, on this basis, identify your communicative intentions – that you are communicating your frustration.

Like all forms of figurative meaning, irony is a prominent manifestation of the fact that all language involves inferential communication (Carapezza & Cuccio, 2018). Different typologies have been provided with respect to the kinds of inferences underlying language comprehension and the debate on this issue is still open – for a review and critical discussion, see Carapezza & Cuccio (2018). The definition of the inferential mechanisms that allow us to deal with symbols and other signs, and the identification of their neural correlates, are fundamental in a comprehensive neurosemiotic approach to language.

Finally, another aspect of any pragmatic account of language is the *definition of language as action*. To speak is never just a mere neutral description of a state of affairs. Speaking always implies carrying out social actions. By using irony, we can ridicule or praise someone; with a declaration, we can start a war, a love affair, or a hearing in the court; with words, we can apologize, get married, and so on. These actions can be carried out only if the right words are uttered, in the right context, by the right person. For example, I can promise so and so only by saying: "I promise so and so." There is no other way of promising. Philosophers of language (Austin, 1962; Searle, 1969) defined these actions carried out through language as *speech acts*. In speech acts theory, meaning is conceived of as a social action. Interestingly, speech acts can be also carried out indirectly. *Indirect speech acts*, which have been the object of experimental investigation (see below), allow us to do something (e.g., placing a request) by uttering something else (e.g., making a statement). Indirect speech acts are an excellent example of figurative language use. Below, we turn to discussing their neural bases.

Figurative language and the brain

Neuroscientific research on figurative language has mainly targeted metaphors (Bambini, 2017; for a discussion, see Cuccio, 2015, 2017, 2018). The present section will, cogently, focus on those same phenomena.

Several studies over the last decades have shown the involvement of the right hemisphere in the comprehension of metaphors and other forms of figurative language (Bambini, 2017; Haggort & Levinson, 2014; Lai et al., 2015). Winner and Gardner (1977) compared the performance of patients with, respectively, left and right brain injury in a picture-recognition task. Participants were required to identify the picture (one of four) that correctly described a metaphorical or a literal sentence. Patients with right hemisphere damage performed significantly worse than those with lesions in the left hemisphere in coupling metaphors with the correct pictures. On these bases, it was advanced the hypothesis that metaphor processing is lateralized to the right hemisphere. However, more recent studies on the brain bases of metaphor comprehension carried out with brain imaging techniques did not confirm the right lateralization hypothesis and allowed the formulation of a more accurate model of the neural infrastructure of metaphor processing (for a review and meta-analysis, see Bohrn et al., 2012; Rapp et al., 2012; Yang, 2014; for a discussion, see Bambini, 2017; Lai et al., 2015).

The neural network recruited by the processing of figurative meaning seems to be bilateral (Figure 8.1) and it includes regions such as the inferior frontal gyrus (IFG, left and right Brodmann's area [BA] 45, left BA 47), the temporal-parietal junction (TPJ, right and left BAs 22 and 39), the right anterior cingulate cortex (ACC, right BAs 24 and 32), and the right dorsolateral prefrontal cortex, specifically the middle frontal gyrus (MFG, right BA 9).

The hypothesis of a bilateral pragmatic network supporting our ability to integrate contextual information and draw inferences has been advanced by authors such as Ferstl et al. (2010), Haggort and Levinson (2014), and Bambini (2017). From this perspective, the bilateral activation of the TPJ is considered to support theory of mind (ToM) functions underpinning our abilities to understand others' mental states and their communicative intentions. The bilateral activation of the IFG is considered to be functional to the integration of background encyclopedic knowledge with co-textual information, which is required for the construction of a high-level representation of the context, needed to disambiguate metaphoric words. The right MFG and the right ACC are considered to implement executive functions needed in the processing of metaphor. Indeed, the comprehension of a metaphor implies the inhibition of literal, non-relevant senses, and the activation of non-literal ones.

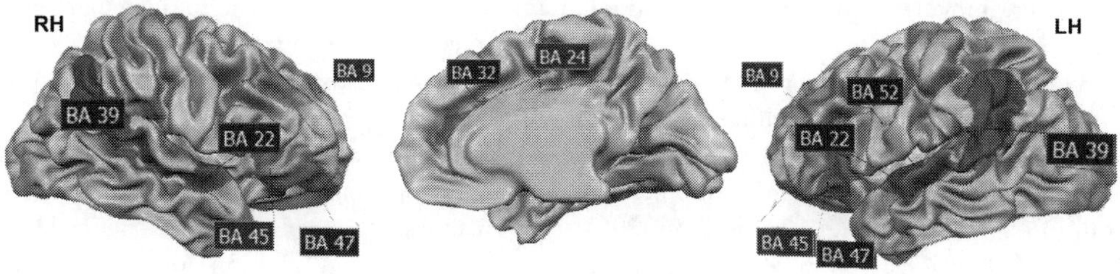

Figure 8.1 The neural network recruited by the processing of figurative meaning

From left to right: a lateral view of the right hemisphere; a sagittal view of the right hemisphere; a lateral view of the left hemisphere. Adapted from Brain Voyager Brain Tutor. Version 2.5. Copyright 2003–2010 Rainer Goebel. See e-book for a full-color version of this figure.

It is worth noting that the processing of metaphors might be affected, among other aspects, by factors such as the conventionality or novelty of the metaphorical expressions. In this regard, Bowdle and Gentner (2005) proposed the *career of metaphor hypothesis*. According to this proposal, over time, each metaphorical expression covers a path from being brand new to become highly conventional. A metaphor is conventional when it is so deeply rooted in our culture that it is no longer considered a comparison between two different domains (e.g., "the table legs"). Novel metaphors are processed as comparisons of the source and target domains (in the above example, respectively, the "butcher" and the "surgeon"), while this might not be the case for conventional and familiar metaphors. In other words, in a novel metaphor, the target is defined thanks to its implicitly drawn analogies with the source domain whereas, when metaphors become conventional, following Bowdle and Gentner's (2005) hypothesis, they are not processed as comparisons anymore. Instead, they determine the creation of new categories – that is, new abstract meanings, now considered as secondary senses of the source domain concept.

The neural correlates of metaphor processing change accordingly, as experimental findings seem to confirm. As Bambini et al. (2011) note, neuropsychological research – at least in its early phase – largely underestimated the *career of metaphor hypothesis*, thus not adequately taking into account the differences in processing, and consequently, in patterns of brain activations, related to metaphors at different stages of their career.

Interestingly, three meta-analyses studies (Bohrn et al., 2012; Rapp et al., 2012; Yang, 2014) examined data on the brain bases of metaphor processing in the light of the degree of novelty/conventionality of the metaphors used in the experiments. In all three studies, the overall metaphors > literal contrast showed activations in both the left and right hemispheres (bilateral IFG, bilateral MFG), whereas the conventional metaphors > literal contrast only produced activation in the left hemisphere (IFG, thalamus, MFG, angular gyrus). Since we know that the left IFG has a role in syntactic processing, the left thalamus has been suggested to work as a central monitor for cortical activities related to the production and execution of language (Klostermann et al., 2013) and the left angular gyrus is involved in semantic processing and word reading (Seghier, 2013). This latter result might indicate that conventional metaphors do not determine an implicit analogy between the source and target domains, which would need a greater inferential effort that would likely be supported by neural structures such as the right IFG.

Instead, as predicted by the *career of metaphor hypothesis*, they might be processed as abstract meanings and accessed as secondary senses of the source domain. In this hypothesis, the right hemisphere might be less recruited in the processing of conventional metaphors since, to make sense of very familiar metaphors, less effort in terms of integration of contextual information and inferential processes may be needed. Abstract meanings, as secondary senses of the source domains, might be stored as lexical entries in the classic language areas of the left hemisphere. The right hemisphere, in this picture, provides an important contribution in terms of the neural substrate to implement pragmatic processes – which, however, are also carried out by left neural infrastructures.

Significantly, some of the areas that constitute the pragmatic network, both in the left and right hemispheres, are typically considered the neural correlates of executive functions (e.g., ACC), attention (e.g., MFG), and ToM (ToM networks include the medial prefrontal cortex [mPFC], the precuneus, the TPJ and the temporal poles: Deuse et al., 2016; Schurz & Perner, 2015). Moreover, both in the Rapp et al. (2012) and Yang (2014) meta-analyses, the novel metaphors > literal contrast showed bilateral activations (bilateral IFG, bilateral MFG, left and right inferior parietal lobe).[1] This seems to suggest that when metaphors are novel, the process of meaning construction is more dependent on the implementation of inferential mechanisms. A greater inferential demand might, then, determine the recruitment of neural structures in the right hemisphere. Importantly, in the literal sentences > overall metaphors contrast none of these three meta-analysis studies showed specific activations to literal meaning. This suggests that both figurative and literal forms of meaning construction recruit a similar network and that the processing of metaphors – especially novel ones – requires an additional processing effort for a more robust integration of contextual information, provided by a stronger involvement of the right hemisphere (for a discussion, see Hartung et al., 2020; Lai et al., 2015).

To explain the different involvement of the right hemisphere in these different conditions – literal sentences, novel, and conventional metaphors (Bohrn et al., 2012; Rapp et al., 2012; Yang, 2014), we must keep in mind that, although in a pragmatic account of language linguistic communication always implies the integration of contextual information and the implementation of inferential processes, the nature of these processes, and consequently the pattern of neural activation supporting them, vary greatly in relation to the utterance we need to understand, to the situation, and to specific task demands. A novel metaphor might be extremely challenging, and might require a conscious and very costly inferential effort – especially if it is not embedded in a supporting context. In the comprehension of conventional metaphors, on the other hand, automatic or semi-automatic, unconscious, and less cognitively costly inferences might be sufficient.

Following this line of thought, Hartung et al. (2020) note that, although context is a key element affecting language processing, many of the studies on metaphor comprehension carried out in the last years used decontextualized stimuli. If language always needs to be contextualized in order to be correctly disambiguated, as is assumed on the bases of pragmatic models of language (as argued above), then in an experimental setting, when linguistic stimuli are embedded in a narrative context, even literal language comprehension should recruit the bilateral pragmatic network that will allow the integration of the sentence in the preceding context. Thus, we can predict that both literal and metaphorical sentences embedded in narrative context recruit inferential processes, which are then reflected by the activation of the bilateral pragmatic network. Greater inferential effort will likely determine a greater involvement of the right hemisphere. In the same line of thought, we can also consider that isolated novel metaphorical sentences are harder to comprehend than both isolated conventional metaphors and isolated literal sentences. This might explain the differences in patterns of neural activation between novel and conventional metaphors and literal sentences discussed by Bohrn et al. (2012), Rapp et al. (2012), and Yang (2014).

Interestingly, Hartung at al. (2020), in order to assess the role of a supporting context – or more precisely, in their study, the role of the co-text – in the interpretation of both literal and novel metaphors, carried out a functional magnetic resonance imaging (fMRI) study where target sentences – novel metaphors and their literal counterparts selected from Cardillo et al. (2018) – were preceded by a meaningful narrative or a jabberwocky context. The latter is a string of syntactically well-formed sentences where content words are replaced by pseudo-words with correct phonological structure. The term "jabberwocky" originates from Lewis Carroll's (1871) poem "Jabberwocky," which is considered a nonsense poem since many of the words in it, although they are syllabically and phonologically plausible in the English language, have no meanings and are made up by the author. The jabberwocky context in Hartung at al.'s (2020) study, differently from the meaningful narrative, did not provide any supporting meaning for the interpretation of the target sentences. Findings from this study showed that the processing of both metaphors and literal sentences embedded in a narrative context, compared with the same sentences embedded in the jabberwocky context, determined the activation of the same bilateral pattern of neural activation comprising the angular gyri, considered a supramodal semantic processing hub, and the anterior temporal poles, middle temporal gyri, and superior temporal sulci that might have a role in semantic processing, inhibiting prototypical responses (anterior and posterior middle temporal gyri), and integrating semantic information (anterior and posterior superior temporal gyri).

According to Hartung et al. (2020), metaphors and literal sentences share neural infrastructures when presented within a narrative context. This might be so because the narrative context provides a support which allows the reader to predict the interpretation of the metaphorical words. This facilitates the metaphorical mapping and minimizes the effect of the violation of expectations. In this view, it is possible to hypothesize that the differences in patterns of brain activations identified in previous studies carried out with isolated literal and metaphorical sentences might reflect prediction violation rather than figurative processing.

The data reviewed in this section allow us to reach some conclusions. The network subserving metaphor processing is bilateral and involves areas such as the left and right IFG; the left and right TPJ; the right ACC and MFG. The recruitment of this network – especially the areas in the right hemisphere – depends on semantic features of the metaphors (their degree of novelty/conventionality, as predicted by the *career of metaphor hypothesis*), on the co-text and context and on the inferential demands posed by the processing of the metaphorical expressions. Below, we consider complementary mechanisms involved in this domain: embodied simulations.

Figurative language and embodied simulation

The biological bases of metaphor have been widely investigated in the embodied approach to language. The latter refers to the hypothesis that the sensorimotor system plays a role in the processing of different types of linguistic information – for a discussion, see Gallese & Cuccio (2018) and Di Cesare et al. (2017). This means linguistic expressions evoking action and perception recruit neural systems for action and perception. For example, the comprehension of the sentence "Mary grasps the glass" will activate hand-related areas in the premotor cortex. Sensorimotor information, in this view, will contribute to the construction of linguistic meaning. This embodied account of language refuses the classical cognitive science view based on the idea that concepts and meanings are represented using amodal and abstract symbols (Fodor, 1983).

Using different experimental techniques, ranging from neuroimaging and electrophysiology to behavioral experiments, thousands of studies have been suggesting that the processing of different aspects of language recruits the sensorimotor system – for a review, see Pulvermüller (2018).

An influential account of the embodied nature of language is crucially based on *embodied simulation*. The latter indicates the activation of action, perception, or emotion neural circuits in the absence of a corresponding action, perception, or emotion (Gallese & Sinigaglia 2011; for a review, see Boulenger et al., 2012). This mechanism is recruited by action observation as well as by other cognitive processes such as mental imagery, the experience of artworks and, most importantly, language comprehension (Gallese & Sinigaglia, 2011). In the last few years, many empirical studies, carried out with different techniques (e.g., Buccino et al., 2005; Glenberg & Kaschak 2002; Glenberg et al., 2008; Hauk, Johnsrude, & Pulvermüller 2004; Kemmerer et al., 2008; Sato et al., 2008; Tettamanti et al., 2005), have shown the involvement of the sensorimotor system in language understanding in a somatotopic manner. The same also holds true for linguistic descriptions of sensations and emotions – in this case, language processing determines the activation of perception- or emotion-related areas of the brain.

These data suggest that language understanding, when language refers to action, emotion, and perception, involves the reactivation of our past bodily experiences. This claim holds true even for the comprehension of bodily metaphors – namely, metaphors based on our bodily experiences (e.g., Boulenger, Hauk, & Pulvermüller, 2009; Boulenger, Shtyrov, & Pulvermüller, 2012; Desai et al., 2011, 2013; for a discussion, see Cuccio, 2015, 2017, 2018). The processing of a metaphorical expression such as "John grasps the idea" will also determine the activation of hand-related areas of the premotor cortex. It has been suggested that, in this example, we comprehend the abstract concept of "understanding" (the target domain of the metaphor) resorting to the physical action of "grasping" (the source domain of the metaphor). Note that, while classic cognitive theories usually described abstract concepts (e.g., "understanding") as amodal and disembodied (Fodor, 1975), these neuroscientific findings support the claim that our bodies directly contribute to the comprehension of both concrete and abstract concepts by means of *embodied simulation* (Cuccio & Caruana, 2019; Cuccio & Gallese, 2018; Gallese & Cuccio, 2018; Gibbs 2003, 2005; Gibbs & Perlman, 2010; Matlock et al., 2005).

Data on the embodiment of metaphors can be interpreted coherently with conceptual metaphor theory (CMT), proposed in the 1980s by Lakoff and Johnson (1980). CMT takes metaphors to be mappings between two conceptual domains (see also Gibbs 2006; Kovecses, 2008). Thanks to these mappings, we typically understand and make sense of abstract concepts by relying on concrete and familiar bodily experiences. "Love is a journey" is a classic example in CMT, in which the abstract concept of "love" is understood and conceptualized via the physical experience of "travelling."

Nevertheless, it is worth noting that divergent findings have also been obtained in another set of studies (e.g., Aziz-Zadeh et al., 2006; Cacciari et al., 2011; Raposo et al., 2009; for a discussion, see Cuccio, 2018). In these studies, the comprehension of figurative and abstract language did not engage *embodied simulation*. Although it is not easy to make a direct comparison between these experiments because they differ in many respects, a meta-analysis suggested that the involvement of the sensorimotor system in non-literal language comprehension depends on semantic features of language stimuli (Yang & Shu, 2016). More specifically, it has also been suggested that the recruitment of the mechanism of simulation, and hence such variability in findings, depends on the level of conventionality of the metaphors used in the studies. The more conventional the metaphor, the less motor activation will be observed in the brain. This might be because, when we use a highly conventional metaphor, we go directly to the abstract meaning without resorting to the bodily based source domain.

In addition to the *career of metaphor hypothesis* (Bowdle & Gentner, 2005; see above for a discussion), a refinement of CMT recently proposed by Gerard Steen (2008, 2011), who introduced the distinction between deliberate and non-deliberate metaphors, can help us to make sense of contrasting results on the role of the sensorimotor system in the processing of bodily metaphors. It is outside the focus of this chapter to discuss deliberate metaphor theory (DMT) in detail. Only the main claim of DMT, which underlines the role of attention in the processing of metaphors, will be presented:

> The central prediction of DMT is about attention (Steen, 2011, 2013): a metaphor is used deliberately when its structure signals that the addressee has to move away their attention momentarily from the target domain of the utterance or even phrase to the source domain that is evoked by the metaphor-related expression. This hypothesis about attention to the source domain is highly specific: it focuses on the mandatory representation of the source domain as part of the situation model in utterance processing (Van Dijk and Kintsch, 1983).
>
> *(Steen 2015: 68)*

In Steen's (2015) view, only deliberate metaphors force us to pay attention to both the source and the target domain during processing. This does not happen when metaphors are not deliberately processed. Steen's (2015) proposal, in other words, highlights the role of attention in metaphor processing – that is, the way we focus our attention on the source and target domains during metaphor comprehension modulates the processing of metaphors. When we pay attention to both the source and the target domains of the metaphor, both will be activated and accessed during online processing, whereas when we just pay attention to the target domain of the metaphor, only a pre-stored meaning will be activated. A mapping will not take place in the latter case. However, following Steen (2015), non-deliberate metaphors can be revitalized by particular linguistic strategies or experimental procedures that can make them deliberately processed again.

Combining Steen's (2015) insights with the *career of metaphor hypothesis*, we can conclude that when we process novel metaphors, both the source and the target domains will be activated and accessed during online processing. Novel metaphors are processed deliberately. In contrast, when we process very familiar and conventional metaphors, only a pre-stored meaning will be activated. These latter metaphors are not processed deliberately; however, they can be revitalized by particular linguistic strategies or experimental procedures. It follows that metaphors can be processed in different ways. If we underestimate this aspect, it will be hard to explain contrasting results in experimental metaphor research.

Furthermore, and very interestingly, this is perfectly in line with data showing that novel metaphors, compared to conventional metaphors and to their literal counterparts, determine an additional inferential effort for a more robust integration of contextual information, reflected by stronger involvement of the right hemisphere.

A crucial problem in this debate is to better define the contribution *embodied simulation* makes to metaphorical meaning and, more generally, to linguistic meaning construction. Currently, this topic is highly debated by philosophers and neuroscientists, with different positions being considered (Shapiro, 2011). How does the body interact with symbols (lexical entries)? This and other issues will be addressed below.

Other forms of figurative meaning

Beyond metaphors, other forms of figurative language, such as irony and indirect speech acts, have been examined in neuroscientific research. Interestingly, the bilateral network implicated in metaphor processing also seems to be partly engaged in these cases. In an fMRI study, Spotorno et al. (2012) observed activations in the bilateral TPJ, precuneus, and mPFC during the comprehension of ironic sentences. Eighteen target sentences were presented, each embedded in two different contexts which made them either ironic or literal. The ironic > literal contrast showed greater activity in both the posterior and ventral parts of the mPFC, the bilateral IFG, the left insula, the bilateral TPJ, the right dorsolateral prefrontal cortex, and the right middle temporal gyrus, suggesting that the comprehension of ironic sentences, compared to their literal counterparts, requires a stronger involvement of the neural infrastructure that underlies our ability to understand other people's mental states. In another fMRI study, van Ackeren et al. (2012) reported the involvement of the ToM network, including the mPFC, the precuneus, and the bilateral TPJ during the comprehension of indirect speech acts – more specifically, indirect requests for action, where the request of an action (e.g., the request to close a window) was advanced, although it was never explicitly encoded in the sentence. Indirect requests for actions recruited motor areas, although no action verbs were mentioned in the sentences (see also Cuccio et al., 2014; Di Cesare et al., 2017; Egorova et al., 2013).

Summarizing, comprehension of metaphors and other forms of figurative language recruit a bilateral network with hubs implicated in executive functions (bilateral mPFC, right MFG, right ACC), attention (MFG), and most of all ToM (TPJ). More particularly, during metaphor processing, the bilateral activation of the IFG seem to underpin the integration of background encyclopedic knowledge with co-textual information. Below, we complement these anatomical findings with insights on relevant temporal dynamics.

The time course of figurative language processing

To understand both literal and figurative language, we need to manage different kinds of information. These include phonological/orthographic, syntactic, and semantic aspects as well as pragmatic information – that is, our encyclopedic background knowledge and our knowledge of other people's mental states. To understand how and when these different kinds of information intervene in the understanding of language, we need to clarify the temporal aspects of the process of language comprehension.

Despite copious attempts to unveil it (Shtyrov et al., 2013), the neural time course of the process of meaning construction is still largely unknown. Two alternative approaches in the debate are afforded by serial/cascaded and parallel processing models (Pulvermüller et al., 2009). Serial and cascaded models posit that different kinds of linguistic information (phonological/orthographic, syntactic, semantic, and pragmatic) are serially accessed whereas parallel models propose that these different pieces of information are simultaneously processed.

According to serial/cascaded models (e.g., Friederici, 2002, 2011), three sequential processing steps can be identified. These have been described thanks to electrophysiological evidence based on event-related potentials (ERP) studies. The early left anterior negativity component, which peaks between 100 and 250 ms after a lexico-syntactic violation, reflects lexico-syntactic processing. At this first stage, information about word categories should be accessed automatically to build a sentence structure. Subsequently, the N400 component, which peaks between 350 and 500 ms after a semantic incongruency, seems to reflect a later and not-automatic stage of semantic processing. The integration of contextual information for single lexical entries should take place here. Finally, the P600 component is considered to reflect a third stage of optional syntactic reanalysis that might occur to solve potential syntactic problems (Friederici, 2002, 2011; for a critical discussion, see Pulvermüller at al., 2009). Differing from the N400, which signals a semantic violation with regard to single words, the syntactic reanalysis reflected by the P600 component seems to suggest a global reanalysis of the structure of the sentence, elicited by pragmatic factors. In this view, the N400 component signals the need to integrate contextual factors in the processing of single words, whereas the P600 seems to reflect the necessity to reanalyse the syntactic structure of full sentences on the basis of the context.

On the contrary, according to parallel models, both in spoken and written language, different kinds of linguistic information (ranging from phonological/orthographic and syntactic to lexical, semantic, and pragmatic) are near-simultaneously accessed very early on, within 100–200 ms after stimulus onset. The recognition point is the earliest moment at which a word is recognized even though the related phonological information is not yet fully available (for a definition of recognition point and discussion of relevant empirical data, see Pulvermüller at al., 2009). As Pulvermüller et al. (2009) note, a growing number of neurophysiological studies firmly indicate that different kinds of linguistic information are early and near-simultaneously processed, within 100–200 ms from the moment when words/sentences are unambiguously identified. From this perspective, many parallel models suggest that later ERP components (e.g., N400 and P600) reflect post-comprehension processes.

For example, in an EEG experiment, Egorova et al. (2013) studied the neural time course of the comprehension of "naming" versus "requesting" (a pragmatic contrast between two kinds of speech acts). Participants were instructed to silently watch short videos displaying a linguistic interaction between two actors. The stimuli differed for two variables: the kind of speech act (naming and requesting) and semantics (hand-related objects and non-hand related objects). Coherently with parallel models, which predict the near-simultaneous processing of both semantic and pragmatic information, a significant main effect of pragmatics emerged between 110 and 130 ms post stimulus onset. That same time window exhibited a near-significant main effect of semantics, which became fully significant between 175 and 185 ms. No significant effects were observed for either factor after the 200 ms mark.

Beyond this evidence, the N400 and P600 effects have been widely replicated in thousands of experiments, which suggests that semantic/pragmatic and syntactic/pragmatic information might be accessed again at later stages of linguistic processing – for a review and discussion, see Pulvermüller at al. (2009). It is thus of paramount importance to deepen our comprehension of the relationship between early and the late psycholinguistic processes. It might be possible that they indicate diverse types of linguistic elaboration taking place at different stages. In other words, whereas proponents of parallel models usually consider late access to linguistic information as reflecting post-comprehension processes, it is here suggested that both early (near-simultaneous) and late processes underpin the understanding of language in functionally different ways. In fact, depending on co-text, context, and task demands, language comprehension might require a different cognitive load in terms of the inferential processes underpinning the construction of meaning. This might be evident especially in the case of new, and unexpected, figurative meanings, where a surplus of inferential processes likely leads to syntactic, semantic, and pragmatic reanalysis at later stages. Interestingly, and coherently with this hypothesis, results of an ERP study (Lai et al., 2009) showed that the amplitudes of the N400 ERP component elicited by the same target word at the end of an anomalous sentence, a novel metaphor, and a conventional metaphor did not differ compared with a literal sentence in an early window (320–440 ms). However, conventional metaphors and literal sentences did not differ in a later window (440–560 ms), whereas they both differed compared with novel metaphors and anomalous sentences. Novel metaphors and anomalous sentences elicited more negative amplitudes. This might suggest that they both required a surplus of inferential activity that determined greater cognitive load.

To clarify this point, I will resort to Evans (2006), who distinguished between lexical concepts and meaning. In Evans' view, lexical entries cannot be considered *per se* as the bearers of meaning:

> While lexical concepts constitute the semantic units conventionally associated with linguistic forms and form an integral part of a language user's individual mental grammar, meaning is a property of situated usage-events, rather than words. That is, meaning is not a function of language *per se*, but arises from language use.
>
> *(Evans, 2006: 491)*

In this account, linguistic meaning is much more than a lexical entry. It is always dependent on contextual factors and, most of all, on the different kinds of inferential processes, which range from quasi-immediate and spontaneous inferences to costly inferential processes that draw on creative resources. Different kinds of inferences are triggered by the demands posed by different tasks, situations, and linguistic expressions (Carapezza & Cuccio, 2018). Thus, inferences underlying language use can be classified according to criteria such as their degree of automaticity, the cognitive load they entail, and the kind of knowledge on which they rely (see Carapezza & Cuccio, 2018; Caruana & Cuccio, 2017; Recanati, 2004; Sperber & Wilson, 2002). For example, automatic, sub-personal[2] inferences take place at the level of language perception (when we identify certain sounds as sounds of a language) and rely on implicit and non-conceptual knowledge. There are also unconscious and automatic inferences, which are very fast, effortless, and very common in language use, and which take place at the personal level. These inferences rely on conceptual knowledge that is unconsciously used in the inferential process, although it can be consciously accessed *ex-post*. If you ask to a friend whether they want a piece of cake and they answer that they are on a diet, you will easily, unconsciously, and automatically, draw the inference that they will not eat the cake. This inference is not consciously drawn, but if someone asks you how you reached that conclusion, you will be able to recall and access your inferential steps. Finally, we also have conscious and non-automatic inferences that are slower and cognitively more demanding, and rely on a conscious and voluntarily controlled access to conceptual knowledge. We resort to this kind of inferences when the understanding of language is problematic and we need additional cognitive effort. This is the case, for example, when we need to comprehend a novel metaphor to which no fixed, conventional meaning is associated (we need to create that meaning *ex novo*) or when two equally plausible interpretations of an utterance are available, as is the case for jokes and irony. In this view, brain responses registered within 200 ms, via an elegant paradigm such as the one used by Egorova et al. (2013), might reflect a process of meaning construction underpinned by quasi-immediate and spontaneous inferences, whereas the N400 and P600 effects might reflect the implementation of more costly and time-consuming inferences. More complex stimuli and task demands will likely determine later access to, and reanalysis of, semantic and syntactic information.

This functional description of language processing, based on the distinction between lexical concepts and meaning, allows us to also discuss the role of *embodied simulation* in figurative meaning comprehension. Lexical entries, from Evans' (2006) perspective, are cues that prompt us to activate our background encyclopaedic knowledge. Both lexical entries and our background encyclopaedic knowledge are thus fundamental elements for the process that leads us to the construction of meaning. Whereas lexical concepts are purely linguistically encoded, our encyclopaedic knowledge includes different kinds of information: sensorimotor knowledge, emotions, and feelings. Simulation routines, which refer to instances of the activation of the mechanism of *embodied simulation*, are among the multi-modal knowledge structures constituting our encyclopaedic knowledge. In this view, simulation routines, being an integral part of our encyclopaedic knowledge, constitutively contribute to the contextually based process of meaning construction. However, this does not commit us to expect an automatic recruitment of simulation mechanisms during the processing of figurative meaning, since this recruitment depends on the linguistic expressions, as predicted by the *career of metaphor hypothesis* and the DMT, as well as on context and task demands.

Summarizing, early and late neurocognitive processes might indicate diverse types of inferential processes during language tasks. In this view, data on the neural time course of linguistic processing can be interpreted in the light of a semiotic distinction between lexical concepts and meaning (Evans, 2006). Within this semiotic framework, serial/cascaded and parallel models can be considered as not mutually exclusive. Furthermore, within this framework, the mechanism of *embodied simulation* also plays a key role in the process of meaning construction, although we are not committed to automatic embodied reactivations when we process metaphors.

Conclusion

In this chapter, the neural correlates and the time course of the processing of figurative language have been presented and discussed in the light of a semiotic account of the process of meaning construction and within the framework of current approaches to metaphorical thinking (CMT, DMT, and the *career of metaphor hypothesis*). We have proposed a neurosemiotic account of language, based on the distinction between lexical concepts and meaning (Evans, 2006), and enriched by a fine-grained typology of the kinds of inferences underlying language comprehension (Carapezza & Cuccio, 2018). This account allows us to reconcile data on the serial/cascaded and parallel models of language processing. Indeed, from this perspective, meaning – differently from lexical concepts – is always the result of a contextually based process, which implies inferences. The latter differ regarding their degree of automaticity, the cognitive load they entail, and the kind of knowledge on which they rely. Different kinds of inferences are triggered by factors such the contextual situation or the semantic features of linguistic expressions. Thus, it has been proposed that early brain responses registered within 200 ms might reflect the processing of linguistic expressions, which entail quasi-immediate and spontaneous inferences, whereas the N400 and P600 effects might reflect the processing of more complex linguistic expressions, which need more costly inferences.

The neurosemiotic account of language presented here, based on the distinction between lexical concepts and meaning (Evans, 2006), also allowed us to deepen our understanding of the role of *embodied simulation* in figurative meaning. *Embodied simulation* is an integral part of our background encyclopaedic knowledge which contributes to the construction of meaning. However, since this semiotic process is contextually based, an automatic recruitment of the mechanism of simulation during the processing of figurative meaning is not predicted, in accordance with theoretical model such as the *career of metaphor hypothesis* or DMT.

Concluding, figurative language is certainly a crucial topic for neurosemiotics, since it makes evident that language is not a code. The "code" perspective does not really explain the mechanisms underlying the construction of meaning and their neural correlates. On the other hand, and complementary, a neurosemiotic perspective is crucial to deepen our understanding of figurative language since this process will greatly benefit from a more general comprehension of the human ability to communicate through signs.

The study of the neural correlates, time course, and embodied nature of figurative uses of language gives us important insights on the brain mechanisms of meaning making as well as on the areas supporting these functional mechanisms. Most of all, the study of the biological bases of metaphor processing makes evident that the recruitment of brain areas and functional mechanisms involved in meaning-making is crucially dependent on contextually situated usage events. A pragmatic view of language thus seems to be central for any neurosemiotic account of our ability to make meaning and use signs. All in all, highlighting the importance of a pragmatic approach in neurosemiotic research is one of the main contributions coming from the study of the biological bases of figurative language.

Notes

1 In the meta-analysis by Bohrn et al. (2012), the novel metaphors > literal contrast showed activations only in the left hemisphere – for a discussion, see Lai et al. (2015).

2 According to Dennett (1969), personal-level phenomena are those mental processes that characterize our lives as subjects while sub-personal phenomena are physical processes that we can describe in mechanical terms.

References

Austin, J. L., & Urmson, J. O. (1962). *How to Do Things with Words*. Oxford: Clarendon Press.

Aziz-Zadeh, L., Wilson, S. M., Rizzolatti, G., & Iacoboni, M. (2006). Congruent embodied representations for visually presented actions and linguistic phrases describing actions. *Current Biology: CB*, *16*(18), 1818–1823. doi: 10.1016/j.cub.2006.07.060

Bambini, V. (2017). *Il cervello pragmatico*. Roma: Carocci.

Bambini, V., Gentili, C., Ricciardi, E., Bertinetto, P. M., & Pietrini, P. (2011). Decomposing metaphor processing at the cognitive and neural level through functional magnetic resonance imaging. *Brain Research Bulletin*, *86*(3–4), 203–216. doi: 10.1016/j.brainresbull.2011.07.015

Bohrn, I. C., Altmann, U., & Jacobs, A. M. (2012). Looking at the brains behind figurative language: A quantitative meta-analysis of neuroimaging studies on metaphor, idiom, and irony processing. *Neuropsychologia*, *50*(11), 2669–2683. doi: 10.1016/j.neuropsychologia.2012.07.021

Boulenger, V., Hauk, O., & Pulvermüller, F. (2009). Grasping ideas with the motor system: Semantic somatotopy in idiom comprehension. *Cerebral Cortex*, *19*(8), 1905–1914. doi: 10.1093/cercor/bhn217

Boulenger, V., Shtyrov, Y., & Pulvermüller, F. (2012). When do you grasp the idea? MEG evidence for instantaneous idiom understanding. *NeuroImage*, *59*(4), 3502–3513. doi: 10.1016/j.neuroimage.2011.11.011

Bowdle, B. F., & Gentner, D. (2005). The career of metaphor. *Psychological Review*, *112*(1), 193–216. doi: 10.1037/0033-295X.112.1.193

Buccino, G., Riggio, L., Melli, G., Binkofski, F., Gallese, V., & Rizzolatti, G. (2005). Listening to action-related sentences modulates the activity of the motor system: A combined TMS and behavioral study. *Cognitive Brain Research*, *24*(3), 355–363. doi: 10.1016/j.cogbrainres.2005.02.020

Cacciari, C., Bolognini, N., Senna, I., Pellicciari, M. C., Miniussi, C., & Papagno, C. (2011). Literal, fictive and metaphorical motion sentences preserve the motion component of the verb: A TMS study. *Brain & Language*, *119*(3), 149–157. doi: 10.1016/j.bandl.2011.05.004

Carapezza, M., & Cuccio V. (2018). Abductive inferences in pragmatic processes. In A. Capone, M. Carapezza, & F. Lo Piparo (Eds.), *Further Advances in Pragmatics and Philosophy. Part 1: From Theory to Practice* (pp. 221–242). New York: Springer.

Cardillo, E. R., McQuire, M., & Chatterjee, A. (2018). Selective metaphor impairments after left, not right, hemisphere injury. *Frontiers in Psychology*, *9*, 2308. doi: 10.3389/fpsyg.2018.02308

Carroll, L. (1872). *Through the Looking Glass and What Alice Found There*. Philadelphia, PA: Henry Altemus.
Caruana, F., & Cuccio, V. (2017). Types of abduction in tool behaviour. *Phenomenology and the Cognitive Sciences, 16*(2), 255–273. doi: 10.1007/s11097-015-9450-y
Cuccio, V. (2015). Embodied simulation and metaphors. On the role of the body in the interpretation of bodily-based metaphors. *Epistemologia, 1*, 99–113. doi: 10.3280/EPIS2015-001007
Cuccio, V. (2017). Body-schema and body-image in metaphor processing. In B. Hampe (Ed.), *Metaphor: From Embodied Cognition to Discourse* (pp. 82–98). Cambridge: Cambridge University Press.
Cuccio, V. (2018). *Attention to Metaphor. From Neurons to Representations*. Amsterdam: John Benjamins.
Cuccio, V., Ambrosecchia, M., Ferri, F., Carapezza, M., Lo Piparo, F., Fogassi, L., & Gallese, V. (2014). How the context matters: Literal and figurative meaning in the embodied language paradigm. *PLoS One, 9*(12), e115381. doi: 10.1371/journal.pone.0115381
Cuccio, V., & Caruana, F. (2019). Rethinking the abstract/concrete concepts dichotomy. Comment on "Words as social tools: Language, sociality and inner grounding in abstract concepts" by Anna M. Borghi et al. *Physics of Life Reviews, 29*, 157–160. doi: 10.1016/j.plrev.2019.04.007
Cuccio, V., & Gallese, V. (2018). A Peircean account of concepts: Grounding abstraction in phylogeny through a comparative neuroscientific perspective. *Philosophical Transactions of the Royal Society of London. Series B, Biological Sciences, 373*(1752), 20170128. doi: 10.1098/rstb.2017.0128
Dennett, D. C. (1969). *Content and Consciousness*. London: Routledge & Kegan Paul.
Desai, R. H., Binder, J. R., Conant, L. L., Mano, Q. R., & Seidenberg, M. S. (2011). The neural career of sensory-motor metaphors. *Journal of Cognitive Neuroscience, 23*(9), 2376–2386. doi: 10.1162/jocn.2010.21596
Desai, R. H., Conant, L. L., Binder, J. R., Park, H., & Seidenberg, M. S. (2013). A piece of the action: Modulation of sensory-motor regions by action idioms and metaphors. *NeuroImage, 83*, 862–869. doi: 10.1016/j.neuroimage.2013.07.044
Deuse, L., Rademacher, L. M., Winkler, L., Schultz, R. T., Gründer, G., & Lammertz, S. E. (2016). Neural correlates of naturalistic social cognition: Brain–behavior relationships in healthy adults. *Social Cognitive and Affective Neuroscience, 11*(11), 1741–1751. doi: 10.1093/scan/nsw094
Di Cesare, G., Errante, A., Marchi, M., & Cuccio, V. (2017). Language for action: Motor resonance during the processing of human and robotic voices. *Brain and Cognition, 118*, 118–127. doi: 10.1016/j.bandc.2017.08.001
Egorova, N., Shtyrov, Y., & Pulvermüller, F. (2013). Early and parallel processing of pragmatic and semantic information in speech acts: Neurophysiological evidence. *Frontiers in Human Neuroscience*, 7, 86. doi: 10.3389/fnhum.2013.00086
Evans, V., & Green, M. J. (2006). *Cognitive Linguistics: An Introduction*. Edinburgh: Edinburgh University Press.
Ferstl, E.C. (2010). The neuroanatomy of discourse comprehension: Where are we now? *Italian Journal of Linguistics, 22*(1), 61–88.
Fodor, J. A. (1975). *Language of Thought*. Cambridge, MA: Harvard University Press.
Fodor, J. A. (1983). *The Modularity of Mind*. Cambridge, MA: MIT Press.
Friederici, A. D. (2002). Towards a neural basis of auditory sentence processing. *Trends in Cognitive Sciences, 6*(2), 78–84. doi: 10.1016/s1364-6613(00)01839-8
Friederici, A. D. (2011). The brain basis of language processing: From structure to function. *Physiological Reviews, 91*(4), 1357–1392. doi: 10.1152/physrev.00006.2011
Gallese, V., & Cuccio, V. (2018). The neural exploitation hypothesis and its implications for an embodied approach to language and cognition: Insights from the study of action verbs processing and motor disorders in Parkinson's disease. *Cortex, 100*, 215–225. doi: 10.1016/j.cortex.2018.01.010
Gallese, V., & Sinigaglia, C. (2011). What is so special about embodied simulation? *Trends in Cognitive Sciences, 15*(11), 512–519. doi: 10.1016/j.tics.2011.09.003
Gibbs, R. W. (1999). *Intentions in the Experience of Meaning*. Cambridge: Cambridge University Press.
Gibbs, R. W. (2003). Embodied experience and linguistic meaning. *Brain Language, 84*(1), 1–15. doi: 10.1016/s0093-934x(02)00517-5
Gibbs, R. W. (2005). *Embodiment and Cognitive Science*. Cambridge: Cambridge University Press.
Gibbs, R. W. (2006). Metaphor interpretation as embodied simulation. *Mind and Language, 21*(3), 434–458. doi: 10.1111/j.1468-0017.2006.00285.x
Gibbs, R. W., & Perlman, M. (2010). Language understanding is grounded in experiential simulations: A response to Weiskopf. Studies in History and *Philosophy of Science, 41*(3), 305–308. doi: 10.1016/j.shpsa.2010.07.004
Glenberg, A. M., & Kaschak, M. P. (2002). Grounding language in action. *Psychonomic Bulletin & Review, 9*(3), 558–565. doi: 10.3758/bf03196313
Glenberg, A. M., Sato, M., Cattaneo, L., Riggio, L., Palumbo, D., & Buccino, G. (2008). Processing abstract language modulates motor system activity. *Quarterly Journal of Experimental Psychology, 61*(6), 905–919. doi: 10.1080/17470210701625550
Grice, H. P. (1957). Meaning. *Philosophical Review, 66*(3), 377–388.

Grice, H. P. (1989). *Studies in the Way of Words*. Cambridge, MA: Harvard University Press.

Hagoort, P., & Levinson, S. C. (2014). Neuropragmatics. In M. S. Gazzaniga, & G. R. Mangun (Eds.), *The Cognitive Neurosciences* (5th ed., pp. 667–674). Cambridge, MA: MIT Press.

Hartung, F., Kenett, Y. N., Cardillo, E. R., Humphries, S., Klooster, N., & Chatterjee, A. (2020). Context matters: Novel metaphors in supportive and non-supportive contexts. *NeuroImage, 212*, Article 116645. doi: 10.1016/j.neuroimage.2020.116645

Hauk, O., Johnsrude, I., & Pulvermüller, F. (2004). Somatotopic representation of action words in human motor and premotor cortex. *Neuron, 41*(2), 301–307. doi: 10.1016/s0896-6273(03)00838-9

Kemmerer, D., Castillo, J. G., Talavage, T., Patterson, S., & Wiley, C. (2008). Neuroanatomical distribution of five semantic components of verbs: Evidence from fMRI. *Brain and Language, 107*(1), 16–43. doi: 10.1016/j.bandl.2007.09.003

Klostermann, F., Krugel, L. K., & Ehlen, F. (2013). Functional roles of the thalamus for language capacities. *Frontiers in Systems Neuroscience*, 7, 1–8. doi: 10.3389/fnsys.2013.00032

Kovecses, Z. (2008). Conceptual metaphor theory: Some criticisms and alternative proposals. *Annual Review of Cognitive Linguistics, 6*, 168–184. doi: 10.1075/arcl.6.08kov

Lai, V. T., Curran, T., & Menn, L. (2009). Comprehending conventional and novel metaphors: An ERP study. *Brain Research,* 1284*,* 145–155. doi: 10.1016/j.brainres.2009.05.088

Lai, V. T., van Dam, W., Conant, L. L., Binder, J. R., & Desai, R. H. (2015). Familiarity differentially affects right hemisphere contributions to processing metaphors and literals. *Frontiers in Human Neuroscience, 9*, 44. doi: 10.3389/fnhum.2015.00044

Lakoff, G., & Johnson, M. (1980). *Metaphors We Live By*. Chicago: University of Chicago Press.

Matlock, T., Ramscar, M., & Boroditsky, L. (2005). On the experiential link between spatial and temporal language. *Cognitive Science, 29*(4), 655–664. doi: 10.1207/s15516709cog0000_17

Pulvermüller, F. (2018). Neural reuse of action perception circuits for language, concepts and communication. *Progress in Neurobiology, 160*, 1–44. doi: 10.1016/j.pneurobio.2017.07.001

Pulvermüller, F., Shtyrov, Y., & Hauk, O. (2009). Understanding in an instant: Neurophysiological evidence for mechanistic language circuits in the brain. *Brain & Language, 110*(2), 81–94. doi: 10.1016/j.bandl.2008.12.001

Raposo, A., Moss, H. E., Stamatakis, E. A., & Tyler, L. K. (2009). Modulation of motor and premotor cortices by actions, action words and action sentences. *Neuropsychologia, 47*(2), 388–396. doi: 10.1016/j.neuropsychologia.2008.09.017

Rapp, A. M., Mutschler, D. E., & Erb, M. (2012). Where in the brain is nonliteral language? A coordinate-based meta-analysis of functional magnetic resonance imaging studies. *NeuroImage, 63*(1), 600–610. doi: 10.1016/j.neuroimage.2012.06.022

Recanati, F. (2004). *Literal Meaning*. Cambridge: Cambridge University Press.

Sato, M., Mengarelli, M., Riggio, L., Gallese, V., & Buccino, G. (2008). Task related modulation of the motor system during language processing. *Brain & Language, 105*(2), 83–90. doi: 10.1016/j.bandl.2007.10.001

Schurz, M., & Perner, J. (2015). An evaluation of neurocognitive models of theory of mind. *Frontiers in Psychology, 6*, 1610. doi: 10.3389/fpsyg.2015.01610

Searle, J. R. (1969). *Speech Acts: An Essay in the Philosophy of Language*. Cambridge: Cambridge University Press.

Seghier, M. L. (2013). The angular gyrus: Multiple functions and multiple subdivisions. *The Neuroscientist: A Review Journal Bringing Neurobiology, Neurology and Psychiatry, 19*(1), 43–61. doi: 10.1177/1073858412440596

Shapiro, L. A. (2011). *Embodied Cognition*. London: Routledge.

Shtyrov, Y., Goryainova, G., Tugin, S., Ossadtchi, A., & Shestakova, A. (2013). Automatic processing of unattended lexical information in visual oddball presentation: Neurophysiological evidence. *Frontiers in Human Neuroscience*, 7, 421. doi: 10.3389/fnhum.2013.00421

Sperber, D., & Wilson, D. (2002). Pragmatics, modularity and mind-reading. *Mind & Language, 17*, 3–23. doi: 10.1111/1468-0017.00186

Spotorno, N., Koun, E., Prado, J., Van Der Henst, J. B., & Noveck, I. A. (2012). Neural evidence that utterance-processing entails mentalizing: The case of irony. *NeuroImage, 63*(1), 25–39. doi: 10.1016/j.neuroimage.2012.06.046

Steen, G. J. (2008). The paradox of metaphor: Why we need a three-dimensional model for metaphor. *Metaphor & Symbol, 23*(4), 213–241. doi: 10.1080/10926480802426753

Steen, G. J. (2011). The contemporary theory of metaphor–now new and improved! *Review of Cognitive Linguistics, 9*(1), 26–64. doi: 10.1075/rcl.9.1.03ste

Steen, G. J. (2013). Deliberate metaphor affords conscious metaphorical cognition. *Journal of Cognitive Semiotics, 5* (1–2), 179–197. doi: 10.1515/cogsem.2013.5.12.179

Steen, G. J. (2015). Developing, testing and interpreting deliberate metaphor theory. *Journal of Pragmatics, 90*, 67–72. doi: 10.1016/j.pragma.2015.03.013

Tettamanti, M., Buccino, G., Saccuman, M. C., Gallese, V., Danna, M., Scifo, P., Fazio, F., Rizzolatti, G., Cappa, S. F., & Perani, D. (2005). Listening to action-related sentences activates fronto-parietal motor circuits. *Journal of Cognitive Neuroscience*, *17*(2), 273–281. doi: 10.1162/0898929053124965

van Ackeren, M. J., Casasanto, D., Bekkering, H., Hagoort, P., & Rueschemeyer, S. A. (2012). Pragmatics in action: Indirect requests engage theory of mind areas and the cortical motor network. *Journal of Cognitive Neuroscience*, *24*(11), 2237–2247. doi: 10.1162/jocn_a_00274

Van Dijk, T. A., & Kintsch, W. (1983). *Strategies of Discourse Comprehension*. New York: Academic Press.

Winner, E., & Gardner, H. (1977). The comprehension of metaphor in brain-damaged patients. *Brain*, *100*(4), 717–729. doi: 10.1093/brain/100.4.717

Yang, J. (2014). The role of the right hemisphere in metaphor comprehension: A meta-analysis of functional magnetic resonance imaging studies. *Human Brain Mapping*, *35*(1), 107–122. doi: 10.1002/hbm.22160

Yang, J., & Shu, H. (2016). Involvement of the motor system in comprehension of non-literal action language: A meta-analysis study. *Brain Topography*, *29*(1), 94–107. doi: 10.1007/s10548-015-0427-5

9

PHARMACOLOGICAL MODULATION OF MEANING ATTRIBUTION

Enzo Tagliazucchi

Introduction

The problem of meaning and its attribution has occupied philosophers, linguists, and scientists for centuries. As in the case of other major outstanding problems – for example, consciousness – the concept of meaning admits multiple interpretations depending on the field of academic inquiry. Philosophers, for example, are concerned with the general relationship between signs and the things they express or signify from different perspectives – such as logical consistency, social constructivism, consensus, and pragmatism, among others (Speaks, 2010). Linguists are concerned with semantics, understood, among other things, as the attribution of meaning depending on syntactic properties and statistical co-occurrence (Steinberg & Jakobovits, 1971). Finally, psychologists and neuroscientists investigate language as a cognitive capacity of human beings, addressing the neural underpinnings of language production and comprehension, and looking at how these biological substrates shape the attribution of meaning to signs and symbols (Croft & Cruse, 2004).

While these different approaches clearly intersect, a coherent and unified account of meaning and its attribution has yet to emerge. An important step forward in this direction is the advancement of neurosemiotics, understood as the neuroscientific investigation of communication, including "the perception of the environment as meaningful, both globally and discretely, and the general capacity to engage in symbolic interactions" (Bouissac, 1987: 204). Neurosemiotics transcends the narrow limitations of formal linguistic approaches towards language and meaning, seeking to bridge the divide between the social and biological processes underlying human communication. This field is concerned with the symbolization and subsequent interpretation of incoming sensory signals, the neural implementation of the landmark features of human language that support its extraordinary expressive power and flexibility, and the detection of personally or socially meaningful stimuli with the subsequent attribution of meaning (Bouissac, 1985).

The field of neurosemiotics benefits from the spectacular methodological advances available to cognitive neuroscience, such as whole-brain imaging and tools for indirect brain stimulation. While these methods have contributed enormously to our understanding of brain structure and function, their non-invasive nature favors insights at the network level, which are difficult to interpret in terms of processes at the molecular and cellular scales. In particular, attempts to investigate meaning attribution at these scales are severely underrepresented in the current literature. In this chapter, we focus on the application of pharmacological stimulation to the field of neurosemiotics, and more

DOI: 10.4324/9781003051817-12

precisely to the question of how different endogenous neurotransmitter systems modulate the process of meaning attribution in the brain. A major advantage of pharmacological studies is the selective activation or inhibition of specific neurochemical pathways by means of drugs with known agonism or antagonism at the corresponding binding sites, respectively. Insofar as the explored compounds have an acceptable safety profile and their acute effects spare core cognitive capacities, they can be combined with experimental paradigms from cognitive neuroscience as well as with neuroimaging methods, with the purpose of understanding the downstream systems-level changes modulating the attribution of meaning (Dawson et al., 1992). A downside of this approach is that neurotransmitter systems are hardly involved in specific functions; therefore, the conclusions available from pharmacological studies tend to be highly non-specific (as indeed are most of the studies discussed in the present chapter).

This chapter is structured as follows. We first present a short overview of the current neuroscientific knowledge of meaning attribution as a two-stage process based on the detection of potentially meaningful stimuli (perceptual salience) and their subsequent incorporation to the social or personal network of semantic concepts. We then describe the available evidence suggesting that these different stages are modulated by dopaminergic and serotonergic transmission, respectively. This discussion leads to an interpretation of certain psychiatric symptoms as deficits in the attribution of meaning. Finally, we discuss how these findings might impact future developments in clinical psychology and psychiatry, both in terms of modeling certain psychotic episodes and for the development of therapeutic options for mood and substance abuse disorders.

Two dimensions of meaning in the brain

As a starting point, we consider that the attribution of meaning by living organisms can be understood from a purely neuroscientific perspective, in the same way as the attribution of meaning by personal computers (or other artificial devices) can be understood from a purely engineering perspective (Dennett, 1987). As in the case of computers, the attribution of meaning by human beings is context-dependent. Humans and other animals navigate a world of highly complex sensory stimuli, of which only a small subset contains information that is meaningful for survival. Perceptual salience refers to the prioritization of sensory information based on the comparison with contextual information – that is, a bias that predisposes subjects to focus their attention on items that are more relevant to them, even if this relevance cannot be captured using objective standards (Cunningham & Turk, 2017). We consider that this juxtaposition between figure and ground represents a first instance where meaning is attributed by living organisms; in turn, discussions of what constitutes figure and what constitutes ground (equivalently, signal, and noise) only make sense in the light of what is relevant to the organism, which ultimately stems from the constraints of natural selection. At this stage, our use of the word "meaning" should not be understood in terms of semantic relationships, but in the sense of significance or relevance, as in the sentence "Animals perceive what is meaningful for their survival."

The construction of meaning in language is related to a delayed form of comparison between percepts or concepts and their contexts. Consider the distributional hypothesis of semantics (Sahlgren, 2008), stating that the similarity between the meaning of two words is related to their statistical co-occurrence in similar linguistic contexts – or, as expressed by Wittgenstein (1953: 49), "the meaning of a word is its use in the language." In other words, according to this view, our attribution of meaning is related to our judgment of concepts in relation to their contexts, which in turn depends on our own past experiences. If we were to ask New Yorkers to construct a semantic map of nouns, we could expect that the word "yellow" would be much closer to "taxi" than "red" or "green"; however, this semantic association would surprise Londoners, for whom taxis are most frequently black. Our use of meaning in this context is understood as what is intended to be (or actually is) expressed by a certain linguistic item.

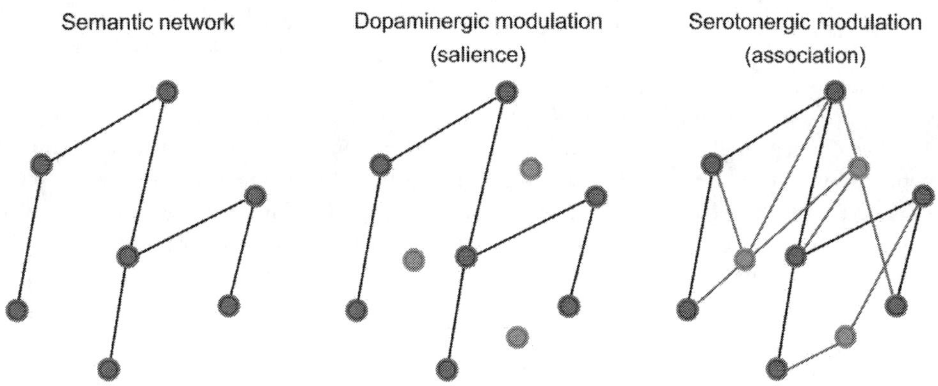

Figure 9.1 Perceptual salience and semantic association

Perceptual salience and semantic association are hypothesized to be modulated by dopaminergic and serotonergic signaling, respectively. Each circle represents a concept in a semantic network, with links between circles indicating similar meaning of the associated concepts. Perceptual salience endows the individual with the capacity to consistently identify novel (apparently) meaningful information in sensory data (red circles), while the relationship of this information with previously available concepts (red lines) is mediated by a process of semantic association. If these processes were modulated by different neurobiological mechanisms and thus could be dissociated, we would expect the possibility of heightened salience to certain percepts that are not embedded within the semantic network (as in the middle panel). See e-book for a full-color version of this figure.

Another way of framing this distinction is in terms of "meaning as salience" vs. "meaning as connectedness." The first case is concerned with perception, identification, and isolation of relevant information from noisy or otherwise uninteresting contexts, and thus depends directly on the *Umwelt* of the organism as shaped by evolution (Von Uexküll, 1921) – that is, the semiotic world of the organism, including all meaningful aspects for its survival and reproduction (Treisman & Gelade, 1980). The second case extends to semantic connections between concepts, equipping humans with symbols to grasp and manipulate information beyond their immediate physical surroundings (see Figure 9.1 for a schematic illustration of both definitions).

From a linguistic point of view, the distinction between salience and semantics may seem unwarranted. It could be the case that our detection of relevant information in the environment depends on how this information is embedded in our personal semantic network. From a neuroscientific stance, however, this distinction would be justified if these two forms of meaning attribution were mediated by different neurobiological mechanisms. In this case, we could expect dissociations to emerge in certain conditions or as a consequence of specific external manipulations – for example, in patients with psychiatric or neurological disorders. In these cases, we could see instances of individuals detecting meaningful information in their environments, without being capable of identifying the semantic content of this information – that is, of connecting it with other well-established concepts. In the following, we review evidence suggesting that this dissociation can indeed occur, and that it depends on signaling by dopamine and serotonin, two neurotransmitters with largely independent (and potentially competing) sets of functions.

Dopaminergic modulation of salience

The detection of salient stimuli is a fundamental first step in the process of meaning attribution. While not necessarily sufficient by itself, perceptual salience is a first filter through which stimuli must pass to be considered meaningful and thus subsequently embedded within a network of semantic associations. Consider, for example, an array of pixels (such as those in a TV screen) undergoing completely random fluctuations. This configuration maximizes the transmission of mathematical information in the sense given by Claude Shannon, but each configuration fails to represent an individual salient or memorable stimulus (Shannon, 1948). As we increase the degree of correlation between the random fluctuations of each pair of pixels, order starts to emerge in the array. Only at an intermediate stage between order (correlations so high that all pixels switch on/off at the same time) and disorder (the initial state of purely random fluctuations) is it possible for humans to recognize an interesting configuration of the system. The main reason is that the statistics of the natural world are typical of visual stimuli at the edge between order and chaos (Zoran & Weiss, 2009). However, even that state will be seen as a sequence of meaningless configurations unless a salient image appears, representing information that is relevant to the receiver when contrasted with its surrounding context (e.g., animals, plants, faces, geometric figures).[1]

Dopamine is an endogenous neurotransmitter that has been implicated in multiple brain functions, from motor execution to learning by reward signals – that is, reinforcement learning (Iversen & Iversen, 2007). One of the most investigated aspects of dopaminergic signaling is its possible role in determining the perceptual salience of incoming stimuli. Activity at midbrain dopaminergic neurons of the ventral tegmental area and substantia nigra pars compacta is related to the processing of salient sensory stimuli, as measured using microdialysis over a timescale of minutes (Heinz et al., 1999). fMRI studies reveal that novel salient stimuli increase activity in the dopaminergic midbrain, even for aversive stimuli (Knolle et al., 2018). These findings have been supported by optogenetic studies with direct stimulation of dopaminergic cells in the dorsal raphe nucleus (Cho et al., 2017). Similar results exist for emotional salience, with activations encompassing the amygdala as well as midbrain structures (Phan et al., 2003). Thus, the attribution of significance to stimuli implicates dopaminergic signaling, especially in those cases relevant for behavioral switching (Shiner et al., 2015). This dopaminergic modulation of perceptual salience can occur regardless of reward anticipation, even though it has been suggested that the novelty of perceptually salient stimuli is by itself rewarding (Berridge & Robinson, 1998).

From these studies, it could be expected that pharmacological blocking or stimulation of dopaminergic circuits modifies behavior in a way consistent with decreased or increased capacity for salience attribution, respectively. This hypothesis has received confirmation from studies using dopamine precursors, reuptake inhibitors, agonists, and antagonists. Levodopa (l-3,4-dihydroxyphenylalanine) is an amino acid that is a precursor to the neurotransmitter dopamine (among others). As such, it is used to treat patients suffering from Parkinson's disease, a neurodegenerative disease affecting dopaminergic motor neurons (Nutl & Fellman, 1984). Thus, levodopa can be used to induce transient increases in the concentration and availability of dopamine in the central nervous system, and thus to investigate the relationship between dopaminergic signaling and cognitive function, including salience attribution. Following this method, Shiner et al. (2015) demonstrated that levodopa facilitated the response to set shifting by increasing the salience of perceptual cues, with increased activity in the ventromedial prefrontal cortex being associated with this effect. Another study established that levodopa increased explicit new word learning, presumably by increasing their semantic salience (Shellshear et al., 2015). Finally, treatment with levodopa can induce some symptoms characteristic of psychoses (Celesia & Barr, 1970), indirectly establishing a link with enhanced dopaminergic transmission and aberrant salience (see below).

Many popular drugs of abuse act by inhibiting the reuptake of dopamine (e.g., cocaine) or by directly activating dopamine receptors (e.g., amphetamine, methamphetamine). In both cases, there is indirect evidence suggesting a modulation of perceptual salience. Lifetime cocaine addiction is linked to functional and structural abnormalities in the salience network (bilateral insula and dorsal anterior cingulate cortex), which can be used to successfully predict relapse (Geng et al., 2017). Another study reported alterations in the functional interaction between the salience and default mode networks in patients with a history of cocaine addiction (Liang et al., 2015); this was replicated in another study on dopamine depletion (Shafiei et al., 2019). Finally, certain drugs linked to dopaminergic function are frequently used as nootropics – that is, drugs aimed to improve cognitive function, including memory, attention, executive function, and motivation. Modafinil, for instance, has been shown to enhance incentive (but not perceptual) salience – in other words, the attribution of a motivational component to a rewarding stimulus (Soskin et al., 2013).

The opposite effect can be elicited by administering dopamine antagonists – drugs that inhibit the activation of dopamine receptors by the neurotransmitter itself. As will be discussed below, some dopamine antagonists (known as antipsychotics) are used to manage psychotic episodes. Several antipsychotic drugs (clozapine, chlorpromazine, risperidone) have been shown to reduce emotional hyperthermia (a biological marker of perceptual salience in rats) in a dose-dependent way (Blessing et al., 2017). As opposed to dopamine agonists and reuptake inhibitors, antipsychotics enhance the functional coupling between the salience and default mode networks (Wang et al., 2017).

The effects of dopaminergic drugs on perceptual salience can be illustrated by anecdotal first-person reports, such as those found in Erowid's experience vaults.[2] For instance, individuals typically exaggerate the salience of small marks in irregular surfaces (such as their own skin), perceiving them as small insects of unspecified kind ("I was seeing bugs everywhere. Thousands of them, around every corner, on every surface – every object morphed into some sort of malicious insects;" "Back in the main room, the knots in the ceiling had turned into beetles and were running all around"). This misperception also affects the auditory sensory modality, with random noises being identified as highly relevant stimuli, such as the individual's own name ("About 45 minutes after taking the extreme dosage I began to have audio hallucinations. Like someone was calling my name, and words just seemed to come out of the air"). At higher doses, users may wrongly infer the presence of other humans or living entities from their surroundings ("I stayed up … screaming at three entities who I could undeniably and clearly see right in front of me").

Perhaps the most compelling argument for an involvement of the dopaminergic system in the process of salience attribution stems from the neurobiology and phenomenology of certain psychiatric conditions resulting in psychotic episodes, such as schizophrenia. A vast literature implicates excessive dopaminergic activation with the emergence of psychotic or psychotic-like episodes (Guillin et al., 2007); this evidence includes the risk of accidentally inducing psychotic episodes by drugs that increase dopaminergic activation (e.g., levodopa, amphetamine, cocaine) (Lieberman et al., 1990), the reduction of psychotic symptoms in patients by drugs that deplete dopamine levels (e.g., reserpine) (Nur & Adams, 2016), the blockage of dopamine D_2 receptors by all currently licensed antipsychotic drugs, the relationship between efficient doses of antipsychotic medications and the affinity for D_2 receptors (Gardner et al., 2005), the post-mortem measurement of heightened dopamine levels in the brains of schizophrenic patients, and the observation of increased plasma and cerebrospinal fluid dopamine metabolite levels in some patients with schizophrenia (Mackay et al., 1982). Positron emission tomography (PET) studies using radiolabeled levodopa have established elevated synthesis of dopamine in schizophrenic patients in vivo (Kumakura et al., 2007). These results are complemented by neuroimaging studies showing abnormal responses of the salience network in patients suffering from schizophrenia (Huang et al., 2019; Palaniyappan et al., 2012; White et al., 2013).

It has been proposed that, as a consequence of genetic predispositions interacting with environmental triggers, the dopaminergic system becomes dysregulated and thus increases dopamine concentration regardless of adaptive cues. In turn, due to the resulting abnormal attribution of salience, endogenously triggered by the aforementioned processes, the patients suffer delusions and hallucinations, including fixed and false beliefs and aberrant perception (Winton-Brown et al., 2014). These symptoms can be understood as the consequence of abnormally high perceptual salience, where everything is imbued with a sense of hidden meaning and novelty, including information that otherwise would be discarded as insignificant or meaningless ("My senses were sharpened. I became fascinated by the little insignificant things around me"; "Sights and sounds possessed a keenness that he had never experienced before"; "I noticed things I had never noticed before"; "Everything is getting a new meaning") (Kapur et al., 2005). Prior to the psychotic episode itself, patients may find themselves in a prodromal stage characterized by an altered sense of meaning and/or significance ("delusional mood") (Kapur et al., 2005) – but in the absence of full-blown delusions of hallucinations, which may eventually appear as the episode progresses. For instance, when facing the noise present in the static of a TV screen, aberrant processing of perceptual salience could lead to the detection of a signal whose content would depend on the expectations of the patient, thus triggering a delusory belief and/or a perceptual hallucination.

Serotonergic modulation of meaning attribution

Sufficiently salient stimuli can be embedded in the network of semantic relationships encoded in human language; this process is not necessarily sequential, as perceptual salience can be aided by temporarily placing the stimulus within this network (Fellbaum, 1998). New concepts can be represented by symbols or combinations of symbols, or by compositions of words with adequate semantic content – for example, the German noun *Kühlschrank* for "fridge": *Kuhl* (cool) + *Schrank* (closet, cupboard). In the same way that the process of salience attribution relies on contrasting a stimulus against its immediate context, humans ultimately attribute meaning by contrasting a new concept with previous knowledge, placing it within a semantic space.

Hyper-associativity refers to an exaggerated capacity to identify semantic relationships between concepts, leading to spurious semantic associations. Ultimately, hyper-associativity can be detrimental to human communication, leading to a form of expression characterized by sudden jumps in the content of speech and hindering the capacity to process and understand the discourse. The reader might be familiar with hyper-associativity from their episodes of rapid eye movement (REM) sleep, in particular in the content of their dreams, which may comprise seemingly natural sequences of events that would be judged as discontinuous or incoherent during wakefulness (Malinowski, 2020).

We propose that the serotonergic system is implicated in the attribution of meaning in the sense of closeness in semantic space (see Figure 9.2 for a specific example, and for the distinction with our hypothesis for dopaminergic signaling). We distinguish between several subtypes of serotonin (5-hydroxytryptamine) receptors and highlight for the purpose of this chapter the sub-type 2A receptor (5-HT_{2A}) (Nichols & Nichols, 2008). These receptors are expressed richly in deep-layer cortical cells (mainly layer V) (Xu & Pandey, 2000), which are abundant in long-range cortical and subcortical projections, and can exert an indirect inhibitory function by activating inhibitory interneurons (Rockland, 2019). PET imaging has been used to show that the density of 5-HT_{2A} receptors is especially high in sensory areas (mainly the visual cortex) and in higher-order transmodal and associative cortical networks, including the precuneus, the thalamus, the temporo-parietal junction, and the frontal lobe (Beliveau et al., 2017) – that is, regions presenting a disproportionately large number of anatomical connections with the rest of the brain (Hagmann et al., 2008).

As expected from the anatomical and functional characteristics of 5-HT_{2A} receptors, their activation is capable of inducing deep modifications in the state of consciousness. Drugs presenting agonism at 5-HT_{2A} receptors are frequently known as psychedelics (Nichols, 2016). As evidenced by a large number of experiments conducted in humans and animals, psychedelic drugs of the tryptamine and phenethylamine families act by agonism at this serotonin receptor subtype (Nichols, 2016). After binding to the 5-HT_{2A} receptor, psychedelics increase the excitability of the target cell. At the molecular scale, the effects of psychedelics are mediated by functional selectivity, where the cascade of intracellular messengers triggered by the binding molecule depends on the final shape of the molecule-receptor complex (González-Maeso et al., 2007). In other words, the shape of the molecule itself is important to determine the functional effect on the neuron, which can explain the differences between the effects of psychedelics, certain 5-HT_{2A} agonists without psychoactive effects (e.g., lisuride), and serotonin itself. The psychoactive properties of psychedelics are also related to the stimulation of a serotonin-glutamate (5-HT_{2A}-mGlu2) receptor complex (González-Maeso et al., 2008); those drugs that are not active at this complex might not elicit typical psychedelic effects

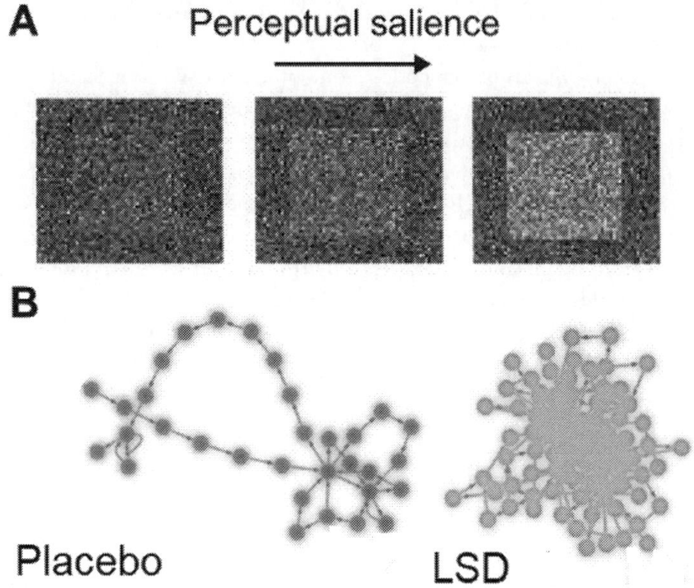

Figure 9.2 Comparison of the effects of dopaminergic stimulants and serotonergic psychedelics

(A) Dopaminergic drugs affect the domain of perceptual salience, enhancing the likelihood of detecting a certain figure within a noisy environment. While this capacity is fundamental for normal cognitive function, when exaggerated it can lead to the misperception of noise as a meaningful signal to be interpreted in terms of the available semantic knowledge. (B) Serotonergic psychedelics lead to semantic hyper-associativity, as shown by speech graphs where nodes represent individual words and arrows indicate their sequential use in speech. Hyper-associativity under the effects of LSD is evidenced by arrows linking a larger proportion of word pairs, regardless of their semantic relatedness. See e-book for a full-color version of this figure.

(Nichols et al., 2016). Relevant to the present discussion, lysergic acid diethylamide (LSD) presents significant agonism at dopaminergic receptors as well, and its effects have been characterized as biphasic – that is, first dominated by serotonergic and then by dopaminergic activation (Marona-Lewicka et al., 2005).

In spite of our highly incomplete knowledge of how psychedelics work in the brain, several theoretical accounts have been put forward that attempt to provide encompassing explanations. The entropic brain hypothesis proposed by Carhart-Harris and colleagues suggests that psychedelics act by increasing the amount of disorder or entropy measured in brain activity signals (Carhart-Harris et al., 2014; Carhart-Harris, 2018). This enhancement of entropy is the objective counterpart of the subjective experience during the psychedelic state, which is perceived as richer and more surprising. More precisely, if the subjective experience induced by psychedelics includes content beyond the repertoire of ordinary wakefulness, then the brain should display a larger repertoire of states to accommodate this increased variability of subjective experiences; this enlargement of the repertoire of brain states can be quantified by entropy metrics. Carhart-Harris also formulated an explanation known as "relaxed beliefs under psychedelics," based on the principle that increased entropy relaxes the precision of high-level priors or beliefs, enhancing bottom-up information flow in the brain (Carhart-Harris & Friston, 2019). Finally, Vollenweider and collaborators have focused on the role of the thalamus in the psychedelic experience (Preller et al., 2019). The thalamic filter model suggests that the principal effects of psychedelics result from thalamic gating deficits, as a consequence of fragmented information processing within cortico-striato-thalamo-cortical feedback loops. These theories are overall consistent with the effects of psychedelics on cognition, which can be summarized as enhanced gating of sensory information, simultaneous with impaired cognitive functions mainly in the domain of attention and decision-making (Bayne & Carter, 2018).

Aldous Huxley's (1954) "Doors of Perception," one of the first written accounts of a psychedelic experience, already highlights the meaning-enhancing properties of these drugs – "objects were all but quivering under the pressure of significance by which they were charged" (Huxley, 1954: 6). Recent research shows that psychedelic experiences can be characterized by a strong and persistent sense of significance. As shown by the group of R. Griffiths, most of those who have psychedelic experiences in a supportive setting consider them to be either one of the five most meaningful experiences of their lives, or the single most meaningful experience (Johnson et al., 2019). Preller and colleagues investigated the neurobiological mechanisms underlying the attribution of personal meaning under the acute effects of LSD, finding that the drug caused participants to attribute personal meaning to stimuli that were previously regarded as meaningless, modulating the processing of meaningful stimuli in cortical midline structures (Preller et al., 2017). Importantly, they showed that these effects depended on 5-HT_{2A} by pre-administering ketanserin (a 2A receptor antagonist) to the participants and showing the absence of significant effects; in other words, the dopaminergic action of LSD was not significant for this dimension of meaning attribution.

Early studies established that psychedelic drugs enhance associativity between words, rendering speech less predictable (Amarel & Cheek, 1965; Landon & Fischer, 1970). This was confirmed by contemporary studies demonstrating increased semantic priming under the acute effects of psychedelics (Family et al., 2016; Spitzer et al., 1996). A recent study investigated the semantic coherence of natural speech under the effects of 75 μg of LSD, finding that the drug increased the average magnitude of jumps in semantic space between consecutive words (Sanz et al., 2020). While loss of coherence in natural speech is documented as a potential marker of schizophrenic psychosis (Elvevåg et al., 2007), Sanz and colleagues showed that LSD induced a state more akin to manic psychosis, with heightened semantic variability coexisting with increased verbosity. Natural language processing tools were also applied to a large number of reports with psychoactive drugs, establishing the highest similarity of psychedelic reports with those of REM dreams (Sanz et al., 2018), thus likening the effects of 5-HT_{2A} stimulation to a well-known hyper-associative state. As in the case of dreams, LSD increased the bizarreness of narratives – that is, a metric designed to capture loss of cohesion due to increased semantic associativity (Kraehenmann et al., 2017.

Is there a more general principle underlying hyper-associativity during the psychedelic state? One of the most pervasive features of the experiences elicited by 5-HT_{2A} stimulation is the blurring of boundaries, not only between the self and the environment (a phenomenon known as "oceanic boundlessness" or "ego dissolution"), but between surrounding objects or concepts (Letheby & Gerrans, 2017; Tagliazucchi et al., 2016). In other words, psychedelics can induce strong feelings of connectedness, an effect hypothesized to underlie some of the possible therapeutic uses of psychedelics, as well as documented improvements in prosocial behavior and in the relationship with nature (Carhart-Harris et al., 2018a). We can hypothesize that psychedelics result in a hyper-associative state by means of increased crosstalk between different brain regions, a more general process that supports the general feeling of connectedness caused by these drugs. This hypothesis is supported by other aspects of the phenomenology of psychedelic experiences, such as synesthesia (the fusion between information from different senses – for example, colored sounds) (Nichols, 2016). Some support also stems from neuroimaging studies showing increased functional connectivity between certain macroscopic brain networks, even though conflicting reports of increased functional segregation also exist (Carhart-Harris et al., 2012, 2016). In particular, it has been shown that both LSD and psilocybin increase the average functional connectivity of regions with high density of 5-HT_{2A} receptors, which coincide with posterior and midline structural hubs of the brain (Tagliazucchi et al., 2016). The large number of long-range anatomical tracts wiring these regions with the rest of the brain could underlie the integrative and hyper-associative action of psychedelic compounds (Hagmann et al., 2008).

Specificity of dopaminergic and serotonergic effects

It is reasonable to question whether the two aforementioned facets of meaning attribution are specifically related to dopaminergic and serotonergic function. This is unlikely, considering the complexity of signaling processes in the human brain and the heterogeneity of pathways and molecules that are involved, even in the specific case of psychedelics (Zamberlan et al., 2018). For instance, the glutamatergic system is also involved in the attribution of salience (Batten et al., 2018; Limongi et al., 2020), and other neurotransmitters could certainly be involved in what we call "meaning as connectedness."

Because of this complexity, it is reasonable to limit our discussion to dopamine and serotonin and ask whether their effects are specific in terms of perceptual salience vs. semantic processing. Experimental data on salience modulation by psychedelic drugs is scarce, with some authors hypothesizing increased salience attribution (Bayne & Carter, 2018). However, this hypothesis contradicts the current literature on the serotonergic modulation of salience. It has been proposed that low serotonergic function enhances salience (in particular, in the emotional domain), constituting a major pathological mechanism underlying major depression (Carver et al., 2009). Neuroimaging data provides indirect evidence of the inverse relationship between salience attribution and serotonergic stimulation, showing that psychedelics decouple the salience network with the rest of the brain, potentially underlying deficits in the efficient and flexible switching between externally and internally oriented cognition under the acute effects of psychedelics (Pasquini et al., 2020). This result is consistent with the more general observation of an opposing effect of dopamine and serotonin in the organization of large-scale functional connectivity networks (Conio et al., 2020). Further evidence of the independence between serotonergic function and salience attribution stems from pharmacological studies in humans showing that the effect of antipsychotic drugs on salience is not mediated by changes in the concentration of serotonin (Amato et al., 2011). Finally, an animal study directly established that a knock-out of the serotonin transporter gene spars incentive salience attribution (Nonkes et al., 2014)

Conversely, previous reports support the suggestion that dopaminergic activation does not lead to enhanced semantic associativity. Levodopa reduces indirect semantic priming and increases reaction times to indirectly related word pairs (Kischka et al., 1996); it also decreases semantic priming for pairs of words where one of them is subordinate to the other (Copland et al., 2003). Overall, this suggests that dopamine restricts the formation of connections in semantic networks. While it is certain that schizophrenia results in less coherent speech, it remains to be shown that this loss of coherence can be attributed directly to enhanced associativity, which seems unlikely considering several reports of impaired semantic priming in schizophrenic patients.

Thus, a picture of meaning attribution emerges with different roles played by these two major neurotransmitter systems. Dopaminergic signaling is important for the detection of salient stimuli, and thus represents a first stage in the attribution of meaning in the environment, in this case heavily mediated by *Umwelt* and thus by evolutionary history. Another dissociable process is modulated by serotonergic function, and consists of embedding those stimuli within a semantic network, where proximity indicates conceptual relatedness. In the same way that serotonin and dopamine are considered competing neurotransmitters, these two roles may unfold independently (and perhaps inhibit mutually), as shown by the possibility of selectively modulating one of them (but not the other) using pharmacological tools.

Therapeutic use of psychedelics and the attribution of personal meaning

The over-attribution of personal meaning is a common feature in psychotic episodes; as such, it is questionable whether psychedelic experiences carry therapeutic value. However, the current literature presents a spectacular validation of the link between the meaning-enhancing properties of psychedelic drugs and their purported therapeutic efficacy for the treatment of certain psychiatric disorders, mostly mood and substance abuse disorders. In particular, it has been shown that the therapeutic effects of psychedelics are strongly mediated by their capacity to induce "mystical-type" experiences characterized by persistent feelings of personal significance and meaningfulness (Johnson et al., 2019).

Psychedelic drugs do not act on isolation, but amplify pre-existent contextual variables known as set and setting (Carhart-Harris et al., 2018b). It has been speculated that psychedelics heighten the placebo response by attributing abnormally high significance to these variables, which is consistent with the dependence of the therapeutic outcome with the specifics of set and setting (Carhart-Harris et al., 2018b). Psychedelic experiences resulting in mystical-type states are also affected by a noetic quality, where the experience seems more real and significant than reality itself (Johnson et al., 2019). This quality could be key to the emergence of spiritual beliefs and magical thinking, which in some cases could contribute to transcending the rigid thought schemes characteristic of mood and addiction disorders (Hartogsohn, 2018). Finally, insofar as hyper-associativity favors creativity and problem-solving, the transient psychedelic state could equip the patients with new mental strategies to cope with and transcend their disorders. In summary, it remains to be investigated how much of the therapeutic potential of psychedelics can be attributed to their meaning-enhancing properties, but the available evidence suggests they play an important (if not critical) role (Hartogsohn, 2018).

Conclusion

Like other problems with similar philosophical pedigree, the problem of meaning can be understood and interpreted in a new light when contextualized in terms of brain structure and function. While it is unlikely that neuroscience can provide the ultimate answer to this problem, it may offer new perspectives and insights that can be developed further from a more integrative perspective. In this chapter, we approached the problem of meaning, drawing a distinction between "meaning as salience" and "meaning as connectedness." While this distinction may appear unwarranted in terms of classical linguistic theory, we showed that this distinction is backed up by our knowledge of two major neurotransmitter systems: dopamine and serotonin. After discussing a wealth of pharmacological and clinical studies, we concluded that these two systems play dissociable (and perhaps competing) roles in the process of meaning attribution. By identifying these potentially orthogonal contributions, we expect future studies will capitalize from more advanced pharmacological and neuroimaging methods to outline the neural circuits related to meaning attribution.

Notes

1 This also underlies the difference between semantic and Shannon's information (Bar-Hillel & Carnap, 1953). The transmission of the latter is maximized when the symbol frequencies are maximally random, while the former depends on the information that is already available to the receiver (e.g., faces are relevant stimuli).

2 See www.erowid.org/experiences

References

Amarel, M., & Cheek, F. E. (1965). Some effects of LSD-25 on verbal communication. *Journal of Abnormal Psychology*, *70*(6), 453–456. doi: 10.1037/h0022773

Amato, D., Natesan, S., Yavich, L., Kapur, S., & Müller, C. P. (2011). Dynamic regulation of dopamine and serotonin responses to salient stimuli during chronic haloperidol treatment. *International Journal of Neuropsychopharmacology*, *14*(10), 1327–1339. doi: 10.1017/S1461145711000010

Bar-Hillel, Y., & Carnap, R. (1953). Semantic information. *The British Journal for the Philosophy of Science*, *4*(14), 147–157. doi: 10.1093/bjps/IV.14.147

Batten, S. R., Pomerleau, F., Quintero, J., Gerhardt, G. A., & Beckmann, J. S. (2018). The role of glutamate signaling in incentive salience: Second-by-second glutamate recordings in awake Sprague-Dawley rats. *Journal of Neurochemistry, 145*(4), 276–286. doi: 10.1111/jnc.14298

Bayne, T., & Carter, O. (2018). Dimensions of consciousness and the psychedelic state. *Neuroscience of Consciousness, 2018*(1), niy008. doi: 10.1093/nc/niy008

Beliveau, V., Ganz, M., Feng, L., Ozenne, B., Højgaard, L., Fisher, P. M., Svarer, C., Greve, D. N., & Knudsen, G. M. (2017). A high-resolution in vivo atlas of the human brain's serotonin system. *Journal of Neuroscience, 37*(1), 120–128. doi: 10.1523/JNEUROSCI.2830-16.2016

Berridge, K. C., & Robinson, T. E. (1998). What is the role of dopamine in reward: Hedonic impact, reward learning, or incentive salience? *Brain Research Reviews, 28*(3), 309–369. doi: 10.1016/s0165-0173(98)00019-8

Blessing, W. W., Blessing, E. M., Mohammed, M., & Ootsuka, Y. (2017). Clozapine, chlorpromazine and risperidone dose-dependently reduce emotional hyperthermia, a biological marker of salience. *Psychopharmacology, 234*(21), 3259–3269. doi: 10.1007/s00213-017-4710-x

Bouissac, P. (1985). Neurosemiotics, a definition. *Recherches Sémiotiques/Semiotics Inquiry, 5*(3), 323–325.

Bouissac, P. (1987). Semiotics in Canada I1. In T. A. Sebeok, & J. Umiker-Sebeok (Eds.), *The Semiotic Web* (p. 191). Berlin: Mouton de Gruyter.

Carhart-Harris, R. L. (2018). The entropic brain – revisited. *Neuropharmacology, 142*, 167–178. doi: 10.1016/j.neuropharm.2018.03.010

Carhart-Harris, R. L., Erritzoe, D., Haijen, E., Kaelen, M., & Watts, R. (2018a). Psychedelics and connectedness. *Psychopharmacology, 235*(2), 547–550. doi: 10.1007/s00213-017-4701-y

Carhart-Harris, R. L., Erritzoe, D., Williams, T., Stone, J. M., Reed, L. J., Colasanti, A., Tyacke, R. J., Leech, R., Malizia, A. L., Murphy, K., Hobden, P., Evans, J., Feilding, A., Wise, R. G., & Nutt, D. J. (2012). Neural correlates of the psychedelic state as determined by fMRI studies with psilocybin. *Proceedings of the National Academy of Sciences, 109*(6), 2138–2143. doi: 10.1073/pnas.1119598109

Carhart-Harris, R. L., & Friston, K. J. (2019). REBUS and the anarchic brain: Toward a unified model of the brain action of psychedelics. *Pharmacological Reviews, 71*(3), 316–344. doi: 10.1124/pr.118.017160

Carhart-Harris, R. L., Leech, R., Hellyer, P. J., Shanahan, M., Feilding, A., Tagliazucchi, E., Chialvo, D. R., & Nutt, D. (2014). The entropic brain: A theory of conscious states informed by neuroimaging research with psychedelic drugs. *Frontiers in Human Neuroscience, 8*, 20. doi: 10.3389/fnhum.2014.00020

Carhart-Harris, R. L., Muthukumaraswamy, S., Roseman, L. … Leech, R. (2016). Neural correlates of the LSD experience revealed by multimodal neuroimaging. *Proceedings of the National Academy of Sciences, 113*(17), 4853–4858. doi: 10.1073/pnas.1518377113

Carhart-Harris, R. L., Roseman, L., Haijen, E., Erritzoe, D., Watts, R., Branchi, I., & Kaelen, M. (2018b). Psychedelics and the essential importance of context. *Journal of Psychopharmacology, 32*(7), 725–731. doi: 10.1177/0269881118754710

Carver, C. S., Johnson, S. L., & Joormann, J. (2009). Two-mode models of self-regulation as a tool for conceptualizing effects of the serotonin system in normal behavior and diverse disorders. *Current Directions in Psychological Science, 18*(4), 195–199. doi: 10.1111/j.1467-8721.2009.01635.x

Celesia, G. G., & Barr, A. N. (1970). Psychosis and other psychiatric manifestations of levodopa therapy. *Archives of Neurology, 23*(3), 193–200. doi: 10.1001/archneur.1970.00480270003001

Cho, J. R., Treweek, J. B., Robinson, J. E., Xiao, C., Bremner, L. R., Greenbaum, A., & Gradinaru, V. (2017). Dorsal raphe dopamine neurons modulate arousal and promote wakefulness by salient stimuli. *Neuron, 94*(6), 1205–1219. doi: 10.1016/j.neuron.2017.05.020

Croft, W., & Cruse, D. A. (2004). *Cognitive linguistics*. Cambridge: Cambridge University Press.

Conio, B., Martino, M., Magioncalda, P., Escelsior, A., Inglese, M., Amore, M., & Northoff, G. (2020). Opposite effects of dopamine and serotonin on resting-state networks: Review and implications for psychiatric disorders. *Molecular Psychiatry, 25*(1), 82–93. doi: 10.1038/s41380-019-0406-4

Copland, D. A., Chenery, H. J., Murdoch, B. E., Arnott, W. L., & Silburn, P. A. (2003). Dopamine enhances semantic salience: Semantic priming evidence from healthy individuals. *Brain and Language, 87*, 103–104. doi: 10.1016/S0093-934X(03) 00220-7

Cunningham, S. J., & Turk, D. J. (2017). Editorial: A review of self-processing biases in cognition. *Quarterly Journal of Experimental Psychology*, 70(6), 987–995. doi: 10.1080/17470218.2016.1276609

Dawson, G. R., Heyes, C. M., & Iversen, S. D. (1992). Pharmacological mechanisms and animal models of cognition. *Behavioural Pharmacology, 3*(4), 285–297.

Dennett, D. C. (1987). Evolution, error, and intentionality. In P. K. Moser & J. D. Trout (Eds.), *Contemporary Materialism* (p. 254). London: Routledge.

Elvevåg, B., Foltz, P. W., Weinberger, D. R., & Goldberg, T. E. (2007). Quantifying incoherence in speech: An automated methodology and novel application to schizophrenia. *Schizophrenia Research, 93*(1–3), 304–316. doi: 10.1016/j.schres.2007.03.001

Family, N., Vinson, D., Vigliocco, G., Kaelen, M., Bolstridge, M., Nutt, D. J., & Carhart-Harris, R. L. (2016). Semantic activation in LSD: Evidence from picture naming. *Language, Cognition and Neuroscience, 31*(10), 1320–1327. doi: 10.1080/23273798.2016.1217030

Fellbaum, C. (1998). A semantic network of English verbs. *WordNet: An Electronic Lexical Database, 3*, 153–178. doi: 10.7551/mitpress/7287.003.0008

Gardner, D. M., Baldessarini, R. J., & Waraich, P. (2005). Modern antipsychotic drugs: A critical overview. *Cmaj, 172*(13), 1703–1711. doi: 10.1503/cmaj.1041064

Geng, X., Hu, Y., Gu, H., Salmeron, B. J., Adinoff, B., Stein, E. A., & Yang, Y. (2017). Salience and default mode network dysregulation in chronic cocaine users predict treatment outcome. *Brain, 140*(5), 1513–1524. doi: 10.1093/brain/awx036

González-Maeso, J., Ang, R. L., Yuen, T., Chan, P., Weisstaub, N. V., López-Giménez, J. F., Zhou, M., Okawa, Y., Callado, L. F., Milligan, G., Gingrich, J. A., Filizola, M., Meana, J., & Gingrich, J. A. (2008). Identification of a serotonin/glutamate receptor complex implicated in psychosis. *Nature, 452*(7183), 93–97. doi: 10.1038/nature06612

González-Maeso, J., Weisstaub, N. V., Zhou, M., Chan, P., Ivic, L., Ang, R., Lira, A., Bradley-Moore, M., Ge, Y., Zhou, Q., Sealfon, S. C., & Sealfon, S. C. (2007). Hallucinogens recruit specific cortical 5-HT2A receptor-mediated signaling pathways to affect behavior. *Neuron, 53*(3), 439–452. doi: 10.1016/j.neuron.2007.01.008

Guillin, O., Abi-Dargham, A., & Laruelle, M. (2007). Neurobiology of dopamine in schizophrenia. *International Review of Neurobiology, 78*, 1–39. doi: 10.1016/S0074-7742(06)78001-1

Hagmann, P., Cammoun, L., Gigandet, X., Meuli, R., Honey, C. J., Wedeen, V. J., & Sporns, O. (2008). Mapping the structural core of human cerebral cortex. *PLoS Biology, 6*(7), e159. doi: 10.1371/journal.pbio.0060159

Hartogsohn, I. (2018). The meaning-enhancing properties of psychedelics and their mediator role in psychedelic therapy, spirituality, and creativity. *Frontiers in Neuroscience, 12*, 129. doi: 10.3389/fnins.2018.00129

Heinz, A., Saunders, R. C., Kolachana, B. S., Jones, D. W., Gorey, J. G., Bachevalier, J., & Weinberger, D. R. (1999). Striatal dopamine receptors and transporters in monkeys with neonatal temporal limbic damage. *Synapse, 32*(2), 71–79. doi: 10.1002/(SICI)1098-2396(199905)32:2<71::AID-SYN1>3.0.CO;2-Q

Huang, H., Botao, Z., Jiang, Y., Tang, Y., Zhang, T., Tang, X., Xu, L., Wang, J., Li, J., Zhenying, Q., Xu, L., Wang, H., Luo, C., Li, C., Xu, J., Goff, D., & Wang, J. (2019). Aberrant resting-state functional connectivity of salience network in first-episode schizophrenia. *Brain Imaging and Behavior*, 1–11. doi: 10.1007/s11682-019-00040-8

Huxley, A. (1954). *The Doors of Perception* (pp. 2–24). London: Chatto and Windus.

Iversen, S. D., & Iversen, L. L. (2007). Dopamine: 50 years in perspective. *Trends in Neurosciences, 30*(5), 188–193. doi: 10.1016/j.tins.2007.03.002

Johnson, M. W., Hendricks, P. S., Barrett, F. S., & Griffiths, R. R. (2019). Classic psychedelics: An integrative review of epidemiology, therapeutics, mystical experience, and brain network function. *Pharmacology & Therapeutics, 197*, 83–102. doi: 10.1016/j.pharmthera.2018.11.010

Kumakura, Y., Cumming, P., Vernaleken, I., Buchholz, H. G., Siessmeier, T., Heinz, A., Kienast, T., Bartenstein, P., & Gründer, G. (2007). Elevated [18F] fluorodopamine turnover in brain of patients with schizophrenia: an [18F] fluorodopa/positron emission tomography study. *Journal of Neuroscience, 27*(30), 8080–8087. doi: 10.1523/JNEUROSCI.0805-07.2007

Kapur, S., Mizrahi, R., & Li, M. (2005). From dopamine to salience to psychosis: Linking biology, pharmacology and phenomenology of psychosis. *Schizophrenia Research, 79*(1), 59–68. doi: 10.1016/j.schres.2005.01.003

Kischka, U., Kammer, T., Maier, S., Weisbrod, M., Thimm, M., & Spitzer, M. (1996). Dopaminergic modulation of semantic network activation. *Neuropsychologia, 34*(11), 1107–1113. doi: 10.1016/0028-3932(96)00024-3

Knolle, F., Ermakova, A. O., Justicia, A., Fletcher, P. C., Bunzeck, N., Düzel, E., & Murray, G. K. (2018). Brain responses to different types of salience in antipsychotic naïve first episode psychosis: An fMRI study. *Translational Psychiatry, 8*(1), 1–13. doi: 10.1038/s41398-018-0250-3

Kraehenmann, R., Pokorny, D., Vollenweider, L., Preller, K. H., Pokorny, T., Seifritz, E., & Vollenweider, F. X. (2017). Dreamlike effects of LSD on waking imagery in humans depend on serotonin 2A receptor activation. *Psychopharmacology, 234*(13), 2031–2046. doi: 10.1007/s00213-017-4610-0

Landon, M., & Fischer, R. (1970). On similar linguistic structures in creative performance and psilocybin-induced experience. *Confinia Psychiatrica, 13*, 115–138.

Letheby, C., & Gerrans, P. (2017). Self unbound: Ego dissolution in psychedelic experience. *Neuroscience of Consciousness, 3*(1). doi: 10.1093/nc/nix016

Liang, X., He, Y., Salmeron, B. J., Gu, H., Stein, E. A., & Yang, Y. (2015). Interactions between the salience and default-mode networks are disrupted in cocaine addiction. *Journal of Neuroscience, 35*(21), 8081–8090. doi: 10.1523/JNEUROSCI.3188-14.2015

Lieberman, J. A., Kinon, B. J., & Loebel, A. D. (1990). Dopaminergic mechanisms in idiopathic and drug-induced psychoses. *Schizophrenia Bulletin, 16*(1), 97–110. doi: 10.1093/schbul/16.1.97

Limongi, R., Jeon, P., Mackinley, M., Das, T., Dempster, K., Théberge, J., Bartha, R., Wong, D., & Palaniyappan, L. (2020). Glutamate and dysconnection in the salience network: Neurochemical, effective-connectivity, and computational evidence in schizophrenia. *Biological Psychiatry*, *88*(3), 273–281. doi: 10.1016/j.biopsych.2020.01.021

Mackay, A. V., Iversen, L. L., Rossor, M., Spokes, E., Bird, E., Arregui, A., Creese, I., & Snyder, S. H. (1982). Increased brain dopamine and dopamine receptors in schizophrenia. *Archives of General Psychiatry*, *39*(9), 991–997. doi: 10.1001/archpsyc.1982.04290090001001

Malinowski, J. (2020). *The Psychology of Dreaming*. London: Routledge.

Marona-Lewicka, D., Thisted, R. A., & Nichols, D. E. (2005). Distinct temporal phases in the behavioral pharmacology of LSD: Dopamine D 2 receptor-mediated effects in the rat and implications for psychosis. *Psychopharmacology*, *180*(3), 427–435. doi: 10.1007/s00213-005-2183-9

Nichols, D. E. (2016). Psychedelics. *Pharmacological Reviews*, *68*(2), 264–355. doi: 10.1124/pr.115.011478

Nichols, D. E., & Nichols, C. D. (2008). Serotonin receptors. *Chemical Reviews*, *108*(5), 1614–1641. doi: 10.1021/cr078224o

Nonkes, L. J., van de Vondervoort, I. I., & Homberg, J. R. (2014). The attribution of incentive salience to an appetitive conditioned cue is not affected by knockout of the serotonin transporter in rats. *Behavioural Brain Research*, *259*, 268–273. doi: 10.1016/j.bbr.2013.11.017

Nur, S., & Adams, C. E. (2016). Chlorpromazine versus reserpine for schizophrenia. *Cochrane Database of Systematic Reviews*, (4). doi: 10.1002/14651858.CD012122.pub2

Nutl, J. G., & Fellman, J. H. (1984). Pharmacokinetics of levodopa. *Clinical Neuropharmacology*, 7(1), 35–50. doi: 10.1097/00002826-198403000-00002

Palaniyappan, L., White, T. P., & Liddle, P. F. (2012). The concept of salience network dysfunction in schizophrenia: From neuroimaging observations to therapeutic opportunities. *Current Topics in Medicinal Chemistry*, *12*(21), 2324–2338. doi: 10.2174/156802612805289881

Pasquini, L., Palhano-Fontes, F., & Araujo, D. B. (2020). Subacute effects of the psychedelic ayahuasca on the salience and default mode networks. *Journal of Psychopharmacology*, *34*(6), 623–635. doi: 10.1177/0269881120909409

Phan, K. L., Taylor, S. F., Welsh, R. C., Decker, L. R., Noll, D. C., Nichols, T. E., Britton, J. C., & Liberzon, I. (2003). Activation of the medial prefrontal cortex and extended amygdala by individual ratings of emotional arousal: A fMRI study. *Biological Psychiatry*, *53*(3), 211–215. doi: 10.1016/s0006-3223(02)01485-3

Preller, K. H., Herdener, M., Pokorny, T., Planzer, A., Kraehenmann, R., Stämpfli, P., Liechti, M. E., Seifritz, E., & Vollenweider, F. X. (2017). The fabric of meaning and subjective effects in LSD-induced states depend on serotonin 2A receptor activation. *Current Biology*, *27*(3), 451–457. doi: 10.1016/j.cub.2016.12.030

Preller, K. H., Razi, A., Zeidman, P., Stämpfli, P., Friston, K. J., & Vollenweider, F. X. (2019). Effective connectivity changes in LSD-induced altered states of consciousness in humans. *Proceedings of the National Academy of Sciences*, *116*(7), 2743–2748. doi: 10.1073/pnas.1815129116

Rockland, K. S. (2019). What do we know about laminar connectivity? *Neuroimage*, *197*, 772–784. doi: 10.1016/j.neuroimage.2017.07.032

Sahlgren, M. (2008). The distributional hypothesis. *Italian Journal of Disability Studies*, *20*, 33–53.

Sanz, C., Pallavicini, C., Carrillo, F., Zamberlan, F., Sigman, M., Mota, N., Copelli, M., Ribeiro, S., Nutt, D., Carhart-Harris, R., & Tagliazucchi, E. (2020). The entropic tongue: Disorganization of natural language under LSD. *Consciousness and Cognition*, *87*, 103070. doi: 10.1016/j.concog.2020.103070

Sanz, C., Zamberlan, F., Erowid, E., & Tagliazucchi, E. (2018). The experience elicited by hallucinogens presents the highest similarity to dreaming within a large database of psychoactive substance reports. *Frontiers in Neuroscience*, *12*, 7. doi: 10.3389/fnins.2018.00007

Shafiei, G., Zeighami, Y., Clark, C. A., Coull, J. T., Nagano-Saito, A., Leyton, M., Dagher, A., & Mišić, B. (2019). Dopamine signaling modulates the stability and integration of intrinsic brain networks. *Cerebral Cortex*, *29*(1), 397–409. doi: 10.1093/cercor/bhy264

Shannon, C. E. (1948). A mathematical theory of communication. *The Bell System Technical Journal*, 27(3), 379–423. doi: 10.1002/j.1538-7305.1948.tb01338.x

Shellshear, L., MacDonald, A. D., Mahoney, J., Finch, E., McMahon, K., Silburn, P., Nathan, P. J., & Copland, D. A. (2015). Levodopa enhances explicit new-word learning in healthy adults: A preliminary study. *Human Psychopharmacology: Clinical and Experimental*, *30*(5), 341–349. doi: 10.1002/hup.2480

Shiner, T., Symmonds, M., Guitart-Masip, M., Fleming, S. M., Friston, K. J., & Dolan, R. J. (2015). Dopamine, salience, and response set shifting in prefrontal cortex. *Cerebral Cortex*, *25*(10), 3629–3639. doi: 10.1093/cercor/bhu210

Soskin, D. P., Holt, D. J., Sacco, G. R., & Fava, M. (2013). Incentive salience: Novel treatment strategies for major depression. *CNS Spectrums*, *18*(6), 307–314. doi: 10.1017/S1092852913000345

Speaks, J. (2010). Theories of meaning. In E. N. Zalta (Ed.), *Stanford Encyclopedia of Philosophy*. Stanford, CA: Stanford University Press.

Spitzer, M., Thimm, M., Hermle, L., Holzmann, P., Kovar, K. A., Heimann, H., Gouzoulis-Mayfrank, E., Kischka, U., & Schneider, F. (1996). Increased activation of indirect semantic associations under psilocybin. *Biological Psychiatry*, *39*, 1055–1057. doi: 10.1016/0006-3223 (95)00418-1

Steinberg, D. D., & Jakobovits, L. A. (Eds.) (1971). *Semantics: An Interdisciplinary Reader in Philosophy, Linguistics and Psychology*. Cambridge: Cambridge University Press.

Tagliazucchi, E., Roseman, L., Kaelen, M., Orban, C., Muthukumaraswamy, S. D., Murphy, K., Laufs, H., Leech, R., McGonigle, J., Crossley, N., Bullmore, E., Williams, T., Bolstridge, M., Feilding, A., Nutt, D. J., & Carhart-Harris, R. (2016). Increased global functional connectivity correlates with LSD-induced ego dissolution. *Current Biology*, *26*(8), 1043–1050. doi: 10.1016/j.cub.2016.02.010

Treisman, A. M., & Gelade, G. (1980). A feature-integration theory of attention. *Cognitive Psychology*, *12*(1), 97–136.

von Uexküll, J. (1921). *Umwelt und innenwelt der tiere*. Berlin: Springer.

Wang, Y., Tang, W., Fan, X., Zhang, J., Geng, D., Jiang, K., Zhu, D., Zhenhua, S., Xiao, Z., & Liu, D. (2017). Resting-state functional connectivity changes within the default mode network and the salience network after antipsychotic treatment in early-phase schizophrenia. *Neuropsychiatric Disease and Treatment*, *13*, 397. doi: 10.2147/NDT.S123598

White, T., Gilleen, J. K., & Shergill, S. S. (2013). Dysregulated but not decreased salience network activity in schizophrenia. *Frontiers in Human Neuroscience*, 7, 65. doi: 10.3389/fnhum.2013.00065

Winton-Brown, T. T., Fusar-Poli, P., Ungless, M. A., & Howes, O. D. (2014). Dopaminergic basis of salience dysregulation in psychosis. *Trends in Neurosciences*, *37*(2), 85–94. doi: 10.1016/j.tins.2013.11.003

Wittgenstein, L. (1953). *Philosophical Investigations* (G. E. M. Anscombe, Trans.). Oxford: Basil Blackwell.

Xu, T., & Pandey, S. C. (2000). Cellular localization of serotonin 2A (5HT2A) receptors in the rat brain. *Brain Research Bulletin*, *51*(6), 499–505. doi: 10.1016/s0361-9230(99)00278-6

Zamberlan, F., Sanz, C., Martínez Vivot, R., Pallavicini, C., Erowid, E., & Tagliazucchi, E. (2018). The varieties of the psychedelic experience: A preliminary study of the association between the reported subjective effects and the binding affinity profiles of substituted phenethylamines and tryptamines. *Frontiers in Integrative Neuroscience*, *12*, 54. doi: 10.3389/fnint.2018.00054

Zoran, D., & Weiss, Y. (2009). Scale invariance and noise in natural images. In *2009 IEEE 12th International Conference on Computer Vision* (pp. 2209–2216). Piscataway, NJ: IEEE. doi: 10.1109/ICCV.2009.5459476

10
HOW GRAMMAR MEANS

Manuel de Vega

Introduction

The current advances of the neuroscience of language are impressive, yet the epistemological approach to language follows the common scientific strategy of "divide and conquer," which we can call a "modular" approach.[1] In this tradition, researchers focus on a specific process, such as word recognition or syntactic processing, designing simple and well-controlled experimental tasks, collecting behavioral or neural measures with isolated individuals, and generating simplified models of the target process (Ibáñez & García, 2018). These models are often contradictory and produce scientific debates that, in turn, generate new experimental hypotheses. Yet, beyond this generative capacity, the modular approach neglects the complex, multisystemic nature of neurolinguistic processes, which generally interact with interoceptive, perceptual, and social contexts rather than being implemented in isolated individuals during simple, repetitive laboratory tasks (Barutta et al., 2011; Ibáñez, 2019).

Whereas modular approaches try to dissociate syntax from other mechanisms of language (e.g., lexico-semantic processing) at both the neural and functional levels, this chapter assumes neurosemiotic principles, proposing an integrative approach to the study of syntax and meaning in communicational contexts. It examines the semantic function of syntax in mapping basic dimensions of human episodic experience; the pragmatic role of syntax, which contributes to the cooperative reference specification between interlocutors in face-to-face communication; and the neural bases of syntax, as based on the reuse of pre-existing, evolutionarily earlier networks. It also proposes that an optimal methodology to examine these functions is applying hyperscanning techniques to interacting speakers. Elaborating on these ideas could contribute to a solid foundation of the neurosemiotic of grammar – leading, as we will see, to new, promising research avenues.

Before describing the neurosemiotic approach defended here, the next section critically summarizes two typically modular approaches in the neuroscience of language, separately concerned with meaning and syntax, respectively. I will argue that, in the standard approach, meaning is generally identified with lexico-conceptual processes, associated with content words (nouns, verbs, and adjectives), while function (syntactic) words and morphology play little or no role in relevant theories. Concerning syntax, the typical methodological and theoretical approaches are extremely modular, focusing on how syntactic structures are encoded or decoded by isolated participants who often receive series of sentences with subtle manipulations that produce rare or anomalous (garden-path, ungrammatical) conditions to test theory-based hypotheses. In the neurolinguistics field, many studies

DOI: 10.4324/9781003051817-13

also have modular goals, such as dissociating the neural networks that implement syntax from the neural networks responsible for semantics. After the critical analysis of conventional approaches, the chapter will present the building blocks for a neurosemiotics of grammar, highlighting the role of syntax in the construction of meaning at the sentence level and its role as pragmatic tool for specifying reference in face-to-face communication.

Conventional approaches to meaning and syntax

Meaning

The traditional approaches to meaning in cognitive psychology and, more recently, in neurosemantics posit that linguistic meaning relies on content words (nouns, verbs, and adjectives), which work as pointers to internal symbols or concepts in a semantic memory network. These theories either disregard or attribute minor roles to function or grammatical words (e.g., prepositions, articles, auxiliary verbs, connectives). The neurosemantic approach inherited this content-word bias and tries to reveal the neural networks underlying word meaning. Neurosemantics was also influenced by the two main theoretical traditions in lexico-semantic studies: embodiment and symbolism. Embodied theories claim that meaning is grounded on perceptual, motor, and emotional processes, and therefore embodied neurosemantics proposes that meaning reuses the very brain structures involved in non-verbal world experience (e.g., Buccino et al. 2016; García & Ibáñez, 2016). Instead, symbolic theories postulate that meaning has an amodal, abstract, and arbitrary format – a sort of inner conceptual language, disconnected from the sensorimotor systems. The neurosemantic version of symbolism searches for a single neural hub in charge of computing meaning independently of modality.

Embodied neurosemantics offers multiple evidence that word meaning is broadly distributed in the brain, comprising content-dependent neural mechanisms in the sensorimotor cortex. For instance, neuroimaging data show that the motor cortex is recruited when people face isolated action verbs, such as *grasp*, *whistle*, or *kick* (Hauk et al., 2004; Pulvermüller et al., 2005). Also, electrophysiological studies reported that mu and beta rhythms – neural markers of motor processes – are desynchronized over fronto-central electrodes when people understand sentences with action verbs (Klepp et al., 2019; Moreno et al., 2013, 2015; van Elk et al., 2010). In the same vein, studies employing single-pulse transcranial magnetic stimulation (TMS) applied to M1 combined with electromyography have shown that understanding manual action verbs, compared with non-action verbs, modulates motor cortical excitability, as measured by motor-evoked potentials in representative hand muscles (Buccino et al., 2005; Papeo et al., 2009). Finally, neuropsychological data indicate that motor disorders, such as Parkinson's disease, are also associated with a selective deficit in naming actions, suggesting that action semantics is partially supported by the motor system (Herrera & Cuetos, 2012). In sum, neuroanatomical, neurophysiological, neuropsychological, and behavioral data point to the role of the motor system in linguistic meaning, which in turn supports embodiment theories.

Symbolic neurosemantics, even accepting that words induce distributed activations, emphasizes the role of high-order semantic hubs. In particular, there is evidence that the anterior temporal lobe (ATL) bilaterally integrates information across sensorimotor networks, which in comparison would play a secondary role in meaning (Lambon Ralph et al., 2009; Patterson et al., 2007). The relevance of the semantic hub is supported by varied data. Patients with semantic dementia suffer a progressive neurodegenerative condition in the ATL and, as a consequence, they show dramatic impairment in a variety of semantic tasks, such as naming pictures; matching words with pictures; verifying whether words refer to pictures; sorting words according to similarity; sorting objects according to similarity; demonstrating the proper use of objects; or recognizing objects based on visual, auditory, somatosensory, or gustatory/olfactory features (Hodges & Patterson, 2007; Lambon Ralph & Patterson, 2008; Mesulam et al., 2013). The use of functional magnetic resonance imaging (fMRI) in healthy participants also reveals significant activity in the ATL (bilaterally) when they perform lexico-conceptual tasks (Binney et al., 2015), and inhibiting ATL by means of low-frequency repetitive TMS (rTMS) impairs performance in such tasks (Pobric et al., 2009). All these data convincingly support the idea that, at some point, meaning processing requires a multimodal conceptual system, with a main hub in the ATL. Nonetheless, this is compatible with the idea that other brain systems (perceptual, motor, emotional) play a functional role for specific linguistic contents, as defended by embodiment scholars.

In conclusion, the embodied approach postulates the relevance of distributed sensorimotor brain networks in processing meaning, whereas the symbolist approach proposes the ATL as a content-free neural hub for computing conceptual meaning. Yet both approaches share a strong bias towards content words, especially nouns and verbs, neglecting semantics at sentence or discourse levels.

Syntax

The neuroscience of syntax employs different disciplinary approaches – that is, neuroanatomy examines *where* syntax is processed in the brain, neurophysiology attempts to reveal *when* syntactic processes occur during the flow of language, and neurocomputation aims to understand *how* neurons compute syntactic structures (Pulvermüller, 2010). There is a great deal of research on these important topics. Neuroimaging studies have confirmed the important role of left perisylvian brain areas (Broca's and Wernicke's areas) in morpho-syntactic processes, although other structures such as the insula, the basal ganglia, and the posterior superior temporal gyrus are also relevant (Friederici, 2017; Kaan & Saab, 2002; Segaert et al. 2012). Furthermore, anatomical and functional connectivity among these structures has been examined by means of diffusion tensor imaging and functional neuroimaging, revealing two dorsal and two ventral pathways connecting Broca's area, Wernicke's area, and other areas that differ grossly in syntactic and semantic functions (Friederici, 2009, 2017). Neurophysiological techniques – electroencephalography (EEG) and magnetoencephalography – provide a high-resolution view of the temporal course of syntactic processes, revealing that some event-related potential (ERP) components are sensitive to syntactic complexity or syntactic violations. For instance, noun–verb agreement violations (e.g., *The athletes is running*) usually elicit an early anterior negativity (ELAN) and a later positivity (P600) – for example, Molinaro et al. (2011). Unfortunately, the "syntactic" character of these components is controversial, as some of them (e.g., ELAN) are confounded with attentional components, while others (e.g., P600) are also sensitive to additional linguistic and non-linguistic factors (Kuperberg, 2007; Pulvermüller, 2010). Finally, a few neurocomputational studies tried to model relevant neural mechanisms. For instance, Pulvermüller and Knoblauch (2009) proposed binary neural assemblies, which are able to compute two-word binding (noun-verb), and Buzsáki (2010) proposed Hebbian-like neural assemblies hierarchically organized to compute syntax. To conclude, neuro-syntax is a very dynamic research field that is improving our knowledge of the anatomical, physiological, and computational processes of grammar.

Interim conclusions

Neurosemantics has intensively studied word meaning, leading to significant advances in theoretical modeling and improving knowledge of language disorders and neurodegenerative diseases. Yet neurosemantics has a lexico-conceptual approach to meaning, focused on content words to the detriment of function words, morphology, and syntax. Therefore, it can hardly explain the meaning of larger linguistic units, such as sentences and discourse. Concerning the neuroscience of syntax, there have been great advances on the neuroanatomy, neurodynamic, neurocomputation, and neuropathology of this fundamental language mechanism. However, most researchers examine syntactic processes in isolated individuals removed from communicational contexts, and they are mainly interested in the processing of syntactical structures *per se*, independent of sentence meaning. In other words, syntax is frequently considered a highly "modular" system, functionally and neuroanatomically dissociated from semantic and communicational processes.

A neurosemiotic approach to syntax should break the modular view of semantics and syntax as functionally separate mechanisms. Both neurosemantic and neurosyntactic studies should assume that language is mainly used for face-to-face communication, and that meaning is constructed cooperatively by speakers, using their linguistic (lexical and syntactical) and non-linguistic resources to align their representations (Garrod & Pickering, 2009) and their neural activity (Hasson et al., 2012; Jiang et al., 2012; Stephens et al., 2010; Stolk et al., 2014). The next section provides some arguments to support an alternative neurosemiotic approach to these topics.

Towards a neurosemiotics of syntactic meaning

What is syntax for? This simple question is seldom asked by researchers, often because of a restricted epistemological focus. The heuristic distinction between the faculty of language in a "narrow sense" and the faculty of language in a "broad sense" (Hauser et al., 2002) is relevant here. Language in a "narrow sense" is just syntax or, more specifically, the syntactic mechanism of recursion – namely, the capability to apply rewriting rules to strings of symbols (e.g., S→NP VP; NP→N; VP→V), which can produce arbitrarily complex embedded structures. Rather, language in a "broad sense" is a functional combination of linguistic processes properly (e.g., lexicon, syntactic recursion) and sensorimotor, conceptual, emotional, and intentional processes. The former approach is typical of formal structural linguistics following Chomsky's tradition, whereas the latter conceives syntactic construals as tools for communicating meaning.

Some psycholinguists and neuroscientists of language seem to accept a modular "narrow sense" of grammar, trying to dissociate syntactic computations from other linguistic functions, like meaning and communication (Willems & Varley, 2010). However, a neurosemiotic approach should respond to a "broad sense" of language by incorporating grammar as part of a multisystemic machinery to compute semantic and pragmatic functions in communicative contexts.

Syntactic constructions convey meaning

The functional dissociation between syntax and semantics advocated by some neuroscientists is misleading. Some animals, like songbirds, show certain competence to combine sounds according to simple (non-recursive) syntactic rules, constructing "phrases." However, songbirds – unlike humans – do not attach this syntactic capacity to their own semantic and communicational systems (Berwick et al., 2011; Hauser & Bever, 2008), and cannot flexibly express an infinite variety of meanings as we do. If recursive capacities in humans were disconnected from their semantic and communication systems, as in birds, our speech would be a system of sophisticated trills. What makes syntax an interesting phenomenon is that grammatical construals guide conceptual binding in online communication.

The functional links between grammar and semantics have been theoretically established by cognitive and functionalist linguistics. Contrary to the modular approaches to syntax, functionalist linguistic theories posit that grammatical tools, including morphological categories, grammatical words (pronouns, articles, conjunctions, prepositions, or auxiliary verbs), and syntactic structures convey crucial conceptual information (e.g., Goldberg, 2019; Jackendoff, 1992; Lakoff, 1987; Talmy, 2000), rather than being purely structural devices. That is, syntactic parsing correlates with conceptual parsing of some informative features in episodic situations. According to Bickerton (1990: 55):

> The relations that grammatical items can express include relative location (above, below, in, on, at, by, next to), relative time (before, after, while, and the various indicators of tense), relative number (many, few, some, the -s of plurality), relative directions (to, from, throughout, left, right, up, down), relative familiarity ("the," for things the speaker thinks the hearer will

> recognize, "a" for things the speaker thinks the hearer won't recognize), relative possibility (can, may, might), and relative contingency (unless, although, until, because), as well as a variety of relationships such as possession (of, possessive -s, have), agency (by), purpose (for), necessity (must, have to), obligation (should, ought to), existence (be), nonexistence (no, none, not) and so on and so forth.

In other words, in most languages a few privileged concepts are grammaticized. Namely, the conceptual features conveyed by morpho-syntactic units appear to be fundamental dimensions of human episodic experience, such as substance, time, space, causality, motion, agency, and intention. The syntactic construals serve to express relationships among concepts, such as who did what to whom, what is where, what is true of what, when it happened, and so on (Pinker, 2010).

Note that this proposal does not imply a strong "universalist" view of syntactic meaning. Instead of a set of biologically pre-wired syntactic rules, we can think that communicational alignment among millions of speakers across generations diachronically induces the emergence of syntactic constructions, as efficient tools for parsing situational parameters (Bohn et al., 2019; Galantucci, 2005; Steels, 2006). However, different communities may come up with slightly different syntactic solutions in their languages. Psycholinguists have reported many of them, related to the syntactic articulation of a given conceptual dimension or to the way that some concepts are conflated in syntactic structures. For instance, languages differ in the spatial perspective induced by their locative markers (Levinson & Levinson, 2003). That is, perspective in English is egocentric by default (e.g., *The cow is behind the fence* involves a speaker's point of view); while in other languages, like Maya Tzeltal, perspective is allocentric or independent of the speaker's point of view (e.g., *The cow is north of the fence*). In addition, motion verbs differ between languages in terms of which information is mandatorily conveyed by the verb and which is optionally referred to by the complement (Slobin, 2003). Thus, in English the mode (M) of motion is in the verb and the direction (D) is optionally in the complement – for example, *She swam* (M) *across* (D) *the river* – whereas the opposite occurs in Spanish – for example, *Ella cruzó* (D) *el río nadando* (M) / *She crossed* (D) *the river swimming* (M). Yet most languages incorporate a few situational concepts in their syntax, such as time, space, causality, ownership, and agency, allowing a fast-track encoding of highly informative parameters of the situations. In other words, syntax is crucial to provide meaning on its own rather than being a module for formal computations.

Syntactic constructions are referential tools

The philosopher W.V. Quine (1960) proposed a thought experiment. A linguist visits a remote tribe, and a native says *gavagai* pointing to a rabbit. According to Quine, this involves a logically unsolvable problem of reference. Does the native refer to the whole rabbit? Maybe she refers to a part of the rabbit, or the rabbit's jump, or a combination of rabbit and ground grass, or the rabbit's shadow, or a fly on the rabbit's ear. Quine was concerned with the indeterminacy of reference in the translation of single words from an unknown language to a familiar one, but indeterminacy is a general problem even among speakers communicating in the same language. For instance, suppose you are with a friend in a library, not surprisingly full of books, and you utter the word *book*. The underspecification of reference is quite similar to that in the *gavagai* case. Even though your friend recognizes the word *book* and automatically activates her conceptual knowledge of books and other associated concepts (types), she probably cannot decide which book you mean (token), or what you expect her to do (intention). Fortunately, speakers can combine content words, morphology, and grammatical words into syntactic construals, to produce informative predicates in a particular communication setting, to specify reference. For instance, if you say *Give me the red book on the table*, probably your friend will have enough contextual and intentional clues to bring you a particular book.

Specifying reference is not a trivial task, even in a simple case like the one mentioned above. In most circumstances, specifying reference is even more challenging, such as when a speaker refers to memory-based objects or events rather than actual perceptual entities, or when describing mental states (beliefs, wishes). For instance, if a friend says to you: "I enjoyed having dinner in the Restaurant Roma last night," she is proposing you to construe a singular episode discriminable from many other similar episodes in your memory, coming from your own experiences of dinners in restaurants, or secondhand experiences from movies, literature, or previous conversations. In addition, your friend is not only informing you about the specific dinner episode, but also about her emotional state of enjoyment. Moreover, reference specification is a multifactorial phenomenon. Referential uncertainty is reduced not only by content words and morpho-syntactic structures, but also by many other cognitive (speakers' shared knowledge, and intentions) as well emotional and paralinguistic (prosody, gestures, gazes, postures, emotional expressions) cues, which are actively used to produce referential alignment (Garrod & Pickering, 2009) or intercognition (Ibáñez & García, 2018).

We can consider three levels of referential problems that differ in their computational demands for the interlocutors in face-to-face communication (Figure 10.1), and are associated with different linguistic and non-linguistic tools (de Vega, 2008). These are (1) online reference, with words and sentences directly referring to perceptual entities in the current situation; (2) displaced reference, with sentences referring to virtual entities in simulated situation models; and (3) decoupled reference, with sentences referring to the speaker's mental states or attitudes (beliefs, wishes) or to hypothetical or unreal events, which frequently requires applying syntactic recursion to produce embedded predicates.

As Figure 10.1 illustrates, online reference occurs when co-present speakers communicate about their current environment, making use of deictic words and gestures, notably pointing, to directly index perceptual entities. Language also provides quite primitive deictic tools, such as demonstratives (*this, that*), pronouns (*I, you*) or adverbs (*now, afterwards, here, there*). In sentences like *give me that* or *now I am here*, the words *me, that, now, I,* and *here* are deictic pointers to persons, objects, or events in the current situation.

Deictic words are semantically very impoverished in that they provide little information about the referent. For instance, in the sentence *give me that*, the word *that* could be almost any object that is visible in the surroundings, and *me* could be any speaker who is talking at a given moment. In spite of this ambiguity, the specification of reference is quite easy because the speaker frequently uses strongly embodied paralinguistic resources. For instance, while saying *give me that*, the speaker could turn her head to the referred object, use a pointing gesture, or gaze at the object to ensure that the listener identifies it. Concurrently, the listener could track the speaker's motions and gaze to figure out which object the speaker is referring to. Online (deictic) reference involves a first-order embodiment, by which the speaker uses their body as an egocentric framework to specify reference. Basically, this first-order embodiment is supported by the sensorimotor system we use when we manipulate objects or navigate in the environment. This system automatically updates spatial relations when we move. Thus, despite our continuous reorientation and navigation in the environment, we manage to keep track of objects' positions in our peripersonal space (de Vega, 2008). Neurological studies confirm the automatic updating of the object-to-body relations after physical motion. For instance, single-neuron studies with monkeys found that the ventral premotor cortex automatically keeps track of the objects' position, even in darkness, allowing automatic updating of the objects' position as the body moves around (Graziano et al., 1997). This updating is not constrained to objects in the visual field, but also applies to hidden objects (e.g., at the back, or occluded), and large-scale environments where landmarks are not immediately perceived (Easton & Sholl, 1995).

Displaced reference occurs when people refer to memory-based entities that are not currently available for perception (Hockett, 1960). Specifying reference in this case requires using more sophisticated linguistic constructions, many of them expressing a figure–ground (F–G) relation. For instance, if your addressee asks you where John's home is, you can use locative constructions which

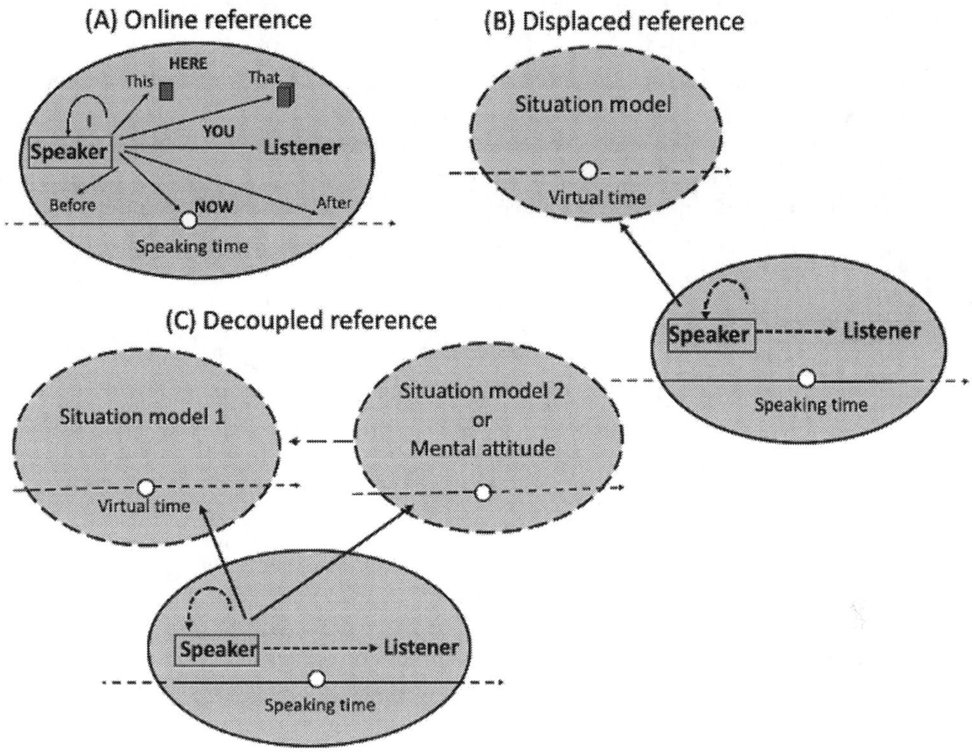

Figure 10.1 Schema of the three levels of referential problems

(A) Online reference to the current perceptual setting (solid line oval), using deictic words (e.g., *I, you, this, here, now*). (B) Displaced reference to entities in virtual situation models (dashed line oval) frequently uses figure–ground (F–G) constructions. (C) Decouple reference to alternative situation models or mental attitudes uses nonfactual constructions. See e-book for a full-color version of this figure.

allow you to refer to the unknown object position with respect to a well-known landmark (e.g., *John's home is behind Saint Patrick's church*). This involves computations that differ from online location by means of deictic expression (e.g., *this*) or gestures. Now you are forced to choose a landmark or "ground" to locate the target object or "figure," must parse the space around in directional categories (front, behind, right, left), and choose the one which better expresses the F-G spatial relationship (de Vega, 2008; Jackendoff & Landau, 1993; Logan & Sandler, 1996; Talmy 2000). The syntactic construals for displaced reference tackle not only spatial location, but also the other fundamental dimensions of the situation, mentioned in the previous section. For instance, *While John was writing a letter, Mary come into the room* (temporal relation); *Mary went to the concert because she loves country music* (causal relation); *Mary has the tickets for the concert* (ownership); or *Mary gave the tickets to John* (transference).

Finally, decoupled reference takes place when people communicate nonfactual events, or mental states, such as wishes or beliefs, introspectively observed in themselves or inferred in others. In some cases, language provides recursive structures for this level of reference, such as mentalist periphrases that govern an embedded predicate. For instance, *John doubts that Mary bought a new pair of shoes*. In this example, the sentence focuses on John's mental attitude rather than on a factual action. Also, there are constructions that refer to nonfactual or hypothetical events, in which the speakers consider two alternative states of the world. Notably, sentential negations (*There is no bread; John does not write novels*) deny an event, object or action, which probably was expected by the speakers (Kaup & Dudschig, 2019). Decoupled reference is even more evident in counterfactual sentences (*If you had bought that lottery ticket you would have won the grand prize*), which invite the listener to consider both the real and the alternative facts (Byrne, 2016).

Note that the linguistic resources of the three levels of reference can be flexibly combined in any situation. F–G constructions can be used with deictics for online communication: *Please bring me this book on the table*. Also, gestures can be associated with displaced reference, as when speakers make symbolic gestures while talking about an episode retrieved from memory (McNeill & Duncan, 2000). Finally, in written narratives, the writer and the reader do not share any communication setting, and yet deictic terms such as *I*, *here*, or *that* are continuously used to refer to virtual entities in a situation model rather than to the current environment.

Interim conclusions

This section proposed an integrative view of grammar, emphasizing its semantic functions and its role in the construal of referential meaning in communicative settings. It argued that syntactic structures convey information on some crucial semantic dimensions, facilitating a fast and automatic parsing of episodic events. Furthermore, it postulated that face-to-face communication is not just a matter of "exchanging concepts" between speakers, but rather involves the pragmatic goal of cooperatively specifying reference. This involves solving some types of computational problems for speakers, depending on whether the entities referred to are present, displaced or decoupled, and grammar provides different tools to do so.

The next section defends that syntax reuses pre-existing structures of the brain as an example of neural embodiment. It also encourages investigating the semantic and referential processes of syntax in communicational contexts and, after reviewing some promising literature on speakers' neural coupling, suggests some new avenues of research focusing on the pragmatic functions of syntax.

Syntactic constructions reuse ancient neural networks

An evolutionary principle of brain organization is the reuse of ancient neural circuits for new functions, while keeping the original functions (Anderson, 2010, 2014). Without a doubt, language is evolutionarily a recent function, and therefore it is likely that syntax reuses pre-existing neural networks. Let us focus on two examples of reuse: Broca's area and the inhibitory control system.

Broca's area

Broca's area is mostly situated in the left inferior frontal gyrus (IFG), and its homologous in non-human primates constitutes a motor control system. In humans, the left IFG is crucial for processing several aspects of speech, such as syntactic sequencing and recursion, while retaining primitive motor control functions (Hamzei et al., 2003; Nishitani et al., 2005; Tettamanti, 2013). In fact, neural reuse benefits from the functional equivalence between new and pre-existing functions, as both involve similar computations although with different purposes (Anderson, 2010, 2014). Therefore, Broca's area would be involved not only in syntax, but also in other tasks involving sequencing, such as action performance, action observation (Hamzei et al., 2003; Olivier et al., 2007), and even music processing (Patel, 2003; Sammler et al., 2013). Current neuroscientific studies confirmed a double function of the left IFG (especially Brodmann areas 44/45) in syntactic parsing and cognitive and motor control (Novick et al., 2010). For instance, when participants learn to parse structures in non-linguistic domains (specifically, hierarchical visuo-spatial events), they activate the same subregion in the IFG (BA 44) as in parsing syntactic structures in natural language (Friederici, 2017).

Recent neurophysiological studies indicate that syntactic sequencing and motor sequencing may share neural mechanisms (Casado et al., 2018, 2020). In these studies, participants were asked to self-pace three-segment sentences with linear structure (*The trees / and the fragrant flowers / blossomed in spring*) or embedded structure (*The trees / where the chicks nested / blossomed in spring*), using either a linear sequence of key pressing with three consecutive fingers of the right hand or using a non-linear sequence in which the middle finger key pressing was replaced by a foot pedal pressing. In half of the sentences, a target verb in the last segment violated syntactic agreement. The results indicated an interaction between motor sequencing and syntactic structure, observed in ERP components associated with syntactic violation. Convergently, there is clinical evidence that motor sequencing and syntax share neural grounds. Specifically, patients with motor disorders due to frontostriatal alterations, such as Parkinson's and Huntington's, show difficulties in syntactic parsing even at early stages of their disease (Birba et al., 2017).

The inhibitory control system

Beyond Broca's area, other neural networks can be actively involved in syntactic processing. The mechanisms of inhibitory control, primarily responsible for motor inhibition, can be reused for particular syntactic operations, such as the processing of sentential negation. In a set of studies, affirmative and negative sentences were presented in the context of motor inhibition tasks (go/no-go or stop-signal), as EEG signals were recorded from participants' scalps. The analysis of brain dynamics revealed that fronto-central theta oscillations – a neural signature of inhibition – were interactively modulated by negation in the context of a motor inhibition task, regardless of the action or non-action content of the sentence (Beltrán et al., 2019; de Vega et al., 2016). Furthermore, stop reaction time and early ERP components associated with inhibition (N1, N2) were modulated by sentential negation during motor inhibition conditions (Beltrán et al., 2018; Liu et al., 2020), and the estimated source for these effects was the right IFG, a main motor inhibition hub. For instance, Figure 10.2 illustrates a study in which affirmative and negative sentences were presented in the context of a stop signal task. In this task, a go signal appears on each trial, prompting participants to press a button, but in some trials a stop signal follows after a variable delay, indicating them to refrain from responding. The delay for go trials with a stop signal is varied individually as to produce about 50 percent successful inhibitions. The results showed that negative sentences modulate the inhibitory N1 component in successful stop signal trials, and the source of this modulation was the right IFG, suggesting that negation shares neural components with response inhibition.

Interim conclusions

This section suggested that the notion of neural reuse can be applied to grammar. First, it briefly reviewed the extensive literature on the multiple functions of Broca's area, which can be characterized as a brain resource for sequencing motor processes, understanding actions, processing music, and, of course, encoding and decoding syntactic structures. Furthermore, it offered evidence that the inhibitory control system, generally employed for suppression of motor responses, is reused to inhibit concepts in the context of sentential negation, as revealed by inhibition-related EEG signatures. The evidence suggests that the neural machinery of grammar is an extensive network that includes ancient structures reused for the new syntactic functions (Friederici, 2017).

Neural coupling in communication

If syntax is a tool for communicating referential meaning, as proposed here, then the most appropriate context for studying the underlying neural processes should be face-to-face communication. Presumably, the neural mechanisms of syntax are coupled and dynamically synchronized across interacting speakers, because they align their cognitive processes at several levels for the reference specification. Recently, there was a growing interest in examining the neural coupling of communicating pairs. The use of hyperscanning techniques allows registration of the brain activity of two interacting

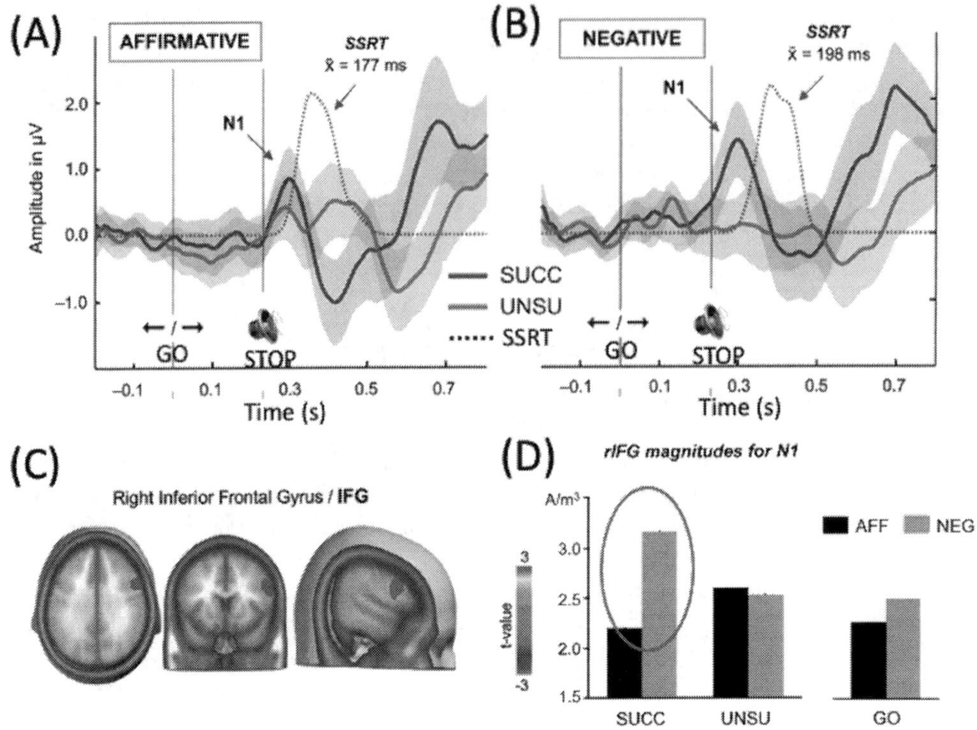

Figure 10.2 Empirical demonstration of the reuse of inhibitory control for linguistic negation

Affirmative (A) and negative (B) sentences differentially modulate the fronto-central inhibitory component N1, in the context of successful stop trials, and also differ in the estimated stop signal reaction time (SSRT). The estimated source of the effect is the right inferior frontal gyrus (IFG), a main structure in the inhibitory control network (C), which shows the largest activity for negative sentences in successful inhibitory trials (D). Figure adapted from Beltrán et al. (2018). See e-book for a full-color version of this figure.

participants at the same time. Some of these studies utilize non-verbal communication games, which provide interesting clues on the neural bases of mentalizing processes employed by communicators when they track the other's intentions and make predictions (Hasson et al., 2012; Krueger et al., 2007; Stolk et al., 2014). These non-verbal games provide a proxy of communication, including the shared goal of reference specification, but they do not tap on the role of language in providing shared reference between communicators.

A few studies have also examined neural coupling between speakers and listeners (Jiang et al., 2012; Schoot et al., 2014; Stephens, et al., 2010). For instance, Stephens et al. (2010) recorded hemodynamic activity of speakers telling a story and, in another moment, of listeners of the story. They found that listeners' brain activity overlapped with that of speakers in most cases, with a temporal delay, but this coupling faded in the absence of comprehension. Stephens et al.'s study did not involve real communication between co-present speakers following a turn-taking procedure. By contrast, Jiang et al. (2012) used functional near-infrared spectroscopy hyperscanning in different communication contexts – including, in some cases, real conversations and gestures. Notably, they demonstrated that brain-to-brain synchrony occurred when speakers conversed face to face, but it diminished when they were sat back to back and/or maintained a monologue, indicating that online social and intentional contexts are crucial to produce neural coupling and alignment. Finally, some fMRI studies exploit the syntactic priming effect observed when speakers influence each other in the choice of syntactic structures (Branigan et al., 2000). For instance, Schoot et al. (2014) asked participants to describe pictures either in a communication or a non-communication context. The results showed that repetition of syntactic structures (either active or passive transitive sentences), compared with novel syntactic structures, induced suppression effects in several syntax-related regions (both for speaker and listener), comprising the bilateral insula and extending to left IFG, middle temporal gyrus, inferior parietal cortex, and precentral gyrus, as well as the bilateral precuneus and supplementary motor area. Importantly, these neural priming effects were observed only in the communication group, although the task was identical in the non-communication group, except for the absence of a real interlocutor. The studies by Jiang et al. (2012) and Schoot et al. (2014) confirmed that face-to-face interaction between interlocutors increases neural coupling, compared with non-communication conditions with equivalent task demands.

Interim conclusions

The above studies on face-to-face verbal communication pioneer a new branch of the neuroscience of language. This branch is challenging because of the difficulty of designing ecologically valid communication contexts under the constraints of hyperscanning techniques while testing non-trivial hypotheses. The neural coupling associated with syntactic priming is a promising finding that supports alignment in face-to-face communication. However, other topics deserve future research (García & Ibáñez, 2014).

The neurosemiotic approach to the semantic and pragmatic functions of grammar advocated here could be tested optimally in communication settings, using hyperscanning to examine the coupling of neural activity in face-to-face verbal communication under different reference specification demands. For instance, in one context, speakers may be asked to communicate the position of objects in a spatial setting visible for the two speakers (online reference), requiring deictic words, gestures, and gazes; whereas in other context speakers may communicate the position of the objects when they are hidden from the addressee (displaced reference), which would demand relational F–G constructions. The neural coupling for online reference would involve more shared sensorimotor resources and less syntactic neural resources than displaced reference, despite sharing the communication goal of locating an object. Other face-to-face contexts can be conceived to induce communication of temporal events, causal relations, and intentionality, among other phenomena, each of them demanding different syntactic resources.

Concluding remarks

This chapter has offered a neurosemiotic approach to grammar and meaning, overcoming the restrictive modular views often found in the literature. It has presented evidence and arguments for an integrative view of grammar as subserving semantic and pragmatic goals in communication. According to this view, syntactic structures are not arbitrary, but reflect basic conceptual dimensions of human episodic experience. Consequently, syntactic parsing is strongly correlated with conceptual parsing, and the construction of meaning is based on grammar as much as on content words.

A core proposal in this chapter is that grammar has pragmatic functions, helping speakers to cooperatively specify referents. It is assumed that communication goes beyond the activation and "exchange" of concepts (types), since interlocutors must be able to identify the specific entities (tokens) that are being referred to. To further that aim, grammar provides various tools for solving the computational problem of reference. That is, online identification of referents relies on deictic words efficiently combined with embodied contextual cues (face expressions, prosody, gestures, gazes), whereas specifying displaced referents requires syntactic tools, such as F-G constructions, for instructing the addressee to create virtual situation models. Finally, decouple reference employs complex constructions to induce alternative situation models and/or provide information on internal states and attitudes.

The chapter posits that grammar hinges on distributed neural networks (Friederici, 2017), some of them with a sensorimotor evolutionary origin. We considered two examples. Broca's area, specialized in sequential motor processes, is reused for syntactic parsing, whereas the inhibitory control system, originally intended to suppress actions, is reused for suppressing concepts in sentential negation. Given the semantic and pragmatic role of grammar, a possible research avenue could be the application of hyperscanning to examine the alignment of neural processes between speakers when cooperatively solving referential problems and activating grammaticized concepts.

The integrative view of grammar developed in this chapter fits well with neurosemiotic principles and can provide guidelines for future research. Additionally, the neurosemiotic framework could be extended to other aspects not considered here, such as the neural interface of grammar with theory of mind, episodic memory, or emotions. Finally, it could be relevant to examine both the role of biological and socio-cultural factors in the origins of syntactic construals. The former could explain the observed similarities between languages, derived from our shared genetics, and neural, bodily, and environmental constraints. The latter could be responsible for the cross-linguistic differences reported by neo-Whorfian relativists. Be that as it may, a neurosemiotic view can help integrate the study of syntax and function words within a general conception of our socio-biological meaning-making capacities.

Note

1 The terms "modular" and "modularity" are used here in a double sense, as "encapsulated" mechanisms (Fodor, 1983) and as paradigm-based methodology.

References

Anderson, M. L. (2010). Neural reuse: A fundamental organizational principle of the brain. *Behavioral and Brain Sciences, 33*(4), 245–266. doi: 10.1017/S0140525X10000853

Anderson, M. L. (2014). *After Phrenology: Neural Reuse and the Interactive Brain*. Cambridge, MA: MIT Press.

Barutta, J., Cornejo, C., & Ibáñez, A. (2011). Theories and theorizers: A contextual approach to theories of cognition. *Integrative Psychological and Behavioral Science, 45*(2), 223–246. doi: 10.1007/s12124-011-9156-9

Beltrán, D., Morera, Y., García-Marco, E., & De Vega, M. (2019). Brain inhibitory mechanisms are involved in the processing of sentential negation, regardless of its content: Evidence from EEG theta and beta rhythms. *Frontiers in Psychology, 10*, 1782. doi: 10.3389/fpsyg.2019.01782

Beltrán, D., Muñetón-Ayala, M., & de Vega, M. (2018). Sentential negation modulates inhibition in a stop-signal task. Evidence from behavioral and ERP data. *Neuropsychologia, 112*, 10–18. doi: 10.1016/j.neuropsycholo gia.2018.03.004

Berwick, R. C., Okanoya, K., Beckers, G. J., & Bolhuis, J. J. (2011). Songs to syntax: The linguistics of birdsong. *Trends in Cognitive Sciences, 15*(3), 113–121. doi: 10.1016/j.tics.2011.01.002

Bickerton, D. (1990). *Language and Species*. Chicago: University of Chicago Press.

Binney, R. J., & Ralph, M. A. L. (2015). Using a combination of fMRI and anterior temporal lobe rTMS to measure intrinsic and induced activation changes across the semantic cognition network. *Neuropsychologia, 76*, 170–181. doi: 10.1016/j.neuropsychologia.2014.11.009

Birba, A., García-Cordero, I., Kozono, G., Legaz, A., Ibáñez, A., Sedeño, L., & García, A. M. (2017). Losing ground: Frontostriatal atrophy disrupts language embodiment in Parkinson's and Huntington's disease. *Neuroscience & Biobehavorial Reviews, 80*, 673–687. doi: 10.1016/j.neubiorev.2017.07.011

Bohn, M., Kachel, G., & Tomasello, M. (2019). Young children spontaneously recreate core properties of language in a new modality. *Proceedings of the National Academy of Sciences, 116*(51), 26072–26077. doi: 10.1073/pnas.1904871116

Branigan, H. P., Pickering, M. J., Stewart, A. J., & McLean, J. F. (2000). Syntactic priming in spoken production: Linguistic and temporal interference. *Memory & Cognition, 28*(8), 1297–1302. doi: 10.3758/BF03211830

Buccino, G., Colagè, I., Gobbi, N., & Bonaccorso, G. (2016). Grounding meaning in experience: A broad perspective on embodied language. *Neuroscience & Biobehavioral Reviews, 69*, 69–78. doi: 10.1016/j.neubiorev.2016.07.033

Buccino, G., Riggio, L., Melli, G., Binkofski, F., Gallese, V., & Rizzolatti, G. (2005). Listening to action-related sentences modulates the activity of the motor system: a combined TMS and behavioral study. *Cognitive Brain Research, 24*(3), 355–363. doi: 10.1016/j.cogbrainres.2005.02.020

Buzsáki, G. (2010). Neural syntax: Cell assemblies, synapsembles, and readers. *Neuron, 68*(3), 362–385. doi: 10.1016/j.neuron.2010.09.023

Byrne, R. M. (2016). Counterfactual thought. *Annual Review of Psychology, 67*, 135–157. doi: 10.1146/annurev-psych-122414-033249

Casado, P., Martín-Loeches, M., León, I., Hernández-Gutiérrez, D., Espuny, J., Muñoz, F., … de Vega, M. (2018). When syntax meets action: Brain potential evidence of overlapping between language and motor sequencing. *Cortex, 100*, 40–51. doi: 10.1016/j.cortex.2017.11.002

Casado, P., Martín-Loeches, M., Muñoz, F., Hernández-Gutiérrez, D., Jiménez-Ortega, L., Sánchez-García, J., … Fondevila, S. (2020). On the interplay between motor sequencing and linguistic syntax: Electrophysiological evidence. *Journal of Neurolinguistics, 53*, 100874. doi: 10.1016/j.jneuroling.2019.100874

de Vega, M. (2008). Levels of embodied meaning: From pointing to counterfactuals. *Symbols and Embodiment. Debates on Meaning and Cognition*, 285–308. doi: 10.1093/acprof:oso/9780199217274.003.0014

de Vega, M., Morera, Y., León, I., Beltrán, D., Casado, P., & Martín-Loeches, M. (2016). Sentential negation might share neurophysiological mechanisms with action inhibition: Evidence from frontal theta rhythm. *Journal of Neuroscience, 36*(22), 6002–6010. doi: 10.1523/JNEUROSCI.3736-15.2016

Easton, R. D., & Sholl, M. J. (1995). Object-array structure, frames of reference, and retrieval of spatial knowledge. *Journal of Experimental Psychology: Learning Memory, and Cognition, 21*, 483–500. doi: 10.1037/0278-7393.21.2.483

Fodor, J. A. (1983). *The Modularity of Mind*. Cambridge, MA: MIT Press

Friederici, A. D. (2009). Pathways to language: Fiber tracts in the human brain. *Trends in Cognitive Sciences, 13*(4), 175–181. doi: 10.1016/j.tics.2009.01.001

Friederici, A. D. (2017). *Language in Our Brain: The Origins of a Uniquely Human Capacity*. Cambridge, MA: MIT Press.

Galantucci, B. (2005). An experimental study of the emergence of human communication systems. *Cognitive Science, 29*(5), 737–767. doi: 10.1207/s15516709cog0000_34

García, A. M., & Ibáñez, A. (2014). Two-person neuroscience and naturalistic social communication: The role of language and linguistic variables in brain-coupling research. *Frontiers in Psychiatry, 5*, 124. doi: 10.3389/fpsyt.2014.00124

García, A. M., & Ibáñez, A. (2016). A touch with words: Dynamic synergies between manual actions and language. *Neuroscience & Biobehavioral Reviews, 68*, 59–95. doi: 10.1016/j.neubiorev.2016.04.022

Garrod, S., & Pickering, M. J. (2009). Joint action, interactive alignment, and dialog. *Topics in Cognitive Science, 1*(2), 292–304. doi: 10.1111/j.1756-8765.2009.01020.x

Goldberg, A. E. (2019). *Explain Me This: Creativity, Competition, and the Partial Productivity of Constructions*. Princeton, NJ: Princeton University Press.

Graziano, M. S., Hu, X. T., & Gross, C. G. (1997). Coding the locations of objects in the dark. *Science, 277*(5323), 239–241. doi: 10.1126/science.277.5323.239

Hamzei, F., Rijntjes, M., Dettmers, C., Glauche, V., Weiller, C., & Büchel, C. (2003). The human action recognition system and its relationship to Broca's area: An fMRI study. *Neuroimage, 19*(3), 637–644. doi: 10.1016/S1053-8119(03)00087-9

Hasson, U., Ghazanfar, A. A., Galantucci, B., Garrod, S., & Keysers, C. (2012). Brain-to-brain coupling: A mechanism for creating and sharing a social world. *Trends in Cognitive Sciences, 16*(2), 114–121. doi: 10.1016/j.tics.2011.12.007

Hauk, O., Johnsrude, I., & Pulvermüller, F. (2004). Somatotopic representation of action words in human motor and premotor cortex. *Neuron, 41*(2), 301–307. doi: 10.1016/S0896-6273(03)00838-9

Hauser, M. D., & Bever, T. (2008). Behavior: A biolinguistic agenda. *Science, 322*(5904) 1057–1059. doi: 10.1126/science.1167437

Hauser, M. D., Chomsky, N., & Fitch, W. T. (2002). The faculty of language: What is it, who has it, and how did it evolve? *Science, 298*(5598), 1569–1579. doi: 10.1126/science.298.5598.1569

Herrera, E., & Cuetos, F. (2012). Action naming in Parkinson's disease patients on/off dopamine. *Neuroscience Letters, 513*(2), 219–222. doi: 10.1016/j.neulet.2012.02.045

Hockett, C. (1960). The origin of speech. *Scientific American, 203*, 89–99.

Hodges, J. R., & Patterson, K. (2007). Semantic dementia: A unique clinicopathological syndrome. *The Lancet Neurology, 6*(11), 1004–1014. doi: 10.1016/S1474-4422(07)70266-1

Ibáñez, A (2019). Insular networks and intercognition in the wild. *Cortex, 115*, 341–344. doi: 10.1016/j.cortex.2019.01.024

Ibáñez, A., & García, A. M. (2018). *Contextual Cognition: The Sensus Communis of a Situated Mind*. Dordrecht: Springer.

Jackendoff, R. (1992). *Semantic Structures* (*Vol. 18*). Cambridge, MA: MIT Press.

Jackendoff, R., & Landau, B. (1993). "What" and "where" in spatial language and spatial cognition. *Behavioral and Brain Sciences, 16*(2), 217–265. doi: 10.1017/S0140525X00029733

Jiang, J., Dai, B., Peng, D., Zhu, C., Liu, L., & Lu, C. (2012). Neural synchronization during face-to-face communication. *Journal of Neuroscience, 32*(45), 16064–16069. doi: 10.1523/JNEUROSCI.2926-12.2012

Kaan, E., & Swaab, T.Y. (2002). The brain circuitry of syntactic comprehension. *Trends in Cognitive Sciences, 6*(8), 350–356. doi: 10.1016/S1364-6613(02)01947-2

Kaup, B., & Dudschig, C. (2019). Understanding negation. Issues on the processing of negation. In V. Deprez, & M.T. Espinal (Eds.), *The Oxford Handbook of Negation*. Oxford: Oxford University Press.

Klepp, A., Van Dijk, H., Niccolai, V., Schnitzler, A., & Biermann-Ruben, K. (2019). Action verb processing specifically modulates motor behaviour and sensorimotor neuronal oscillations. *Scientific Reports, 9*(1), 1–11. doi: 10.1038/s41598-019-52426-9

Krueger, F., McCabe, K., Moll, J., Kriegeskorte, N., Zahn, R., Strenziok, M., … Grafman, J. (2007). Neural correlates of trust. *Proceedings of the National Academy of Sciences, 104*(50), 20084–20089. doi: 10.1073/pnas.0710103104

Kuperberg, G. R. (2007). Neural mechanisms of language comprehension: Challenges to syntax. *Brain Research, 1146*, 23–49. doi: 10.1016/j.brainres.2006.12.063

Lakoff, G. (1987). *Women, Fire, and Dangerous things. What Categories Reveal About the Mind*. Chicago: University of Chicago Press.

Lambon Ralph, M. A., & Patterson, K. (2008). Generalization and differentiation in semantic memory: Insights from semantic dementia. *Annals of the New York Academy of Sciences, 1124*(1), 61–76. doi: 10.1196/annals.1440.006

Lambon Ralph, M. A., Pobric, G., & Jefferies, E. (2009). Conceptual knowledge is underpinned by the temporal pole bilaterally: Convergent evidence from rTMS. *Cerebral Cortex, 19*(4), 832–838. doi: 10.1093/cercor/bhn131

Levinson, S. C., & Levinson, S. C. (2003). *Space in Language and Cognition: Explorations in Cognitive Diversity*. Cambridge: Cambridge University Press.

Liu, B., Gu, B., Beltrán, D., Wang, H., & de Vega, M. (2020). Presetting an inhibitory state modifies the neural processing of negated action sentences: An ERP study. *Brain and Cognition, 143*, 105598. doi: 10.1016/j.bandc.2020.105598

Logan, G. D., & Sandler, D. D. (1996). A computational analysis of the apprehension of spatial relations. In P. Bloom et al. (Eds.), *Language and Space* (pp. 493–529). Cambridge, MA: MIT Press.

McNeill, D., & Duncan, S. D. (2000). Growth points in thinking-for-speaking. *Language and Gesture, 141*, 161. doi: 10.1017/CBO9780511620850.010

Mesulam, M. M., Wieneke, C., Hurley, R., Rademaker, A., Thompson, C. K., Weintraub, S., & Rogalski, E. J. (2013). Words and objects at the tip of the left temporal lobe in primary progressive aphasia. *Brain, 136*(2), 601–618. doi: 10.1093/brain/aws336

Molinaro, N., Barber, H. A., & Carreiras, M. (2011). Grammatical agreement processing in reading: ERP findings and future directions. *Cortex, 47*(8), 908–930. doi: 10.1016/j.cortex.2011.02.019

Moreno, I., de Vega, M., & León, I. (2013). Understanding action language modulates oscillatory mu and beta rhythms in the same way as observing actions. *Brain and Cognition, 82*(3), 236–242. doi: 10.1016/j.bandc.2013.04.010

Moreno, I., De Vega, M., León, I., Bastiaansen, M., Lewis, A. G., & Magyari, L. (2015). Brain dynamics in the comprehension of action-related language: A time-frequency analysis of mu rhythms. *NeuroImage, 109*, 50–62. doi: 10.1016/j.neuroimage.2015.01.018

Nishitani, N., Schurmann, M., Amunts, K., & Hari, R. (2005). Broca's region: From action to language. *Physiology, 20*(1), 60–69. doi: 10.1152/physiol.00043.2004

Novick, J. M., Trueswell, J. C., & Thompson-Schill, S. L. (2010). Broca's area and language processing: Evidence for the cognitive control connection. *Language and Linguistics Compass, 4*(10), 906–924. doi: 10.1111/j.1749-818X.2010.00244.x

Olivier, E., Davare, M., Andres, M., & Fadiga, L. (2007). Precision grasping in humans: From motor control to cognition. *Current Opinion in Neurobiology, 17*(6), 644–648. doi: 10.1016/j.conb.2008.01.008

Papeo, L., Vallesi, A., Isaja, A., & Rumiati, R. I. (2009). Effects of TMS on different stages of motor and non-motor verb processing in the primary motor cortex. *PloS One, 4*(2), e4508. doi: 10.1371/journal.pone.0004508

Patel, A. D. (2003). Language, music, syntax and the brain. *Nature Neuroscience, 6*(7), 674–681. doi: 10.1038/nn1082

Patterson, K., Nestor, P. J., & Rogers, T. T. (2007). Where do you know what you know? The representation of semantic knowledge in the human brain. *Nature Reviews Neuroscience, 8*(12), 976–987. doi: 10.1038/nrn2277

Pinker, S. (2010). The cognitive niche: Coevolution of intelligence, sociality, and language. *Proceedings of the National Academy of Sciences, 107*(Supp. 2), 8993–8999. doi: 10.1073/pnas.0914630107

Pobric, G., Ralph, M. A. L., & Jefferies, E. (2009). The role of the anterior temporal lobes in the comprehension of concrete and abstract words: rTMS evidence. *Cortex, 45*(9), 1104–1110. doi: 10.1016/j.cortex.2009.02.006.

Pulvermüller, F. (2010). Brain embodiment of syntax and grammar: Discrete combinatorial mechanisms spelt out in neuronal circuits. *Brain and Language*, *112*(3), 167–179. doi: 10.1016/j.bandl.2009.08.002

Pulvermüller, F., Hauk, O., Nikulin, V.V., & Ilmoniemi, R. J. (2005). Functional links between motor and language systems. *European Journal of Neuroscience*, *21*(3), 793–797. doi: 10.1038/nrn1706.

Pulvermüller, F., & Knoblauch, A. (2009). Discrete combinatorial circuits emerging in neural networks: A mechanism for rules of grammar in the human brain? *Neural Networks*, *22*(2), 161–172. doi: 10.1016/j.neunet.2009.01.009

Quine, W.V. O. (2013 [1960]). *Word and Object*. Cambridge, MA: MIT Press.

Sammler, D., Koelsch, S., Ball, T., Brandt, A., Grigutsch, M., Huppertz, H. J., ... & Friederici, A. D. (2013). Co-localizing linguistic and musical syntax with intracranial EEG. *NeuroImage*, *64*, 134–146. doi: 10.1016/j.neuroimage.2012.09.035

Schoot, L., Menenti, L., Hagoort, P., & Segaert, K. (2014). A little more conversation: The influence of communicative context on syntactic priming in brain and behavior. *Frontiers in Psychology*, *5*, 208. doi: 10.3389/fpsyg.2014.00208

Segaert, K., Menenti, L., Weber, K., Petersson, K. M., & Hagoort, P. (2012). Shared syntax in language production and language comprehension: An fMRI study. *Cerebral Cortex*, *22*(7), 1662–1670. doi: 10.1093/cercor/bhr249

Slobin, D. I. (2003). Language and thought online: Cognitive consequences of linguistic relativity. In D. Genter, & S. Goldin-Meadow (Eds.), *Language in Mind: Advances in the Study of Language and* Thought (pp. 157–191). Cambridge, MA: MIT Press.

Steels, L. (2006). Experiments on the emergence of human communication. *Trends in Cognitive Sciences*, *10*(8), 347–349. doi: 10.1016/j.tics.2006.06.002

Stephens, G. J., Silbert, L. J., & Hasson, U. (2010). Speaker–listener neural coupling underlies successful communication. *Proceedings of the National Academy of Sciences*, *107*(32), 14425–14430. doi: 10.1073/pnas.1008662107

Stolk, A., Noordzij, M. L., Verhagen, L., Volman, I., Schoffelen, J. M., Oostenveld, R., ... Toni, I. (2014). Cerebral coherence between communicators marks the emergence of meaning. *Proceedings of the National Academy of Sciences*, *111*(51), 18183–18188. doi: 10.1073/pnas.1414886111

Talmy, L. (2000). *Toward a Cognitive Semantics*. Cambridge, MA: Cambridge University Press.

Tettamanti, M. (2013). A research program in neuroimaging for an evolutionary theory of syntax. *Language and Cognition*, *5*(2–3), 157–166. doi: 10.1515/langcog-2013-0010

van Elk, M., van Schie, H. T., Zwaan, R. A., & Bekkering, H. (2010). The functional role of motor activation in language processing: Motor cortical oscillations support lexical semantic retrieval. *NeuroImage*, *50*(2), 665–677. doi: 10.1016/j.neuroimage.2009.12.123

Willems, R. M., & Varley, R. A. (2010). Neural insights into the relation between language and communication. *Frontiers in Human Neuroscience*, *4*, 203. doi: 10.3389/fnhum.2010.00203

11

DISCOURSE AND THE BRAIN

Capturing meaning in the wild

Nicholas Riccardi and Rutvik H. Desai

Introduction

Husband: "Hey, how was your day at work?"

Wife: "It felt so long. I had to speak with five different clients, and one of them is that stubborn one I've complained about before. The only break I had was when I walked to lunch with Susan; it was such a nice day out. When I get home, I just want to sit on the couch, eat some ice cream, and watch TV. How was yours?"

This semifictional phone conversation between a husband and his wife is just one example of "language in the wild," or natural language. It begins with a question prompt, to which the wife responds by telling the story of her day. The husband, as an active listener, must then process the arbitrary speech signs and symbols produced by his wife, convert them to meaningful messages, and understand them within larger contexts such as prior knowledge (e.g., the "stubborn client" she had complained about before) and future plans (e.g., relax and watch TV). In interpreting linguistic and nonlinguistic signs, the husband and wife are semioticians, like the rest of us.

Understanding how the brain derives meaning from language's arbitrary symbolic structure is foundational to neurosemiotics. The brain must not only extract meaning from isolated signs and symbols (e.g., individual sounds/words), but it must also interpret their meanings in the context of the information around them. The meaning of signs depends not just on the sign, but also on what is going on around the sign. A "thumbs up" sign means "everything is ok" or "I am with you" in many cultures. In scuba diving, though, it means "end the dive and rise to the surface." This is also the case with linguistic signs such as words. If the wife in the above example is a doctor, then "client" refers to individuals with health problems. If the wife is a lawyer, then clients are individuals involved in legal disputes and nothing is implied about their health status. This surrounding information that helps construct meaning takes many forms, including prior words in a sentence and discourse, the tone of the speaker (likely exasperated in the given example), nonverbal gestures, and knowledge that has been communicated to us previously (Susan is a friend or coworker of the wife). How does the brain represent this information?

Over the past two decades, a rich body of research has examined the neural basis of representation of meaning expressed in language. Using neuroimaging, brain stimulation, and lesion methods, it has revealed a distributed set of regions forming a complex network that dynamically represents

 DOI: 10.4324/9781003051817-14

various aspects of meanings of words and sentences (Binder & Desai, 2011; Binder et al., 2009; Desai & Riccardi, 2021). Most studies have relied on carefully selected word-, phrase-, and sentence-level stimuli. This choice is motivated by the fact that words have many psycholinguistic properties that are partly correlated with each other. To disentangle and pinpoint brain bases of any particular variable of interest (e.g., high imageability), it is necessary to control for myriad other variables (e.g., frequency, number of phonemes, orthographic and phonological neighbors) and to minimize the complex influence of context. This approach has provided fundamental and novel insights into how concepts are represented and processed in the brain, with wide-ranging theoretical and clinical implications (e.g., Lambon-Ralph et al., 2017). However, language in the wild does not often consist of single words or sentences that are not part of a larger discourse or narrative, defined here as language that is above sentence level. Naturalistic language takes multiple forms, many of which have distinct purposes. Narrative and expository genres are commonly distinguished (Clinton et al., 2020). Despite the variety, the main goal of virtually all natural language is to transfer information from one brain to another, a process sometimes referred to as "brain-to-brain coupling" (Hasson et al., 2012). To accomplish this coupling, multiple cognitive processes are required, including linking sentences together, integrating new information into the existing context, and learning relationships between concepts or characters within the discourse.

A growing body of research is aimed at examining not only how these discourse-level tasks are accomplished, but also the neural basis of lexical semantics and related psycholinguistic variables when language is processed in relatively naturalistic contexts (Kemmerer, 2021). This work is complementary to the traditional single-word and sentence-level approach and is essential to expanding our understanding of the representation of concepts in a more ecologically valid context, a topic of central importance to neurosemiotics. Here, we provide a brief overview of this research, focusing on fMRI studies – for a review of magnetoencephalographic and electroencephalographic studies, see Alday (2019). First, we discuss findings related to lexical semantics and related variables such as frequency and surprisal when words are processed in discourse context. Combinatorial operations and discourse-level processes are addressed next, followed by a discussion of the possible roles of major areas that are consistently implicated in discourse semantics. We conclude with cautions, caveats, and suggestions for future research.

Lexical processing in discourse context

Words have numerous psycholinguistic properties that have been studied using behavioral and neuroimaging methods. An interesting question is how or whether discourse context affects these variables. Here, we review some of the work that examines lexical variables in naturalistic context. Figure 11.1 shows activation peaks from several studies that parametrically examined some variables related to semantics (see also Table 11.1).

Word frequency

Different words are encountered at different rates in natural language. For example, the word "shop" happens much more often than the word "hippopotamus." Word frequency refers to how often a given word occurs in language, measured by counting occurrences in large text and speech corpora. It is a central psycholinguistic variable that has salient effects in both comprehension and production, and it explains the most variance in standard psycholinguistic tasks, such as lexical decision, picture naming, and word naming (Adelman et al., 2014; Balota et al., 2004; Benkí, 2003). Neuroimaging research using single-word stimuli has found that low frequency words are typically associated with greater activity than high frequency words in areas such as the inferior frontal gyrus (IFG), the anterior insula, the intraparietal sulcus (IPS), and the visual wordform area (VWFA), with this activity

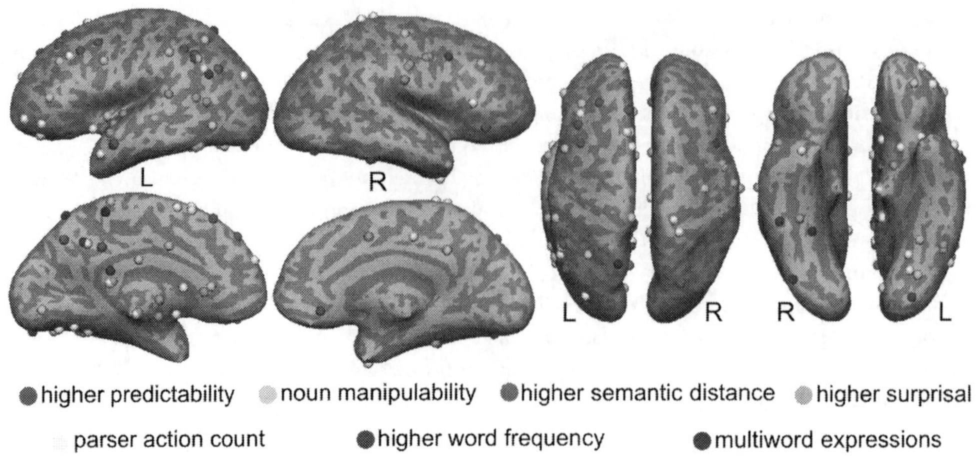

Figure 11.1 Activation peaks for several lexical variables studied in a discourse context

Taken from Bhattasali et al. (2018), Desai et al. (2018), Frank and Willems (2017), Willems et al. (2016), and Desai et al. (2016). See e-book for a full-color version of this figure.

Table 11.1 Variables associated with major regions implicated in naturalistic language studies. AG: angular gyrus; ATL: anterior temporal lobe; pCu/pCi: precuneus/posterior cingulate

Area	*Predictability*	*Semantic distance*	*Parser action count*	*Word frequency*	*Surprisal*	*Multiword expressions*
AG	Π	Π	Π	Π		
ATL		Π	Π		Π	
pCu/pCi		Π	Π	Π	Π	Π

often being attributed to higher phonological, orthographic, or executive demands (Graves et al., 2010; Hauk et al., 2008; Yarkoni et al., 2008). Effects of higher frequency are more controversial, with several studies finding no effects and a few studies finding increased activation in temporal and inferior parietal areas associated with semantics (e.g., Graves et al., 2010). Behavioral studies indicate that higher frequency words have richer semantic representations, measured by several variables such as the number of semantic neighbors, number of features, contextual diversity, and number of associates (Pexman et al., 2007; Reilly & Desai, 2017). Stronger automatic activation of this information may be expected for higher frequency words.

To investigate effects of frequency in naturalistic contexts, Desai et al. (2020) used concurrent fMRI and eye-tracking while participants silently read 22 paragraphs of text. Co-registration of fMRI signal and fixations from eye-tracking allowed extraction of word-specific responses. Rapid serial visual presentation is often used in studies with sentence and discourse stimuli, where presentation rate of words is controlled experimentally. Allowing participants to read entire paragraphs presented on the screen provides a more naturalistic scenario, as the participant controls fixation duration on each word, can re-fixate, or can skip words entirely, closely approximating natural reading. Frequency was modeled as a predictor, controlling for the psycholinguistic confounds of concreteness, number of letters and syllables, and lexical and syntactic surprisal. Higher frequency was correlated with greater activity in areas commonly associated with semantic processing, including the bilateral angular gyrus (AG), the precuneus/posterior cingulate (pCu/pCi), and the anterior temporal lobe (ATL). The authors interpreted these findings as an extensive and automatic activation of the semantic system due to high frequency words having greater semantic richness, a relationship enhanced by the semantic depth of a naturalistic context. This suggests that in some single-word studies, task-specific factors (e.g., the need to make a word/nonword response in a lexical decision task) may partially suppress this spread of activation, resulting in weaker positive correlations with frequency.

More strongly differing from single-word studies, this research showed relatively low levels of negatively correlated activity. The commonly seen activation in the IFG was missing. Lower frequency was correlated with greater activity in the left IPS and posterior supramarginal gyrus (SMG), which the authors attributed to attentional and phonological demands, respectively. Additionally, negatively correlated activity was reduced and a large cluster in the medial superior frontal gyrus (SFG) was eliminated after controlling for lexical and syntactic surprisal, suggesting that predictive processes during naturalistic reading may lower the neural costs of encountering low-frequency words. Methodologically, this study demonstrated that by using simultaneous eye-tracking and fMRI, a high temporal resolution signal can be extracted that enables study of word-level variables during naturalistic, self-paced narrative reading. This study also illustrates one dimension along which well-established results from single-word studies may differ when words are considered within the context of a narrative.

The above evidence reveals some effects of frequency on processing of linguistic symbols, and its interaction with context. These findings align with the basic semiotic insight that signs' meanings can vary with context. Due to richer semantic content (including both associations and features), a more extensive set of neuroanatomical areas is recruited to represent frequent signs. Effects of frequency are enhanced with naturalistic context, as deeper neural representation of individual symbols leads to more efficient textual integration and richer situation models.

Surprisal and entropy

The brain is constantly predicting what it will encounter next (Bubic et al., 2010), a feature that plays an important role in natural language processing. Multiple types of information are used during discourse to predict upcoming words and aid comprehension, including knowledge about the structure of the language (e.g., English has a subject-verb-object structure) and about the world (e.g., associated concepts). In an fMRI study, Willems et al. (2016) examined two aspects of prediction, surprisal and entropy, while participants passively listened to novel excerpts and their reverse as a control condition. Briefly, surprisal is defined as the probability of the current word given the previously encountered words (e.g., a word with high surprisal deviates significantly from what was expected). Entropy is defined as the probability distribution of all *upcoming* words at a given timepoint during a sentence. High entropy indicates that many different words are possible (low predictability), while low entropy means relatively few words are likely (high predictability). The authors used a computational model to give each content word in the novel a surprisal and entropy rating to reveal the neural correlates of these measures, while controlling for word frequency. High surprisal was associated with greater activity in the left VWFA, the bilateral STG and ATL, and the right IFG. Considering that the VWFA is sensitive to word forms and the STG comprises the primary and secondary auditory cortices, the authors interpreted activity in these areas as being related to lower-level auditory or wordform predictions that must be updated when encountering a surprising word. The bilateral ATL activity may be due to lexical-semantic integration demands, which are likely to increase in the event of high surprisal.

Low entropy was associated with increased activity in the right IFG, the left middle frontal gyrus (MFG), and the left AG. The authors speculated that the AG, which has been implicated as a semantic "convergence zone" (Binder & Desai, 2011; Bonner et al., 2013), may be involved in predicting the semantic content of the upcoming word. The IFG and MFG, on the other hand, have been associated with top-down domain-general processing. Here, their sensitivity to highly predictable words perhaps reflects their involvement in priming word representations that engage widely distributed in other brain areas.

These studies demonstrate that the brain constantly uses previous signs and symbols to predict what is coming next. When a word has high surprisal, indicating an unsuccessful prediction, multiple areas are recruited to update and integrate that unexpected symbol into the larger context. When a word is easily predicted (e.g., low entropy), spreading activation can ignite relevant features of the word before it is encountered, enabling efficient integration into context.

Semantic features

A vast body of literature has been devoted to understanding how semantic content is represented in the brain. This research has shown that the semantic system is widely distributed neuroanatomically, and that some parts of that system are preferentially involved in the representation of specific semantic features, while others are sensitive to many features. Broadly, studies have shown that the set of brain regions activated during naturalistic discourse is very similar to the lexical-semantic system that has been revealed by single-word or sentence studies. For example, in one of the earliest neuroimaging studies of narrative speech, Crinion et al. (2003) examined which brain areas were active while adult participants listened to children's stories. The control condition was listening to the story played in reverse, which makes the stories unintelligible while maintaining acoustic complexity and voice qualities of the narrator. When stories were contrasted with reversed stories, there was significant activation in the left ventral IFG and posterior STG, as well as the bilateral ATL extending posteriorly towards the middle temporal gyri and the STG. Following this, multiple neuroimaging investigations of narrative processing have found similar activation patterns (e.g., Awad et al., 2007; Choi et al., 2014; Crinion et al., 2006; Frank & Willems, 2017; Wang et al., 2015; Willems et al., 2016; Xu et al., 2005), with the addition of other regions such as the bilateral AG, MFG, pCi, and medial prefrontal cortex. These areas are well-established parts of the lexical-semantic system. Figure 11.2 shows activation peaks from three such studies. However, relatively coarse contrasts, such as speech versus reversed speech, do not allow for more detailed analysis of how individual semantic features are represented during discourse. Here, more specific analyses will be briefly discussed.

One such study by Wehbe et al. (2014), examined how brain activity was modulated by a set of syntactic, semantic, and discourse-level features while participants read a novel excerpt presented

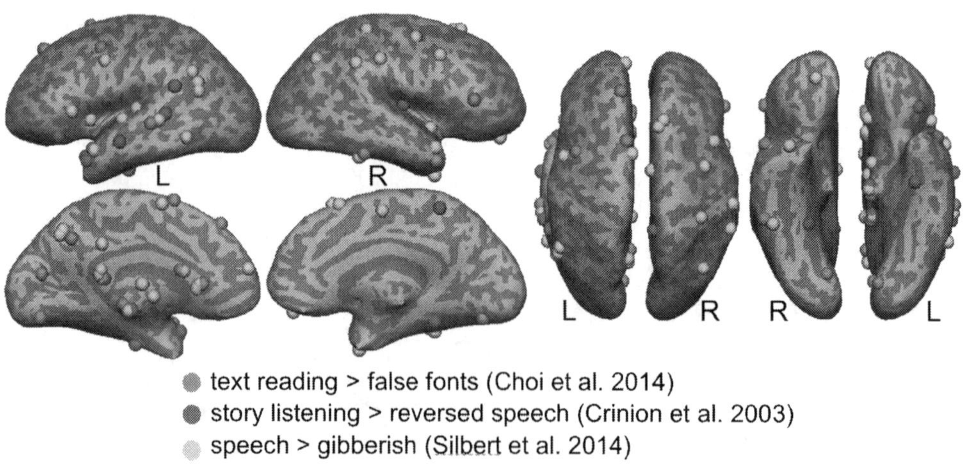

Figure 11.2 Activation peaks from three selected studies

These studies that have reported discourse processing relative to a low-level baseline, such as false fonts or reversed speech. Most peaks represent large surrounding clusters. See e-book for a full-color version of this figure.

word by word. They trained a computational model to predict brain activity in response to a set of 195 features (100 of which were related to semantic content) that were assigned to each word within the story. They found that the semantic features of words were encoded by neural activity in the left IFG and STG as well as the bilateral MTG and AG. At a finer-grained level, they found that words pertaining specifically to physical motions of story characters were represented in the left posterior STG and the left AG (areas implicated in biological motion perception and action), and that the identities of specific characters could be distinguished by activity within the right posterior STG/ MTG – an area associated with theory of mind (Saxe, 2006).

In a related study, Huth et al. (2016) recorded brain activity while participants listened to two hours of stories. They trained a model to predict the voxel-wise BOLD signal associated with the semantic features of individual words and found that semantic content of words was encoded by extensive bilateral activity in the frontal, temporal, and parietal lobes. Using dimension-reduction, the words were weighted according to 12 major semantic categories, such as emotional, social, visual, and numeric. Results suggested that the previously mentioned areas of the cortex comprised semantic "tiles," wherein certain sub-regions are uniquely selective for specific semantic features. For example, areas proximal to the AG were selective for social concepts, while surrounding areas in the parietal cortex were selective for numeric, visual, and tactile concepts. Tiles within the temporal and frontal lobes were selective for other semantic features, such as tactile or violent associations. These semantic tiles were largely consistent across individual participants, demonstrating that either innate neurobiological principals or shared cultural experiences may influence the organization of semantic feature representations in the brain.

This study is an outstanding example of leveraging a large dataset combined with sophisticated analyses to enable examination of lexical semantics during natural speech, for thousands of words simultaneously. A lack of consideration given to potential confounds is a limitation. The authors included only word rate, phoneme rate, and phonemes as covariates. Yet words have many psycholinguistic properties that affect their processing (e.g., frequency, contextual diversity, age of acquisition, associative and taxonomic semantic neighborhoods, phonological neighborhood, to name a few major ones), in addition to many semantic dimensions and other more specialized variables (such as clustering coefficient, biphone/triphone frequency, number of senses, cumulative frequency, and consistency) – let alone their phrase-, sentence-, and discourse-level properties. If such variables are even mildly differentially correlated with semantic categories, the results can be misleading. This is a potential reason why extensive bilateral activation was found in this study, including many perplexing results. For example, it is difficult to explain why the right MFG – an area strongly associated with executive processes such as monitoring and sustained attention – contains a tile representing tactile concepts. Some of the activation, especially in frontal and parietal areas, may represent a mix of conceptual representations, executive processing, and psycholinguistic confounds.

Another important question in naturalistic contexts pertains to how the brain represents and integrates the semantic content of words that are thematically related, but taxonomically dissimilar. For example, in the sentence "the man drank the water," none of the content words have similar meanings, yet they are thematically related, making the sentence readily comprehensible. In an fMRI study, Frank and Willems (2017) examined this by generating semantic vector representations for each content word from novel excerpts presented auditorily to participants. Within each sentence, the associative semantic distance between the content words and the preceding words was calculated and then correlated with the BOLD signal, controlling for word frequency and surprisal. They found that higher semantic distance was associated with increased activity in the left ATL, the pCu, and the bilateral AG. This suggests that these areas may be involved not only in representing semantic features, but also in the higher-level process of establishing thematic relationships between semantically dissimilar words – for a review, see Mirman et al. (2017).

In a similar vein, during discourse processing, information is sometimes encountered that is not only semantically dissimilar from previous words in a sentence but globally inconsistent with the information that has been given previously (e.g., a "twist" in a story). Ferstl et al. (2005) examined this as participants listened to stories that provided either chronological or emotional information. Half the stories were globally consistent, while the other half contained a word or phrase at the end that contradicted what had been learned throughout the story (e.g., the first five sentences described a character in a happy situation, but the sixth sentence stated that the character felt sad). Participants were instructed to pay close attention for inconsistencies. By comparing emotional versus chronological conditions regardless of (in)consistency, they found that the pCu, the IPS, and the temporoparietal junction (TPJ) were more active for chronological stories, while the ventromedial prefrontal cortex and the amygdala were associated with emotional ones. This corroborates previous studies showing that certain brain areas are preferentially involved in comprehension depending on the type of semantic information being processed. Then, by comparing consistent versus inconsistent stories at the onset of the target word (collapsed across story type), the authors found that right ATL activity was significantly higher for the inconsistent than consistent condition. This suggests that the right ATL is recruited when encountering unexpected lexical-semantic information, perhaps reflecting increased processing demands when there is a sudden need to update the preceding context.

These studies show how different features of objects or signs, such as perceptual or emotional characteristics, are represented in brain areas that are both information-specific and information-general, and which regions are involved in updating and integrating this information in light of context.

Embodiment

Considerable evidence suggests that conceptual processing relies, at least in part, on brain areas that are involved in physical action or perception (Binder & Desai, 2011), a finding couched in "embodied" or "grounded" theories of cognition. Under this framework, primary or secondary action/perception brain areas functionally contribute to the representation of corresponding semantic features – for example, comprehending action concepts such as "kick" would involve portions of action network (Desai et al., 2015; Johari et al., 2021; Riccardi et al., 2019, 2020). Although many single-word and sentence studies address the relationship between action/perception circuits and conceptual representation, far fewer studies examine this relationship in the context of natural discourse.

Desai et al. (2016) explored the neural correlates of noun manipulability during natural reading using simultaneous eye-tracking and fMRI while participants silently read short passages. Using eye-fixation timepoints, they correlated noun manipulability ratings with the BOLD signal while controlling for number of letters, word frequency, and concreteness. Higher manipulability was associated with greater activity in the bilateral inferior parietal lobe, including the SMG and the AG, as well as the left inferior temporal sulcus. Importantly, these areas have been implicated in the actual use of tools in fMRI and neuropsychological studies. This suggests that, during naturalistic reading, conceptual representation of manipulability recruits action/perception circuits.

Further evidence comes from Birba et al. (2020a), who used transcranial direct current stimulation (tDCS) to examine how stimulation of the primary motor cortex (M1) might affect action-content processing during naturalistic narratives. Participants received tDCS over the left M1, sham stimulation of M1, or stimulation of the left ventrolateral prefrontal cortex. After stimulation, they listened to action texts (ATs, stories that were highly action-related) and neutral texts (NTs, stories lacking action associations), and then answered questions about information either relevant to the verbs in the stories or about circumstances (locative or chronological details). They found that, for the AT condition, M1 stimulation selectively decreased performance in the verb-related questions compared to the circumstantial questions. Importantly, this effect was specific to M1 group (no such effects was found in the other two groups) and it survived after controlling for working memory and vocabulary skills.

In a similar study, this time using electroencephalography, Birba et al. (2020b) recorded brain activity while bilingual participants read ATs and NTs in their first and second languages (L1, L2).

When reading in L1, the AT condition (compared to NT) was associated with increased connectivity between electrodes that have been traditionally implicated in action-related processes. While this group-level effect was not found in the L2 condition, the authors found that greater action-related connectivity for AT was associated with greater L2 proficiency and earlier age of L2 acquisition. These findings suggest that action language processing involves functional connections between action-related brain areas, and that the strength of this connectivity is associated with how consolidated the language is. Taken together, these investigations corroborate single word studies demonstrating a relationship between processing the meanings of linguistic symbols and action/perception circuits, and they show that this relationship remains important for semantic representation even in naturalistic contexts.

Combinatorial and compositional processing

Discourse comprehension requires the combination of smaller symbols into a larger whole at multiple levels. For example, at a relatively low level, individual words must be combined into meaningful phrases. At higher levels, the meanings conveyed through phrases, sentences, and paragraphs must be linked to create a cohesive narrative. Understanding the anatomical organization of how units of information are combined is a vital goal for neurosemiotics, as encountering single words in isolation is relatively rare in everyday life. Here, we briefly review some investigations of the neural bases of combination and composition.

Bhattasali et al. (2018) examined the neural correlates of combination and retrieval at the phrase level using fMRI while participants listened to a story. They used a computational model to identify "multi-word expressions" (MWEs), or word sequences that are better treated as a single unit instead of multiple smaller units that need to be combined. They also used a parser-action counter to measure the compositional complexity of word sequences, with the intention of measuring brain activity associated with having to build a phrase from the bottom up. They hypothesized that MWEs, which may not require as much bottom-up composition, would be associated with memory processes, while composition would rely more on brain areas typically associated with combinatorial processes. After controlling for word frequency and the intensity and frequency of the auditory stimulus, they found that the presence of MWEs was associated with greater activity in the right pCu. Composition, on the other hand, was associated with many brain areas, including the bilateral ATL, IFG, and TPJ, as well as the left posterior STG/MTG and the right AG. In a second analysis, MWEs were rated based on their "cohesiveness" (more cohesive MWEs are more likely to be memorized than less cohesive ones). More cohesive MWEs were associated with right pCu activity, while less cohesive MWEs were associated with left-lateralized AG, MTG, ATL, and IFG activity. pCu is implicated in episodic memory, supporting the authors' claim that MWE processing is supported by memory. Composition, on the other hand, relies on a variety of areas bilaterally which have been implicated in semantic and syntactic representation and combination.

Brennan and Pylkkanen (2012) investigated compositional processes by using magnetoencephalography to record brain activity while participants read *Sleeping Beauty* (presented one word at a time). Magnetoencephalography is a powerful method for naturalistic language research, as it provides good spatial resolution while also allowing for millisecond-level temporal resolution. They compared activity for words in the narrative condition to a control condition where the words were presented in scrambled order. They found that, for the narrative condition, ATL activity significantly increased 250 ms after word onset, which they attributed to sentence-level compositional and combinatorial processes.

In another investigation of composition, Hsu et al. (2019) used simultaneous eye-tracking and fMRI to study brain activity while participants read passages from scientific texts. They used word order to operationally define the processes of composition and integration. Earlier content words were considered to be important for composition, as they are involved in the initial building of the meaning of the sentence. Later words were considered to be measuring integrative processes, where new information is added to the context built by previous words. Earlier words were associated with greater activity in the bilateral pCu/pCi, the anterior cingulate (ACC), the right insula, and the left posterior fusiform gyrus. Later words were associated with activity in areas such as the left AG, SMG, and MTG, as well as the bilateral pCu and IFG. This suggests that different brain areas might be more involved in the initial building of the information structure compared to later integrative processes. They also examined neural activity associated with the texts' knowledge structure, a graph theoretical measure of how well associations between concepts are communicated by the text. Texts with optimal knowledge structure allow for more efficient composition and integration of the provided information. Optimal knowledge structure was associated with greater activity in the left MTG, STG, and dorsolateral prefrontal cortex, while suboptimal knowledge structure was associated with greater activity in the bilateral ACC and the left IFG. This suggests that when information is more difficult to combine into a coherent whole, the brain may recruit areas related to executive processes, such as dual-tasking and attention.

Xu et al. (2005) examined how brain activity was modulated as participants progressed through the beginning, middle, and end of a collection of fables presented via text. This allowed for a broad investigation of the neural correlates associated with synthesizing narrative elements into a coherent whole. By comparing the beginning of the story to the control condition of randomly presented words, they found that initial story composition was associated with a largely left-lateralized network of regions including the IFG, the ATL, and the AG. However, when directly contrasting the end of the story with the beginning, they found that the activity had shifted to become more bilateral, including areas such as the right ATL, AG, pCu, and IFG. This suggests that, as narrative elements are integrated into a complete story, right hemisphere areas are recruited to aid in the possibly richer representation of the narrative and connect it to prior experience, knowledge, and beliefs.

These studies explored how the brain combines and integrates linguistic symbols at phrase, sentence, and narrative levels. At the phrase level, different brain areas are preferentially recruited depending on whether the phrases are very common or fixed (likely relying on memory processes) or more unique (requiring meaning to be built from the ground-up). At sentence and narrative levels, different brain areas are more involved in processing early information, when the sentence or story is first being built, compared to later information, which requires integration to the already existing knowledge structure.

Regions involved in semantics of discourse processing

As we have seen, many cognitive processes are required to successfully make meaning from linguistic symbols in naturalistic contexts, ranging from relatively low-level lexical-semantic retrieval of single words, to combinatorial processes, all the way up to higher-level functions such as contextual integration, creation of situation models, and inferring thoughts, emotions, and motivations of actors within the narrative. Several brain regions are consistently implicated in the semantics of naturalistic discourse processing and can be thought of as neurosemiotic "hubs." We now discuss possible roles of these regions, relating them to cognitive processes involved in interpretation of signs.

Anterior temporal lobe

The ATL is one of the most common regions activated during naturalistic language processing. A large body of research implicates the ATL in lexical access (Mesulam et al., 2013), semantic knowledge (Lambon-Ralph et al., 2017), combinatorial processes (Brennan et al., 2012), and social-emotional processing (Olson et al., 2013), all of which are part of discourse comprehension. Given the previously discussed evidence, it is possible that the ATL plays a special role in combining and integrating lexical-semantic information, perhaps especially so when that information is unexpected or difficult to synthesize. Naturalistic language studies have found that ATL activity is associated with high surprisal (Willems et al., 2016), semantic distance (Frank & Willems, 2017), and compositional demands (Bhattasali et al., 2018) at the sentence-level. The right ATL was also activated in response to encountering a word that was inconsistent with the previous context (Ferstl et al., 2005). All of these processes required the combination and integration of new, and sometimes unexpected, lexical-semantic items into an existing context.

The ATL has also been implicated in syntactic structure building (e.g., Brennan & Pylkkanen, 2012, 2017). For example, using magnetoencephalography, Brennan and Pylkkanen (2017) found that ATL activity was associated with the amount of syntactic structure being processed during naturalistic listening – see also Henderson et al. (2016). The investigation of composition by Bhattasali et al. (2018), discussed previously, could also be interpreted as measuring syntactic structure building, as their measure of composition was parser-action count. However, as noted by Brennan et al. (2012), it is difficult to disentangle syntactic from semantic processes during natural language comprehension, given that as syntactic structure is being built, semantic content is also being processed.

Here we briefly suggest a novel hypothesis: that the role of lateral ATL in language processing is *lexical* rather than semantic or syntactic. ATL may represent units that connect (orthographic and phonological) lexical forms to their meaning. It contains both long-term and short-term memory (STM) for unique items (such as words). This hypothesis can explain why unexpected or semantically distant words lead to greater activation in ATL, as the prior context needs to be kept active longer in STM in order to re-evaluate and integrate the unexpected item. This interpretation is also consistent with the syntactic structure building account, as new nodes in the syntactic tree place greater demands on STM. At the discourse level, STM is used to link various components of discourse and for anaphora resolution, leading to greater involvement for discourse over sentences. This hypothesis differs from the semantic hub view in that, for our account, the ATL is not responsible for storing coherent concepts themselves, but instead points to the distributed semantic representations elsewhere. Deficits in language tasks after ATL damage arise from impairments in *access* to semantic content rather than to semantic content itself. Thus, the ATL is a critical neurosemiotic hub that connects the sign to its object (or what is signified), when the relationship between the two is largely arbitrary or symbolic. This hypothesis awaits further experimental examination.

Angular gyrus

The AG is another important part of the neurosemiotic system. This structure has been implicated in functions such as semantic representation, especially for concrete concepts (Wang et al., 2010), as well as episodic memory and attention – for a review, see Seghier (2013). It is also part of the default mode network (DMN), a group of brain areas that are active when participants are at "rest" (i.e., not actively attending to stimuli or performing an explicit task in the scanner). Interestingly, DMN activity has been attributed to mind-wandering or daydreaming (Kucyi & Davis, 2014) and has a large contribution from semantics, as participants may be thinking about past, future, or hypothetical events, including people, objects, and relations in the events. This is a state of mind that shares many similarities with naturalistic language processing.

Naturalistic language studies suggest that the AG may serve as a high-level semantic convergence zone that not only represents specific semantic features, but might also prime semantic representations, including events that engage mechanisms elsewhere in the brain (Binder & Desai, 2011). Evidence that the AG subserves processing of specific semantic features in discourse comes from Desai et al. (2016) and Wehbe et al. (2014), who found that AG activity was associated with noun manipulability and physical motions of characters, respectively. Other studies provided evidence that the AG is involved in semantic representation at an even higher level. For example, Wehbe et al. (2014) demonstrated that the AG encodes semantic features of words, while Desai et al. (2020) and Willems et al. (2016) associated AG activity with the representation of rich semantic contexts, larger semantic neighborhoods, and priming of the larger semantic system when upcoming words are strongly predicted. This also meshes with its role in representing thematic relationships between concepts (Schwartz et al., 2011). Frank and Willems (2017) found that AG activity was associated with words that were semantically dissimilar from previous words in the sentence, a situation which would require thematic relationships to be built between semantically unrelated concepts (e.g., *the man drank the water*). Additionally, studies showing that AG activity increases towards the end of sentences (Hsu et al., 2019) or stories (Xu et al., 2005) could be interpreted as evidence of greater thematic processing, or "semantic structure building," as more complex relationships between characters or concepts are established. Thus, AG may have role in integration of distributed features to form coherent lexical concepts, as well as integration across time spanning phrase, sentence, and discourse-level scales to form event concepts.

Precuneus and posterior cingulate

The pCu and pCi are frequently activated but less well understood hubs of conceptual activity. They are sensitive to lexical semantic variables such as concreteness (Binder et al., 2009), but are also active during higher-level processes such as daydreaming, internally-directed cognition, episodic memory, emotion, and theory of mind – for reviews, see Cavanna and Trimble (2006) and Leech and Sharp (2014). They are also part of the DMN and are highly functionally connected to multiple brain networks. This has led to suggestions that these areas are involved in "tuning" or coordinating activity in distributed areas of the brain. It is possible that in naturalistic language processing, the pCu and pCi are involved in building and maintaining "situation models," which comprise information about characters, events, and settings within the discourse (Kemmerer, 2021). Support for this account comes from studies demonstrating that these regions become more active as sentences and stories progress (Hsu et al. 2019; Xu et al. 2005), perhaps reflecting the updating of situation model content. Activity in these regions is also associated with "event boundaries" in narratives, where information about characters, time, events, and locations is changed (Speer et al., 2007). Further evidence comes from Ferstl et al. (2005), who found that the left pCu was activated in response to stories containing chronological information, which is an important part of the situation model. Two functional divisions of the pCu/pCi territory have been suggested (Cavanna & Trimble, 2006). The anterior section, including the pCi and retrosplenial cortex, would be associated with mental imagery and spatial navigation especially for egocentric processing, with higher activation for concrete concepts. The posterior region would be more involved in episodic memory retrieval, exhibiting greater activity for abstract concepts (Desai et al., 2018b). Thus, this large territory as a whole may play a central role in updating situation models involved in discourse, through episodic memory with both concrete/spatial and abstract components. A better understanding of how the pCu and pCi are involved in building and integrating linguistic symbols into situation models will be important for a complete neurosemiotic model.

Bilaterality

Although it is agreed that the brain's language systems are at least partially bilateral, most traditional language studies find largely left-lateralized activity with limited involvement of the right hemisphere (Binder et al., 2009), and neuropsychological studies have shown that patients with right hemisphere brain damage usually have better language-related outcomes than those with left hemisphere damage. In contrast to these observations, many of the investigations described above found highly bilateral activity associated with naturalistic language processing. This raises the important question of how the right hemisphere is contributing to discourse comprehension (Beeman & Chiarello, 2013).

One possibility is that the right hemisphere is contributing to "paralinguistic" processes – that is, aspects of communication that are not directly related to language. For example, research has shown that the right hemisphere is involved in nonverbal semantic processing, speech prosody, pragmatics (use of language in context), and understanding subtle linguistic or social cues (Lehman Blake et al., 2013). Paralinguistic information is an important part of effective communication, and hence is important for understanding how different types of signs contribute to meaning-making. These paralinguistic processes could be expected to play a more significant role in naturalistic language than in single-word or sentence studies, leading to greater bilateral activity. Another possibility, as suggested by Ferstl et al. (2005), is that the right hemisphere is recruited in response to increased processing demands associated with naturalistic language processing. Under this hypothesis, the heightened conceptual, compositional, and integrative demands of discourse lead to the activation of homologous right hemisphere areas to support functions that usually could be handled by the left hemisphere. Future studies should seek to reveal how right hemisphere areas functionally contribute to the neural representation of signs, their objects, and their interpretations.

Neurosemiotics and language in the wild

The studies discussed here represent initial steps into the neurosemiotic quest for understanding brain bases of representation and processing of signs. The "good news" is that, at least for some psycholinguistic variables, the wealth of insight that has been accumulated from studies of relatively isolated signs and symbols is applicable to their processing in naturalistic contexts as well. At the same time, the evidence from the naturalistic language research discussed in this chapter can both inform, and be informed by, neurosemiotic perspectives of meaning and comprehension. Perhaps most significantly, the findings help delineate the neuroanatomy of specific semiotic processes, such as connecting the sign to its object, representing and interpreting the meaning of the object, and combining smaller symbols into a coherent whole. These anatomical findings also give credence to a holistic and dynamic view of symbol processing, much in line with neurosemiotic perspectives. That is, the results show that the anatomical representations of symbol processing change dynamically within the larger context of a narrative, due to complex interactions between many different types of signs and symbols (i.e., both linguistic and paralinguistic).

Naturalistic language research in cognitive neuroscience, on the other hand, can be informed and inspired by the more holistic neurosemiotic perspective. Traditional neuroscientific research tends to be highly modular, with the goal of investigating a single, specific process (e.g., syntax, semantics). Conversely, semiotic perspectives underscore the fact that these processes interact with each other in dynamic, highly complex ways in order to build meaning out of a combination of linguistic, paralinguistic, and social/contextual signs and symbols. A clear goal for the field is to delineate how these factors influence the ways in which the brain represents meaning.

Cautions, caveats, and future directions

Naturalistic language research is essential for a more complete understanding of neurosemiotics. However, similar to single-word studies, it comes with inherent limitations and difficulties, which must be addressed. First, it is difficult (and sometimes impossible) to disentangle specific cognitive processes, including the broad categories of syntax and semantics, and many sub-processes within, when using naturalistic stimuli. This limits the strength of conclusions that can be drawn pertaining to the contributions of individual brain areas. Relatedly, using low-level control conditions such as reversed speech or pseudoword passages allows for only coarse conclusions regarding discourse processing, and does not shed light on specific components of this process. When examining any particular component of meaning, the issue of confounds and correlated variables is also non-trivial. The number of psycholinguistic variables that affect processing of just single words is virtually unlimited. Over 200 psycholinguistic variables are currently known and have been used, and this list is continually increasing. It can be argued that the traditional approach of studying a particular variable by matching conditions on all other variables is misleading and provides a false sense of security, because there are always other variables that are not accounted for. Some argue that the solution to this problem is to collect a large amount of data and not worry about controlling for potential confounds. We disagree with such an approach, which advocates for simply ignoring confounds. It is true that perfect matching of lexical (or phrase and sentence level) variables is virtually impossible; however, it does not mean that not accounting for any or few variables is somehow better than controlling for as many major variables as possible. Through decades of psycholinguistic research, several salient lexical variables have been identified (e.g., frequency, contextual diversity, letter and phoneme length, consistency, and imageability/concreteness, as well as orthographic, phonological, and semantic neighborhoods). Further contributions come from sentence and discourse-level variables, such as surprisal and entropy, verb argument structure, and sentence type. This knowledge from past research should be used while acknowledging that any list of variables is never complete. Collecting large amounts of data can ensure that words typically occur in multiple contexts, and this can limit effects of any specific context. However, this does not automatically solve the problem of confounds. If anything, it can exacerbate it, because with a large *n*, even small correlations become significant. Control conditions with randomized sentences and word lists (as opposed to nonspeech or similar low-level controls) can possibly provide a better "out" from the conundrum of matching for psycholinguistic variables.

The study of naturalistic language is advancing in a number of fruitful directions – see Newman-Norlund et al. (2021) for a description of an ongoing, large-scale investigation that includes discourse and naturalistic language measures. These include: (1) better control for lexical and sentence-level variables either through randomized presentation or matching; (2) combining methods to leverage their unique strengths (e.g., fMRI and eye-tracking, or fMRI and electroencephalography); (3) carefully manipulating discourse content to isolate specific components of discourse processing; (4) studying structural and functional connectivity and its modulation during discourse; (5) studying oscillatory activity at different time scales; and (6) using brain stimulation methods to address roles of specific regions in discourse processing. Studies that use naturalistic materials, while certainly being demanding, promise to pay rich dividends in advancing neurosemiotics.

Conclusion

In this chapter, we have provided a brief review of neuroscientific studies investigating how the brain derives meaning from language in naturalistic contexts, a question at the heart of neurosemiotics. The findings revealed a distributed network of brain areas that work together dynamically to build, maintain, and update information communicated via naturalistic language. Viewing this research through the holistic perspective of semiotics reveals exciting new directions for investigations devoted to the neural representations of meaning. A goal of the field is to pioneer novel methods and experiment designs to shed light on the complex interplay between linguistic, paralinguistic, and social/contextual information in the brain, which will provide a more complete understanding of the biological bases of meaning in the wild.

References

Adelman, J. S., Sabatos-DeVito, M. G., Marquis, S. J., & Estes, Z. (2014). Individual differences in reading aloud: A mega-study, item effects, and some models. *Cognitive Psychology, 68*, 113–160. doi: 10.1016/j.cogpsych.2013.11.001

Alday, P. M. (2019). M/EEG analysis of naturalistic stories: A review from speech to language processing. *Language, Cognition and Neuroscience, 34*(4), 457–473. doi: 10.1080/23273798.2018.1546882

Awad, M., Warren, J. E., Scott, S. K., Turkheimer, F. E., & Wise, R. J. (2007). A common system for the comprehension and production of narrative speech. *Journal of Neuroscience, 27*(43), 11455–11464. doi: 10.1523/JNEUROSCI.5257-06.2007

Balota, D. A., Cortese, M. J., Sergent-Marshall, S. D., Spieler, D. H., & Yap, M. (2004). Visual word recognition of single-syllable words. *Journal of Experimental Psychology. General, 133*(2), 283–316. doi: 10.1037/0096-3445.133.2.283

Beeman, M., & Chiarello, C. (2013). *Right Hemisphere Language Comprehension: Perspectives from Cognitive Neuroscience*. Hillsdale, NJ: Lawrence Erlbaum.

Benkí, J. R. (2003). Quantitative evaluation of lexical status, word frequency, and neighborhood density as context effects in spoken word recognition. *Journal of the Acoustical Society of America, 113*(3), 1689–1705. doi: 10.1121/1.1534102

Bhattasali, S., Fabre, M., Luh, W-M., Al Saied, H., Constant, M., Pallier, C. R., Brennan, J. R., Spreng, N., & Hale, J. (2018). Localising memory retrieval and syntactic composition: An fMRI study of naturalistic language comprehension. *Language, Cognition and Neuroscience, 34*(4), 491–510. doi: 10.1080/23273798.2018.1518533

Binder, J. R., & Desai, R. H. (2011). The neurobiology of semantic memory. *Trends in Cognitive Sciences, 15*(11), 527–536. doi: 10.1016/j.tics.2011.10.001

Binder, J. R., Desai, R. H., Graves, W. W., & Conant, L. L. (2009). Where is the semantic system? A critical review and meta-analysis of 120 functional neuroimaging studies. *Cerebral Cortex, 19*(12), 2767–2796. doi: 10.1093/cercor/bhp055

Birba, A., Beltran, D., Martorell Caro M., Trevisan, P., Kogan, B., Sedeño, L., Ibáñez, A., & García., A. (2020b). Motor-system dynamics during naturalistic reading of action narratives in first and second language. *NeuroImage, 216,* 116820. doi: 10.1016/j.neuroimage.2020.116820

Birba, A., Vitale, F., Padrón, I., Dottori, M., de Vega, M., Zimerman, M., Sedeño, L., Ibáñez, A., & García, A. M. (2020a). Electrifying discourse: Anodal tDCS of the primary motor cortex selectively reduces action appraisal in naturalistic narratives. *Cortex, 132,* 460–472. doi: 10.1016/j.cortex.2020.08.005

Bonner, M. F., Peelle, J. E., Cook, P. A., & Grossman, M. (2013). Heteromodal conceptual processing in the angular gyrus. *NeuroImage, 71,* 175–186. doi: 10.1016/j.neuroimage.2013.01.006

Brennan, J., Nir, Y., Hasson, U., Malach, R., Heeger, D. J., & Pylkkänen, L. (2012). Syntactic structure building in the anterior temporal lobe during natural story listening. *Brain and Language, 120*(2), 163–173. doi: 10.1016/j.bandl.2010.04.002

Brennan, J., & Pylkkänen, L. (2012). The time-course and spatial distribution of brain activity associated with sentence processing. *NeuroImage, 60*(2), 1139–1148. doi: 10.1016/j.neuroimage.2012.01.030

Brennan, J. R., & Pylkkänen, L. (2017). MEG evidence for incremental sentence composition in the anterior temporal lobe. *Cognitive Science, 41*(6), 1515–1531. doi: 10.1111/cogs.12445

Bubic, A., von Cramon, D. Y., & Schubotz, R. I. (2010). Prediction, cognition and the brain. *Frontiers in Human Neuroscience, 4,* 25. doi: 10.3389/fnhum.2010.00025

Cavanna, A. E., & Trimble, M. R. (2006). The precuneus: A review of its functional anatomy and behavioural correlates. *Brain, 129*(Pt 3), 564–583. doi: 10.1093/brain/awl004

Choi, W., Desai, R. H., & Henderson, J. M. (2014). The neural substrates of natural reading: A comparison of normal and nonword text using eyetracking and fMRI. *Frontiers in Human Neuroscience, 8,* 1–11. doi: 10.3389/fnhum.2014.01024

Clinton, V., Taylor, T., Bajpayee, S., Davison, M. L., Carlson, S. E., & Seipel, B. (2020). Inferential comprehension differences between narrative and expository texts: A systematic review and meta-analysis. *Reading and Writing, 33*(9), 2223–2248. doi: 10.1007/s11145-020-10044-2

Crinion, J. T., Lambon-Ralph, M. A., Warburton, E. A., Howard, D., & Wise, R. J. (2003). Temporal lobe regions engaged during normal speech comprehension. *Brain, 126*(5), 1193–1201. doi: 10.1093/brain/awg104

Crinion, J. T., Warburton, E. A., Lambon-Ralph, M. A., Howard, D., & Wise, R. J. (2006). Listening to narrative speech after aphasic stroke: The role of the left anterior temporal lobe. *Cerebral Cortex, 16*(8), 1116–1125. doi: 10.1093/cercor/bhj053

Desai, R. H., Choi, W., & Henderson, J. M. (2020). Word frequency effects in naturalistic reading. *Language, Cognition and Neuroscience, 35*(5), 583–594. doi: 10.1080/23273798.2018.1527376

Desai, R. H., Choi, W., Lai, V. T., & Henderson, J. M. (2016). Toward semantics in the wild: Activation to manipulable nouns in naturalistic reading. *Journal of Neuroscience, 36*(14), 4050–4055. doi: 10.1523/JNEUROSCI.1480-15.2016

Desai, R. H., Herter, T., Riccardi, N., Rorden, C., Fridriksson, J. (2015). Concepts within reach: Action performance predicts action language processing in stroke. *Neuropsychologia, 71,* 217–224. doi: 10.1016/j.neuropsychologia.2015.04.006

Desai, R. H., Reilly, M., & van Dam, W. (2018b). The multifaceted abstract brain. *Philosophical transactions of the Royal Society of London. Series B, Biological Sciences, 373*(1752), 20170122. doi: 10.1098/rstb.2017.0122

Ferstl, E. C., Rinck, M., & von Cramon, D. Y. (2005). Emotional and temporal aspects of situation model processing during text comprehension: An event-related fMRI study. *Journal of Cognitive Neuroscience, 17*(5), 724–739. doi: 10.1162/0898929053747658

Frank, S. L., & Willems, R. M. (2017). Word predictability and semantic similarity show distinct patterns of brain activity during language comprehension. *Language, Cognition and Neuroscience, 32*, 1192–1203. doi: 10.1080/23273798.2017.1323109

Graves, W. W., Desai, R., Humphries, C., Seidenberg, M. S., & Binder, J. R. (2010). Neural systems for reading aloud: A multiparametric approach. *Cerebral Cortex, 20*(8), 1799–1815. doi: 10.1093/cercor/bhp245

Hasson, U., Ghazanfar, A. A., Galantucci, B., Garrod, S., & Keysers, C. (2012). Brain-to-brain coupling: A mechanism for creating and sharing a social world. *Trends in Cognitive Sciences, 16*(2), 114–121. doi: 10.1016/j.tics.2011.12.007

Hauk, O., Davis, M. H., & Pulvermüller, F. (2008). Modulation of brain activity by multiple lexical and word form variables in visual word recognition: A parametric fMRI study. *NeuroImage, 42*(3), 1185–1195. doi: 10.1016/j.neuroimage.2008.05.054

Henderson, J. M., Choi, W., Lowder, M. W., & Ferreira, F. (2016). Language structure in the brain: A fixation-related fMRI study of syntactic surprisal in reading. *NeuroImage, 132*, 293–300. doi: 10.1016/j.neuroimage.2016.02.050

Hsu, C. T., Clariana, R., Schloss, B., & Li, P. (2019). Neurocognitive signatures of naturalistic reading of scientific texts: A fixation-related fMRI study. *Scientific Reports, 9*(1), 10678. doi: 10.1038/s41598-019-47176-7

Huth, A., de Heer, W., Griffiths, T., Theunissen, F., Gallant, J. L. (2016). Natural speech reveals the semantic maps that tile human cerebral cortex. *Nature, 532*, 453–458 doi: 10.1038/nature17637

Johari, K., Riccardi, N., Malyutina, S., Modi, M., Desai, R. H. (2021). HD-tDCS over motor cortex facilitates figurative and literal action sentence processing. *Neuropsychologia, 159*, 107955. doi: 10.1016/j.neuropsychologia.2021.107955

Kemmerer, D. (2021). *Cognitive Neuroscience of Language*. Hove: Psychology Press

Kucyi, A., & Davis, K. D. (2014). Dynamic functional connectivity of the default mode network tracks daydreaming. *NeuroImage, 100*, 471–480. doi: 10.1016/j.neuroimage.2014.06.044

Lambon-Ralph, M. A., Jefferies, E., Patterson, K., & Rogers, T. T. (2017). The neural and computational bases of semantic cognition. *Nature Reviews Neuroscience, 18*(1), 42–55. doi: 10.1038/nrn.2016.150

Leech, R., & Sharp, D. J. (2014). The role of the posterior cingulate cortex in cognition and disease. *Brain, 137*(Pt 1), 12–32. doi: 10.1093/brain/awt162

Lehman Blake, M., Frymark, T., & Venedictov, R. (2013). An evidence-based systematic review on communication treatments for individuals with right hemisphere brain damage. *American Journal of Speech-Language Pathology, 22*(1), 146–160. doi: 10.1044/1058-0360(2012/12-0021)

Mesulam, M. M., Wieneke, C., Hurley, R., Rademaker, A., Thompson, C. K., Weintraub, S., & Rogalski, E. J. (2013). Words and objects at the tip of the left temporal lobe in primary progressive aphasia. *Brain, 136*(Pt 2), 601–618. doi: 10.1093/brain/aws336

Mirman, D., Landrigan, J. F., & Britt, A. E. (2017). Taxonomic and thematic semantic systems. *Psychological Bulletin, 143*(5), 499–520. doi: 10.1037/bul0000092

Newman-Norlund, R. D., Newman-Norlund, S. E., Sayers, S., Nemati, S., Riccardi, N., Rorden, C., Fridriksson, J. (2021). The aging brain cohort (ABC) repository: The University of South Carolina's multimodal lifespan database for studying the relationship between the brain, cognition, genetics and behavior in healthy aging. *Neuroimage: Reports, 1*(1), 100008. doi: 10.1016/j.ynirp.2021.100008

Olson, I. R., McCoy, D., Klobusicky, E., & Ross, L. A. (2013). Social cognition and the anterior temporal lobes: A review and theoretical framework. *Social Cognitive and Affective Neuroscience, 8*(2), 123–133. doi: 10.1093/scan/nss119

Pexman, P. M., Hargreaves, I. S., Edwards, J. D., Henry, L. C., & Goodyear, B. G. (2007). The neural consequences of semantic richness: When more comes to mind, less activation is observed. *Psychological Science, 18*(5), 401–406. doi: 10.1111/j.1467-9280.2007.01913.x

Reilly, M., & Desai, R. H. (2017). Effects of semantic neighborhood density in abstract and concrete words. *Cognition*, 169, 46–53. doi: 10.1016/j.cognition.2017.08.004

Riccardi, N., Yourganov, G., Rorden, C., Fridriksson, J., & Desai, R. H. (2019). Dissociating action and abstract verb comprehension post-stroke. *Cortex, 120*, 131–146. doi: 10.1016/j.cortex.2019.05.013

Riccardi, N., Yourganov, G., Rorden, C., Fridriksson, J., & Desai, R. (2020). Degradation of praxis brain networks and impaired comprehension of manipulable nouns in stroke. *Journal of Cognitive Neuroscience, 32*(3), 467–483. doi: 10.1162/jocn_a_01495

Saxe, R. (2006). Uniquely human social cognition. *Current Opinion in Neurobiology, 16*(2), 235–239. doi: 10.1016/j.conb.2006.03.001

Schwartz, M. F., Kimberg, D. Y., Walker, G. M., Brecher, A., Faseyitan, O. K., Dell, G. S., Mirman, D., & Coslett, H. B. (2011). Neuroanatomical dissociation for taxonomic and thematic knowledge in the human brain. *Proceedings of the National Academy of Sciences of the United States of America, 108*(20), 8520–8524. doi: 10.1073/pnas.1014935108

Seghier, M. L. (2013). The angular gyrus: Multiple functions and multiple subdivisions. *The Neuroscientist: A Review Journal Bringing Neurobiology, Neurology and Psychiatry, 19*(1), 43–61. doi: 10.1177/1073858412440596

Speer, N. K., Zacks, J. M., & Reynolds, J. R. (2007). Human brain activity time-locked to narrative event boundaries. *Psychological Science, 18*(5), 449–455. doi: 10.1111/j.1467-9280.2007.01920.x

Wang, J., Conder, J. A., Blitzer, D. N., & Shinkareva, S. V. (2010). Neural representation of abstract and concrete concepts: A meta-analysis of neuroimaging studies. *Human Brain Mapping, 31*(10), 1459–1468. doi: 10.1002/hbm.20950

Wang, X., Yang, J., Yang, J., Mencl, W. E., Shu, H., & Zevin, J. D. (2015). Language differences in the brain network for reading in naturalistic story reading and lexical decision. *PloS ONE, 10*(5), e0124388. doi: 10.1371/journal.pone.0124388

Wehbe, L., Murphy, B., Talukdar, P., Fyshe, A., Ramdas, A., Mitchell, T. (2014) Simultaneously uncovering the patterns of brain regions involved in different story reading subprocesses. *PLoS One*, *9*(11), e112575. doi: 10.1371/journal.pone.0112575

Willems, R. M., Frank, S. L., Nijhof, A. D., Hagoort, P., & van den Bosch, A. (2016). Prediction during natural language comprehension. *Cerebral Cortex, 26*(6), 2506–2516. doi: 10.1093/cercor/bhv075

Xu, J., Kemeny, S., Park, G., Frattali, C., & Braun, A. (2005). Language in context: Emergent features of word, sentence, and narrative comprehension. *NeuroImage, 25*(3), 1002–1015. doi: 10.1016/j.neuroimage.2004.12.013

Yarkoni, T., Speer, N. K., Balota, D. A., McAvoy, M. P., & Zacks, J. M. (2008). Pictures of a thousand words: Investigating the neural mechanisms of reading with extremely rapid event-related fMRI. *NeuroImage, 42*(2), 973–987. doi: 10.1016/j.neuroimage.2008.04.258

12

WORDS, MEANINGS, AND THE BILINGUAL BRAIN

Nicola del Maschio, Jubin Abutalebi and Daniela Perani

Introduction

Neurosemiotics is an emergent field devoted to the study of the neural bases of communicative behavior from a multi- and cross-disciplinary perspective. In particular, the discipline targets the neurobiological mechanisms that underlie our general capacity to engage in symbolic interactions, with special reference to the emergence and situated transmission of meaning in interactive contexts (see García et al., 2020: 92–97). Accordingly, far from being restricted to the abstract conceptualization of verbal signs, neurosemiotic approaches aim to account for the role of cognitive (non-linguistic), contextual, and experiential factors in shaping meaningful communicative exchanges.

A largely understudied model to investigate communicative behavior from a neurosemiotic perspective is represented by bilingualism, here intended as the routine use of two or more languages, at whatever level of proficiency in either language. In contrast with first language (L1) acquisition, second language (L2) learning comes in multiple different forms, and bilingualism encompasses a broad typology of speakers. Looking at data from a bilingual population at one specific point in time, individuals may differ, for example, in how proficient they are in their L2, in the age and context of acquisition of the L2, in the relative degree of exposure to the L1 and the L2, as well as in motivational, attitudinal, and identification factors (e.g., Birdsong, 2018: 1–17). Dimensions of bilingual experience also change over time, frequently as a direct response to environmental demands. For instance, in increasingly common contexts of bilingualism and immigration, immigrant individuals who are immersed in a L2 environment may gradually reduce their L1 use, and eventually exhibit changes or loss in their L1, a phenomenon known as language attrition (Schmid, 2011; Schmid & Kopke, 2019: 63–72). In this case, the non-use of the L1, as well as the growing influence of the L2 on the L1, are typically associated with a shift in language dominance (i.e., the relative proficiency and/or use in two languages): the immigrants' native language – formerly dominant – recedes, whereas the language of the host country – formerly non-dominant – becomes the immigrants' dominant language.

The natural variation that characterizes bilingual experience not only imposes sociolinguistic differences among bilingual individuals, but also impacts linguistic and non-linguistic processing in the bilingual brain (Costa & Sebastián-Gallés, 2014: 336–345; Perani & Abutalebi, 2005: 202–206). Although the neural circuitry housing a bilingual's two languages is similar, the degree of neural overlap between the two languages is modulated by factors such as language proficiency and use,

 DOI: 10.4324/9781003051817-15

as well as L2 age of acquisition (AoA). Moreover, some brain structures show differential activity in bilinguals and monolinguals, arguably resulting from increased processing demands for the former group. Substantial evidence has been provided that when initiating speech, listening, or reading in a single language, bilinguals activate representations from both of their languages (for reviews: Kroll & Gollan, 2014: 165–181; Titone et al., 2016: 11–46). The co-activation of both languages has been suggested to give rise to cross-language competition that must be solved to ensure that the right language is used in each communicative context (e.g., Hermans et al., 1998: 213–229; Marian & Spivey, 2003: 97–115; but see Costa, 2005: 308–325). The context-dependent use of a target language, in the face of the co-activation and potential competition between languages, has been associated with the recruitment of a set of executive (cognitive) processes collectively known as "language control" (Green, 1986: 210–223, 1998: 67–81). Language control emerges from the integration of separable cortical and subcortical neural networks associated with domain-general executive functions (Abutalebi & Green, 2016: 689–698; see Figure 12.1). The structures and connections that mediate the specific demands of bilingual language processing thus extend beyond the classic left perisylvian language areas, and engage regions associated with language control in different interactional contexts.

Overall, the ability to communicate in two languages affords the opportunity to investigate issues concerning the dynamic interplay between brain, language, cognition, and environment that otherwise might remain unexplored in monolingual speakers. A multidimensional approach to bilingual communication is offered by neurosemiotics, a discipline devoted to the investigation of the neural and experiential continuities of communicative behavior by integrating current insights from natural and social sciences (Ibáñez et al., 2017). In the field of bilingualism research, especially amenable to scrutiny within a neurosemiotic framework is the topic of the representation and control of the bilingual lexicon,[1] which targets the way bilinguals construe word meaning. It is generally assumed that bilinguals have a single conceptual system from which activity flows onto distinct but integrated lexicons (e.g., Dijkstra & Van Heuven, 1998: 189–225, 2002: 175–197; Kroll & Stewart, 1994: 149–174). But how do linguistic and non-linguistic (control) processes interact during lexical selection for accurate production in the intended language? And to what extent do experiential and contextual factors modulate this process?

The present chapter is structured as follows. First, rather than focusing on classic models of the bilingual lexicon (e.g., Dijkstra & Van Heuven, 1998: 189–225; Kroll & Stewart, 1994: 149–174), extensively reviewed and revised elsewhere (e.g., Dijkstra et al., 2019: 657–679; Kroll & Ma, 2018: 294–319), we provide an overview of current models of bilingual speech production, with

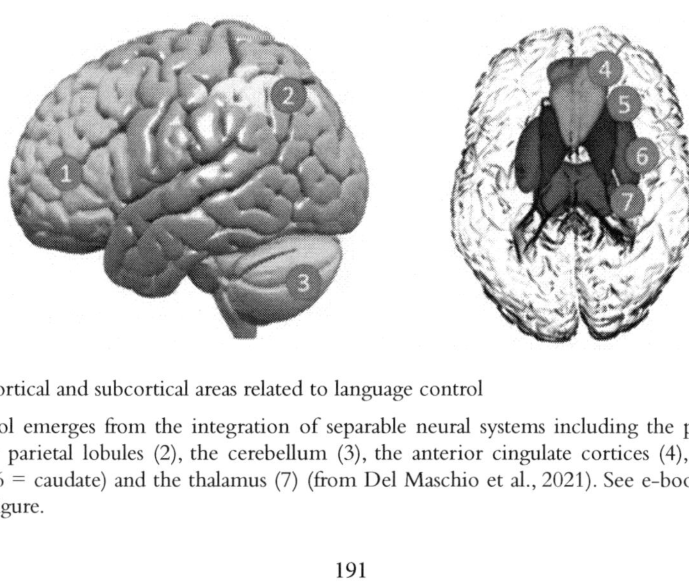

Figure 12.1 Cortical and subcortical areas related to language control

Language control emerges from the integration of separable neural systems including the prefrontal cortices (1), the inferior parietal lobules (2), the cerebellum (3), the anterior cingulate cortices (4), the basal ganglia (5 = putamen; 6 = caudate) and the thalamus (7) (from Del Maschio et al., 2021). See e-book for a full-color version of this figure.

special reference to the relationship between representations and control during lexical selection. Second, by focusing on recent meta-analytic results from our lab, we discuss what neuroimaging data reveal about bilinguals' ability to process and control lexico-semantic functions. In both sections, we highlight the relevance of addressing some of the findings discussed within the emerging field of neurosemiotics. Finally, an integrative section is proposed in which we highlight opportunities for cross-fertilization between neurosemiotics, embodied approaches to language, and neuroemergentist approaches to bilingualism.

Bilingual word production: Activation, competition, and control

With reference to language production, a critical issue is how bilinguals manage to avoid potential interference from the language not in use when translating thoughts into meaningful speech. Imagine a face-to-face conversation in a multilingual environment. To address their interlocutor in an intended language, a bilingual speaker must establish and maintain the task goal of speaking in that language and not another. A face-to-face conversation is inherently multimodal – that is, the linguistic signal is accompanied by visual and acoustic information that contributes to utterance and meaning construction (Vigliocco et al., 2014:1–7). Whereas a variety of perceptual cues (e.g., the addressee's voice, facial expressions, and manual gestures) may support speaking in the intended language, other cues (e.g., the voices of other speakers talking in the other language) may activate the goal of speaking in the language not in use, leading to potential interference between languages in the speaker's mind. From a neurosemiotic perspective, a similar scenario can be described in terms of the relationship between perceived communicative signs (i.e., the pattern of linguistic and non-linguistic environmental cues) and the resulting cognitive representation in the interpretant's mind (Peirce, 1955: 98–119), as reflected in neural activation (e.g., Wolf et al., 2018: 1–16). In this context, interference from the language not in use may be portrayed as an interpretive conflict due to incongruence between perceived communicative signs – some supporting the current language goal, others triggering selection of the language not in use – resulting in additional processing demands and interference on the speaker's executive control system.

Traditionally, two groups of models have been proposed that address the issue of activation, competition, and control during language production: language-specific selection models and language-non-specific selection models. These groups of models conceptualize lexical access differently and make different predictions about the engagement of control mechanisms that allow bilinguals to keep production separate in each language. According to language-specific selection models (e.g., Costa & Caramazza, 1999: 231–244; Costa et al., 1999: 365–397; Finkbeiner et al., 2006: 1075–1089; La Heij, 2005: 289–307), lexical access is restricted to the intended language, with no cross-language competition involved in the lexical selection process. Specifically, the intention to speak in one language would set the activation level higher for candidates in that language, without considering potential competitors in the other language. Within this framework, La Heij (2005: 289–307) proposed that the intended language is specified at the conceptual level as part of the preverbal message. A language cue would ensure that the activation spreading from a given concept only reaches the corresponding lexical representation in the intended language, with no additional activation or inhibition needed during lexical selection. In this way, lexical retrieval in bilinguals and monolinguals would be mediated by similar selection mechanisms. This specific proposal, however, seems to contrast with the psycholinguistic evidence that both languages are activated even when only one language is in use (e.g., Colomé, 2001; Hermans et al., 1998; Morales et al., 2011; Thierry & Wu, 2007). To account for this aspect, a different proposal within the framework of language-specific selection models identified the lexical level, rather than the conceptual level, as the locus of lexical selection (see Costa, 2005). In particular, capitalizing on behavioral findings from a series of picture-word interference tasks (e.g., Costa et al., 1999; Costa et al., 2000), Costa and colleagues suggested that the lexical representations of both languages may indeed be activated during lexical selection. However, the selection mechanism would only be sensitive to the activated representations of the intended language, with no need to actively suppress the activated translation equivalents from the other language. To provide some context, in picture-word interference tasks a target picture must be named while ignoring a superimposed word distractor. The word distractor can be either semantically related to the target picture (e.g., *school* and *teacher*) or not (e.g., *school* and *leopard*). A standard finding of these tasks is semantic interference: the picture is named more slowly when the word distractor is semantically related to the target picture. Semantic interference is also found when the picture must be named in a language (e.g., English: *school*) that differs from the language in which the distractor is presented (e.g., Italian: *insegnante* [teacher]). To account for this finding, Costa et al. (1999) proposed that, since the distractor in the unintended language (*insegnante*) also activates its translation in the intended language (*teacher*), a delay in the selection of the name of the target picture (*school*) could be induced by the translation of the distractor (*teacher*) rather than by the distractor itself (*insegnante*). That is, semantic interference would stem from within-language competition in the lexicon of the intended language, and not from cross-language competition between the distractor word of the unintended language and the picture name of the intended language. This latter hypothesis, on the other hand, has been sustained by proponents of non-language-specific selection models.

Non-language-specific selection models differ from the former group of models primarily on competition for selection. Specifically, based on several findings of cross-language effects at different word levels (for review, see Paolieri et al., 2018), non-language-specific selection models claim that the intention to plan speech in one language is not enough to restrict activation to that language (De Bot, 1992; Green, 1986, 1998; Poulisse, 1997). For accurate production to proceed, lexical candidates of the intended language actively compete with alternatives from the unintended language, and bilinguals must use top-down control mechanisms to suppress those alternatives. The most widely known non-language-specific selection model is the inhibitory control model (IC) by Green (1986, 1998). Although formally proposed in the late 1990s, the hypotheses of the IC model continue to stimulate debate in bilingual studies. The IC model explicitly includes multiple levels of inhibition in the mechanisms that support bilingual language processing. In particular, both linguistic (task schemas) and non-linguistic (supervisory attentional system) control mechanisms are contemplated. The model assumes that: (1) lexical representations are selected in the intended language if their level of activation surpasses that of other lexical representations in both languages; and (2) inhibition is proportional to the level of activation of the lexical representations to be suppressed. A paradigm extensively used to support the claim that inhibitory processes are used in bilinguals' lexico-semantic control is language switching (e.g., Abutalebi & Green, 2008; Costa & Santesteban, 2004; Meuter & Allport, 1999). In brief, in language switching procedures, bilingual participants are asked to name items in L1 and L2 depending on a cue. Each item can be named in the same language as its previous trial (non-switch trial condition), or in the opposite language to its previous trial (switch trial condition). The critical task measure is the switch cost (i.e., mean naming latencies on switch trial condition minus mean naming latencies on non-switch trial condition). Language switching studies usually reveal asymmetric switch costs between languages. Specifically, increased naming latencies have been reported for L2–L1 vs. L1–L2 switching – that is, switching to the dominant language (i.e., typically the L1) is more costly than switching to the weaker language (i.e., typically the L2). Based on the IC model assumptions, the use of L2 would lead to greater inhibition of L1, so that later switching to L1 is more costly because of the need to overcome greater inhibition. A still open question, however, is whether inhibition *per se*, rather than specific inhibitory mechanisms or other mechanisms altogether, might be responsible for the asymmetry in bilinguals' language switching (see e.g., Bobb & Wodniecka, 2013; Santesteban & Schwieter, 2020). Whereas for language-specific selection models lexical access does not explicitly entail involvement of domain-general executive control functions, the IC model includes both linguistic processes and non-linguistic control mechanisms. Crucially, as partly anticipated, processing costs during language switching are influenced by various factors, both participant- and task-related (e.g., Gollan & Ferreira, 2009; Guo et al., 2013; Philipp et al., 2007; Verhoef et al., 2009). Much research has focused on proficiency and language dominance, showing that the higher the proficiency in the L2, the smaller the asymmetry in switch costs between the two languages (e.g., Costa et al., 2006; Meuter & Allport, 1999). The impact of individual differences in language proficiency on switch costs has been related to a differential recruitment of language control strategies by highly versus low-proficient bilinguals (e.g., Calabria et al., 2012). Of note, additional factors can interact with proficiency in shaping switch costs and mechanisms of language control, such as the context of language use (e.g., Green & Abutalebi, 2013; Hartanto & Yang, 2016) and the frequency of language switching (e.g., Prior & Gollan, 2011). Recently, by comparing Italian-English bilinguals and Italian-Sardinian bilinguals on a language switching task, Bonfieni et al. (2019) reported that switch costs are also affected by L2 daily exposure. In particular, higher L2 exposure predicted reduced switch costs in L1. The authors interpreted this finding as indicating that more exposure to the L2 alleviates the cognitive burden of suppressing the (dominant) L1, making it easier for bilinguals to access and switch between languages.

Speaking one language rather than another involves the selection, retrieval, and articulation of words that meet the speaker's intended meaning. The way this process is controlled seems to depend on multiple interacting factors, including dimensions of bilingual experience (e.g., language dominance) and contexts of bilingual language use (e.g., switching vs. non-switching contexts). Translating thoughts into meaningful speech, however, may be influenced by other variables that are rarely contemplated by psycholinguistic models of bilingual language production. For instance, motivational and emotional mechanisms may be relevant (e.g., Dornyei & Skehan, 2003; Liu & Huang, 2011), as well as psychosocial factors such as contextual attitude (Huensch & Thompson, 2017) and mentalizing abilities (Tiv, O'Regan & Titone, 2021). Some of these variables have been examined in specific subfields of bilingualism research (e.g., L2 learning and pronunciation studies), but little attempts have been made to integrate individual differences within these domains into more comprehensive approaches to bilingual language production. As far as emotion-language coupling is concerned, there is evidence for weakened emotional responses while processing an L2, as indexed, for example, by reduced electrodermal reactivity to L2 emotion-laden words (e.g., Harris, 2004). Emotional differences between first and second language might depend on the different embodiment that the languages have, which in turn may affect the emotional resonance of the language (Pavlenko, 2012). Not surprisingly, such differences are moderated by factors that are linked in reciprocal relationships such as AoA, proficiency, and (emotional) context of learning (see Caldwell-Harris, 2015).

By tracking the convergences of the neural, perceptual, cognitive, and emotional processes that jointly shape our efforts to extract meaning from social interactions, a neurosemiotic outlook may foster a holistic understanding of bilinguals' communication from the speaker's perspective.

Lexico-semantic processing in the bilingual brain

The results of functional neuroimaging studies agree with the hypothesis that there are similar principles of semantic representation across languages, and that bilinguals show similar activation patterns while they are processing lexico-semantic representations in their L1 and L2. When differences across languages emerge, they are more likely to be attributed to the recruitment of control mechanisms to regulate cross-language competition rather than to differences in the actual representation of the two languages (e.g., Abutalebi et al., 2005: 497–515; Del Maschio & Abutalebi, 2019: 197–213). The recruitment of such mechanisms, in turn, is sculpted by experiential and contextual constraints. For instance, the functional connectivity both within and between perisylvian and executive control networks is modulated by the individual and interactive effects of L2 age of acquisition, L2 proficiency, and relative amount of L1/L2 input or exposure, the main quantifiable dimensions in which bilingual experience is usually partitioned (e.g., DeLuca et al., 2019: 7565–7574; Sulpizio et al., 2020a: 1–11). Recently, Sulpizio et al. (2020b: 834–853) used meta-analytic data to enucleate systems involved in the processing and control of different types of linguistic knowledge – including lexico-semantics – in bilinguals' L1 and L2. Given the study's aim, both production and comprehension tasks were included in the analyses. Results for *lexico-semantic processing in L1* showed a widespread pattern of bilateral activation in cortical and subcortical regions that largely overlaps with the semantic network reported by meta-analytic studies on monolingual language processing (e.g., Binder et al., 2009: 2767–2796). In particular, at the cortical level, significant clusters of activation were found in left temporal structures, bilateral portions of the parietal cortex, and frontal regions (e.g., the inferior frontal gyrus). At the subcortical level, lexico-semantic processing was associated with the activation of the right caudate, the left thalamus, and the left amygdala. The aforementioned cortical structures are known to be associated with the storing and processing of semantic knowledge (temporal cortex: see Binder et al., 2009: 2767–2796; Cappa, 2012: 427–431), with lexical efficiency and vocabulary learning (parietal lobe: e.g., Grogan et al., 2012: 1347–1352; Lee et al., 2007: 1184–1189; Mechelli et al., 2004), and with lexical selection and semantic decisions (frontal regions: e.g., Noppeney et al., 2004: 1269–1280; Thompson-Schill et al., 1999: 513–522). The activation of the caudate and thalamic regions, on the other hand, is arguably linked to semantic control processes (e.g., Canini et al., 2016: 4179–4196; Cousins et al., 2017: 45–54). Results *for lexico-semantic processing in L2* showed a smaller set of additional activated regions, which mainly involved subcortical and cerebellar structures: the bilateral globus pallidus, the right insula, and the right cerebellum. These regions are not usually reported as part of the semantic network, and their recruitment is arguably to be attributed to control-related functions. According to Green's IC model (see also Abutalebi & Green, 2007: 242–275), language control is likely to recruit phylogenetically earlier systems such as subcortical and cerebellar structures that subserve the domain-general control of action. The globus pallidus has been proposed to play a role in lexical selection and production monitoring (e.g., Liu et al., 2010: 75–82). The right insula, only sporadically associated with L2 semantic processing, has been suggested to support various language control functions, especially in cognitively demanding contexts (Wager et al., 2005: 323–340; Vigneau et al., 2011: 577–593). Cerebellar structures, on the other hand, have been implicated in bilinguals' ability to resist speech interference from a dominant L1 while comprehending an utterance in L2 (Filippi et al., 2011: 10732–10740, 2020: 1–13). Notably, there was a diminished recruitment of the amygdala in L2 versus L1, possibly attributable to the stronger link between cognitive and affective processes that individuals are supposed to experience in their native language (see Caldwell-Harris, 2015: 214–219; Pavlenko, 2008: 147–164).

The finding of a larger set of activated regions in L1 than L2 is not necessarily an argument against an integrated bilingual lexicon (with shared semantic representations) of the sort assumed by classic psycholinguistic models. Some models of bilingual speech production, such as the Revised Hierarchical Model (RHM) by Kroll and Stewart (1994: 149–174), assume the L1 lexicon to be larger than that of L2, and the connections between L1 concepts to be stronger than those between L2. However, since some previous studies have reported a reversed pattern of activation (i.e., a larger set of activated regions for L2 than L1), further experimental indication is needed to clarify which specific combination of factors moderates the interplay between the semantic representations and control of lexico-semantic processing in L1 and L2.

Importantly, when Sulpizio et al. (2020b: 834–853) separately investigated the activation patterns in early and late proficient bilinguals, the subcortical activity associated with L2 processing was detected especially in the latter group (see Figure 12.2). This finding is in line with results of other meta-analytic studies of bilingual language processing (Cargnelutti et al., 2019: 1–19; Liu & Cao, 2016: 68–73), and may suggest that the age of L2 onset acquisition modulates brain function irrespective of the high level of proficiency attained. L2 AoA plays a prominent role in L2 learning (Birdsong, 1999) and modulates language dominance (Birdsong, 2014: 374–392). Since the brain displays a heightened sensitivity to acquire instructive and adaptive signals from the environment during development, having an early contact with an L2 may have long-term effects on the cross-talk

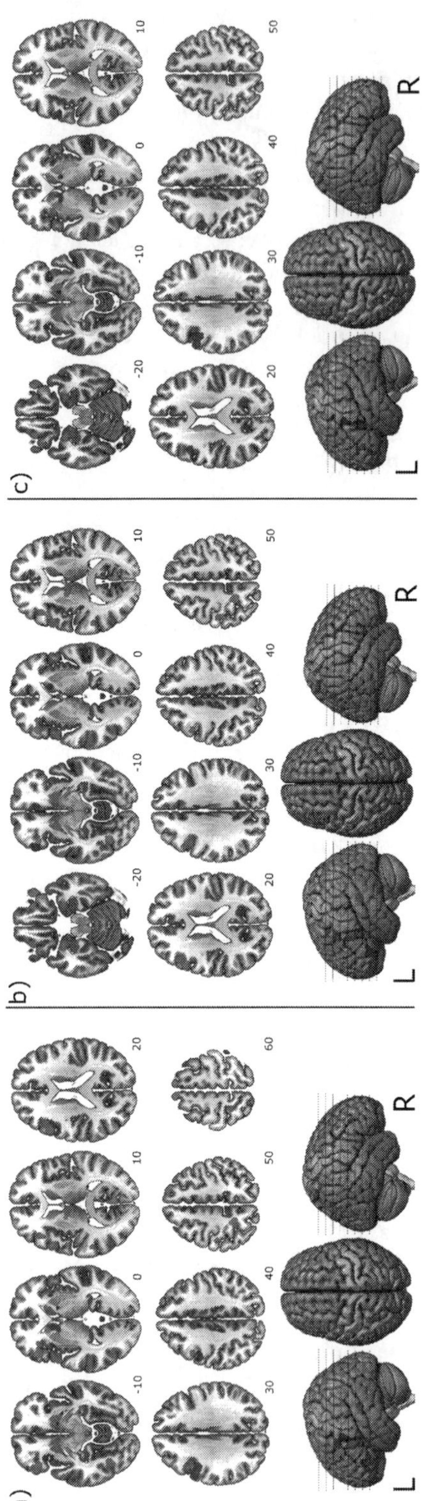

Figure 12.2 Functional activation areas involved in lexical-semantic processing in L1 and L2

(a) Functional activations collapsed over age of acquisition (AoA); red = L1 > L2, blue = L2 > L1; b) Functional activations for early (red) and late (blue) bilinguals (L1 > L2); c) Functional activations for early (red) and late (blue) bilinguals (L2 > L1) (from Sulpizio et al., 2020b). See e-book for a full-color version of this figure.

between semantic and control networks. Partial evidence to this claim comes from functional connectivity analysis on bilinguals' resting-state networks. For example, Berken et al. (2016: 1165–1172) found that simultaneous versus sequential bilinguals had a stronger connectivity between the left inferior frontal gyrus and its right counterpart, as well as between the inferior frontal gyrus and the right dorsolateral prefrontal cortex, the bilateral inferior parietal lobule, and the cerebellum. Similar effects of L2 AoA have been reported by Gullifer et al. (2018: 123–134) on the inter-hemispheric connectivity of frontal regions.

Since Lambert et al. (1959: 77–82)'s definition of bilinguals as a small group of speakers with perfect knowledge in both of their languages, the conceptualization of bilingualism has expanded to include speakers with different language background and varying degrees of proficiency. The findings here reported on the neural basis of bilinguals' lexico-semantic processing further highlight the importance of modeling bilingualism as a multidimensional and continuous construct (Baum & Titone, 2014: 857–894; Luk & Bialystok, 2013: 605–621; Sulpizio et al., 2020a: 1–11).

Towards an integrative view of bilingual communication

A neurosemiotic perspective on (bilinguals') communicative behavior may resonate with embodied and emergentist approaches to human language and bilingualism.

According to embodied theories of language (e.g., Barsalou, 2008: 617–645; Gallese & Lakoff, 2005: 455–479; Glenberg, 2010: 586–596; Pulvermüller & Fadiga, 2016: 311–324; Zwaan, 2004: 35–62), the meaning of linguistic expressions is fundamentally rooted in our experiences – that is, embodied. The meaningful building blocks of language (e.g., words) relate to the sensorimotor and emotional experiences we had with the world, and the same neural structures involved in making sensorimotor and emotional experiences are also involved in interpreting the linguistic material related to those experiences – see, for discussion, Meteyard et al. (2012: 788–804). Linguistic communication and meaningful exchanges would thus be possible because the construction and interpretation of meaning is grounded in shared (or shareable) individual experiences (Buccino et al., 2016: 69–78).

The basis of emergentism is the study of complex systems (e.g., Aziz-Alaoui & Bertelle, 2009). Complexity theory suggests that the patterns of a complex system emerge from the interaction and joint activities of the system's components and cannot be predicted from the behavior of any of such components. According to (neuro)emergentist theories of language learning (Bates et al., 1979; Behrens, 2009: 383–411; Elman et al., 1996) and bilingualism (Hernandez et al., 2005: 220–225; Hernandez et al., 2019: 214–223), the complexity of human language should be understood in terms of the interaction of more basic non linguistic variables, such as perceptual mechanisms, learning capabilities, processing capacity, and experiential and contextual factors.

The theoretical premises of neurosemiotic, embodied, and emergentist approaches to communicative behavior stand in marked contrast to the "classical view" of language as an abstract and a-modal computational system underpinned by specifically dedicated neural structures (e.g., Fodor, 1975; Pylyshyn, 1984). One the one hand, both embodiment and neurosemiotic approaches emphasize the importance of sensory, motor, and affective experience for (bilinguals') communicative behavior, as well as the relevance of conceptualizing (bilinguals') meaningful communication as the result of different multimodal semiotic resources. On the other hand, (neuro)emergentism shares with neurosemiotics the representation of a dual-language system as a non-linear system arising from the dynamic interaction of smaller elements across time, as well as the need for integrative research that systematically tracks developmental changes in conjunction with brain activity and non-linguistic cognitive processes over the lifespan.

In what follows, we will introduce a topic that can potentially bring together insights from the three approaches mentioned: iconicity in bilingual language processing.

Iconicity in bilingual language processing

Traditional views about the construction of lexical meaning are dominated by the idea that words exhibit a purely arbitrary form-to-meaning relationship. However, a growing amount of computational and experimental evidence across spoken and signed modalities suggests that arbitrariness is not the only referential mechanism that supports the learning and processing of lexical items (Lockwood & Dingemanse, 2015: 1–14; Perniss & Vigliocco, 2014: 1–13). Non-arbitrary mappings are generally defined as *iconic*, an *icon* being "a sign which stands for something merely because it resembles it" (Peirce 1931–1936: 3, 362), linguistic *iconicity* being a sensory perceived resemblance between properties of linguistic form and properties of meaning (Taub, 2001). Iconicity is a multifaceted phenomenon that manifests itself at various degrees in linguistic communication. The visuo-spatial modality of signed languages allows for an abundance of iconic visual-to-visual mappings across various levels of linguistic processing (Perniss et al., 2010: 1–15). In speech, the degree of iconicity is notoriously limited to specific classes of words (e.g., onomatopoeic words), arguably due to the reduced amount of experience that can be iconically represented in the oral-aural channel. Despite being underrepresented in the lexicon of spoken languages, iconic items such as onomatopoeic forms have been shown to be most prevalent in early child-directed speech and in children's early productions, and to be learnt more easily by children relative to non-iconic forms (e.g., Motamedi, et al., 2020; see also Imai et al., 2008: 54–65). In adults, iconicity has been recently reported to provide a benefit to visual word recognition (Sidhu et al., 2020: 164–181) and a processing advantage in aphasic patients (Meteyard et al., 2015: 264–275).

As a counterweight to the abundant literature on iconicity in monolingual language processing, very little is reported in the context of bilingual studies. However, some data have emerged for specific groups of bilinguals (e.g., bimodal bilinguals), and we will briefly mention them here. Casey and Emmorey (2009: 290–312), for instance, investigated the effects of knowledge of sign language on co-speech gesture by comparing the spontaneous gestures of bimodal bilinguals (native users of ASL and English) and non-signing native English speakers. Relative to monolingual speakers, bimodal bilinguals produced more iconic gestures, a finding that was interpreted as reflecting the interaction between the ASL language production system (and the iconicity present therein) and the co-speech gesture system. Increased iconic gesturing was also reported in novice adult signers after one year of ASL study, despite no significant change in the production rate of other non-iconic gesture types (Casey et al., 2012: 677–686). These results suggest that even short-term exposure to the iconic contents of sign language can influence co-speech gesture production in adult L2 learners. Of interest, Ortega and colleagues found that, even if the semantic contents of iconic signs are easily learned and recalled by adult sign language learners, their articulation is typically less accurate than that of more arbitrary signs (e.g., Ortega, 2013; Ortega & Morgan, 2015: 660–688). This may occur because the similarity in form between iconic signs and co-speech gestures interfere with adult sign learning. To further account for this gestural interference, the authors proposed that adult L2 learners of sign language may initially acquire signs in their co-speech gesture system, rather than in sign language as a completely separate system.

According to Perniss and Vigliocco (2014: 1–13), arbitrariness and iconicity coexist to bring distinct advantages for learning words and using them to convey meaningful messages. In particular, arbitrariness would enable efficient transmission of an unbounded array of concepts; iconicity would be instrumental in mapping language onto human experience as the content of linguistic communication. Whether and to what extent iconic mechanisms mediate the acquisition and use of a dual lexico-semantic system are key questions for future investigation in bilingual studies.

Overall, this chapter should be considered in light of a number of limitations. Among others, the omission of high-temporal resolution evidence and the exclusive focus on lexico-semantic processing (leaving aside other critical aspects of bilingual language processing such as phonological and syntactic processing). In addition, both the architecture of the executive control system (as specified in its multiple interweaving subfunctions) and the different forms of bilingual language control proposed in the literature (e.g., proactive vs. reactive) were necessarily oversimplified to make the chapter easily accessible to its potential readership.

Conclusions

Communicative behavior relies on extended neural networks that support the integration of semantic information from multiple expressive channels and cues in orchestrated ways. "The perception of the environment as meaningful, both globally and discretely, and the general capacity to engage in symbolic interactions" (Bouissac, 1986: 204–206) are the object of inquiry of neurosemiotics, which aims to integrate socio-biological perspectives on meaning and communication. In this chapter, we have focused on the representation and control of the lexico-semantic system in the bilingual brain as a research subfield that may be profitably framed within a neurosemiotic perspective. Increasingly widespread and inherently variable, bilingualism represents a natural model for investigating our efforts to construe meaning in everyday interactions, considering the interplay of cognitive functions, experiential factors, and the interpretation of social perceptual features of the environment.

In the first section, we focused on the relationship between representations and control during bilingual speech production, with reference to the experiential and contextual factors that may affect lexico-semantic processing. As shown by the meta-analytic results discussed, bilinguals who perform lexico-semantic tasks in L1 versus L2 may differentially recruit brain systems involved in language control (with stronger cognitive effort associated with L2 processing), especially when the second language is learned after early childhood. Accounting for the multidimensional quality of bilingual experience, recent functional connectivity studies suggest that L2 AoA interact with proficiency and exposure in shaping the interplay between semantic- and control-related networks. As detailed in the last section of this chapter, neuroimaging and psycholinguistic data as well as embodied and emergentist approaches to bilingual language communication may be fruitfully integrated in the broader agenda of neurosemiotics.

Note

1 A *lexicon* can be defined as a repository of meaningful linguistic expressions (e.g., words) from which more complex expressions are built; a *mental lexicon* is typically referred to as a particular user's knowledge of their own vocabulary; *lexical access* is seen as the act of retrieving a word from the mental lexicon, given a lexical concept to be expressed; *lexical selection* is the mechanism by which a word is chosen (during recognition or production) for further processing; *lexical semantics* loosely refers to the study of word meaning (Murphy, 2010).

References

Abutalebi, J., Cappa, S. F., & Perani, D. (2005). What can functional neuroimaging tell us about the bilingual brain (497–515). In: J. F. Kroll and A. M. B. De Groot (Eds.), *Handbook of Bilingualism: Psycholinguistic Approaches*. Oxford: Oxford University Press.

Abutalebi, J., & Green, D. (2007). Bilingual language production: The neurocognition of language representation and control. *Journal of Neurolinguistics*, *20*, 242–275.

Abutalebi, J., & Green, D. W. (2008). Control mechanisms in bilingual language production: Neural evidence from language switching studies. *Language and Cognitive Processes*, *23*(4), 557–582.

Abutalebi, J., & Green, D. W. (2016). Neuroimaging of language control in bilinguals: neural adaptation and reserve. *Bilingualism: Language and Cognition*, *19*(4), 689–698.

Aziz-Alaoui, M., & Bertelle, C. (Eds.). (2009). *From System Complexity to Emergent Properties*. Luxembourg: Springer.

Barsalou, L. W. (2008). Grounded cognition. *Annual Review of Psychology*, *59*, 617–645.

Bates, E.A. Benigni, L., Bretherton, I., Camaioni, L., Volterra, V. (1979). *The Emergence of Symbols: Cognition and Communication in Infancy*. New York: Academic Press.

Baum, S., & Titone, D. (2014). Moving toward a neuroplasticity view of bilingualism, executive control, and aging. *Applied Psycholinguistics*, *35*(5), 857–894.

Behrens, H. (2009). Usage-based and emergentist approaches to language acquisition. *Linguistics*, *47*(2), 383–411.

Berken, J. A., Chai, X., Chen, J. K., Gracco, V. L., & Klein, D. (2016). Effects of early and late bilingualism on resting-state functional connectivity. *Journal of Neuroscience*, *36*(4), 1165–1172.

Binder, J. R., Desai, R. H., Graves, W. W., & Conant, L. L. (2009). Where is the semantic system? A critical review and meta-analysis of 120 functional neuroimaging studies. *Cerebral Cortex*, *19*(12), 2767–2796.

Birdsong, D. (1999). *Second Language Acquisition and the Critical Period Hypothesis.* Hillsdale, NJ: Lawrence Erlbaum.

Birdsong, D. (2014). Dominance and age in bilingualism. *Applied Linguistics*, *35*(4), 374–392.

Birdsong, D. (2018). Plasticity, variability and age in second language acquisition and bilingualism. *Frontiers in Psychology*, *9*, 81.

Bobb, S., & Wodniecka, Z. (2013). Language switching in picture naming: What asymmetric switch costs (do not) tell us about inhibition in bilingual speech planning. *Journal of Cognitive Psychology, 25*(5), 568–585.

Bonfieni, M., Branigan, H. P., Pickering, M. J., & Sorace, A. (2019). Language experience modulates bilingual language control: The effect of proficiency, age of acquisition, and exposure on language switching. *Acta Psychologica*, *193*, 160–170.

Bouissac, P. (1986). Semiotics in Canada I. In T. A. Sebeok & D. J. Umiker-Sebeok (Eds.), *The Semiotic Web* (191–252). Berlin: Mouton de Gruyter.

Buccino, G., Colagè, I., Gobbi, N., & Bonaccorso, G. (2016). Grounding meaning in experience: A broad perspective on embodied language. *Neuroscience & Biobehavioral Reviews*, *69*, 69–78.

Calabria, M., Hernández, M., Branzi, F. M., & Costa, A. (2012). Qualitative differences between bilingual language control and executive control: Evidence from task-switching. *Frontiers in Psychology*, *2*, 399.

Caldwell-Harris, C. L. (2015). Emotionality differences between a native and foreign language: Implications for everyday life. *Current Directions in Psychological Science*, *24*(3), 214–219.

Canini, M., Della Rosa, P. A., Catricalà, E., Strijkers, K., Branzi, F. M., Costa, A., & Abutalebi, J. (2016). Semantic interference and its control: A functional neuroimaging and connectivity study. *Human Brain Mapping*, *37*(11), 4179–4196.

Cappa, S. F. (2012). Imaging semantics and syntax. *NeuroImage*, *61*(2), 427–431.

Cargnelutti, E., Tomasino, B., & Fabbro, F. (2019). Language brain representation in bilinguals with different age of appropriation and proficiency of the second language: A meta-analysis of functional imaging studies. *Frontiers in Human Neuroscience*, *13*, 154.

Casey, S., & Emmorey, K. (2009). Co-speech gesture in bimodal bilinguals. *Language and Cognitive Processes*, *24*(2), 290–312.

Casey, S., Emmorey, K., & Larrabee, H. (2012). The effects of learning American Sign Language on co-speech gesture. *Bilingualism: Language and Cognition* 15, 677–686.

Colomé, À. (2001). Lexical activation in bilinguals' speech production: Language-specific or language-independent?. *Journal of Memory and Language*, *45*(4), 721–736.

Costa, A. (2005). Lexical access in bilingual production. In J. F. Kroll and A. M. B. De Groot (Eds.), *Handbook of Bilingualism: Psycholinguistic Approaches* (pp. 308–325). Oxford: Oxford University Press.

Costa, A., & Caramazza, A. (1999). Is lexical selection in bilingual speech production language-specific? Further evidence from Spanish-English and English-Spanish bilinguals. *Bilingualism: Language and Cognition*, *2*, 231–244.

Costa, A., Caramazza, A., & Sebastián-Gallés, N. (2000). The cognate facilitation effect: Implications for models of lexical access. *Journal of Experimental Psychology: Learning, Memory, and Cognition*, *26*, 1283–1296.

Costa, A., Miozzo, M., & Caramazza, A. (1999). Lexical selection in bilinguals: Do words in the bilingual's two lexicons compete for selection? *Journal of Memory and Language*, *41*(3), 365–397.

Costa, A., & Santesteban, M. (2004). Lexical access in bilingual speech production: Evidence from language switching in highly proficient bilinguals and L2 learners. *Journal of Memory and Language*, *50*, 491–511.

Costa, A., Santesteban, M., & Ivanova, I. (2006). How do highly proficient bilinguals control their lexicalization process? Inhibitory and language-specific selection mechanisms are both functional. *Journal of Experimental Psychology: Learning, Memory, and Cognition*, *32*(5), 1057.

Costa, A., & Sebastián-Gallés, N. (2014). How does the bilingual experience sculpt the brain? *Nature Reviews Neuroscience*, *15*(5), 336–345.

Cousins, K.A., Ash, S., Irwin, D.J., Grossman, M., (2017). *Dissociable substrates underlie the production of abstract and concrete nouns. Brain and Language*, *165*, 45–54.

De Bot, K. (1992). A bilingual production model: Levelt's speaking model adapted. *Applied Linguistics*, *13*, 1–24.

Del Maschio, N., & Abutalebi, J. (2019). Language organization in the bilingual and multilingual brain. In: J. W. Schwieter (Ed.). *The Handbook of the Neuroscience of Multilingualism* (pp. 197–213). Chichester: John Wiley & Sons.

Del Maschio, N., Fedeli, D., & Abutalebi, J. (2021). Bilingualism and aging: Why research should continue. Linguistic Approaches to *Bilingualism*, *11*(4), 505–519.

DeLuca, V., Rothman, J., Bialystok, E., & Pliatsikas, C. (2019). Redefining bilingualism as a spectrum of experiences that differentially affects brain structure and function. *Proceedings of the National Academy of Sciences, 116*(15), 7565–7574.

Dijkstra, A., & Van Heuven, W.J.B. (1998). The BIA-model and bilingual word recognition. In J. Grainger, J. & A. Jacobs (Eds.), *Localist Connectionist Approaches to Human Cognition* (pp. 189–225). Hillsdale, NJ: Lawrence Erlbaum.

Dijkstra, A., & Van Heuven, W.J.B. (2002). The architecture of the bilingual word recognition system: From identification to decision. *Bilingualism: Language and Cognition, 5*, 175–197

Dijkstra, T., Wahl, A., Buytenhuijs, F., Van Halem, N., Al-Jibouri, Z., De Korte, M., & Rekké, S. (2019). Multilink: a computational model for bilingual word recognition and word translation. *Bilingualism: Language and Cognition, 22*(4), 657–679.

Dörnyei, Z., and Skehan, P. (2003). Individual differences in second language learning. In C. J. Doughty & M. H. Long (Eds.), *The Handbook of Second Language Acquisition* (pp. 589–630). Malden, MA: Blackwell.

Elman, J. L., Bates, E. A., & Johnson, M. H., Karmiloff-Smith, A., Parisi, D., Plunkett, K. (1996). *Rethinking Innateness: A Connectionist Perspective on Development*. Cambridge, MA: MIT Press.

Filippi, R., Periche Tomas, E., Papageorgiou, A., & Bright, P. (2020). A role for the cerebellum in the control of verbal interference: Comparison of bilingual and monolingual adults. *PloS One, 15*(4), e0231288.

Filippi, R., Richardson, F. M., Dick, F., Leech, R., Green, D. W., Thomas, M. S., & Price, C. J. (2011). The right posterior paravermis and the control of language interference. *Journal of Neuroscience, 31*(29), 10732–10740.

Finkbeiner, M., Almeida, J., Janssen, N., & Caramazza, A. (2006). Lexical selection in bilingual speech production does not involve language supression. *Journal of Experimental Psychology: Learning, Memory, and Cognition, 32*(5), 1075.

Fodor, J. A. (1975). *The Language of Thought*. Cambridge, MA: Harvard University Press.

Gallese, V., & Lakoff, G. (2005). The brain's concepts: The role of the sensory-motor system in conceptual knowledge. *Cognitive Neuropsychology, 22*(3–4), 455–479.

García, A. M., Franco-O'Byrne, D., & Ibáñez, A. (2020). Neurosemiotics: Blurbing a field beyond the "two cultures divide". In L. Lacková, C. Rodríguez & K. Kull (Eds.), *Gatherings in Biosemiotics XX* (pp. 92–97). Tartu: University of Tartu Press.

Glenberg, A. M. (2010). Embodiment as a unifying perspective for psychology. *Wiley Interdisciplinary Reviews: Cognitive Science, 1*(4), 586–596.

Gollan, T. H., & Ferreira, V. S. (2009). Should I stay or should I switch? A cost-benefit analysis of voluntary language switching in young and aging bilinguals. *Journal of Experimental Psychology. Learning, Memory, and Cognition, 35*(3), 640.

Green, D. W. (1986). Control, activation, and resource: A framework and a model for the control of speech in bilinguals. *Brain and Language, 27*(2), 210–223.

Green, D. W. (1998). Mental control of the bilingual lexico-semantic system. *Bilingualism: Language and Cognition, 1*, 67–81.

Green, D. W., & Abutalebi, J. (2013). Language control in bilinguals: The adaptive control hypothesis. *Journal of Cognitive Psychology, 25*(5), 515–530.

Grogan, A., Jones, Ō. P., Ali, N., Crinion, J., Orabona, S., Mechias, M. L., … Price, C. J. (2012). Structural correlates for lexical efficiency and number of languages in non-native speakers of English. *Neuropsychologia, 50*(7), 1347–1352.

Gullifer, J. W., Chai, X. J., Whitford, V., Pivneva, I., Baum, S., Klein, D., & Titone, D. (2018). Bilingual experience and resting-state brain connectivity: Impacts of L2 age of acquisition and social diversity of language use on control networks. *Neuropsychologia, 117*, 123–134.

Guo, T., Liu, F., Chen, B., & Li., S. (2013). Inhibition of non-target languages in multilingual word production: Evidence from Uighur-Chinese-English trilinguals. *Acta Psychologica, 143*, 277–283.

Harris, C. L. (2004). Bilingual speakers in the lab: Psychophysiological measures of emotional reactivity. *Journal of Multilingual and Multicultural Development, 25*(2–3), 223–247.

Hartanto, A., & Yang, H. (2016). Disparate bilingual experiences modulate task-switching advantages: A diffusion-model analysis of the effects of interactional context on switch costs. *Cognition, 150*, 10–19.

Hermans, D., Bongaerts, T., de Bot, K., & Schreuder, R. (1998). Producing words in a foreign language: Can speakers prevent interference from their first language? *Bilingualism: Language and Cognition, 1*(3), 213–229.

Hernandez, A. E., Claussenius-Kalman, H. L., Ronderos, J., Castilla-Earls, A. P., Sun, L., Weiss, S. D., & Young, D. R. (2019). Neuroemergentism: A framework for studying cognition and the brain. *Journal of Neurolinguistics, 49*, 214–223.

Hernandez, A., Li, P., & MacWhinney, B. (2005). The emergence of competing modules in bilingualism. *Trends in Cognitive Sciences, 9*(5), 220–225.

Huensch, A., & Thompson, A. S. (2017). Contextualizing attitudes toward pronunciation: Foreign language learners in the United States. *Foreign Language Annals*, *50*(2), 410–432.

Ibáñez, A., Sedeño, L., & García, A. M. (2017). *Neuroscience and Social Science: The Missing Link*. New York: Springer.

Imai, M., Kita, S., Nagumo, M., & Okada, H. (2008). Sound symbolism facilitates early verb learning. *Cognition*, *109*(1), 54–65.

Kroll, J. F., & Gollan, T. H. (2014). Speech planning in two languages: What bilinguals tell us about language production. In M. Goldrick, V. Ferreira, & M. Miozzo (Eds.), *The Oxford Handbook of Language Production* (pp. 165–181). Oxford: Oxford University Press.

Kroll, J. F., & Ma, F. (2018). The bilingual lexicon. In E. M. Fernández and H. S. Cairns (Eds.), *The Handbook of Psycholinguistics* (pp. 294–319). Hoboken, NJ: Wiley Blackwell.

Kroll, J. F., & Stewart, E. (1994). Category interference in translation and picture naming: Evidence for asymmetric connections between bilingual memory representations. *Journal of Memory and Language*, *33*(2), 149–174.

La Heij, W. (2005). Selection processes in monolingual and bilingual lexical access. In J. F. Kroll & A. M. B. De Groot (Eds.), *Handbook of Bilingualism: Psycholinguistic Approaches* (pp. 289–307). Oxford: Oxford University Press.

Lambert, W. E., Havelka, J., Gardner, R. C. (1959). Linguistic manifestations of bilingualism. *The American Journal of Psychology*, *72*(1), 77–82.

Lee, H., Devlin, J. T., Shakeshaft, C., Stewart, L. H., Brennan, A., Glensman, J., Pitcher, K., Crinion, J., Mechelli, A., Frackowiak, R. S. J., Green, D. W., & Price, C. J. (2007). Anatomical traces of vocabulary acquisition in the adolescent brain. *Journal of Neuroscience*, *27*(5), 1184–1189.

Liu H, & Cao, F. (2016). L1 and L2 processing in the bilingual brain: A meta-analysis of neuroimaging studies. *Brain and Language*, *159*, 60–73.

Liu, H., Hu, Z., Guo, T., & Peng, D. (2010). Speaking words in two languages with one brain: Neural overlap and dissociation. *Brain Research*, *1316*, 75–82.

Liu, M., & Huang, W. (2011). An exploration of foreign language anxiety and English learning motivation. *Education Research International*, 12(5), 1–8.

Lockwood, G., and Dingemanse, M. (2015). Iconicity in the lab: A review of behavioural, developmental, and neuroimaging research into sound-symbolism. *Frontiers in Psychology*, *6*, 1246.

Luk, G., & Bialystok, E. (2013). Bilingualism is not a categorical variable: Interaction between language proficiency and usage. *Journal of Cognitive Psychology*, *25*(5), 605–621.

Marian, V., & Spivey, M. (2003). Competing activation in bilingual language processing: Within-and between-language competition. *Bilingualism: Language and Cognition*, *6*(2), 97.

Mechelli, A., Crinion, J. T., Noppeney, U., O'Doherty, J., Ashburner, J., Frackowiak, R. S., & Price, C. J. (2004). Structural plasticity in the bilingual brain. *Nature*, *431*(7010), 757.

Meteyard, L., Cuadrado, S. R., Bahrami, B., & Vigliocco, G. (2012). Coming of age: A review of embodiment and the neuroscience of semantics. *Cortex*, *48*(7), 788–804.

Meteyard, L., Stoppard, E., Snudden, D., Cappa, S. F., & Vigliocco, G. (2015). When semantics aids phonology: A processing advantage for iconic word forms in aphasia. *Neuropsychologia*, *76*, 264–275.

Meuter, R. F., & Allport, A. (1999). Bilingual language switching in naming: Asymmetrical costs of language selection. *Journal of Memory and Language*, *40*(1), 25–40.

Morales, L., Paolieri, D., & Bajo, T. (2011). Grammatical gender inhibition in bilinguals. *Frontiers in Psychology*, *2*, 284.

Motamedi, Y., Murgiano, M., Perniss, P., Wonnacott, E., Marshall, C., Goldin-Meadow, S., & Vigliocco, G. (2020). Linking language to sensory experience: onomatopoeia in early language development. *Developmental Science*, 24(3), e13066.

Murphy, M. L. (2010). *Lexical Meaning*. Cambridge: Cambridge University Press.

Noppeney, U., Phillips, J., & Price, C. (2004). The neural areas that control the retrieval and selection of semantics. *Neuropsychologia*, *42*(9), 1269–1280.

Ortega, G. (2013). Acquisition of a Signed Phonological System by Hearing Adults: The Role of Sign Structure and Iconicity (Doctoral dissertation), University College of London.

Ortega, G., & Morgan, G. (2015). Phonological development in hearing learners of a sign language: The influence of phonological parameters, sign complexity, and iconicity. *Language Learning*, *65*(3), 660–688.

Paolieri, D., Morales, L., & Bajo, T. (2018). Production in bilingual and multilingual speakers. In E. M. Fernández and H. S. Cairns (Eds.). *The Handbook of Psycholinguistics* (pp. 82–110). Hoboken, NJ: Wiley Blackwell.

Pavlenko, A. (2008). Emotion and emotion-laden words in the bilingual lexicon. *Bilingualism: Language and Cognition*, *11*(2), 147–164.

Pavlenko, A. (2012). Affective processing in bilingual speakers: Disembodied cognition? *International Journal of Psychology*, *47*(6), 405–428.

Peirce, C. S. (1931–1936). Volumes 1–6. In C. Hartshorne and P. Weiss (Eds.), *The Collected Papers*. Cambridge, MA: Harvard University Press.

Peirce, C. S. (1955). Logic as semiotic: the theory of signs (98–119). In J. Buchler (Ed.), *Philosophical Writings of Peirce*. New York: Dover.

Perani, D., & Abutalebi, J. (2005). The neural basis of first and second language processing. *Current Opinion in Neurobiology, 15*(2), 202–206.

Perniss, P., Thompson, R., & Vigliocco, G. (2010). Iconicity as a general property of language: Evidence from spoken and signed languages. *Frontiers in Psychology, 1*, 227.

Perniss, P., & Vigliocco, G. (2014). The bridge of iconicity: From a world of experience to the experience of language. *Philosophical Transactions of the Royal Society B: Biological Sciences, 369*(1651), 20130300

Philipp, A.M., Gade, M., and Koch, I. (2007). Inhibitory processes in language switching: Evidence from switching language-defined response sets. *European Journal of Cognitive Psychology, 19*(3), 395–416.

Poulisse, N. (1997). Language production in bilinguals. In A. M. B. de Groot, & J. F. Kroll (Eds.), *Tutorials in Bilingualism: Psycholinguistic Perspectives* (pp. 201–224). Hillsdale, NJ: Lawrence Erlbaum.

Prior, A., & Gollan, T. H. (2011). Good language-switchers are good task-switchers: Evidence from Spanish-English and Mandarin-English bilinguals. *Journal of the International Neuropsychological Society, 17*(4), 682–691.

Pulvermüller, F., and Fadiga, L. (2016). Brain language mechanisms built on action and perception. In G. Hickok and S. Small (Eds.), *Neurobiology of Language* pp. 311–324). Cambridge, MA: Academic Press.

Pylyshyn, Z. W. (1984). *Computation and Cognition: Toward a Foundation for Cognitive Science*. Cambridge, MA: MIT Press.

Santesteban, M., & Schwieter, J. W. (2020). Lexical selection and competition in bilinguals. In R. Heredia & A. Cieślicka (Eds.), *Bilingual Lexical Ambiguity Resolution* (pp.126–157). Cambridge: Cambridge University Press.

Schmid, M. (2011). *Language Attrition*. Cambridge: Cambridge University Press.

Schmid, M., & Kopke, B. (Eds.) (2019). *The Oxford Handbook of Language Attrition*. Oxford: Oxford University Press.

Sidhu, D. M., Vigliocco, G., & Pexman, P. M. (2020). Effects of iconicity in lexical decision. *Language and Cognition, 12*(1), 164–181.

Sulpizio, S., Del Maschio, N., Del Mauro, G., Fedeli, D., & Abutalebi, J. (2020a). Bilingualism as a gradient measure modulates functional connectivity of language and control networks. *NeuroImage, 205*, 116306.

Sulpizio, S., Del Maschio, N., Fedeli, D., & Abutalebi, J. (2020b). Bilingual language processing: A meta-analysis of functional neuroimaging studies. *Neuroscience & Biobehavioral Reviews, 108*, 834–853.

Taub, S. F. (2001). *Language from the Body: Iconicity and Metaphor in American Sign Language*. Cambridge: Cambridge University Press.

Thierry, G., & Wu, Y. J. (2007). Brain potentials reveal unconscious translation during foreign-language comprehension. *Proceedings of the National Academy of Sciences, 104*(30), 12530–12535.

Thompson-Schill, S. L., D'Esposito, M., & Kan, I. P. (1999). Effects of repetition and competition on activity in left prefrontal cortex during word generation. *Neuron, 23*(3), 513–522.

Titone, D, Whitford V, Lijewska A, & Itzhak I (2016). Bilingualism, executive control, and eye movement measures of reading: A selective review and re-analysis of bilingual vs. multilingual reading data (11–46). In J. Schwieter (Ed.), *Cognitive Control and Consequences in the Multilingual Mind*. Amsterdam: John Benjamins.

Tiv, M., O'Regan, E., & Titone, D. (2021). In a bilingual state of mind: Investigating the continuous relationship between bilingual language experience and mentalizing. *Bilingualism: Language and Cognition*, 24(5), 918–931.

Verhoef, K., Roelofs, A., & Chwilla, D. J. (2009). Role of inhibition in language switching: Evidence from event-related brain potentials in overt picture naming. *Cognition, 110*, 84–99.

Vigliocco, G., Perniss, P., & Vinson, D. (2014). Language as a multimodal phenomenon: implications for language learning, processing and evolution. *Philosophical Transactions of the Royal Society B: Biological Sciences, 369*, 20130292.

Vigneau, M., Beaucousin, V., Hervé, P.Y., Jobard, G., Petit, L., Crivello, F., … Tzourio-Mazoyer, N. (2011). What is right-hemisphere contribution to phonological, lexico-semantic, and sentence processing? Insights from a meta-analysis. *NeuroImage, 54*(1), 577–593.

Wager, T. D., Sylvester, C. Y. C., Lacey, S. C., Nee, D. E., Franklin, M., & Jonides, J. (2005). Common and unique components of response inhibition revealed by fMRI. *NeuroImage, 27*(2), 323–340.

Wolf, D., Mittelberg, I., Rekittke, L. M., Bhavsar, S., Zvyagintsev, M., Haeck, A., Cong, F., Klasen, M., & Mathiak, K. (2018). Interpretation of social interactions: Functional imaging of cognitive-semiotic categories during naturalistic viewing. *Frontiers in Human Neuroscience, 12*, 296.

Zwaan, R.A. (2004). The immersed experiencer: Toward an embodied theory of language comprehension. In B. H. Ross (Ed.), *The Psychology of Learning and Motivation* (pp. 35–62). New York: Academic Press.

13

HOW DO SIGN LANGUAGES MEAN?

Ruth Campbell

Introduction

The notion that meanings can be communicated beyond language is a foundational semiotic insight. In communities and groups where spoken language is not used, such as hunting groups or silent religious communities, meanings are transmitted between people by a variety of means, but especially through gestures – based on bodily positions, face and head actions, and especially manual actions (Sebeok, 2001). Sign languages (SLs), however, have a different basis. SLs of deaf people are structured, have stable components, and can communicate infinite novel meaning combinations to those who use them. How might this happen? What are the implications for understanding brain networks that support the emergence of meanings? A neurosemiotic standpoint requires that we take account of all the experiences – external and endogenous – that an organism may encounter, in order to understand and communicate events that mean. Therefore, whether these gestures should be considered to be the domain of (neuro)linguistics or gesture studies is somewhat moot from a neurosemiotic perspective. A truly synergistic view of the phenomenon should transcend disciplinary boundaries.

These issues are the focus of this chapter. First, I sketch some aspects of meaningful communication that are seen in deaf children born into hearing families without a SL and the cortical correlates of their later exposure to SL. Then, I briefly summarize how SL manifests in the cortical networks engaged by deaf people who are exposed to a SL early in life – especially when compared with neurolinguistic findings in hearing people exposed to spoken language. In considering some "easy-to-see" manual dispositions and actions, further cortical networks are implicated. I then consider why, in skilled SL users, and despite their ubiquity in all SLs, such iconic SL elements fail to impact differentially on core language networks in the brain. I conclude that while prevalent in all SLs, iconicity takes on different roles in the acquisition of a SL in contrast to its skilled usage. I then delve into a possible biological source for this key role of iconic gesture in developing meaningful communication: a neurosemiotic proposal. This speculation builds on the discovery of functional specificity in two distinct signal processing networks in the brain – a dorsal pathway, implicating fronto-parietal structures; and a ventral pathway, implicating lateral temporo-frontal structures. These pathways can map manual dispositions and manual actions to support different types of meaning related to handshapes and actions in SL, as well as in gestures accompanying speech (emblems and pantomimes).

 DOI: 10.4324/9781003051817-16

I conclude that biological evolution has shaped these pathways in order to distinguish between two forms of meaningful biological event: *acts* (dorsal) and *things* (ventral), which have evolved into human linguistic systems as well as in nonverbal communication systems. A neurosemiotic viewpoint allows these inferences to emerge and points to further exploration of how brains may process and develop meaningful communication, whether these are considered "language" or "gesture."

Early signs: The role of homesign in the development of signed communication

Homesign: A way into language through iconicity

At least 90 percent of children born deaf are born to hearing families, and they are not exposed to a spoken language except via lipreading. What means of communication might develop under these conditions? A deaf child in a hearing family can develop gestural, largely manual, communication with their family: homesign (Goldin-Meadow, 2003, 2017). While the gestures used vary from family to family, homesign has language-like features, including stable meanings for particular items (a lexicon), stable forms for such gestures (consistency in meaning), and ways to modify a message, such as requests or negation. In describing an event, the homesigner typically uses a handshape to indicate an object and a manual movement to describe what is done with or to it – a grammar-like construction. These constructions are used systematically. While users of a spoken language use (manual) gestures to modify their utterances, they rarely use the manual form in such systematic ways: an indication that homesigners are not basing their repertoire on imitation of co-speech gestures used by hearing users of a spoken language (Goldin-Meadow & Yang, 2017). What do homesigners use to share meanings with their hearing caregivers and friends? How do they achieve a level of symbolic competence in the absence of language exposure? One answer is that they seek out resemblances in the experienced world that can be captured in a manual gesture or series of gestures. These are shared experiences available to the hearing talker and to the deaf child: iconic resemblances. Pointing is a universal type of gesture, possibly originating in aiming to touch the object of interest (O'Madagain et al., 2019). A head turn or shake to indicate negation may have originated in the infant refusing food (Darwin, 1872). Indicating the size or shape of an object by placing the hands close together or apart is an iconic feature that is readily mapped and widely used by non-signers. The linking of such gestures into gesture sequences is seen in homesign, allowing more complex reference to emerge. The stability of such gestural forms suggests a basic psychological process allowing for the development of symbols that can be shared between (sighted) participants: a socio-biological basis for semiotic function.[1]

What neural processes are implicated in homesign? Adult Deaf[2] people who learned a SL as older children, usually in Deaf schools, are characterized as late sign learners (LSLs) and were likely homesigners before coming to school. LSLs show different patterns of cortical recruitment compared with signers who acquired a SL early in life, usually from SL parents or a SL community, where the SL is better established. In particular, LSLs show more diffuse patterns of cortical activation than early signers, and less evidence of recruitment of core (perisylvian) language regions in the left hemisphere (LH). The neural connections between the posterior (superior temporal and parieto-temporal) and anterior (frontal and prefrontal) hubs of the core language system are less developed in LSLs than in early signers, and visual brain regions are activated to a greater extent in LSLs (Cheng et al., 2019; Emmorey et al., 2003; Ferjan Ramirez et al., 2013; Leonard et al., 2012; Malaia et al., 2020; Mayberry et al., 2018; Pénicaud et al., 2013; Simon, Campbell, et al., 2020; Woll, 2018). Functionally, while LSLs can show deficits in syntactic processing of a SL (Cheng & Mayberry, 2020; Mayberry et al., 2018; Mayberry & Fischer, 1989), they do not appear to have difficulty acquiring or using lexical information: new meanings for specific things or acts continue to be acquired and used efficiently even when language is learned late (Lieberman et al., 2015).

Sign languages are born – and made – by Deaf people

SLs emerge where Deaf people – especially Deaf children – congregate. Unlike homesign, which involves the participation of a hearing person, SLs are used by Deaf people to communicate with each other (although, of course, hearing people who learn a SL can also be involved). Every SL has all the design features of any spoken language, except that they are neither spoken nor heard. All SLs are grammatically structured. They use componential structures and arbitrary, non-iconic forms, allowing complex and abstract meanings to be communicated in real time, including events displaced from the interaction itself (Hockett, 1958; and for SL, see Liddell, 2003). While some SLs have a centuries-old historical pedigree which is not limited to the geographical place of origin (Power et al., 2020), many have a lifespan that reflects the community in which they emerge and evolve, and which may be transient or recent. Therefore, SLs are not always mutually comprehensible, although they share common features that can be readily mastered if one is already a SL user. These features offer clues concerning how meanings may be communicated efficiently using a visual manual system. These are iconic: the relationship between the sign and what is signified is evident as long as participants have sensory, cognitive, and cultural experiences of the world enabling such resemblances to be mapped effectively (Emmorey, 2014). While all SLs are highly iconic (Brentari, 2019), this need not imply a clear one-to-one relationship between a sign in every SL and a specific gesture: for example, the sign BABY[3] can vary across different SLs. Some indicate the contours of a small child; others represent "baby" as a cradling movement of the arms and body (DiNapoli, 2017). Both are iconic, yet the signs carry different conceptual weight depending on the specific SL. Which iconic aspect of an event is embodied will depend on the SL.

How sign languages work: Iconicity, language, and gesture

Some aspects of meaning, which may not be obvious in spoken language, become clearer in SL and when non-signers view signed communications. Take telicity. In (American) SL, the manually signed distinction between telic verbs (DECIDE – an action with a defined endpoint) and non-telic verbs (THINK – a continuous action) can be reliably interpreted for telicity by non-signers. Telic verbs are produced with a visible "end" manual gesture, which is absent for non-telic verbs; it is a direct link between a linguistic feature and an action pattern produced by the hands (Malaia & Wilbur, 2012; Strickland et al., 2015). Note that the full meaning of the sign is opaque to someone unfamiliar with the particular SL. Iconicity delivers a feature of meaning, but may not stand in for the symbol – the sign – itself.

Signs that resemble their referents are acquired early by Deaf infants (Meier, 2016; Thompson et al., 2012); they are learnt more easily by hearing people learning a SL as a second language (e.g., Campbell et al., 1992; see Ortega, 2017). They are more prevalent in the early stages of evolution of a new SL than in an established one (Coppola & Senghas, 2017; Pyers & Senghas, 2020). However, within all SLs, hand and body position can be used to express spatial relationships, whether abstract ("higher up in the league") or concrete ("the cat is under the table") – *topographic* reference. SLs also abound in *classifiers*, specific combinations of hand configurations (with static or changing location) that can modify both an entity and its movement over a complete phrase (Emmorey, 2003; Morgan & Woll, 2007). Classifiers can recapitulate formal imagistic properties of the referent – a single finger pointing up can indicate any of a range of long thin objects in British Sign Language – and also functional imagistic aspects (a hooked finger action pattern may indicate drinking or picking something up).

The hands constitute just one channel for delivering information; other body parts can also be used simultaneously to impart the message. Just as hearing users of spoken languages use manual gestures to modulate the verbal message, facial actions modulate manual articulations. Facial actions carry a multitude of functions in SL. They can be used to ask questions, to indicate agreement or disagreement, to modify action patterns and descriptions of things, to indicate events in the scene, or to afford ready mapping to emotional and mental state conditions, such as ANGRY or WORRIED (Baker & Padden, 1978). Face parts, such as movements of the eye or mouth regions (Boyes Breaem & Sutton-Spence, 2001; Dachkovsky & Sandler, 2009), may be implicated, as well as whole-face actions alongside head and body dispositions.

Language and/or gesture: Neurolinguistic and neurosemiotic considerations

Manual actions to depict spatial relations as well as non-manual (i.e., facial) actions to depict a variety of meanings are ubiquitous in SLs. Whether they should be classed as "language" or as "gesture" is an issue for sign linguists and gesture theorists (Cormier et al., 2013; Goldin-Meadow & Brentari, 2017). A semiotic approach, which takes a "meaning-first" view of communicative processes, may partially sidestep these issues. Similarly, the neurolinguist and the neurosemiotician take different pathways to understanding how meanings are instantiated in the brain. The neurolinguist may want to know to what extent such actions function as linguistic elements – phonological, morphological, syntactic – and, if so, where they can be found in specific subnetworks of the core language system. Meanings emerge from such componential processes interfacing with widely distributed semantic brain networks, especially within fronto-temporal circuits in both hemispheres (Wright et al., 2012). Instead, the neurosemiotician wants to know how different neural networks may support mappings from both external events and internal plans and procedures ("signals") that can deliver meanings.

Most neuroscientific research exploring meanings in SL comes from skilled SL users who are Deaf, and is compared with hearing users of a spoken language. That is, most studies to date have controlled for language skill and have come under the microscope of the sign linguist. While this contrast may address neurolinguistic concerns, it may be less helpful for neurosemiotics.

Pivoting from neurolinguistics to neurosemiotics

First it needs to be established whether SL users and spoken language users have "similar brains." This is not easy, since deafness and SL are separate though heavily interacting factors that affect brain development and function (Campbell et al., 2014). We have noted that LSLs show reduced connectivity between perisylvian regions, and somewhat variable and diffuse patterns of activation when presented with SL stimuli. Skilled Deaf SL users, by contrast, show very marked structural and functional brain similarities to hearing non-signers. In both skilled Deaf SL users and hearing users of a spoken language, the core language regions of the brain, around the sylvian fissure of the LH, are similar in extent and are activated similarly by language-structured stimuli (Cardin et al., 2013; Emmorey, 2002; Emmorey, Grabowski, et al., 2003; MacSweeney et al., 2006; MacSweeney et al., 2004; MacSweeney et al., 2002; Neville et al., 1997; Newman et al., 2015; Sakai et al., 2005) (see Figure 13.1). Additionally, in hearing users of a spoken language, speech accompanied by non-speech bodily gestures also activates this core left perisylvian language network (Dick et al., 2009; Dick et al., 2014; Jouravlev et al., 2019; Özyürek, 2014), leading to the suggestion that such a network is better conceptualized as a core communication network (Xu et al., 2009).

Does this mean that bodily gestures, like (and with) vocal articulations, must engage the core language system of the LH to evoke meaning? When the core language regions are damaged by LH insult or by surgical separation of the cortical hemispheres (commissurotomy), the ability to communicate meanings need not be lost (e.g., Göksun et al., 2015; Kita & Lausberg, 2008), an insight that was apparent to proponents of neurosemiotics before functional neuroimaging (Grzybek, 1993; Ivanov, 1994).

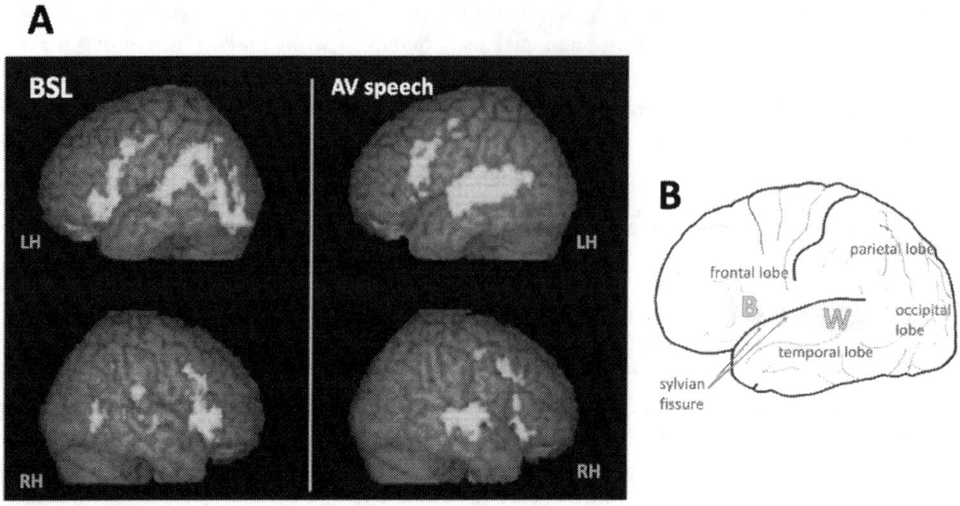

Figure 13.1 Neural aspects of sign language processing

A. Regions activated by BSL sentence comprehension in deaf native signers and audiovisual (AV) spoken sentences by hearing English non-signers. LH – left hemisphere, RH – right hemisphere. These show the similar patterns of activation for each modality, with LH perisylvian activation as the major finding. These activations were contrasted with a baseline condition in which the model was seen at rest (voxelwise $p<0.00005$). Activation up to 5 mm beneath the cortical surface is displayed. Adapted from MacSweeney et al, 2002, with permission. B. Schematic of left hemisphere showing perisylvian regions B (Broca's area, left inferior frontal gyrus) and W (Wernicke's area, left superior temporal gyrus). See e-book for a full-color version of this figure.

How – and when – do iconic features function in SL?

In skilled SL users, iconic features of the language, such as topographic relations, SL classifiers, and facial actions, all show activation in visual (inferior occipital) and visuospatial (frontoparietal) brain regions over and beyond activation in perisylvian regions of the LH (Campbell et al., 2011; Capek et al., 2009; Emmorey et al., 2005; MacSweeney et al., 2002). Despite this, paradoxically, when investigated directly by contrasting sign stimuli judged iconic with those which are arbitrary, iconic SL stimuli are not processed differently from non-iconic stimuli with respect to their cortical activation in skilled SL users (Emmorey et al., 2004).

In a major electrophysiological study exploring time course and amplitude of cortical waveforms related to sign comprehension, iconicity failed to affect speed or amplitude of the neural response, unlike sign-frequency and sign-concreteness, which showed specific effects relatively early in processing, indicative of lexical access to a sign's meaning. A weak effect was noted late in processing, suggestive of post-lexical, strategic, conscious awareness of the iconicity of the sign (Emmorey et al., 2020; McGarry et al., 2021). Iconicity can go some way towards accounting for specific aspects of SLs and their semiotic significance. However, in SLs, as in spoken languages, it cannot get us all the way (Dingemanse et al., 2015).

Iconicity has its greatest impact on the early stages of SL acquisition, as in homesign. Iconic signs are learned earlier by signing infants in signing households and they are evident in the emergence and evolution of a new SL where Deaf children from non-signing backgrounds come together in a Deaf school (Meier, 2016; Pyers & Senghas, 2020). The effects of iconicity on cortical systems can be seen in (hearing) non-signers learning a SL for the first time, where the P3a component – an electrophysiological marker of semantic access – has greater amplitude for signs that can resemble gestures than for signs that do not. As the authors note,

> nonsigners generate expectations about the form of iconic signs never seen before based on their implicit knowledge of gestures … Learners thus draw from any available semiotic resources when acquiring a second language, and not only from their linguistic experience …
>
> *(Ortega, Özyürek, & Peeters, 2020: 403)*

What might be termed "the retreat from iconicity" as the language develops and is mastered may be a better fit with the classical linguistic insight that elements of language are essentially arbitrary, and that meaning is processed via componential, syntactically constructed processes. In terms of neural function, we should predict that language mastery correlates with the maturation of the core language system in left perisylvian regions. It does appear that the pattern of more diffuse cortical processing in LSLs can be modified by exposure to a SL in late childhood, as the critical period for language acquisition may extend into adolescence, with a shift to LH perisylvian processing (Ferjan Ramirez et al., 2016).

Is the core language system necessary for meaning processing in SL users?

Comparing LSLs and early SL users of a signed language can illuminate the extent to which different elements may or may not be captured by the core language system. SL classifiers are processed similarly by LSLs and early SL users, unlike well-established syntactic features of a SL, such as word order, which show delayed neural responses over core language regions in LSLs (Malaia et al., 2020). Meanings are instantiated in brains that may lack a core language system – or where a new language is developing. Gestural categories, including emblems (such as a thumbs-up sign) and pantomimes (gestures that imitate familiar actions), can be processed at little cognitive cost (Malaia et al., 2020). The same may be true for non-manual actions (Box 13.1).

Box 13.1 Headshake-NOT: An illustration of how an iconic gesture is realized in brain systems

Head movements play a number of critical roles in face-to-face communication in hearing people, including semantic as well as pragmatic and discourse functions (McClave, 2000). In British Sign Language, as in many sign languages (SLs), headshake-NOT is an obligatory sign to indicate negation, and has been ascribed a syntactic function (Quer, 2012). If that gesture requires syntactic processing in order to deliver its meaning it should be impaired in patients with left hemisphere (LH) lesions and damage to the core language network. However, in a case-series study of three signing patients with LH lesions and three with right hemisphere (RH) lesions, when asked to match a picture to a signed utterance that could include a headshake-NOT, the sign for negation was interpreted correctly in the aphasic LH lesion patients – and not in the RH patients, whose language abilities were intact (Atkinson et al., 2004). In the intact brain of a SL user, the visual information from inferior occipito-temporal, posterior temporal, and temporo-parietal regions around the angular gyrus can be relayed to LH core language networks for full linguistic analysis (Campbell et al., 2011). The patients' responses show that this is not required for understanding the headshake gesture, which can be processed in the undamaged, language-less RH.

A neurosemiotic standpoint emphasizes that the meaning of "negation" need not be confined to a syntactic process, but reflects further cultural, symbolic, and biological processes. Darwin speculated that the origins of the headshake, a universal gesture of negation, may lie in the infant's refusal of the mother's breast, just as the (also universal) nod of agreement may reflect the infant's forward movement of the head towards the breast. These gestures appear to be endogenous rather than learned, since they are evident in both blind people (who are unlikely to have observed and copied the gesture) and in people who lack other cognitive and linguistic capacities (Darwin, 1872).

To conclude, Deaf sign-language users show a more varied pattern of (SL) acquisition than hearing users of a spoken language, allowing a peek into the origins and sustainability of language and communication within a language community. As with a spoken language, when the SL is acquired early in a signing home, the core language network in LH perisylvian regions is activated to a similar extent and shows similar structural properties with respect to both anatomy of the specific regions and their interconnections. Command of the language is secure, with highly developed syntactic skills. In the skilled SL user, topographic and classifier aspects, as well as non-manual features, are retained in communication, and have been described linguistically. LSLs do not show the same developmental pattern. Yet in both cases, the meanings of gestural actions of others are acquired readily and easily – via iconic resemblance between a sign in the SL and its referent. Brain regions that are specialized for visuospatial processing and for the processing of bodily actions, in occipito-temporal and occipito-parietal brain networks, are implicated in both LSLs and skilled SL users. Understanding the meanings of a gesture produced by a SL user may sometimes require the core language network – but sometimes not (as in headshake-NOT negation). However, these considerations are somewhat perfunctory: what types of meaning may be processed and delivered by which cortical networks? This is surely a concern for neurosemiotics. We now turn to that issue in relation to SL.

A deeper dive: The extraction of meaning types through dual processing streams

Orientation: A sketch of brain regions and functions

Three functions can be adduced in all descriptions of cortical processes and their locations: (1) sensory processes (i.e., primary auditory and primary visual regions) which deliver information to brain regions that integrate across modalities; (2) associative and componential processes that develop "higher order," often amodal, descriptions that relate the signal to the experienced environment (lateral temporal and parietal regions); and (3) command and control processes that effect a coherent model of the world when integrated with the first two processes, and which are implicated in motor behavior and planning – frontal and prefrontal regions (e.g., see Kandel, 2013; Luria, 1966; Mody, 2017). The white matter tracts that connect frontal and posterior regions are critical to these processes, enabling network approaches to offer further insights (Anderson et al., 2013). None of these functions, on its own, can be said to be the source or site of semiotic functions. However, it is within the amodal and multimodal regions of the superior temporal and inferior parietal regions, and their connections, that integrative processes that deliver meaning may be sought.

Dual processing streams for visual (and auditory) signals

For vision, two input processing streams, originating in the visual cortex in the occipital lobe, can be outlined. One route projects to superior parietal and then superior prefrontal regions via the superior longitudinal fasciculus and the arcuate fasciculus – a dorsal route. The other projects via inferior temporal to superior temporal regions and inferior frontal via the uncinate tracts – a ventral route. The functional distinction between the routes first formalized as a *where* pathway (dorsal) and a *what* pathway (ventral) (Ungerleider & Mishkin, 1982) was amended by Goodale and Milner (1992), who described the dorsal pathway as a *how* pathway for analyzing visual events. For communicative events as manual displays, there is a similar distinction. Damage to the ventral pathway impacts especially on *emblem* gestures such as thumbs-up or crossed fingers for luck, while dorsal pathway damage affects the ability to comprehend *pantomime* gestures, such as hammering or brushing teeth (Schwartz et al., 1998). Each route appears to be specialized for processing functionally different types of visual events.

Rauschecker (2018), noting that both visual and auditory pathways show a dorsal/ventral distinction, suggests that the ventral pathway – in either modality – is specialized to support identification of meaningful objects in the external world. The dorsal pathway supports processing that can parse dynamic events in space and time, especially in relation to the observer. The distinction between telic and non-telic action patterns, mentioned previously, which can be understood both by non-signers and signers, may be an example of how dorsal pathways process the manner of the manual gesture. A smooth manual action punctuated by an abrupt end (telic) is readily interpreted as "an event with a discrete endpoint," mapping onto a range of known action patterns that share this feature (Malaia & Wilbur, 2010), suggesting that this feature is retained and retrievable in the semantic representation of such action patterns.

In distinction to models of processing that are driven by sensory-specific hierarchical inputs (bottom-up), Rauschecker's account equally emphasizes components of the inferior frontal and prefrontal regions that utilize prediction models based on pre-occurring event processing (top-down) (Lupyan & Clark, 2015). Activation in the network itself modulates and sustains the achieved percept: a sensory-motor model of action/perception. Thus, within the anterior (ventral) stream, descending neural excitation predicts and maintains specific representations, supporting working memory for items and their meanings. The descending posterior (dorsal) stream, by controlling componential analysis of the signal, can deliver a variety of elements and meanings, depending on the parsing of the dynamically structured input. Meanings can be carried in both streams, with a role for the ventral stream in semantic processing for specific discrete events, but also involvement of, and integration with, dorsal processing networks which manage dynamic aspects of the signal, enabling a range of semantic and syntactic operations (Matchin & Hickok, 2019). Within these streams, specific nodes constitute key integrative sites. Around the angular gyrus, the inferior parietal lobule (IPL), lying just posterior to posterior superior temporal sulcus (Figure 13.2), receives projections from the ventral stream but is itself part of the dorsal stream. It may be a key locus for representing pantomime-type actions (*show me how you brush your teeth*). In patients with IPL damage, this function is impaired (Niessen et al., 2014; Pizzamiglio et al., 2019; Rothi et al., 1986). The LH dorsal route is implicated not only in SL production (Emmorey et al., 2007; Shum et al., 2020), but also in processing specific SL components, including topographic and classifier constructions (MacSweeney et al., 2006; MacSweeney et al., 2008; MacSweeney et al., 2002).

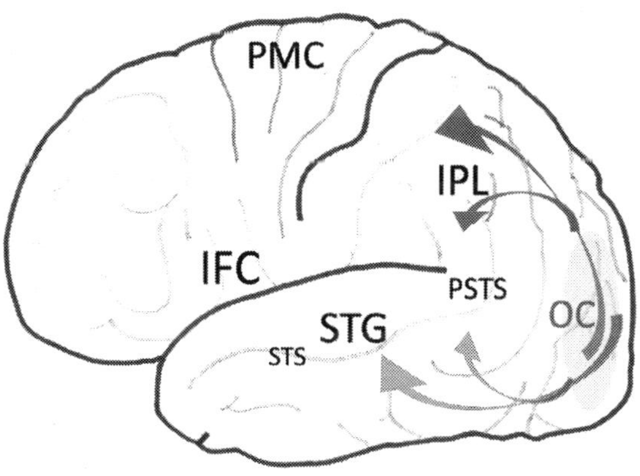

Figure 13.2 Schematic of major visual input streams

Shaded region indicates location of primary occipital (visual) cortex OC. Ventral stream: red; dorsal stream: blue. IFC: inferior frontal cortex, PMC: premotor cortex, STG: superior temporal gyrus, STS: superior temporal sulcus, PSTS: posterior superior temporal sulcus; IPL: inferior parietal lobule. The figure does not indicate predictive (top-down) pathways within frontal, fronto-parietal and fronto-temporal regions, which are critically important in sustained network activation. See e-book for a full-color version of this figure.

Actions (pantomimes) and things (emblems): Functional differentiation of gesture follows dual routes

Frontoparietal activation underpins a range of functions inherent in SL processing, including the meanings of dynamic actions (as in pantomimes). In contrast to pantomimes, which embody meaningful actions ("sewing," "boxing"), emblems have an agreed meaning within a particular language community. Emblems function like words in the established lexicon ("content" words, especially nouns and adjectives). Discrete sign utterances ("lists of signs"), whose lexical meaning can be grasped in the absence of a syntactic or discourse framework, can utilize this route (MacSweeney et al., 2006; Stroh et al., 2019). Emblems engage the ventral system (Andric et al., 2013). However, pantomimic gestures can resemble productive action terms, which often become meaningful in combination with other items in the utterance – that is, transitive gestures (Shetreet et al., 2010; Yang et al., 2015).

While partial and necessarily sketchy, this conception of the major neurosemiotic streams suggests that gesture, SL, and spoken language show commonalities of cortical processing based on how they depict events in the world, while at the same time those depictions can be of two different types. The identification and classification of discrete entities and their associations utilize the ventral processing network. The processing of dynamic actions, whose spatiotemporal characteristics can be controlled and moderated via frontal lobe activation, requires the dorsal pathway (Andric et al., 2013; Vigliocco et al., 2020; Yang et al., 2015). The lateralization of these processes may then reflect the extent to which the gestural patterns are processed linguistically.

Hand shapes and hand actions: Discrete sensitivities in sensory networks

Are there signal properties of seen gesture that could account for this pattern, both within a SL and more generally? Within the visual system in infero-temporal and occipital regions, there is further functional specialization relevant to semiotic processing. Regions that are most sensitive to seen movement of hands and arms are in *posterior* parts of the superior temporal lobe, often including IPL, adjacent to the supramarginal gyrus, and in dorsal route processing (Grosbras et al., 2012). By contrast, the perception of hand and finger positions is less dependent on movement characteristics. Finger and hand positions preferentially activate specific regions in *inferior* temporal cortex (Bracci et al. , 2010; Downing et al., 2006), with projections to more anterior regions of the superior temporal lobe (Pelphrey et al., 2005). This differentiation of signal information maps conveniently onto distinctions in SL. Finger and hand positions are more critical to interpretation of items that are in the established sign lexicon and may show greater activation in more anterior parts of the superior temporal gyrus (see McCullough et al., 2012; Okada et al., 2016). By contrast, manual *manner* of movement (i.e., fast or slow, shaky or smooth) and *path* (direction of movement) is reflected in activation along frontoparietal networks, including the IPL, preferentially accessing the dorsal processing stream (see, e.g., Campbell et al., 2011; MacSweeney et al., 2002). This latter pattern can be construed as relatively specialized for the processing of action terms in SL. A similar distinction may be made with respect to the brain bases for emblem gestures (ventral) and pantomime gestures (dorsal) in hearing people using a spoken language (Dick et al., 2014; Okada et al., 2016). What may be important neurosemiotically, in searching for the origins of different types of communicative gesture and the evolution of SLs, is that the patterning of the different gesture types maps readily onto known cortical pathways and networks which have distinct semantic functions. A neurosemiotic perspective allows insights such as these to emerge naturally in considering how gestures can signal meaning in brain systems.

Conclusion

In contrast to a syntax-based approach to understanding language processes and their brain correlates, a neurosemiotic account delineates the ways in which meaningful experiences effect symbolic mappings from sensorimotor events to comprehension in cortical systems, embedding them in the cultural and biological environment of the users. These mappings can clearly be seen in homesign and in SLs, with their very special conditions of acquisition and development. In considering aspects of skilled SL processing that are absent in spoken language (i.e., spatial features and non-manual gestures), the functional "ground plan" for understanding the variety of communicative meanings of seen gestures extends beyond the core perisylvian language network, which is the focus of neurolinguistic research, and makes special use of iconic resemblances between observed bodily actions and plausible events. Distinct, separable cortical systems are involved, connecting frontal and posterior regions, around multimodal hubs in superior temporal and inferior parietal cortices of both hemispheres (Newman et al., 2010; Simon, Lazzouni, et al., 2020).

The propensity for a core language network to develop primarily within a single brain hemisphere is the signature of human language abilities, including the manual language abilities of Deaf people. Neurosemiotics goes beyond this, showing that meaning through visible bodily gesture is implicated both at the root of understanding each other's intentions as well as the development and evolution of language, however manifested. It makes apparent that the human brain is structured to process communicative features of heads, hands, and bodies, and to capture their meanings.

Acknowledgements

I am grateful to Bencie Woll for comments and corrections on a draft of this chapter in relation to SL structures and processes, and for her friendship.

Notes

1 Pidgin languages serve a similar function, as users of different languages meet their need to communicate. However, users of pidgin are already skilled own-language users. The insight from homesign is that this communication mode, with the range of meanings it expresses, can develop spontaneously in the absence of a language model, and is often initiated by the deaf child (Morford & Goldin Meadow, 1997).

2 Deaf (upper case D) is used to denote membership of communities and individuals that self-define as users of a SL as a primary means of communication. The use of "deaf" (lower-case d) is often confined to describing people from an audiological perspective as having impaired hearing. They may or may not be SL users.

3 Here and elsewhere in this chapter, the use of SMALL CAPS denotes an SL item.

References

Anderson, M. L., Kinnison, J., & Pessoa, L. (2013). Describing functional diversity of brain regions and brain networks. *NeuroImage*, *73*, 50–58. doi: 10.1016/j.neuroimage.2013.01.071

Andric, M., Solodkin, A., Buccino, G., Goldin-Meadow, S., Rizzolatti, G., & Small, S. L. (2013). Brain function overlaps when people observe emblems, speech, and grasping. *Neuropsychologia*, *51*(8), 1619–1629. doi: 10.1016/j.neuropsychologia.2013.03.022

Atkinson, J., Campbell, R., Marshall, J., Thacker, A., & Woll, B. (2004). Understanding "not": Neuropsychological dissociations between hand and head markers of negation in BSL. *Neuropsychologia*, *42*(2), 214–229. doi: 10.1016/s0028-3932(03)00186-6

Baker, C., & Padden, C. (1978). Focussing on the non-manual components of ASL. In P. Siple (Ed.), *Understanding Language Through Sign Language Research* (pp. 27–57). New York: Academic Press.

Boyes Breaem, P., & Sutton-Spence, R. (Eds.). (2001). *The Hands are the Head of the Mouth: The Mouth as Articulator in Sign Language*. Hamburg: Signum.

Bracci, S., Ietswaart, M., Peelen, M. V., & Cavina-Pratesi, C. (2010). Dissociable neural responses to hands and non-hand body parts in human left extrastriate visual cortex. *Journal of Neurophysiology*, *103*(6), 3389–3397. doi: 10.1152/jn.00215.2010

Brentari, D. (2019). *Sign Language Phonology*. New York: Cambridge University Press.

Campbell, R., Capek, C. M., Gazarian, K., MacSweeney, M., Woll, B., David, A. S., … Brammer, M. J. (2011). The signer and the sign: Cortical correlates of person identity and language processing from point-light displays. *Neuropsychologia*, *49*(11), 3018–3026. doi: 10.1016/j.neuropsychologia.2011.06.029

Campbell, R., MacSweeney, M., & Woll, B. (2014). Cochlear implantation (CI) for prelingual deafness: The relevance of studies of brain organization and the role of first language acquisition in considering outcome success. *Frontiers in Human Neuroscience, 8*, 834. doi: 10.3389/fnhum.2014.00834

Campbell, R., Martin, P., & White, T. (1992). The recognition of signs: Does learning BSL improve memory for hand posture? *Applied Linguistics, 13*, 185–201.

Capek, C. M., Grossi, G., Newman, A. J., McBurney, S. L., Corina, D., Roeder, B., & Neville, H. (2009). Brain systems mediating semantic and syntactic processing in deaf native signers: biological invariance and modality specificity. *Proceedings of the National Academy of Sciences of the United States of America, 106*(21), 8784–8789. doi: 10.1073/pnas.0809609106

Cardin, V., Orfanidou, E., Rönnberg, J., Capek, C. M., Rudner, M., & Woll, B. (2013). Dissociating cognitive and sensory neural plasticity in human superior temporal cortex. *Nature Communications, 4*, 1473. doi: 10.1038/ncomms2463

Cheng, Q., & Mayberry, R. I. (2020). When event knowledge overrides word order in sentence comprehension: Learning a first language after childhood. *Developmental Science, 24*(5) e13073. doi: 10.1111/desc.13073

Cheng, Q., Roth, A., Halgren, E., & Mayberry, R. I. (2019). Effects of early language deprivation on brain connectivity: Language pathways in deaf native and late first-language learners of American Sign Language. *Frontiers in Human Neuroscience, 13*, 320. doi: 10.3389/fnhum.2019.00320

Coppola, M., & Senghas, A. (2017). Is it language (yet)? The allure of the gesture-language binary. *Behavioral and Brain Sciences, 40*, e50. doi: 10.1017/S0140525X1500285X

Cormier, K., Schembri, A., & Woll, B. (2013). Pronouns and pointing in sign languages. *Lingua, 137*, 230–247. doi: 10.1016/j.lingua.2013.09.010

Dachkovsky, S., & Sandler, W. (2009). Visual intonation in the prosody of a sign language. *Language and Speech, 52*(Pt 2–3), 287–314. doi: 10.1177/0023830909103175

Darwin, C. (1872). *The Expression of the Emotions in Man and Animals*. London: John Murray.

Dick, A. S., Goldin-Meadow, S., Hasson, U., Skipper, J. I., & Small, S. L. (2009). Co-speech gestures influence neural activity in brain regions associated with processing semantic information. *Human Brain Mapping, 30*(11), 3509–3526. doi: 10.1002/hbm.20774

Dick, A. S., Mok, E. H., Raja Beharelle, A., Goldin-Meadow, S., & Small, S. L. (2014). Frontal and temporal contributions to understanding the iconic co-speech gestures that accompany speech. *Human Brain Mapping, 35*(3), 900–917. doi: 10.1002/hbm.22222

DiNapoli, D. (2017). Iconicity chains in sign languages. In C. Bowern, L. Horn, & R. Zanuttini (Eds.), *On Looking Into Words (and Beyond)* (pp. 517–546). Berlin: Language Science Press.

Dingemanse, M., Blasi, D. E., Lupyan, G., Christiansen, M. H., & Monaghan, P. (2015). Arbitrariness, iconicity, and systematicity in language. *Trends in Cognitive Sciences, 19*(10), 603–615. doi: 10.1016/j.tics.2015.07.013

Downing, P. E., Peelen, M. V., Wiggett, A. J., & Tew, B. D. (2006). The role of the extrastriate body area in action perception. *Social Neuroscience, 1*(1), 52–62. doi: 10.1080/17470910600668854

Emmorey, K. (2002). *Language, Cognition, and the Brain: Insights from Sign Language Research*. Hillsdale, NJ: Lawrence Erlbaum.

Emmorey, K. (2003). *Perspectives on Classifer Constructions in Sign Language*. Hillsdale, NJ: Lawrence Erlbaum.

Emmorey, K. (2014). Iconicity as structure mapping. *Philosophical Transactions of the Royal Society B: Biological Sciences, 369*(1651), 20130301. doi: 10.1098/rstb.2013.0301

Emmorey, K., Allen, J. S., Bruss, J., Schenker, N., & Damasio, H. (2003). A morphometric analysis of auditory brain regions in congenitally deaf adults. *Proceedings of the National Academy of Sciences of the United States of America, 100*(17), 10049–10054. doi: 10.1073/pnas.1730169100

Emmorey, K., Grabowski, T., McCullough, S., Damasio, H., Ponto, L., Hichwa, R., & Bellugi, U. (2003). Neural systems underlying lexical retrieval for sign language. *Neuropsychologia, 41*(1), 85–95. doi: 10.1016/s0028-3932(02)00089-1

Emmorey, K., Grabowski, T., McCullough, S., Damasio, H., Ponto, L., Hichwa, R., & Bellugi, U. (2004). Motor-iconicity of sign language does not alter the neural systems underlying tool and action naming. *Brain and Language, 89*(1), 27–37. doi: 10.1016/S0093-934X(03)00309-2

Emmorey, K., Grabowski, T., McCullough, S., Ponto, L. L., Hichwa, R. D., & Damasio, H. (2005). The neural correlates of spatial language in English and American Sign Language: A PET study with hearing bilinguals. *NeuroImage, 24*(3), 832–840. doi: 10.1016/j.neuroimage.2004.10.008

Emmorey, K., Mehta, S., & Grabowski, T. J. (2007). The neural correlates of sign versus word production. *NeuroImage, 36*(1), 202–208. doi: 10.1016/j.neuroimage.2007.02.040

Emmorey, K., Winsler, K., Midgley, K. J., Grainger, J., & Holcomb, P. J. (2020). Neurophysiological correlates of frequency, concreteness, and iconicity in American Sign Language. *Neurobiology of Language, 1*(2), 249–267. doi: 10.1162/nol_a_00012

Ferjan Ramirez, N., Leonard, M. K., Davenport, T. S., Torres, C., Halgren, E., & Mayberry, R. I. (2016). Neural language processing in adolescent first-language learners: Longitudinal case studies in American Sign Language. *Cerebral Cortex*, *26*(3), 1015–1026. doi: 10.1093/cercor/bhu273

Ferjan Ramirez, N., Leonard, M. K., Torres, C., Hatrak, M., Halgren, E., & Mayberry, R. I. (2013). Neural language processing in adolescent first-language learners. *Cerebral Cortex*. doi: 10.1093/cercor/bht137

Goldin-Meadow, S. (2003). *The Resilience of Language: What Gesture Creation in Deaf Children can Tell us About How All Children Learn Language*. New York: Psychology Press.

Goldin-Meadow, S. (2017). What the hands can tell us about language emergence. *Psychonomic Bulletin & Review*, *24*(1), 213–218. doi: 10.3758/s13423-016-1074-x

Goldin-Meadow, S., & Brentari, D. (2017). Gesture and language: Distinct subsystem of an integrated whole. *Behavioral and Brain Sciences*, *40*, e74. doi: 10.1017/S0140525X1600039X

Goldin-Meadow, S., & Yang, C. (2017). Statistical evidence that a child can create a combinatorial linguistic system without external linguistic input: Implications for language evolution. *Neuroscience & Biobehavioral Review*, *81*(Pt B), 150–157. doi: 10.1016/j.neubiorev.2016.12.016

Goodale, M. A., & Milner, A. D. (1992). Separate visual pathways for perception and action. *Trends in Neurosciences*, *15*(1), 20–25. doi: 10.1016/0166-2236(92)90344-8

Grosbras, M. H., Beaton, S., & Eickhoff, S. B. (2012). Brain regions involved in human movement perception: A quantitative voxel-based meta-analysis. *Human Brain Mapping*, *33*(2), 431–454. doi: 10.1002/hbm.21222

Grzybek, P. (1993). *Psychosemiotik, Neurosemiotik = Psychosemiotics, neurosemiotics*. Bochum: Brockmeyer.

Göksun, T., Lehet, M., Malykhina, K., & Chatterjee, A. (2015). Spontaneous gesture and spatial language: Evidence from focal brain injury. *Brain and Language*, *150*, 1–13. doi: 10.1016/j.bandl.2015.07.012

Hockett, C. F. (1958). *A Course in Modern Linguistics*. New York: Macmillan.

Ivanov, V. (1994). Neurosemiotics and neurobiology (Review of Gazzaniga 1988 (book) *Mind matters: How mind and brain interact to create our conscious lives*, Boston 1988). *Semiotica*, *1/2*, 103–121.

Jouravlev, O., Zheng, D., Balewski, Z., Le Arnz Pongos, A., Levan, Z., Goldin-Meadow, S., & Fedorenko, E. (2019). Speech-accompanying gestures are not processed by the language-processing mechanisms. *Neuropsychologia*, *132*, 107132. doi: 10.1016/j.neuropsychologia.2019.107132

Kandel, E. R. (2013). *Principles of Neural Science* (5th edn). New York: McGraw-Hill.

Kita, S., & Lausberg, H. (2008). Generation of co-speech gestures based on spatial imagery from the right-hemisphere: Evidence from split-brain patients. *Cortex*, *44*(2), 131–139. doi: 10.1016/j.cortex.2006.04.001

Leonard, M. K., Ferjan Ramirez, N., Torres, C., Travis, K. E., Hatrak, M., Mayberry, R. I., & Halgren, E. (2012). Signed words in the congenitally deaf evoke typical late lexicosemantic responses with no early visual responses in left superior temporal cortex. *The Journal of Neuroscience*, *32*(28), 9700–9705. doi: 10.1523/JNEUROSCI.1002-12.2012

Liddell, S. K. (2003). *Grammar, Ggesture, and Meaning in American Sign Language*. Cambridge: Cambridge University Press.

Lieberman, A. M., Borovsky, A., Hatrak, M., & Mayberry, R. I. (2015). Real-time processing of ASL signs: Delayed first language acquisition affects organization of the mental lexicon. *Journal of Experimental Psychology: Learning, Memory, and Cognition*, *41*(4), 1130–1139. doi: 10.1037/xlm0000088

Lupyan, G., & Clark, A. (2015). Words and the world: Predictive coding and the language-perception-cognition interface. *Current Directions in Psychological Science*, *24*(4), 279–284. doi: 10.1177/0963721415570732

Luria, A. (1966). *Higher Cortical Functions in Man*. Boston: Springer.

MacSweeney, M., Campbell, R., Woll, B., Brammer, M. J., Giampietro, V., David, A. S., … & McGuire, P. K. (2006). Lexical and sentential processing in British Sign Language. *Human Brain Mapping*, *27*(1), 63–76. doi: 10.1002/hbm.20167

MacSweeney, M., Campbell, R., Woll, B., Giampietro, V., David, A. S., McGuire, P. K., … Brammer, M. J. (2004). Dissociating linguistic and nonlinguistic gestural communication in the brain. *NeuroImage*, *22*(4), 1605–1618. doi: 10.1016/j.neuroimage.2004.03.015

MacSweeney, M., Capek, C. M., Campbell, R., & Woll, B. (2008). The signing brain: The neurobiology of sign language. *Trends in Cognitive Sciences*, *12*(11), 432–440. doi: 10.1016/j.tics.2008.07.010

MacSweeney, M., Woll, B., Campbell, R., Calvert, G. A., McGuire, P. K., David, A. S., … Brammer, M. J. (2002). Neural correlates of British Sign Language comprehension: Spatial processing demands of topographic language. *Journal of Cognitive Neuroscience*, *14*(7), 1064–1075. doi: 10.1162/089892902320474517

Malaia, E., Krebs, J., Roehm, D., & Wilbur, R. B. (2020). Age of acquisition effects differ across linguistic domains in sign language: EEG evidence. *Brain and Language*, *200*, 104708. doi: 10.1016/j.bandl.2019.104708

Malaia, E., & Wilbur, R. (2010). Sign languages: Contribution to neurolinguistics from cross-modal research. *Lingua*, *120*(12), 2704–2706. doi: 10.1016/j.lingua.2010.03.014

Malaia, E., & Wilbur, R. B. (2012). Kinematic signatures of telic and atelic events in ASL predicates. *Language and Speech*, *55*(Pt 3), 407–421.

Matchin, W., & Hickok, G. (2019). The cortical organization of syntax. *Cerebral Cortex*, 30(3), 1481–1498. doi: 10.1093/cercor/bhz180

Mayberry, R. I., Davenport, T., Roth, A., & Halgren, E. (2018). Neurolinguistic processing when the brain matures without language. *Cortex*, *99*, 390–403. doi: 10.1016/j.cortex.2017.12.011

Mayberry, R. I., & Fischer, S. D. (1989). Looking through phonological shape to lexical meaning: The bottleneck of non-native sign language processing. *Memory & Cognition*, *17*(6), 740–754.

McClave, E. (2000). Linguistic functions of head movement in the context of speech. *Journal of Pragmatics*, *32*(7), 855–878. doi: 10.1016/S0378-2166(99)00079-X

McCullough, S., Saygin, A. P., Korpics, F., & Emmorey, K. (2012). Motion-sensitive cortex and motion semantics in American Sign Language. *NeuroImage*, *63*(1), 111–118. doi: 10.1016/j.neuroimage.2012.06.029

McGarry, M. E., Mott, M., Midgley, K. J., Holcomb, P. J., & Emmorey, K. (2021). Picture-naming in American Sign Language: An electrophysiological study of the effects of iconicity and structured alignment. *Language Cognition and Neuroscience*, *36*(2), 199–210. doi: 10.1080/23273798.2020.1804601

Meier, R. (2016). Sign language acquisition. *Oxford Handbooks Online: Scholarly Research Reviews*. doi: 10.1093/oxfordhb/9780199935345.013.19

Mody, M. (2017). *Neural Mechanisms of Language Innovations in Cognitive Neuroscience*. New York: Springer.

Morford, J. P. & Goldin-Meadow, S. (1997). From here and now to there and then: the development of displaced reference in homesign and English. *Child Development*, *68*(3), 420–435.

Morgan, G., & Woll, B. (2007). Understanding sign language classifiers through a polycomponential approach. *Lingua*, *117*(7), 1159–1168. doi: 10.1016/j.lingua.2006.01.006

Neville, H. J., Coffey, S. A., Lawson, D. S., Fischer, A., Emmorey, K., & Bellugi, U. (1997). Neural systems mediating American Sign Language: Effects of sensory experience and age of acquisition. *Brain and Language*, *57*(3), 285–308. doi: 10.1006/brln.1997.1739

Newman, A. J., Supalla, T., Fernandez, N., Newport, E. L., & Bavelier, D. (2015). Neural systems supporting linguistic structure, linguistic experience, and symbolic communication in sign language and gesture. *Proceedings of the National Academy of Sciences of the United States of America*, *112*(37), 11684–11689. doi: 10.1073/pnas.1510527112

Newman, A. J., Supalla, T., Hauser, P. C., Newport, E. L., & Bavelier, D. (2010). Prosodic and narrative processing in American Sign Language: An fMRI study. *NeuroImage*, *52*(2), 669–676. doi: 10.1016/j.neuroimage.2010.03.055

Niessen, E., Fink, G. R., & Weiss, P. H. (2014). Apraxia, pantomime and the parietal cortex. *NeuroImage: Clinical*, *5*, 42–52. doi: 10.1016/j.nicl.2014.05.017

O'Madagain, C., Kachel, G., & Strickland, B. (2019). The origin of pointing: Evidence for the touch hypothesis. *Science Advances*, *5*(7), eaav2558. doi: 10.1126/sciadv.aav2558

Okada, K., Rogalsky, C., O'Grady, L., Hanaumi, L., Bellugi, U., Corina, D., & Hickok, G. (2016). An fMRI study of perception and action in deaf signers. *Neuropsychologia*, *82*, 179–188. doi: 10.1016/j.neuropsychologia.2016.01.015

Ortega, G. (2017). Iconicity and sign lexical acquisition: A review. *Frontiers in Psychology*, *8*, 1280. doi: 10.3389/fpsyg.2017.01280

Ortega, G., Özyürek, A., & Peeters, D. (2020). Iconic gestures serve as manual cognates in hearing second language learners of a sign language: An ERP study. *Journal of Experimental Psychology: Learning, Memory, and Cognition*, *46*(3), 403–415. doi: 10.1037/xlm0000729

Özyürek, A. (2014). Hearing and seeing meaning in speech and gesture: insights from brain and behaviour. *Philosophical Transactions of the Royal Society B: Biological Sciences*, *369*(1651), 20130296. doi: 10.1098/rstb.2013.0296

Pelphrey, K. A., Morris, J. P., Michelich, C. R., Allison, T., & McCarthy, G. (2005). Functional anatomy of biological motion perception in posterior temporal cortex: An FMRI study of eye, mouth and hand movements. *Cerebral Cortex*, *15*(12), 1866–1876. doi: 10.1093/cercor/bhi064

Pizzamiglio, G., Zhang, Z., Kolasinski, J., Riddoch, J. M., Passingham, R. E., Mantini, D., & Rounis, E. (2019). A role for the action observation network in apraxia after stroke. *Frontiers in Human Neuroscience*, *13*, 422. doi: 10.3389/fnhum.2019.00422

Power, J. M., Grimm, G. W., & List, J.-M. (2020). Evolutionary dynamics in the dispersal of sign languages. *Royal Society Open Science*, 7(1), 191100. doi: 10.1098/rsos.191100

Pyers, J., & Senghas, A. (2020). Lexical Iconicity is differentially favored under transmission in a new sign language: The effect of type of iconicity. *Sign Language & Linguistics*, *23*(1–2), 73–95. doi: 10.1075/sll.00044.pye

Pénicaud, S., Klein, D., Zatorre, R. J., Chen, J. K., Witcher, P., Hyde, K., & Mayberry, R. I. (2013). Structural brain changes linked to delayed first language acquisition in congenitally deaf individuals. *NeuroImage*, *66*, 42–49. doi: 10.1016/j.neuroimage.2012.09.076

Quer, J. (2012). Negation. In R. Pfau, M. Steinbach, & B. Woll (Eds.), *Sign Language: An International Handbook* (pp. 316–339). Berlin: De Gruyer Mouton.

Rauschecker, J. P. (2018). Where, when, and how: Are they all sensorimotor? Towards a unified view of the dorsal pathway in vision and audition. *Cortex, 98*, 262–268. doi: 10.1016/j.cortex.2017.10.020

Rothi, L. J., Mack, L., & Heilman, K. M. (1986). Pantomime agnosia. *Journal of Neurology, Neurosurgery & Psychiatry, 49*(4), 451–454. doi: 10.1136/jnnp.49.4.451

Sakai, K. L., Tatsuno, Y., Suzuki, K., Kimura, H., & Ichida, Y. (2005). Sign and speech: Amodal commonality in left hemisphere dominance for comprehension of sentences. *Brain, 128*(Pt 6), 1407–1417. doi: 10.1093/brain/awh465

Schwartz, R. L., Barrett, A. M., Crucian, G. P., & Heilman, K. M. (1998). Dissociation of gesture and object recognition. *Neurology, 50*(4), 1186–1188. doi: 10.1212/wnl.50.4.1186

Sebeok, T. A. (2001). *Signs: An Introduction to Semiotics* (2nd edn). Toronto: University of Toronto Press.

Shetreet, E., Friedmann, N., & Hadar, U. (2010). Cortical representation of verbs with optional complements: The theoretical contribution of fMRI. *Human Brain Mapping, 31*(5), 770–785. doi: 10.1002/hbm.20904

Shum, J., Fanda, L., Dugan, P., Doyle, W. K., Devinsky, O., & Flinker, A. (2020). Neural correlates of sign language production revealed by electrocorticography. *Neurology, 95*(21), e2880-e2889. doi: 10.1212/WNL.0000000000010639

Simon, M., Campbell, E., Genest, F., MacLean, M. W., Champoux, F., & Lepore, F. (2020). The impact of early deafness on brain plasticity: A systematic review of the white and gray matter changes. *Frontiers in Neuroscience, 14*, 206. doi: 10.3389/fnins.2020.00206

Simon, M., Lazzouni, L., Campbell, E., Delcenserie, A., Muise-Hennessey, A., Newman, A. J., ... Lepore, F. (2020). Enhancement of visual biological motion recognition in early-deaf adults: Functional and behavioral correlates. *PLoS One, 15*(8), e0236800. doi: 10.1371/journal.pone.0236800

Strickland, B., Geraci, C., Chemla, E., Schlenker, P., Kelepir, M., & Pfau, R. (2015). Event representations constrain the structure of language: Sign language as a window into universally accessible linguistic biases. *Proceedings of the National Academy of Sciences of the United States of America, 112*(19), 5968–5973. doi: 10.1073/pnas.1423080112

Stroh, A. L., Rösler, F., Dormal, G., Salden, U., Skotara, N., Hänel-Faulhaber, B., & Röder, B. (2019). Neural correlates of semantic and syntactic processing in German Sign Language. *NeuroImage, 200*, 231–241. doi: 10.1016/j.neuroimage.2019.06.025

Thompson, R. L., Vinson, D. P., Woll, B., & Vigliocco, G. (2012). The road to language learning is iconic: evidence from British Sign Language. *Psychological Science, 23*(12), 1443–1448. doi: 10.1177/0956797612459763

Ungerleider, L., & Mishkin, M. (1982). Two cortical visual systems. In D. Ingle, M. Goodale, & R. Mansfield (Eds.), *Analysis of visual behaviour* (pp. 549–586). Cambridge, MA: MIT Press

Vigliocco, G., Krason, A., Stoll, H., Monti, A., & Buxbaum, L. J. (2020). Multimodal comprehension in stroke patients. *Cortex, 133*, 309–327. doi: 10.1016/j.cortex.2020.09.025

Woll, B. (2018). The consequences of very late exposure to BSL as an L1. *Bilingualism: Language and Cognition, 21*(5), 936–937. doi: 10.1017/S1366728918000238

Wright, P., Stamatakis, E. A., & Tyler, L. K. (2012). Differentiating hemispheric contributions to syntax and semantics in patients with left-hemisphere lesions. *The Journal of Neuroscience, 32*(24), 8149–8157. doi: 10.1523/JNEUROSCI.0485-12.2012

Xu, J., Gannon, P. J., Emmorey, K., Smith, J. F., & Braun, A. R. (2009). Symbolic gestures and spoken language are processed by a common neural system. *Proceedings of the National Academy of Sciences of the United States of America, 106*(49), 20664–20669. doi: 10.1073/pnas.0909197106

Yang, J., Andric, M., & Mathew, M. M. (2015). The neural basis of hand gesture comprehension: A meta-analysis of functional magnetic resonance imaging studies. *Neuroscience & Biobehavioral Reviews, 57*, 88–104. doi: 10.1016/j.neubiorev.2015.08.006

PART III

The neurosemiotics of social dynamics

14
EMPATHY, MEANING, AND THE HUMAN BRAIN

Konrad Lehmann and Philipp Kanske

Introduction

Imagine yourself out having dinner with a friend, when suddenly her cell phone rings and she answers. Abruptly, she starts asking a couple of questions in a frantic way and then becomes quieter, fights back her tears, and eventually starts crying. Although you do not immediately share exactly the same responses as your friend, you do feel her suffering and probably feel somewhat saddened yourself. This feeling or process of resonating with or vicariously sharing others' emotions has been referred to as empathy (de Vignemont & Singer, 2006; Decety & Cowell, 2014), a term that is originally derived from the Greek *empatheia*, which literally means "feeling into" (Pinotti, 2010: 93–98). In social science, the label "empathy" is frequently stretched beyond the pure sharing of others' emotions (i.e., affective empathy) towards the cognitive understanding of others' emotions, desires, thoughts, intention, goals, and motives (Frith & Frith, 2005; Premack & Woodruff, 1978). The latter is described as "cognitive empathy," theory of mind, or mentalizing – which we will use throughout this chapter for reasons of demarcation and clarity (Kanske, 2018; Kanske et al., 2015). Returning to our example from the beginning, mentalizing will allow you to understand that your friend is sad even if you do not resonate with their emotion and do not feel saddened yourself. Mentalizing thus gives us an abstract understanding of the inner states of others while empathy furnishes us with an immediate affective or emotional grasp of these inner states. Although these processes can be well distinguished, they do seem to interact in more complex social situations (Schurz et al., 2020). Both empathy and mentalizing are effective tools in the interpretation of communicative behaviors, which consequently makes them compelling concepts in the field of neurosemiotics as "the scientific investigation of the neurological processes underlying communicative behavior in all its forms as well as the prerequisites for such behavior" (Bouissac, 2018). Our inferences about the inner states of others largely condition the ways we construe meaning during our social encounters.

In this chapter, we outline the cognitive and neural mechanisms of both empathy and mentalizing, starting with observational contexts as the most common source of our scientific understanding of these processes. However, since the explanatory value of these contexts is limited regarding the construal of meaning during natural, dynamic, and embedded social interactions "in the wild," we move to the role and morphology of empathy and mentalizing in these complex interactions in the second part of this chapter. Lastly, we consider how empathy and mentalizing help us to construe meaning within our social lives.

DOI: 10.4324/9781003051817-18

Empathy

As mentioned above, empathy allows us to access the inner state of others by sharing their emotional state (de Vignemont & Singer, 2006; Decety & Cowell, 2014), which means we effectively experience the observed emotion vicariously – or in a first-person manner. An important additional aspect to this definition is that we know the other person is the source of our feeling (Singer & Klimecki, 2014). Consequently, on an algorithmic level, in order to meet the definition of empathy, resonating with another person's emotion first requires us to somehow detect (not necessarily explicitly) a mismatch between our own state and that of the other person. We then need to adapt our internal milieu to attain a similar embodied feeling as experienced by the other person.

The neural architecture enabling us to carry out these steps, hence leading to the experience of empathy, has been thoroughly investigated and mapped to the anterior cingulate cortex (ACC) and anterior insula (AI) (Kanske et al., 2015; Lamm et al., 2011; Preckel et al., 2018), which is commonly summarized as the salience network (Seeley et al., 2007). Specifically, via its bidirectional noradrenergic projections with the locus coeruleus, the ACC most likely computes the fluctuation between the sender's and receiver's emotional or bodily states, as this region is involved in tracking volatility (Lau et al., 2020; Parr & Friston, 2018; Sales et al., 2019). The AI, on the other hand, has been implicated in the computation of errors between predicted and observed bodily states and in the adaptation of the internal milieu through top-down set point modulation (Barrett & Simmons, 2015; Gu et al., 2013). Studies employing resting-state functional magnetic resonance imaging showed relations between connectivity within the salience network and heart rate variability (Chang et al., 2013), vagal tone (Guo et al., 2016), and muscle nerve activity (Taylor et al., 2015). Likewise, gray matter volume within the salience network is associated with heart rate variability (Wei & Wu, 2020) and with empathy (Valk et al., 2017).

Interestingly, both the ACC and the AI are furnished with large spindle-shaped neurons (von Economo neurons), which are particularly suitable for conveying information over longer distances, such as from the brain to the rest of the body (Allman et al., 2005, 2011). Accordingly, atrophy in von Economo neurons in the AI and ACC, as seen in behavioral variant frontotemporal dementia (Kim et al., 2012; Seeley, 2010; Seeley et al., 2006), is accompanied by a loss of empathy and self-conscious emotions while cognitive functions mostly remain intact (Baez et al., 2014; Rankin et al., 2006; Sturm et al., 2006).

Importantly, the proneness to empathize with another person and the amount of empathy are highly context dependent (Keysers & Gazzola, 2014; Zaki, 2014). This contextual variation is particularly pronounced when comparing ingroup versus outgroup targets (Cikara & Paluck, 2013; Gutsell & Inzlicht, 2010). For example, Hein et al. (2010) showed that soccer fans exhibit less empathic concern when seeing the suffering of a fan of a rival team compared with a fan from their own team. Empathic concern and neural responses in the AI predicted the motivation to relieve an ingroup member from their suffering.

Besides group affiliation, a professional context largely modulates the engagement to empathize with others. For example, physicians underestimate the degree of pain in patients (Marquié et al., 2003), which is accompanied by diminished corresponding neural responses (Decety et al., 2010). Furthermore, potential costs in terms of money (Andreoni et al., 2017) or time (Cameron & Payne, 2011), as well as emotional (Cameron et al., 2016) or cognitive (Cameron et al., 2019) resources, constitute motivational factors that strongly influence proneness to show empathy.

The motivational and contextual effects on empathy clearly point to the pragmatic value of sharing others' emotions. When empathic sharing could have detrimental consequences (e.g., for professionals practicing their jobs) or hinder a desired outcome (e.g., helping a rival), we avoid resonating with another person's emotions. The emotion of empathy could convey a bodily feeling, informing us about whether we can or want to sympathize with another individual. In this sense, it might deliver a homeostatic informational gain, signaling whether an affiliative response is in line with maintaining internal stability (Barrett & Simmons, 2015). In a neurosemiotic reading, our feelings in respect to others help us categorize the context of the relationship towards the other person, constituting a "frame of sense" (Salvatore & Venuleo, 2008). This frame is implicit to the affordances we experience when acting towards other people. As mentioned, some contexts invite us to resonate with someone while other contexts require us to focus on other situational aspects, depending on our relation to a person in a given context. Affordances have been argued to constitute a description of a relationship between organisms and the environment, rendering the perceived affordance a sign-relation (Campbell et al., 2019).

On a higher level, our bodily feelings in respect to another person also constitute a potent source for interpretational mechanisms. They might be considered Peirce-signals, being described as a sign when something is interpreted as such. For example, my bodily feelings may signal a motivation to approach a friend and comfort her. Such pre-reflective impulses, when they reach awareness, and thus a more abstract representational level, are associated, interpreted, and integrated to give meaning to our interpersonal lives; not for nothing do we rely on our bodily or gut feelings when reflecting on our interpersonal relationships.

Mentalizing

While empathizing furnishes us with an embodied feeling, mentalizing rather supplies an abstract understanding of mental states that could be considered more cognitively informed. Inherent to the concept of mentalizing is the assumption that, by themselves, mental or inner states are not directly observable but need to be reversely inferred from observable actions (Tamir & Thornton, 2018). However, the actions (including facial expressions, utterances, and so on) are not unambiguously indicative of inner states; rather, the relation between these two layers entails uncertainties. For example, when you see a stranger running down the street, their motion could be motivated by the gleeful anticipation of seeing their partner or by a fearful attempt to escape an intrusive and shady stranger, or by something completely different. In order to gain more certainty about others' inner states, additional informational sources need to be consulted. Here, contextual information gives us the opportunity to narrow down possible alternatives to more precisely estimate the internal state of another person. Provided with rich contextual information, we may have the impression that we can observe mental states directly because the additional information delivers prior assumptions that narrow down our hypothetical alternatives – for a debate, see de Bruin & Strijbos (2015), Gallagher (2008), Michael & de Bruin (2015), and Zahavi (2011). For example, if we see the woman running down the street waving to a bus driver 30 meters ahead, we might feel we have collected enough evidence to assume that the woman is in a rush to catch the bus.

At a neural level, mentalizing is commonly associated with activity in the default mode network (DMN), including the medial prefrontal cortex (MPFC), the temporoparietal junction (TPJ), the superior temporal sulcus, the temporal poles, and the precuneus (Bzdok et al., 2012; Kanske et al., 2016; Schurz et al., 2014, 2021). These brain regions have also been implied in processes such as episodic memory (Sestieri et al., 2011), episodic prospection (Spreng & Grady, 2009), and mindwandering (Schooler et al., 2011). What these processes share is a common core of counterfactual thinking or simulation (Buckner, 2012; Hassabis & Maguire, 2009; Van Hoeck et al., 2015) – that is, thinking about how the world would look if something were different. In respect to mental states, counterfactual simulations could be a central process in narrowing down possible alternatives to arrive at an adequate estimation about a possible inner state. For example, when your boss asks you for a meeting next week without giving a hint about the possible content, but they have a broad grin on their face, you may engage in counterfactual simulation to find out whether you should be afraid in the face of the upcoming encounter. Thinking about your boss grinning while they are planning to tell you something that affects you negatively (e.g., your contract is not being extended) would indicate that they are somehow malevolent. However, when you then consider that your boss is usually pretty benevolent, you might gain certainty that they have something in mind that will affect you positively.

Given that the relations between observable actions and mental states are not one to one, and considering that mental states are also subject to fluctuations, counterfactual simulations are necessary in order to gain a satisfactory degree of certainty. Of course, these simulations do not necessarily have to reach consciousness, but possibly happen largely implicitly (Low & Perner, 2012). However, both explicit and implicit forms of mental state inference serve to reduce uncertainty to reach more precise predictions about the social environment (Tamir & Thornton, 2018). In a neurosemiotic sense, counterfactually reducing the uncertainty about another's mental state delivers the contextual frame or sign relation about how observable actions might be read; it helps to select a sense out of an infinite number of possible senses. This process can be construed as an interpretive mechanism or a semiotic resource (Leeuwen, 2005) for constructing meaning from our environment. By mentally embedding observable behaviors within a reference frame, be it contextual information or hypothetical alternatives, our reading of the behaviors becomes meaningful. As the American scientist Arthur Asa Berger put it: "Meaning is relational. Nothing means anything in itself, and everything means something because of some kind of relationship in which it is embedded" (Berger, 1989: 173).

Empathy and mentalizing during complex social interactions in the wild

Insights into the socio-affective and socio-cognitive mechanisms described above mainly come from spectatorial paradigms. As such, they are limited in their explanatory value regarding the construal of meaning during interactions "in the wild." In contrast to most neuroscience studies, actual interactions are characterized as dynamic, complex, and embedded in contextually rich environments (Ibáñez, 2019; Ibáñez & García, 2018). Here, we rehearse critical points regarding spectatorial paradigms and make an attempt to illuminate empathy and mentalizing in embedded situations and how these processes might help us to engage in symbolic interactions (Bouissac, 2018) and navigate in our social environment.

Empathy and mentalizing are commonly conceived as domains that enable social interaction – for a debate regarding the role of mentalizing, see Froese & Gallagher (2012) and Reddy & Morris (2004). However, the gap between the laboratory assessment – where participants are put in an isolated and passive spectator perspective – and actual social interaction is seldomly crossed, especially in the investigation of the underlying neural mechanisms. The application of a passive spectator perspective is based on assumptions of a cognitivistic tradition that views mental processes in a linear fashion from receiving stimuli to processing these stimuli (in mainly context-invariant neural modules) to generating responses (Engel et al., 2013). However, recent claims and discussions, spanning philosophy, experimental psychology and neuroscience, have often criticized this approach as being detached and not ecologically valid, since observation and actual interaction are assumed to be fundamentally different (e.g., Becchio et al., 2010; De Jaegher et al., 2010; Lehmann et al., 2019; Schilbach et al., 2013; Shamay-Tsoory & Mendelsohn, 2019; Wheatley et al., 2019). These claims are very well aligned with developments in the field of neurosemiotics, based on the fact that "communication is a real-time social process which must be understood at the level of dyadic interactions" (Galantucci, 2009). During real social interaction, the implicitly adopted linear relationship between stimuli, mental processes, and reaction is resolved or rather transformed to a circular relationship where every action conditions new sensory input to be handled (Gomez-Marin & Ghazanfar, 2019). Semiotically speaking, the level of description is extended from an individual level of interpreting signs towards an intersubjective level of coupled sense-makers that both send and receive signs.

The circular relationship or bidirectional information flow in the context of social interaction has major consequences for empathy and mentalizing, as these processes become nested, recursive, and more dynamic (Palmer et al., 2015). When I am not only making inferences about the mental states of another person from a detached spectator perspective but the other person is doing the same about me, I integrate their inference process into mine. For example, when a colleague is standing in your office chatting with you, you might be inclined not to look at your watch since you expect that this could be conceived as a subtle signal for them to leave. Similarly, talking with a friend about a stranger sitting at the next table in a restaurant leads to monitoring that the stranger does not hear the content of the conversation. These reciprocal inferences have been argued to play a role in the emergence of societal norms (Theriault et al., 2021) and culture (Veissière et al., 2020). Nested recursion during interactions largely increases the complexity of mental state inferences, and thus the amount of uncertainty. The DMN is a likely candidate that could reduce accrued uncertainty. Studies that report neural correlates of social interaction versus social observations can indicate such an involvement of the DMN. This has been observed when participants exchange verbal messages with another person (Alkire et al., 2018) or engage in mutual eye contact (Cavallo et al., 2015). Several studies found DMN activity when playing a dyadic game like "rock, paper, scissors" or the ultimatum game against a human versus a computer opponent (Chaminade et al., 2012; Rilling et al., 2004). Interestingly, the DMN activity is not only modulated dichotomously (human versus computer), but also by the degree to which an opponent is perceived as having a mind, which also influences how variable a person is changing their tactics against the perceived opponent (Takahashi et al., 2014). Further substantiating the notion of counterfactual uncertainty reduction in the DMN, computational modeling in interpersonal competitive decision-making also mapped recursivity of learning and decision processes on DMN activity (Hampton et al., 2008; Hill et al., 2017). When the neural activity in the right TPJ as part of the DMN is disrupted via transcranial magnetic stimulation, the ability to integrate recursive thinking in the own decision and the connectivity between TPJ and MPFC are diminished (Hill et al., 2017).

Besides the impact of embedded second-person situations on mentalizing, the investigation of empathy is also largely affected by such a contextual shift. While in spectatorial paradigms participants only receive information about feeling states of another person and are asked to adapt to it, in second-person situations the adaptation becomes mutual as participants both receive and send information (Figure 14.2). This means that my adaption to a change in your feeling state consequently has an impact on your adaptation to the change in my feeling state, and so on. Ultimately, this leads to a co-regulated adaptation or coupling (De Jaegher et al., 2010), which might proceed infinitely. Interestingly, at a neural level, the AI and ACC – both involved in the bodily regulations within the requirements of the external world (Petzschner et al., 2017) – receive a vastly higher demand. This is due to the increasing complexity of regulatory processes within conjugated loops (Figure 14.1) – that is, one loop between and one loop within each interaction partner) as compared to a single regulatory loop within a person receiving input from the outside (Thomas, 1978). Accordingly, neuroscientific studies provided evidence for an involvement of the AI and the ACC during reciprocal interaction (Alkire et al., 2018; Cavallo et al., 2015; Pfeiffer et al., 2014; Redcay et al., 2010) while plain receiving of messages without the opportunity to influence the interaction partner does not evoke such an activation (Rice & Redcay, 2016).

Although the described situations might not fulfill common layperson perceptions of empathy as the feeling with a suffering person, it most likely captures a more subtle resonating with another person and a vicarious sharing of embodied processes. In this line, studies could show a synchrony of bodily processes, such as facial temperature variation between mother and child (Ebisch et al., 2012), shared heart rate dynamics during interaction (Fusaroli et al., 2016), or synchrony in brain activity (Nguyen et al., 2020). Several studies also reported significant correlations between the level of synchrony of a psychophysiological measure such as skin conductance or heart rate and the subjective rating of empathy (e.g., Järvelä et al., 2014; Messina et al., 2013; for a review see Palumbo et al., 2017).

Interestingly, empathy during reciprocal interaction emerges through interlocked processes between intrapersonal *and* interpersonal feedback loops, which renders empathy a dialectical and intersubjective product living between individuals. This has consequences in the consideration of

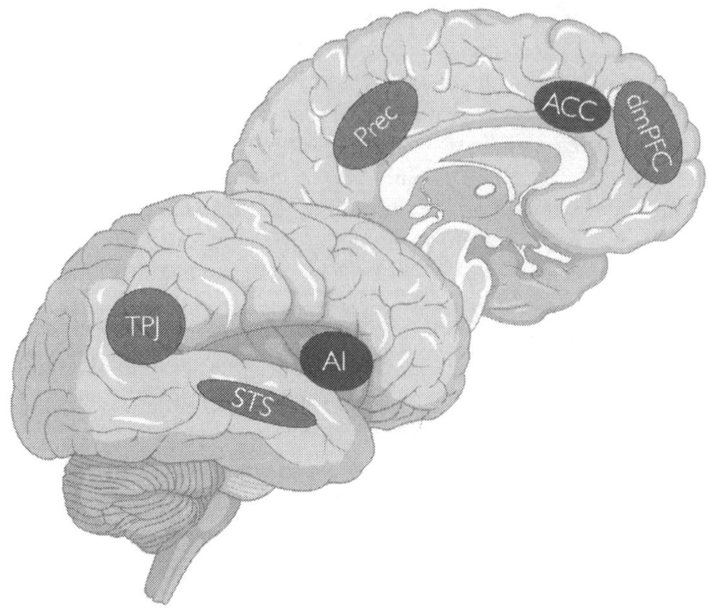

Figure 14.1 Brain networks relevant for empathy and mentalizing

Bubbles represent brain networks important for empathy (dark grey/red) and mentalizing (light grey/blue). AI: anterior insula, ACC: anterior cingulate cortex, dmPDC: dorsomedial prefrontal cortex, Prec: Precuneus, STS: superior temporal sulcus, TPJ: temporoparietal junction. Image created with BioRender (biorender.com). See e-book for a full-color version of this figure.

psychopathology, such as in the case of autism. Prominent theories – for example, the double empathy problem (Milton, 2012) or the dialectical misattunement hypothesis (Bolis et al., 2017) – consider communication and empathy deficits in autism as not residing in the individual but in the misfit between two individuals. Indeed, the lack of empathy is not just ascribed to a person with autism spectrum disorder (ASD), but also to a neurotypical person who shows diminished empathy with a person diagnosed with ASD. Likewise, in the case of behavioral variant frontotemporal dementia, which is characterized by a loss of empathy, caregivers show more distancing, anger, and use of negative emotional words during their interaction with the patient (Ascher et al., 2010; Oyebode et al., 2013).

The misfit in resonating with the feelings of another person can have multiple sources in the picture of interlocked feedback loops between one's and others regulatory bodily circuits and their relation (Figure 14.2). For example, in the neurodegenerative disorder pure autonomic failure, patients exhibit a very specific disability to regulate their internal bodily state (arrows pointing downward in Figure 14.2), as their sympathetic and parasympathetic pathways become denervated, resulting in a difficulty to adequately modulate heart rate or blood pressure to external demands (Critchley et al., 2001; Magnifico et al., 1998). Strikingly, within the complex loops of interpersonal attunement, this specific alteration has been found to accompany blunted empathic responses (Chauhan et al., 2008).

Summarizing the relevance of empathy and mentalizing in the construal of meaning

In the previous sections, we depicted empathy as an embodied feeling that – to a certain degree – is in resonance with the feeling states of another person. This process is largely influenced by contextual

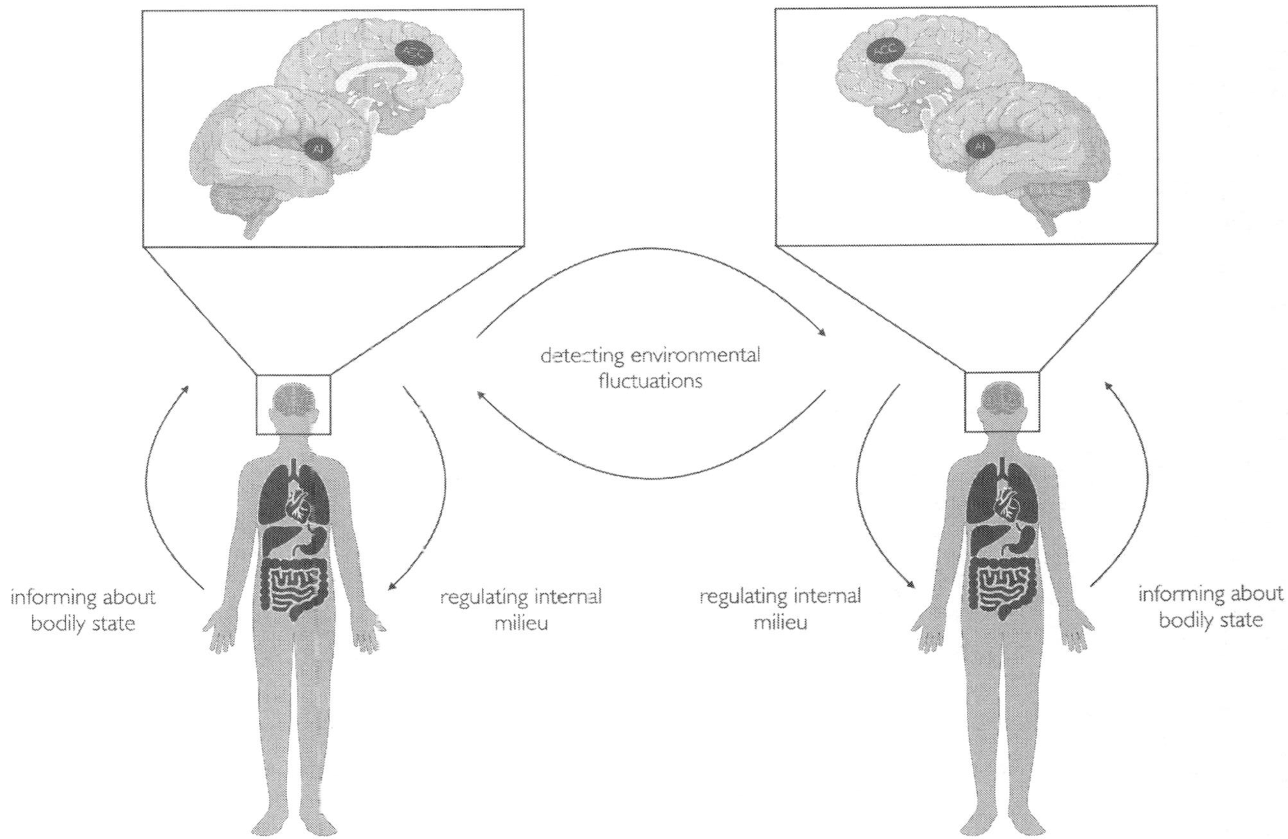

Figure 14.2 Mutual adaptation within a second-person situation

The anterior cingulate cortex (ACC) and the anterior insula (AI) play a role in (1) regulating the internal milieu, (2) receiving input from the internal milieu, and (3) detecting fluctuations within the environment (e.g., between the own and another person's bodily states). Image created with BioRender (biorender.com). See e-book for a full-color version of this figure.

factors, such as group affiliation or a professional environment, as well as motivational factors – for example, whether empathizing could be costly for oneself. In this way, empathy as resonating with someone else acts as a signal that shapes our first-person experience of an interpersonal situation and delivers an affective subjective frame, which conditions the way we interpret a certain situation or, put differently, how we construe meaning. As such, this affective subjective frame or "frame of sense" (Salvatore & Venuleo, 2008) serves the neurosemiotic function of categorizing the relationship towards another person. When we empathize with or feel into someone, we tend to share their interpretation of a situation. A timely example is the question of whether you welcome refugees to your homeland or not. If you feel with their suffering when you see pictures of refugees in dinghies in distress at sea, then you are probably more inclined to relieve them from their suffering and also engage in prosocial activities (Klimecki et al., 2016). Beyond that, our bodily feelings in respect to others may also serve as (Peirce-)signals, as soon as these feelings serve as a basis for interpretation when reflecting on an interpersonal relationship.

In contrast to empathizing, mentalizing offers an abstract or cognitive understanding of another person's states. We argued that observable actions are not unambiguously indicative of inner states, but need to be mentally embedded within a reference frame through the process of counterfactual thinking or simulation. This reference frame then delivers guiding principles on how to interpret or read behaviors, and thus helps us in the construction of meaning. Regarding our refugee example, mentalizing would make you understand their situation, but it does not follow that you will necessarily engage in prosocial activities to improve their situation.

We further showed that, in contrast to observational research, studies adopting a second-person approach demand a higher allocation of empathizing and mentalizing resources from the individual. While engaging in empathy and mentalizing from an observational stance can certainly be seen as a "prerequisite for communicative behavior," only engaging in real dynamic interaction can satisfy the full definition of neurosemiotics as it deals with the "general capacity to engage in symbolic interactions." We contended that the higher demand on empathizing and mentalizing during the engagement in interactions is attributable to the introduction of nested recursion and an increased dynamics. Here, we identified the salience and default mode network as crucial hubs for processing and creating sign relations in the interpersonal domain. This is critical in the agenda of neurosemiotics, striving for the identification of physiological processes that give rise to sign relations. Importantly, approaching interpersonal behavior from a dynamic and dyadic stance also lives up to experimental semiotics, arguing that human communication has to be investigated in interaction (Galantucci, 2009; Galantucci & Garrod, 2011). Complex interactions engender a historicity in the exchange of signals that inhabits its own evolved meaning. Becoming reciprocally coupled to another person expands the role from the mere observer receiving external signals towards a bidirectional signal exchange, which we argued is also supported by mentalizing and empathizing capacities in their respective neural networks. Integrating a neurosemiotic perspective in the study of empathy bears great potential for a synergistic framework, illuminating physiological underpinnings of intersubjective sign relations connecting people.

References

Alkire, D., Levitas, D., Warnell, K. R., & Redcay, E. (2018). Social interaction recruits mentalizing and reward systems in middle childhood. *Human Brain Mapping*, *39*(10), 3928–3942. doi: 10.1002/hbm.24221

Allman, J. M., Tetreault, N. A., Hakeem, A.Y., Manaye, K. F., Semendeferi, K., Erwin, J. M., Park, S., Goubert, V., & Hof, P. R. (2011). The von Economo neurons in fronto-insular and anterior cingulate cortex. *Annals of the New York Academy of Sciences*, *1225*, 59–71. doi: 10.1111/j.1749-6632.2011.06011.x

Allman, J. M., Watson, K. K., Tetreault, N. A., & Hakeem, A.Y. (2005). Intuition and autism: A possible role for Von Economo neurons. *Trends in Cognitive Sciences*, *9*(8), 367–373. doi: 10.1016/j.tics.2005.06.008

Andreoni, J., Rao, J. M., & Trachtman, H. (2017). Avoiding the ask: A field experiment on altruism, empathy, and charitable giving. *Journal of Political Economy*, *125*(3), 625–653. doi: 10.1086/691703

Ascher, E. A., Sturm, V. E., Seider, B. H., Holley, S. R., Miller, B. L., & Levenson, R. W. (2010). Relationship satisfaction and emotional language in frontotemporal dementia and Alzheimer's disease patients and spousal caregivers. *Alzheimer Disease and Associated Disorders*, *24*(1), 49–55. doi: 10.1097/WAD.0b013e3181bd66a3

Baez, S., Manes, F., Huepe, D., Torralva, T., Fiorentino, N., Richter, F., Huepe-Artigas, D., Ferrari, J., Montañes, P., Reyes, P., Matallana, D., Vigliecca, N. S., Decety, J., & Ibanez, A. (2014). Primary empathy deficits in frontotemporal dementia. *Frontiers in Aging Neuroscience*, *6*, 262. doi: 10.3389/fnagi.2014.00262

Barrett, L. F., & Simmons, W. K. (2015). Interoceptive predictions in the brain. *Nature Reviews Neuroscience*, *16*(7), 419–429. doi: 10.1038/nrn3950

Becchio, C., Sartori, L., & Castiello, U. (2010). Toward you: The social side of actions. *Current Directions in Psychological Science*, *19*(3), 183–188. doi: 10.1177/0963721410370131

Berger, A. A. (1989). *Signs in Contemporary Culture: An Introduction to Semiotics*. Salem, WI: Sheffield.

Bolis, D., Balsters, J., Wenderoth, N., Becchio, C., & Schilbach, L. (2017). Beyond autism: Introducing the dialectical misattunement hypothesis and a Bayesian account of intersubjectivity. *Psychopathology*, *50*(6), 355–372. doi: 10.1159/000484353

Bouissac, P. (2018). Semiotics in Canada I. In T. A. Sebeok & D. J. Umiker-Sebeok (Eds.), *The Semiotic Web* (pp. 191–252). Berlin: Mouton de Gruyter.

Buckner, R. L. (2012). The serendipitous discovery of the brain's default network. *NeuroImage*, *62*(2), 1137–1145. doi: 10.1016/j.neuroimage.2011.10.035

Bzdok, D., Schilbach, L., Vogeley, K., Schneider, K., Laird, A. R., Langner, R., & Eickhoff, S. B. (2012). Parsing the neural correlates of moral cognition: ALE meta-analysis on morality, theory of mind, and empathy. *Brain Structure and Function*, *217*(4), 783–796. doi: 10.1007/s00429-012-0380-y

Cameron, C. D., Harris, L. T., & Payne, B. K. (2016). The emotional cost of humanity: Anticipated exhaustion motivates dehumanization of stigmatized targets. *Social Psychological and Personality Science*, 7(2), 105–112. doi: 10.1177/1948550615604453

Cameron, C. D., Hutcherson, C. A., Ferguson, A. M., Scheffer, J. A., Hadjiandreou, E., & Inzlicht, M. (2019). Empathy is hard work: People choose to avoid empathy because of its cognitive costs. *Journal of Experimental Psychology: General*, *148*(6), 962–976. doi: 10.1037/xge0000595

Cameron, C. D., & Payne, B. (2011). Escaping affect: How motivated emotion regulation creates insensitivity to mass suffering. *Journal of Personality and Social Psychology*, *100*(1), 1–15. doi: 10.1037/a0021643

Campbell, C., Olteanu, A., & Kull, K. (2019). Learning and knowing as semiosis: Extending the conceptual apparatus of semiotics. *Sign Systems Studies*, *47*(3–4), 352–381. doi: 10.12697/SSS.2019.47.3-4.01

Cavallo, A., Lungu, O., Becchio, C., Ansuini, C., Rustichini, A., & Fadiga, L. (2015). When gaze opens the channel for communication: Integrative role of IFG and MPFC. *NeuroImage*, *119*, 63–69. doi: 10.1016/j.neuroimage.2015.06.025

Chaminade, T., Rosset, D., Da Fonseca, D., Nazarian, B., Lutcher, E., Cheng, G., & Deruelle, C. (2012). How do we think machines think? An fMRI study of alleged competition with an artificial intelligence. *Frontiers in Human Neuroscience*, *6*, 103. doi: 10.3389/fnhum.2012.00103

Chang, C., Metzger, C. D., Glover, G. H., Duyn, J. H., Heinze, H.-J., & Walter, M. (2013). Association between heart rate variability and fluctuations in resting-state functional connectivity. *NeuroImage*, *68*, 93–104. doi: 10.1016/j.neuroimage.2012.11.038

Chauhan, B., Mathias, C. J., & Critchley, H. D. (2008). Autonomic contributions to empathy: Evidence from patients with primary autonomic failure. *Autonomic Neuroscience*, *140*(1), 96–100. doi: 10.1016/j.autneu.2008.03.005

Cikara, M., & Paluck, E. L. (2013). When going along gets you nowhere and the upside of conflict behaviors. *Social and Personality Psychology Compass*, 7(8), 559–571. doi: 10.1111/spc3.12047

Critchley, H. D., Mathias, C. J., & Dolan, R. J. (2001). Neuroanatomical basis for first- and second-order representations of bodily states. *Nature Neuroscience*, *4*(2), 207–212. doi: 10.1038/84048

de Bruin, L., & Strijbos, D. (2015). Direct social perception, mindreading and Bayesian predictive coding. *Consciousness and Cognition*, *36*, 565–570. doi: 10.1016/j.concog.2015.04.014

De Jaegher, H., Di Paolo, E., & Gallagher, S. (2010). Can social interaction constitute social cognition? *Trends in Cognitive Sciences*, *14*(10), 441–447. doi: 10.1016/j.tics.2010.06.009

de Vignemont, F., & Singer, T. (2006). The empathic brain: How, when and why? *Trends in Cognitive Sciences*, *10*(10), 435–441. doi: 10.1016/j.tics.2006.08.008

Decety, J., & Cowell, J. M. (2014). Friends or foes: Is empathy necessary for moral behavior? *Perspectives on Psychological Science: A Journal of the Association for Psychological Science*, *9*(5), 525–537. doi: 10.1177/1745691614545130

Decety, J., Yang, C.-Y., & Cheng, Y. (2010). Physicians down-regulate their pain empathy response: An event-related brain potential study. *NeuroImage*, *50*(4), 1676–1682. doi: 10.1016/j.neuroimage.2010.01.025

Ebisch, S. J., Aureli, T., Bafunno, D., Cardone, D., Romani, G. L., & Merla, A. (2012). Mother and child in synchrony: Thermal facial imprints of autonomic contagion. *Biological Psychology*, *89*(1), 123–129. doi: 10.1016/j.biopsycho.2011.09.018

Engel, A. K., Maye, A., Kurthen, M., & König, P. (2013). Where's the action? The pragmatic turn in cognitive science. *Trends in Cognitive Sciences, 17*(5), 202–209. doi: 10.1016/j.tics.2013.03.006

Frith, C., & Frith, U. (2005). Theory of mind. *Current Biology, 15*(17), R644–R645. doi: 10.1016/j.cub.2005.08.041

Froese, T., & Gallagher, S. (2012). Getting interaction theory (IT) together: Integrating developmental, phenomenological, enactive, and dynamical approaches to social interaction. *Interaction Studies, 13*(3), 436–468. doi: 10.1075/is.13.3.06fro

Fusaroli, R., Bjørndahl, J. S., Roepstorff, A., & Tylén, K. (2016). A heart for interaction: Shared physiological dynamics and behavioral coordination in a collective, creative construction task. *Journal of Experimental Psychology: Human Perception and Performance, 42*(9), 1297–1310. doi: 10.1037/xhp0000207

Galantucci, B. (2009). Experimental semiotics: A new approach for studying communication as a form of joint action. *Topics in Cognitive Science, 1*(2), 393–410. doi: 10.1111/j.1756-8765.2009.01027.x

Galantucci, B., & Garrod, S. (2011). Experimental semiotics: A review. *Frontiers in Human Neuroscience, 5,* 11. doi: 10.3389/fnhum.2011.00011

Gallagher, S. (2008). Direct perception in the intersubjective context. *Consciousness and Cognition, 17*(2), 535–543. doi: 10.1016/j.concog.2008.03.003

Gomez-Marin, A., & Ghazanfar, A. A. (2019). The life of behavior. *Neuron, 104*(1), 25–36. doi: 10.1016/j.neuron.2019.09.017

Gu, X., Hof, P. R., Friston, K. J., & Fan, J. (2013). Anterior insular cortex and emotional awareness. *Journal of Comparative Neurology, 521*(15), 3371–3388. doi: 10.1002/cne.23368

Guo, C. C., Sturm, V. E., Zhou, J., Gennatas, E. D., Trujillo, A. J., Hua, A. Y., Crawford, R., Stables, L., Kramer, J. H., Rankin, K., Levenson, R. W., Rosen, H. J., Miller, B. L., & Seeley, W. W. (2016). Dominant hemisphere lateralization of cortical parasympathetic control as revealed by frontotemporal dementia. *Proceedings of the National Academy of Sciences, 113*(17), E2430–E2439. doi: 10.1073/pnas.1509184113

Gutsell, J. N., & Inzlicht, M. (2010). Empathy constrained: Prejudice predicts reduced mental simulation of actions during observation of outgroups. *Journal of Experimental Social Psychology, 46*(5), 841–845. doi: 10.1016/j.jesp.2010.03.011

Hampton, A. N., Bossaerts, P., & O'Doherty, J. P. (2008). Neural correlates of mentalizing-related computations during strategic interactions in humans. *Proceedings of the National Academy of Sciences, 105*(18), 6741–6746. doi: 10.1073/pnas.0711099105

Hassabis, D., & Maguire, E. A. (2009). The construction system of the brain. *Philosophical Transactions of the Royal Society B, 364,* 1263–1271. doi: 10.1098/rstb.2008.0296

Hein, G., Silani, G., Preuschoff, K., Batson, C. D., & Singer, T. (2010). Neural responses to ingroup and outgroup members' suffering predict individual differences in costly helping. *Neuron, 68*(1), 149–160. doi: 10.1016/j.neuron.2010.09.003

Hill, C. A., Suzuki, S., Polania, R., Moisa, M., O'Doherty, J. P., & Ruff, C. C. (2017). A causal account of the brain network computations underlying strategic social behavior. *Nature Neuroscience, 20*(8), 1142–1149. doi: 10.1038/nn.4602

Ibáñez, A. (2019). Insular networks and intercognition in the wild. *Cortex, 115,* 341–344. doi: 10.1016/j.cortex.2019.01.024

Ibáñez, A., & García, A. M. (2018). With context in mind, with mind in context. In A. Ibáñez, & A. M. García (Eds.), *Contextual Cognition: The Sensus Communis of a Situated Mind* (pp. 1–5). Heidelberg: Springer. doi: 10.1007/978-3-319-77285-1_1

Järvelä, S., Kivikangas, J. M., Kätsyri, J., & Ravaja, N. (2014). Physiological linkage of dyadic gaming experience. *Simulation & Gaming, 45*(1), 24–40. doi: 10.1177/1046878113513080

Kanske, P. (2018). The social mind: Disentangling affective and cognitive routes to understanding others. *Interdisciplinary Science Reviews, 43*(2), 115–124. doi: 10.1080/03080188.2018.1453243

Kanske, P., Böckler, A., Trautwein, F.-M., Parianen Lesemann, F. H., & Singer, T. (2016). Are strong empathizers better mentalizers? Evidence for independence and interaction between the routes of social cognition. *Social Cognitive and Affective Neuroscience, 11*(9), 1383–1392. doi: 10.1093/scan/nsw052

Kanske, P., Böckler, A., Trautwein, F.-M., & Singer, T. (2015). Dissecting the social brain: Introducing the EmpaToM to reveal distinct neural networks and brain-behavior relations for empathy and Theory of Mind. *NeuroImage, 122,* 6–19. doi: 10.1016/j.neuroimage.2015.07.082

Keysers, C., & Gazzola, V. (2014). Dissociating the ability and propensity for empathy. *Trends in Cognitive Sciences, 18*(4), 163–166. doi: 10.1016/j.tics.2013.12.011

Kim, E.-J., Sidhu, M., Gaus, S. E., Huang, E. J., Hof, P. R., Miller, B. L., DeArmond, S. J., & Seeley, W. W. (2012). Selective frontoinsular von economo neuron and fork cell loss in early behavioral variant frontotemporal dementia. *Cerebral Cortex, 22*(2), 251–259. doi: 10.1093/cercor/bhr004

Klimecki, O. M., Mayer, S. V., Jusyte, A., Scheeff, J., & Schönenberg, M. (2016). Empathy promotes altruistic behavior in economic interactions. *Scientific Reports*, *6*(1), 31961. doi: 10.1038/srep31961

Lamm, C., Decety, J., & Singer, T. (2011). Meta-analytic evidence for common and distinct neural networks associated with directly experienced pain and empathy for pain. *NeuroImage*, *54*(3), 2492–2502. doi: 10.1016/j.neuroimage.2010.10.014

Lau, T., Gershman, S. J., & Cikara, M. (2020). Social structure learning in human anterior insula. *ELife*, *9*, e53162. doi: 10.7554/eLife.53162

Leeuwen, T.V. (2005). *Introducing Social Semiotics*. Bristol: Psychology Press.

Lehmann, K., Maliske, L., Böckler, A., & Kanske, P. (2019). Social impairments in mental disorders: Recent developments in studying the mechanisms of interactive behavior. *Clinical Psychology in Europe*, *1*(2), e33143. doi: 10.32872/cpe.v1i2.33143

Low, J., & Perner, J. (2012). Implicit and explicit theory of mind: State of the art. *British Journal of Developmental Psychology*, *30*(1), 1–13. doi: 10.1111/j.2044-835X.2011.02074.x

Magnifico, F., Misra, V. P., Murray, N. M. F., & Mathias, C. J. (1998). The sympathetic skin response in peripheral autonomic failure: Evaluation in pure autonomic failure, pure cholinergic dysautonomia and dopamine-beta-hydroxylase deficiency. *Clinical Autonomic Research*, *8*(3), 133–138. doi: 10.1007/BF02281117

Marquié, L., Raufaste, E., Lauque, D., Mariné, C., Ecoiffier, M., & Sorum, P. (2003). Pain rating by patients and physicians: Evidence of systematic pain miscalibration. *Pain*, *102*(3), 289–296. doi: 10.1016/S0304-3959(02)00402-5

Messina, I., Palmieri, A., Sambin, M., Kleinbub, J. R., Voci, A., & Calvo, V. (2013). Somatic underpinnings of perceived empathy: The importance of psychotherapy training. *Psychotherapy Research*, *23*(2), 169–177. doi: 10.1080/10503307.2012.748940

Michael, J., & De Bruin, L. (2015). How direct is social perception? *Consciousness and Cognition*, *36*, 373–375. doi: 10.1016/j.concog.2015.08.005

Milton, D. E. M. (2012). On the ontological status of autism: The "double empathy problem." *Disability & Society*, *27*(6), 883–887. doi: 10.1080/09687599.2012.710008

Nguyen, T., Bánki, A., Markova, G., & Hoehl, S. (2020). Studying parent–child interaction with hyperscanning. *Progress in Brain Research*, *254*, 1–24. doi: 10.1016/bs.pbr.2020.05.003

Oyebode, J. R., Bradley, P., & Allen, J. L. (2013). Relatives' experiences of frontal-variant frontotemporal dementia. *Qualitative Health Research*, *23*(2), 156–166. doi: 10.1177/1049732312466294

Palmer, C. J., Seth, A. K, & Hohwy, J. (2015). The felt presence of other minds: Predictive processing, counterfactual predictions, and mentalising in autism. *Consciousness and Cognition*, *36*, 376–389. doi: 10.1016/j.concog.2015.04.007

Palumbo, R. V., Marraccini, M. E., Weyandt, L. L., Wilder-Smith, O., McGee, H. A., Liu, S., & Goodwin, M. S. (2017). Interpersonal autonomic physiology: A systematic review of the literature. *Personality and Social Psychology Review*, *21*(2), 99–141. doi: 10.1177/1088868316628405

Parr, T., & Friston, K. J. (2018). The anatomy of inference: Generative models and brain structure. *Frontiers in Computational Neuroscience*, *12*, 90. doi: 10.3389/fncom.2018.00090

Petzschner, F. H., Weber, L. A. E., Gard, T., & Stephan, K. E. (2017). Computational psychosomatics and computational psychiatry: Toward a joint framework for differential diagnosis. *Biological Psychiatry*, *82*(6), 421–430. doi: 10.1016/j.biopsych.2017.05.012

Pfeiffer, U. J., Schilbach, L., Timmermans, B., Kuzmanovic, B., Georgescu, A. L., Bente, G., & Vogeley, K. (2014). Why we interact: On the functional role of the striatum in the subjective experience of social interaction. *NeuroImage*, *101*, 124–137. doi: 10.1016/j.neuroimage.2014.06.061

Pinotti, A. (2010). Empathy. In H. R. Sepp, & L. Embree (Eds.), *Handbook of Phenomenological Aesthetics* (pp. 93–98). Heidelberg: Springer. doi: 10.1007/978-90-481-2471-8_18

Preckel, K., Kanske, P., & Singer, T. (2018). On the interaction of social affect and cognition: Empathy, compassion and theory of mind. *Current Opinion in Behavioral Sciences*, *19*, 1–6. doi: 10.1016/j.cobeha.2017.07.010

Premack, D., & Woodruff, G. (1978). Does the chimpanzee have a theory of mind? *Behavioral and Brain Sciences*, *1*(4), 515–526. doi: 10.1017/S0140525X00076512

Rankin, K. P., Gorno-Tempini, M. L., Allison, S. C., Stanley, C. M., Glenn, S., Weiner, M. W., & Miller, B. L. (2006). Structural anatomy of empathy in neurodegenerative disease. *Brain*, *129*(11), 2945–2956. doi: 10.1093/brain/awl254

Redcay, E., Dodell-Feder, D., Pearrow, M. J., Mavros, P. L., Kleiner, M., Gabrieli, J. D. E., & Saxe, R. (2010). Live face-to-face interaction during fMRI: A new tool for social cognitive neuroscience. *NeuroImage*, *50*(4), 1639–1647. doi: 10.1016/j.neuroimage.2010.01.052

Reddy, V., & Morris, P. (2004). Participants don't need theories: Knowing minds in engagement. *Theory & Psychology*, *14*(5), 647–665. doi: 10.1177/0959354304046177

Rice, K., & Redcay, E. (2016). Interaction matters: A perceived social partner alters the neural processing of human speech. *NeuroImage*, *129*, 480–488. doi: 10.1016/j.neuroimage.2015.11.041

Rilling, J. K., Sanfey, A. G., Aronson, J. A., Nystrom, L. E., & Cohen, J. D. (2004). The neural correlates of theory of mind within interpersonal interactions. *NeuroImage*, *22*(4), 1694–1703. doi: 10.1016/j.neuroimage.2004.04.015

Sales, A. C., Friston, K. J., Jones, M. W., Pickering, A. E., & Moran, R. J. (2019). Locus Coeruleus tracking of prediction errors optimises cognitive flexibility: An active inference model. *PLOS Computational Biology*, *15*(1), e1006267. doi: 10.1371/journal.pcbi.1006267

Salvatore, S., & Venuleo, C. (2008). Understanding the role of emotion in sense-making: A semiotic psychoanalytic oriented perspective. *Integrative Psychological & Behavioral Science*, *42*(1), 32–46. doi: 10.1007/s12124-007-9039-2

Schilbach, L., Timmermans, B., Reddy, V., Costall, A., Bente, G., Schlicht, T., & Vogeley, K. (2013). Toward a second-person neuroscience. *Behavioral and Brain Sciences*, *36*(4), 393–414. doi: 10.1017/S0140525X12000660

Schooler, J. W., Smallwood, J., Christoff, K., Handy, T. C., Reichle, E. D., & Sayette, M. A. (2011). Meta-awareness, perceptual decoupling and the wandering mind. *Trends in Cognitive Sciences*, *15*(7), 319–326. doi: 10.1016/j.tics.2011.05.006

Schurz, M., Maliske, L., & Kanske, P. (2020). Cross-network interactions in social cognition: A review of findings on task related brain activation and connectivity. *Cortex*, *130*, 142–157. doi: 10.1016/j.cortex.2020.05.006

Schurz, M., Radua, J., Aichhorn, M., Richlan, F., & Perner, J. (2014). Fractionating theory of mind: A meta-analysis of functional brain imaging studies. *Neuroscience and Biobehavioral Reviews*, *42*, 9–34. doi: 10.1016/j.neubiorev.2014.01.009

Schurz, M., Radua, J., Tholen, M. G., Maliske, L., Margulies, D. S., Mars, R. B., Sallet, J., & Kanske, P. (2021). Toward a hierarchical model of social cognition: A neuroimaging meta-analysis and integrative review on empathy and theory of mind. *Psychological Bulletin*, *147*(3), 293–327. doi: 10.1037/bul0000303

Seeley, W. W. (2010). Anterior insula degeneration in frontotemporal dementia. *Brain Structure and Function*, *214*(5), 465–475. doi: 10.1007/s00429-010-0263-z

Seeley, W. W., Carlin, D. A., Allman, J. M., Macedo, M. N., Bush, C., Miller, B. L., & DeArmond, S. J. (2006). Early frontotemporal dementia targets neurons unique to apes and humans. *Annals of Neurology*, *60*(6), 660–667. doi: 10.1002/ana.21055

Seeley, W. W., Menon, V., Schatzberg, A. F., Keller, J., Glover, G. H., Kenna, H., Reiss, A. L., & Greicius, M. D. (2007). Dissociable intrinsic connectivity networks for salience processing and executive control. *Journal of Neuroscience*, *27*(9), 2349–2356. doi: 10.1523/JNEUROSCI.5587-06.2007

Sestieri, C., Corbetta, M., Romani, G. L., & Shulman, G. L. (2011). Episodic memory retrieval, parietal cortex, and the default mode network: Functional and topographic analyses. *Journal of Neuroscience*, *31*(12), 4407–4420. doi: 10.1523/JNEUROSCI.3335-10.2011

Shamay-Tsoory, S. G., & Mendelsohn, A. (2019). Real-life neuroscience: An ecological approach to brain and behavior research. *Perspectives on Psychological Science*, *14*(5), 841–859. doi: 10.1177/1745691619856350

Singer, T., & Klimecki, O. M. (2014). Empathy and compassion. *Current Biology*, *24*(18), R875-R878. doi: 10.1016/j.cub.2014.06.054

Spreng, R. N., & Grady, C. L. (2009). Patterns of brain activity supporting autobiographical memory, prospection, and theory of mind, and their relationship to the default mode network. *Journal of Cognitive Neuroscience*, *22*(6), 1112–1123. doi: 10.1162/jocn.2009.21282

Sturm, V. E., Rosen, H. J., Allison, S., Miller, B. L., & Levenson, R. W. (2006). Self-conscious emotion deficits in frontotemporal lobar degeneration. *Brain*, *129*(9), 2508–2516. doi: 10.1093/brain/awl145

Takahashi, H., Terada, K., Morita, T., Suzuki, S., Haji, T., Kozima, H., Yoshikawa, M., Matsumoto, Y., Omori, T., Asada, M., & Naito, E. (2014). Different impressions of other agents obtained through social interaction uniquely modulate dorsal and ventral pathway activities in the social human brain. *Cortex*, *58*, 289–300. doi: 10.1016/j.cortex.2014.03.011

Tamir, D. I., & Thornton, M. A. (2018). Modeling the predictive social mind. *Trends in Cognitive Sciences*, *22*(3), 201–212. doi: 10.1016/j.tics.2017.12.005

Taylor, K. S., Kucyi, A., Millar, P. J., Murai, H., Kimmerly, D. S., Morris, B. L., Bradley, T. D., & Floras, J. S. (2015). Association between resting-state brain functional connectivity and muscle sympathetic burst incidence. *Journal of Neurophysiology*, *115*(2), 662–673. doi: 10.1152/jn.00675.2015

Theriault, J. E., Young, L., & Barrett, L. F. (2021). The sense of should: A biologically-based framework for modeling social pressure. *Physics of Life Reviews*, *36*, 100–136. doi: 10.1016/j.plrev.2020.01.004

Thomas, R. (1978). Logical analysis of systems comprising feedback loops. *Journal of Theoretical Biology*, *73*(4), 631–656. doi: 10.1016/0022-5193(78)90127-3

Valk, S. L., Bernhardt, B. C., Böckler, A., Trautwein, F.-M., Kanske, P., & Singer, T. (2017). Socio-cognitive phenotypes differentially modulate large-scale structural covariance networks. *Cerebral Cortex*, *27*(2), 1358–1368. doi: 10.1093/cercor/bhv319

Van Hoeck, N., Watson, P. D., & Barbey, A. K. (2015). Cognitive neuroscience of human counterfactual reasoning. *Frontiers in Human Neuroscience*, *9*, 420. doi: 10.3389/fnhum.2015.00420

Veissière, S. P. L., Constant, A., Ramstead, M. J. D., Friston, K. J., & Kirmayer, L. J. (2020). Thinking through other minds: A variational approach to cognition and culture. *Behavioral and Brain Sciences*, *43*, 1–75. doi: 10.1017/S0140525X19001213

Wei, L., & Wu, G.-R. (2020). Structural covariance of the salience network associated with heart rate variability. *Brain Imaging and Behavior*. doi: 10.1007/s11682-020-00298-3

Wheatley, T., Boncz, A., Toni, I., & Stolk, A. (2019). Beyond the isolated brain: The promise and challenge of interacting minds. *Neuron*, *103*(2), 186–188. doi: 10.1016/j.neuron.2019.05.009

Zahavi, D. (2011). Empathy and direct social perception: A phenomenological proposal. *Review of Philosophy and Psychology*, *2*(3), 541. doi: 10.1007/s13164-011-0070-3

Zaki, J. (2014). Empathy: A motivated account. *Psychological Bulletin*, *140*(6), 1608–1647.

15

BIOLOGICAL BASES OF MORAL COGNITION AND THEIR ROLE IN THE CONSTRUAL OF MEANING

Sandra Baez

Introduction

Most human acts have moral repercussions, with judgments about right and wrong depending on complex interactions between cognitive, emotional, and motivational mechanisms (Moll & Schulkin, 2009) shaped through cultural exposure (Zeki et al., 2004). Morality is a system of norms and values guiding our behavior in a community. Therefore, the evaluation of another agent's actions or our own actions, made with respect to these norms and values, is central to daily functioning (Heekeren et al., 2005). Given that linguistic communication and symbol-mediated cognition are integrated into every aspect of our lives (Deacon, 2016), morality is shaped by social interaction mediated by signs. Thus, morality is not a naturally occurring universal concept; rather, it is dependent on non-verbal cues, words, language, and forms of discourse that are socioculturally specific (Tappan, 1997). The classical study of semiotics has focused on the properties of signs (e.g., reference, symbolism, indication, metaphor, analogy), eventually incorporating aspects of interpersonal communication that are sensitive to social dynamics and cultural niches (García et al., 2020). More recently, neurosemiotics has emerged as an epistemological domain that includes the scientific investigation of the neurological processes underlying communicative behavior (Bouissac, 1987). Thus, neurosemiotics aims to study communication from a perspective that is both social and biological, and that involves multiple aspects of neurocognitive mechanisms that underlie the emergence and exchange of explicit and implicit meanings during human activity. This includes language, facial expressions, gestures, bodily movements, visceral processes, and images of any kind (García et al., 2020), all of which are highly relevant for moral cognition processes.

In this chapter, I describe several subdomains of moral cognition and their links with neurosemiotics, and I review their biological basis. First, I address the links between moral cognition and neurosemiotics. Then I review the neural, genetic, and endocrine factors associated with moral cognition. I focus on evidence from neuroimaging research and from behavioral studies on the moral profile of patients with neuropsychiatric disorders. I then describe neurocognitive models of moral cognition processes, emphasizing the relevance of context processing for such complex social cognitive domains. Finally, I highlight the importance of implementing a multilevel approach that integrates semiotics, social, psychological, neural, genetic, and endocrine factors for a deeper understanding of moral cognition.

DOI: 10.4324/9781003051817-19

Moral cognition and neurosemiotics

Semiotics, in the most popular sense, is the study of signs (Saussure, 2011). Semiotics deals with the understanding of signs, which are the fundamental elements and minimal units necessary to construct the human mind and culture. Semiosis, the generation and use of signs, is a fundamental component of life. Signs and meanings exist in all living systems (Barbieri, 2009). Indeed, codes and conventions are the basis of our social life. Words, language, and forms of discourse are crucial because they constitute the semiotic systems that are necessary for the communication, collaboration, and interaction that characterize social processes (Wertsch et al., 1995), including morality.

Social interactions arise from patterns of communicative signs, whose perception and interpretation require the interaction of multiple cognitive functions. It is through our social interactions that we form judgments about morality (Turiel, 2008). Although social interactions comprise several interwoven multimodal cues, a behavioral pattern as a whole acts as a communicative sign, and can thus be described using sign theory (semiotics) (Wolf et al., 2018). One of the most influential contributions to the field of semiotics was introduced by Charles Peirce (Peirce & Buchler, 1955). This semiotic theory is compatible with cognitive and social neuroscience approaches since it emphasizes the perspective of the interpreting mind (Peirce & Buchler, 1955), represented by the observer's brain activity. In particular, for the study of moral cognition, this framework may describe the relationship between perceived signs (e.g., verbal and non-verbal cues from social interactions) and the interpretant (Peirce & Buchler, 1955).

The emergent field of neurosemiotics has focused on the investigation of the neural processes underlying communicative behavior, including the perception of the environment as meaningful, and the general capacity to engage in symbolic interactions (Bouissac, 1987: 204–206). Accordingly, "neurosemiotics aims to study communication from a perspective that is both social and biological, going far beyond the abstract conceptualization of signs" (García et al,, 2020: 93). This cross-disciplinary field targets the neurocognitive mechanisms that underlie the emergence and exchange of meanings during human interactions. Beyond verbal domains, more recent approaches have concentrated on the biological underpinnings of our efforts to construe meaning in everyday interactions, considering the role of emotions, empathy, theory of mind, and moral cognition.

Morality can be considered the degree of adherence to the customs and values accepted by a social group (Moll et al., 2005). Moral cognition consists of using such codes to guide culturally adequate social behavior. Accordingly, moral cognition comprises all the mental processes underlying our discernment of acceptable and inacceptable actions. This broad construct encompasses different but interrelated subdomains, including moral sensitivity, moral reasoning, and moral judgment. Moral sensitivity represents the first stage of a moral decision, which is associated with an instant feeling of approval or disapproval when we witness a morally laden scenario (Haidt, 2001). This detection typically happens prior to moral reasoning and moral judgment. Moral reasoning, a controlled process leading to moral judgments (Moll et al., 2005), includes the laborious steps of deductive reasoning and cost-benefit analyses. Finally, moral judgment refers to an evaluative judgment that is based on assessments of the adequacy of one's own and others' behaviors based on socially shaped ideas of right and wrong (Moll et al., 2005).

Making a moral judgment is fundamentally a neurosemiotically mediated action. For an action to be considered right or wrong, a particular meaning must be associated with it (Tappan, 1997). This holds whether that action is "instinctive" (e.g., rushing out into busy traffic to rescue a child), or "deliberative" (e.g., weighing the pros and cons of euthanasia). In either case, moral judgment is an interpretation of the action in question, based on the shared assumptions and understandings that constitute culture (Tappan, 1997). Thus, moral judgment, considered as mediated action, entails both the agent (the person who is doing the acting) and relevant "cultural tools" or "mediational means."

Usually, the tools employed in mediating moral cognition are words, language, and forms of discourse, which enable the individual to think, feel, and act in a way that, in their particular sociocultural context, is understood to be "moral" (Tappan, 2006).

Consistent with this view, a sociocultural perspective proposes that moral development entails the internalization of semiotically and linguistically mediated social relations, as external speech becomes inner speech (Vygotsky, 1978). Children first begin to learn from parents, grandparents, and caregivers about social rules and standards of behavior. This learning occurs primarily in the context of conversation (Dunn, 1987). Over the course of several years, communication with others regarding rules, standards, and the consequences of their transgression gradually becomes communication with oneself regarding what one should and not do in a given situation (Tappan, 2006). Thus, as a symbolic domain, language allows people to articulate their experiences in a meaningful way. At one level, one may conceive of these forms in terms of "symbols and referents," but at a deeper level, everyday cultural discourse provides a novel language – "a language of morals through which children come to understand what it means to be human" (Bhatia, 2000: 164).

The moral agent cannot be understood simply as an individual actor; instead, it should be considered an "individual-acting-with-mediational-means" (Tappan, 1997: 85). Consistent with the semiotic perspective, moral cognition can be considered essentially social, founded on community and knowledge intersubjectively distributed beyond the boundaries of the individual (Paolucci, 2012). Indeed, moral values – that is, concepts that represent principles, standards, goals, or attitudes held by individuals or groups (Kvaran & Sanfey, 2010) – are socially and culturally shaped. Concepts such as loyalty, justice, honor, and fairness are common examples of moral values, which clearly involve symbolically mediated shared values. Often, our moral judgments are strongly shaped by our moral values and by what others in our community believe (Baumeister & Leary, 1995). In fact, when people have a "moral mandate" – when they think they are defending an important moral issue – they behave differently and are more willing to justify improper behavior than when they have no moral mandate (Skitka, 2002).

Actions with moral content are imbued with specific sociocultural meaning and significance, which distinguishes them from other types of actions. They are interpreted in specific ways and framed by moral languages and forms of moral discourse. Making moral judgments requires a contextualization of one's own or others' actions both in terms of cultural and social dimensions and in terms of a shared system of values that frames the intentionality of actions (Paolucci, 2012). Understanding others largely depends on our tendency to attribute meaning and intentions to their actions. This ability to infer the beliefs, intentions, and emotions of others – known as theory of mind (Baron-Cohen et al., 1985) – is critical to predict the subjective consequences of our actions and to judge how people might react to them. Indeed, moral cognition processes are influenced by inferences regarding the intentional or accidental nature of the agent's action (Cushman, 2008; Young & Saxe, 2009a).

Typically, moral judgment is determined primarily by the agent's intention rather than the outcome of the action (Cushman, 2008). However, when intention and outcome are in conflict, moral judgments rely on the consideration of the agent's mental state and the harmfulness of their actions (Young & Saxe, 2008; 2009a). In fact, individuals who inflict harm on others are usually exculpated insofar as their actions are deemed accidental (Cushman, 2008; Treadway et al., 2014). Such a morally loaded decision requires a robust representation of tacit intentions to override a preponderant negative response to the outcome (Young & Saxe, 2009a), an ability that relies heavily on theory of mind. Understanding others' intentions, in turn, involves a semiotic process based on both spoken language and non-verbal communication.

Construing the meaning of others' intentions and applying moral judgment to their actions depends on a variety of modalities and contextual factors (Baez, García, & Ibáñez, 2018). During social interactions, a multitude of auditory and visual cues interact to convey meaning. These cues range from spoken words and manual gestures to facial expressions, eye gaze, body orientation, and body movements (Lotze et al., 2006; Schilbach et al., 2006). The interpretation of these cues depends on a variety of contextual factors and a network of different brain structures that drive an interplay of cognitive functions. Thus, moral cognition relies on extended neural networks, but also on the interaction of other biological factors such as genetics and hormones. In the next sections, I review neural, endocrine, and genetic factors associated with moral cognition.

Biological bases of moral cognition

Neural bases

Knowledge about the neural bases of moral cognition has derived mainly from neuroimaging studies as well as behavioral/neuropsychological evidence of moral impairments in patients with psychiatric and neurological conditions (Baez, García, & Santamaría-García, 2017; Pascual et al., 2013). Studies using fMRI (e.g., Greene et al., 2001; Moll et al., 2003; Young & Saxe, 2009b) have revealed that moral cognition engages a distributed network, the main hubs of which include the ventromedial prefrontal cortex (vmPFC), the orbitofrontal cortex (OFC), the ventrolateral prefrontal cortex, the amygdala, the superior temporal sulcus, the precuneus, and the temporoparietal junction (TPJ) (see Figure 15.1).

The vmPFC seems to play multiple roles in processes supporting moral cognition. For instance, it biases moral judgment by associating external stimuli with socio-emotional values and is involved in mentalizing and empathy (D'Argembeau et al., 2008; Moll et al., 2008). The vmPFC is also crucial for processing intention and outcome information during moral judgments (Ciaramelli et al., 2007; Young & Saxe, 2008). Indeed, patients with damage to this region judge harmful intentions in the absence of harmful outcomes as more morally permissible when compared with healthy controls (Young et al., 2010).

The OFC and the ventrolateral prefrontal cortex are implicated in the inhibition of automatic or impulsive responses and in processing social prompts (Baxter et al., 2000; Roelofs et al., 2009). The OFC is engaged by stimuli conveying rewards and punishments, and by tasks requiring the integration of cognitive processes with affective values (Amodio & Frith, 2006). This region also contributes to the moral decision-making process itself, by encoding signals that inform an individual about what action to take (O'Doherty, 2007). Patients with lesions involving the OFC often develop changes in their interpersonal emotional skills, while displaying disproportionate impairments in social behavior (Moll et al., 2005) and a reduced experience of moral emotions (Funayama et al., 2019).

The amygdala is involved in moral learning and responses to threats. Through stimulus–reinforcement learning, the amygdala enables the association of actions that harm others with the aversive reinforcement of the victims' distress (Blair, 2007). Furthermore, the amygdala contributes to automatic emotional evaluations of morally salient actions (Shenhav & Greene, 2014). Perceiving an individual who intentionally hurts another person triggers an early increase in amygdalar activation, which plays a critical role in evaluating actual or potential threats (Hesse et al., 2016; Phelps, 2006). Individuals with psychopathy show reduced amygdala activity when judging the acceptability of frightening others and impaired judgment regarding the moral acceptability of causing fear to others (Marsh & Cardinale, 2014).

The precuneus subserves the processing of mental states (Baez et al., 2016; Koster-Hale et al., 2013) and integration of self-referential stimuli in the broader emotional or moral context of the self (Northoff & Bermpohl, 2004). Finally, the TPJ is involved in inferencing others' mental states (Saxe & Kanwisher, 2003). The right TPJ is particularly implicated in judging accidental harms. When individuals are judging such events, this area shows distinct spatial patterns of responses, and an increase in its activation is correlated with greater consideration of exculpating agents (Young & Saxe, 2009b). Consistently, participants who receive transcranial direct current stimulation in the right TPJ assign

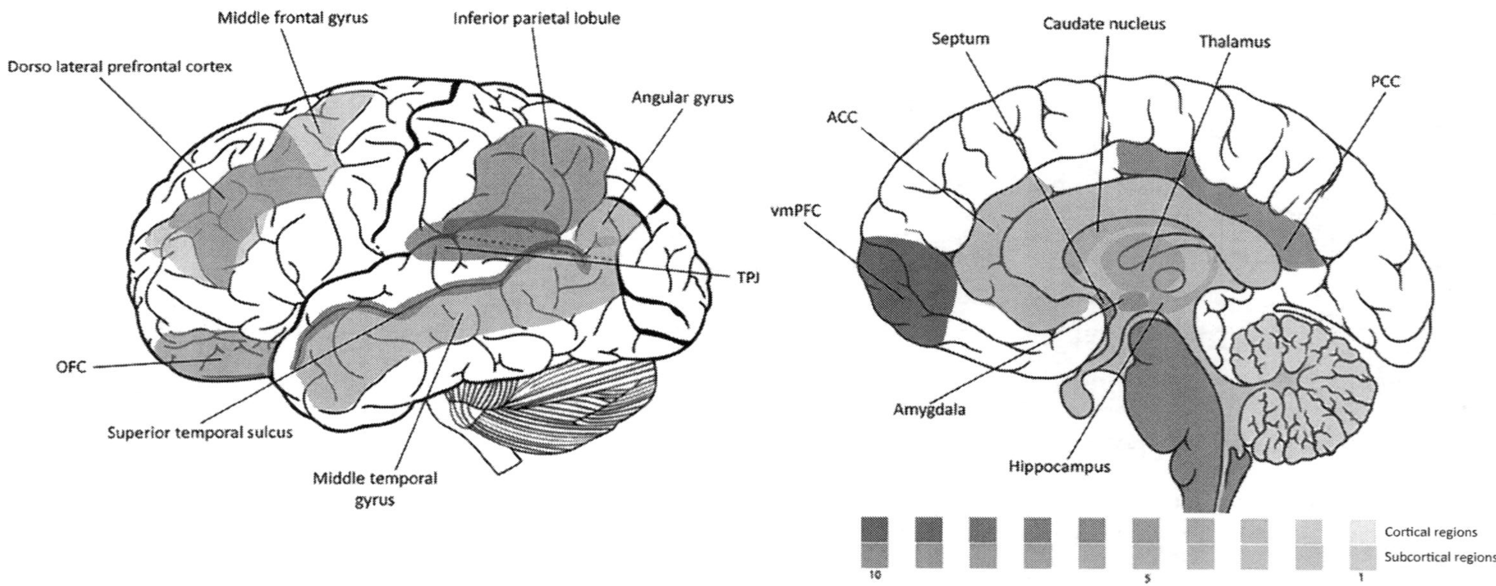

Figure 15.1 Brain regions implicated in moral cognition

This figure shows the density of moral neuroscience studies. The intensity of the color is proportional to the number of the citations of the corresponding region in the article. The left panel shows the main cortical regions involved in moral cognition, while the right panel shows the subcortical ones. Reproduced with authorization from Pascual et al. (2013). See e-book for a full-color version of this figure.

less blame to accidental harms (Sellaro et al., 2015). Together, these findings support the critical role of the TPJ in mediating belief attribution for moral judgment.

All these particular areas play an important role in judging moral situations. However, recent calls (Baez et al., 2016; Baez, García, & Ibáñez, 2017; Baez, García, & Santamaría-García, 2017; Ibáñez & Manes, 2012; Moll et al., 2008) suggest that high-level social processes, such as moral cognition, should be interpreted in terms of the functioning of complex brain networks that integrate context-dependent representations. In the next section, I describe relevant neurocognitive models supporting this view.

Neurocognitive network models of moral cognition

Social interactions occur in context-rich settings (Ibáñez & Manes, 2012), which modulate all aspects of cognition, from basic perception to interpersonal domains. Adequate social and moral behaviors require the integration of explicit and implicit contextual factors, which depends on the functioning of extended brain networks. Few neurocognitive models have attempted to explain how specific mechanisms and brain regions contribute to contextual modulations in social cognitive domains, including moral cognition. The first model to address this issue was the event-feature-emotion complex model (Moll et al., 2005), which proposes that moral cognition emerges from the integration of content and context-dependent representations in cortical-limbic networks. The model postulates three sequential moral cognition mechanisms: (1) the prefrontal cortex provides contextual event representations; (2) the temporal cortex contributes social perceptual features of the environment; and (3) limbic regions underlie emotional states. According to the event-feature-emotion complex model, moral emotions and moral judgments would result from interactions among values, norms, and contextual aspects of social situations (Moll et al., 2005).

The social context network model (Ibáñez & Manes, 2012), a more recent approach, describes the influence of context on social cognitive processing. This model is not focused on moral cognition, but it explains how context modulates social cognition domains in general. According to this model, a cortical network engaging frontal, temporal, and insular regions mediates contextual associations during social situations (see Figure 15.2). Frontal regions (e.g., the OFC, the lateral prefrontal cortex, and the

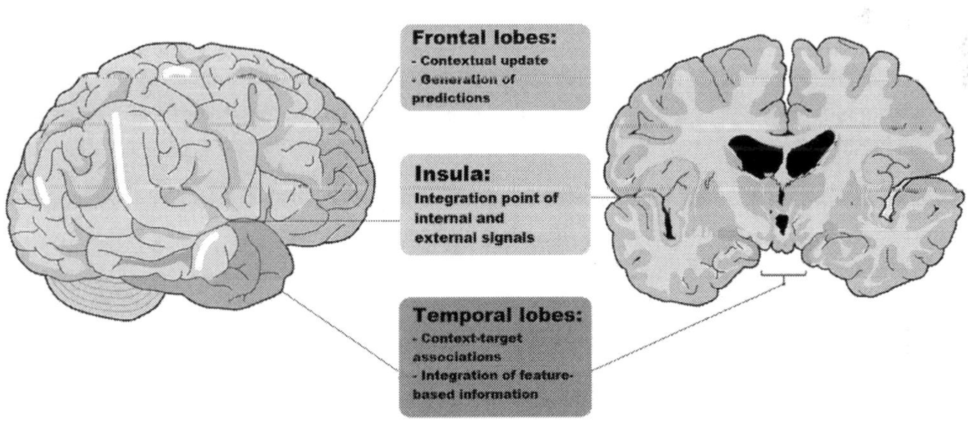

Figure 15.2 The brain network proposed by the social context network model (SCNM)

This model proposes that social contextual cues are processed by a specific brain network. This network comprises frontal (light blue), temporal (orange), and insular (green) regions and their connections. Prefrontal areas would be involved in the generation of focused predictions by updating associations among representations in a specific context. Target-context associations subserved by temporal regions would be integrated with feature-based information processed in frontal regions. The insular cortex would support the convergence of emotional and cognitive states related to the coordination between external and internal milieus. Reproduced with authorization from (Baez, García, & Ibáñez, 2018). See e-book for a full-color version of this figure.

superior orbital sulcus) are involved in the updating of ongoing contextual information and its association with episodic memory. Temporal circuits connecting with the amygdala, the hippocampus, and the perirhinal and parahippocampal cortices index the value of target-context associations. Finally, the insula coordinates internal and external milieus to trigger internal motivational states.

As mentioned above, although particular brain areas play an important role in moral cognition, such complex social cognitive domains should be interpreted in terms of the functioning of frontotemporal networks. Future research may strengthen the neurocognitive models outlined in this section by providing more evidence on brain networks and processes critically involved in contextual modulation of moral cognition. In addition, given that genetic and neuroendocrine factors have also been proven to play a central role in regulating moral cognition mechanisms, more comprehensive models integrating these factors promise a deeper understanding of moral cognition compared with research that focuses exclusively on behavioral responses and associated brain regions (Haidt & Kesebir, 2010). In the next sections, I outline the evidence on the influence of hormonal and genetic factors on moral cognition.

Hormonal bases

Neuromodulators such as hormones modify neuronal dynamics, excitability, and synaptic functions, influencing moral cognition (Chen et al., 2016). Several studies have investigated the role of hormones in moral cognition, paying particular attention to testosterone, cortisol, and oxytocin.

Testosterone has been involved in a diverse array of human social and emotional behaviors (Gong et al., 2017), including moral judgments. High salivary testosterone levels are associated to utilitarian judgments that result in harm to others. For instance, individuals with higher baseline testosterone levels rate impersonal moral dilemmas as more permissible (Gong et al., 2017), and are more likely to make utilitarian decisions (Carney & Mason, 2010). Moreover, a study using a placebo-controlled within-subject design (Chen et al., 2016) showed that testosterone administration in females elicited more utilitarian responses to moral dilemmas. Moreover, a lower ratio between the length of the index and ring fingers (2D:4D ratio), reflecting higher prenatal testosterone exposure, was related to more utilitarian responses. These findings provide evidence to support that prenatal sex-hormone priming could prove important for early neurodevelopment, which plays a crucial role in the manifestations of testosterone on moral judgment. A more recent study (Brannon et al., 2019) explored the effect of testosterone on moral dilemma judgments using a double-blind administration of testosterone or placebo to both males and females. Unexpectedly, results showed that higher levels of endogenous testosterone measured at baseline were associated with lower sensitivity to moral norms, whereas administration of exogenous testosterone increased participants' sensitivity to moral norms. These results show that the role of testosterone in moral judgments is more complex than previously suggested and should be studied further in future investigations.

Cortisol levels can also modulate moral cognition. Overall, higher cortisol levels are associated with more deontological moral decisions (Singer et al., 2017; Starcke et al., 2011; Zhang et al., 2018). For instance, healthy individuals exposed to acute stress situations make more altruistic decisions regarding moral dilemmas, and these decision tendencies are positively associated with their cortisol levels (Singer et al., 2017). Additional evidence suggests that higher stress and cortisol levels are related to increased general preference to opt out of action in moral dilemmas (Hermans et al., 2017). Stress impairs individuals' cognitive control, diminishes their confidence in making optimal decisions, and reduces their willingness to engage in the action (Gawronski et al., 2017). However, cortisol levels are not always related to deontological decisions. It seem that the need for closure moderates the association between cortisol and moral decisions (Kossowska et al., 2016). Cortisol levels are associated with more utilitarian judgments in in-group dilemmas for individuals with a considerable need for closure. For individuals with less need for closure, high cortisol levels are associated with more deontological decisions than utilitarian ones (Kossowska et al., 2016). In sum, current findings suggest that both acute stress exposure and cortisol levels may have prosocial effects on everyday moral decision-making.

Moral cognition is further influenced by oxytocin. De Dreu et al. (2010) were the first to explore the effects of this hormone on moral decisions and intergroup relations. Using moral dilemmas, these authors found that intranasal oxytocin administration makes subjects more likely to sacrifice a different-race individual in order to save race-unspecified others than they were to sacrifice a same-race individual in the same circumstances. In line with these findings, it has been suggested that oxytocin might promote empathy and prosocial behavior, but only for in-group members, reducing prosocial behavior towards the out-group (De Dreu et al., 2010). Intranasal oxytocin administration has also been found to bias behavioral responses towards the endorsement of moral dilemmas involving self-benefit in men, to decrease behavioral endorsement of self-benefit scenarios in moral dilemmas in women (Scheele et al., 2014), and to reduce neural responses to moral dilemmas (Preckel et al., 2015). When judging scenarios of criminal intent, oxytocin administration increased men's ratings of harm caused to victims, but it did not influence their judgment that the criminal offenders deserved punishment (Krueger et al., 2012). Consistently, another study (Goodyear et al., 2016) investigating the effects of intranasal oxytocin on intuitions about the relationship between free will and moral responsibility found that, under placebo, participants held the offender more morally responsible when acting in an indeterministic universe as opposed to a deterministic one. Under oxytocin, however, participants rated the offender's actions with greater leniency and assigned less moral responsibility in both universes. A more recent study (Zhang et al., 2020) revealed that individuals who receive oxytocin make more moral goodness judgments of good intentions than those in the control condition (i.e., placebo). Specifically, oxytocin enhanced the moral goodness judgment of a dictator with hyperfair intention, regardless of outcomes, while it did not affect the judgment of a dictator with unknown or unfair intention.

Although further research is needed, existing evidence supports the idea that neuroendocrine factors can influence moral cognition by regulating brain activity in areas that have been associated with moral judgments.

Genetic factors

As stated above, moral cognition depends on the coordinated interaction of multiple neural systems. These systems depend critically on specific neurotransmitters such as dopamine, serotonin, and oxytocin. Genes that produce or regulate these neurotransmitters may influence moral judgment phenotypes (Bernhard et al., 2016).

Genetic variations in oxytocin receptor genes are associated to individual differences in moral judgment. For instance, Walter et al. (2012) found that carriers of at least one C-allele of the rs2268498 oxytocin gene judged accidental harms as significantly more blameworthy than non-carriers, indicating that the former reduces the relative weight placed on intention versus outcome (Walter et al., 2012). Furthermore, more copies of the C-allele of rs237889 – the oxytocin receptor gene – are associated with a higher frequency of utilitarian judgments in moral dilemmas (Bernhard et al., 2016). A more recent study (Palumbo et al., 2020) explored the potential effects on moral choices of three single polymorphisms and their combinations (rs53576, rs2268498, and rs1042770) in male insurance brokers compared with controls. Results showed that insurance brokers expressed the utilitarian attitude phenotype more than the controls did. When analyzed individually, none of the selected variants influenced the responses to moral dilemmas. However, a composite genetic profile that potentially increases oxytocin activity was associated with higher moral acceptability in brokers. Together, the findings described suggest that moral variations in the oxytocin receptor gene influence moral judgment and, more generally, that genetic polymorphisms can influence complex social cognition processes.

Polymorphisms in the dopamine pathway genes, which potentiate the dopaminergic neurotransmission, also seem to be involved in moral cognition. For example, Pellegrini et al. (2017) genotyped five genetic variants of the dopaminergic pathway [rs1800955 in the dopamine receptor D4 (*DRD4*) gene, *DRD4 48 bp* variable number of tandem repeat (*VNTR*), solute carrier family 6 member 3 (*SLC6A3*), 40 bpVNTR, rs4680 in the catechol-O-methyl transferase (*COMT*) gene, and rs1800497 in the ankyrin repeat and kinase domain containing 1 (*ANKK1*) gene in 200 subjects who were requested to answer moral dilemmas. They found that no individual variant showed any significant effects on moral dilemma responses. However, the genotype combinations that improve dopaminergic signaling selectively increased moral acceptability in females, enhancing the cognitive and reducing the emotional components of moral decision-making in females, making their responses more similar to those provided by males (Pellegrini et al., 2017). Another study also investigated the extent to which the Val158Met polymorphism of the *COMT* gene contributes to individual differences in moral permissibility (Ru et al., 2017). The results showed that individuals with the Val/Val genotype, associated with lower levels of dopamine, endorsed impersonal harm as more impermissible. Together, these findings support the link between dopaminergic pathways and moral cognition.

The neuromodulator serotonin influences a wide range of functions involved in both behavior and cognition. Polymorphisms in the serotonin transporter gene have also been associated with individual differences in moral judgment. Endogenous serotonin neurotransmission is influenced by a polymorphism of the serotonin transporter (5-HTT) in the serotonin transporter gene *SLC6A4*, called 5-HTTLPR. Compared to carriers of the long form of the polymorphism, carriers of the short form show reduced transcription, expression and function of 5-HTT, which influences serotonin reuptake (Marsh et al., 2011). In moral judgment tasks, relative to long (L) allele homozygotes, carriers of the short (S) allele show particular reluctance to endorsing utilitarian actions resulting in foreseen harm to an innocent individual. Individuals with LL genotype judge perpetrating unintentional harm as more acceptable than SL or SS genotype individuals (Marsh et al., 2011). Similarly, 5-HTTLPR short-allele carriers are less compliant with harming another person even when harm or death would inevitably occur to this other individual anyway (Martínez et al., 2020). These results indicate that inherited variants in a genetic polymorphism that influences serotonin neurotransmission influence moral judgments, and suggest that the short allele is associated with elevated emotional responsiveness.

Briefly, genetically informed research of phenotypes related to moral cognition has proliferated rapidly in the last few years. Ensuing findings have sparked paradigm shifts from theories based solely on socialization toward those integrating biological influences.

Towards an integrative view of moral cognition

Making a moral judgment, it has been argued, constitutes a neurosemiotically mediated action. It requires an interpretation of the action in question, which is based on the shared assumptions and understandings that constitute culture (Tappan, 1997). In line with this view, the sociocultural perspective proposes that moral development entails the internalization of semiotically and linguistically mediated social relations (Vygotsky, 1978). Accordingly, everyday cultural discourse provides children with a novel language of morals through which they come "to understand what it means to be human" (Bhatia, 2000: 164). Thus, moral cognition can be considered essentially social, founded on community and knowledge, intersubjectively distributed beyond the boundaries of the individual (Paolucci, 2012). Indeed, actions with moral content are imbued with specific sociocultural meanings that set them apart from other types of actions. They are interpreted in terms of a shared system of values that frames the intentionality of actions. In turn, our efforts to construe meaning in everyday interactions are informed by our inferences about the inner states and intentions of the individuals with whom we interact. Construing the meaning of others' intentions and applying moral judgment to their actions depends on the interpretation of a variety of signs and contextual cues (i.e., from spoken words and manual gestures to facial expressions, eye gaze, body orientation, and body movements). The interpretation and integration of such cues depends on semiotically mediated mechanisms relying on extended the neural networks, and the hormonal and genetic factors described above.

The evidence reviewed in this chapter highlights the influence of cultural, social, psychological, neural, endocrine, and genetic factors on the mechanisms subserving moral cognition and supports the emergence of a multilevel approach. This integrative view promises a deeper understanding of moral cognition compared with research that focuses exclusively on behavioral responses and associated brain regions (Haidt & Kesebir, 2010). Moving forward, this integrative approach requires the overcoming of the artificially imposed schism between social and biological or physical aspects of our existence (Ibáñez et al., 2017). A new integrative framework must be conceived to transcend the segregation between theoretical and methodological traditions, exploit their common grounds, and produce new knowledge in a variety of arenas (García et al., 2020). This is a core mission of neurosemiotics (García et al., 2020). The very premises of the field pave the way for a truly synergistic framework capable of forging new theoretical and empirical vistas beyond classical differentiations between the natural and the social sciences.

Conclusion

For an action to be considered right or wrong, a particular meaning must be associated with that action. Construing this meaning depends on a variety of cultural and contextual factors, as well as on the interaction of extended neural networks, alongside genetic and hormonal factors. Available evidence highlights the relevance of considering the influence of contextual, cultural, and biological factors to understand the mechanisms subserving moral cognition. Future research may strengthen current models by providing more refined evidence on meaning construction processes, as well as neural, genetic, and neuroendocrine factors critically involved in moral cognition. A multilevel approach that integrates semiotics, psychology, neuroscience, and biology promises a deeper understanding of the complex domain of moral cognition. This integrative approach would be capable of forging new theoretical and empirical vistas beyond classical differentiations between the natural and the social sciences.

Acknowledgments

The author acknowledges financial support provided by the Vice Presidency for Research & Creation publication fund at the Universidad de los Andes.

References

Amodio, D. M., & Frith, C. D. (2006). Meeting of minds: The medial frontal cortex and social cognition. *Nature Reviews Neuroscience*, 7(4), 268–277.

Baez, S., García, A. M., & Ibáñez, A. (2017). The social context network model in psychiatric and neurological diseases. *Current Topics in Behavioral Neurosciences*, *30*, 379–396.

Baez, S., Kanske, P., Matallana, D., Montañes, P., Reyes, P., Slachevsky, A., Matus, C., Vigliecca, N. S., Torralva, T., Manes, F., & Ibáñez, A. (2016). Integration of intention and outcome for moral judgment in frontotemporal dementia: Brain structural signatures. *Neuro-Degenerative Diseases*, *16*(3–4), 206–217.

Baez, S., García, A. M., & Ibáñez, A. (2018). How does social context influence our brain and behavior? *Frontiers for Young Minds*, *6*, 3.

Baez, S., García, A. M., & Santamaría-García, H. (2017). Moral cognition and moral emotions. In *Neuroscience and Social Science* (pp. 169–197). New York: Springer.

Barbieri, M. (2009). A short history of biosemiotics. *Biosemiotics*, *2*, 221–245.

Baron-Cohen, S., Leslie, A. M., & Frith, U. (1985). Does the autistic child have a "theory of mind"? *Cognition*, *21*(1), 37–46.

Baumeister, R. F., & Leary, M. R. (1995). The need to belong: Desire for interpersonal attachments as a fundamental human motivation. *Psychological Bulletin*, *117*(3), 497–529.

Baxter, M. G., Parker, A., Lindner, C. C., Izquierdo, A. D., & Murray, E. A. (2000). Control of response selection by reinforcer value requires interaction of amygdala and orbital prefrontal cortex. *Journal of Neuroscience, 20*(11), 4311–4319.

Bernhard, R. M., Chaponis, J., Siburian, R., Gallagher, P., Ransohoff, K., Wikler, D., Perlis, R. H., & Greene, J. D. (2016). Variation in the oxytocin receptor gene (OXTR) is associated with differences in moral judgment. *Social Cognitive and Affective Neuroscience, 11*(12), 1872–1881.

Bhatia, S. (2000). Language socialisation and the construction of socio-moral meanings. *Journal of Moral Education, 29*(2), 149–166.

Blair, R. J. R. (2007). The amygdala and ventromedial prefrontal cortex in morality and psychopathy. *Trends in Cognitive Sciences, 11*(9), 387–392.

Bouissac, P. (1987). Semiotics in Canada I. In T. Sebeok, & J. Umiker-Sebeok (Ed.), *The semiotic web 1987* (pp. 191–252). Berlin: De Gruyter Mouton.

Brannon, S. M., Carr, S., Jin, E. S., Josephs, R. A., & Gawronski, B. (2019). Exogenous testosterone increases sensitivity to moral norms in moral dilemma judgements. *Nature Human Behaviour, 3*(8), 856–866.

Carney, D. R., & Mason, M. F. (2010). Decision making and testosterone: When the ends justify the means. *Journal of Experimental Social Psychology, 46*(4), 668–671.

Chen, C., Decety, J., Huang, P.-C., Chen, C.-Y., & Cheng, Y. (2016). Testosterone administration in females modulates moral judgment and patterns of brain activation and functional connectivity. *Human Brain Mapping, 37*(10), 3417–3430.

Ciaramelli, E., Muccioli, M., Làdavas, E., & Di Pellegrino, G. (2007). Selective deficit in personal moral judgment following damage to ventromedial prefrontal cortex. *Social Cognitive and Affective Neuroscience, 2*(2), 84–92.

Cushman, F. (2008). Crime and punishment: Distinguishing the roles of causal and intentional analyses in moral judgment. *Cognition, 108*(2), 353–380.

D'Argembeau, A., Xue, G., Lu, Z.-L., Van der Linden, M., & Bechara, A. (2008). Neural correlates of envisioning emotional events in the near and far future. *Neuroimage, 40*(1), 398–407.

De Dreu, C. K., Greer, L. L., Handgraaf, M. J., Shalvi, S., Van Kleef, G. A., Baas, M., Ten Velden, F. S., Van Dijk, E., & Feith, S. W. (2010). The neuropeptide oxytocin regulates parochial altruism in intergroup conflict among humans. *Science, 328*(5984), 1408–1411.

Deacon, T. W. (2016). On Human (Symbolic) Nature: How the word became flesh. In G. Etzelmüller & C. Tewes (Eds.), *Embodiment in evolution and culture* (pp. 129–150). Tübingen: Mohr Siebeck GmbH and Co. KG.

Dunn, J. (1987). The beginnings of moral understanding: Development in the second year. In J. Kagan, & S. Lamb (Eds.), *The Emergence of Morality in Young Children*, (pp. 91–112). Chicago: University of Chicago Press.

Funayama, M., Koreki, A., Muramatsu, T., Mimura, M., Kato, M., & Abe, T. (2019). Impairment in judgement of the moral emotion guilt following orbitofrontal cortex damage. *Journal of Neuropsychology, 13*(3), 550–563.

García, A. M., Franco-O'Byrne, D., & Ibáñez, A. (2020). Neurosemiotics: Blurbing a field beyond the "two cultures divide." In L. Lacková, C. Rodríguez & K. Kull (Eds.), *Gatherings in biosemiotics XX*, (pp. 92–97). Tartu: University of Tartu Press.

Gawronski, B., Armstrong, J., Conway, P., Friesdorf, R., & Hütter, M. (2017). Consequences, norms, and generalized inaction in moral dilemmas: The CNI model of moral decision-making. *Journal of Personality and Social Psychology, 113*(3), 343.

Gong, P., Fang, P., Yang, X., Ru, W., Wang, B., Gao, X., & Liu, J. (2017). The CAG polymorphism in androgen receptor (AR) gene impacts the moral permissibility of harmful behavior in females. *Psychoneuroendocrinology, 80*, 74–79.

Goodyear, K., Lee, M. R., O'Hara, M., Chernyak, S., Walter, H., Parasuraman, R., & Krueger, F. (2016). Oxytocin influences intuitions about the relationship between belief in free will and moral responsibility. *Social Neuroscience, 11*(1), 88–96.

Greene, J. D., Sommerville, R. B., Nystrom, L. E., Darley, J. M., & Cohen, J. D. (2001). An fMRI investigation of emotional engagement in moral judgment. *Science, 293*(5537), 2105–2108.

Haidt, J. (2001). The emotional dog and its rational tail: A social intuitionist approach to moral judgment. *Psychological Review, 108*(4), 814–834.

Haidt, J., & Kesebir, S. (2010). Morality. In S. T. Fiske, D. T. Gilbert, & G. Lindzey (Eds.), *Handbook of Social Psychology* (pp. 797–832). Hoboken, NJ: John Wiley & Sons.

Heekeren, H. R., Wartenburger, I., Schmidt, H., Prehn, K., Schwintowski, H.-P., & Villringer, A. (2005). Influence of bodily harm on neural correlates of semantic and moral decision-making. *NeuroImage, 24*(3), 887–897.

Hermans, E. J., Henckens, M. J. A. G., Joëls, M., & Fernández, G. (2017). Time-dependent shifts in neural systems supporting decision-making under stress. In J.-C. Dreher & L. Tremblay (Eds.), *Decision Neuroscience: An Integrative Perspective* (pp. 371–385). Cambridge, MA: Elsevier.

Hesse, E., Mikulan, E., Decety, J., Sigman, M., Garcia, M. del C., Silva, W., Ciraolo, C., Vaucheret, E., Baglivo, F., & Huepe, D. (2016). Early detection of intentional harm in the human amygdala. *Brain, 139*(1), 54–61.

Ibáñez, A., & Manes, F. (2012). Contextual social cognition and the behavioral variant of frontotemporal dementia. *Neurology*, *78*(17), 1354–1362.

Ibáñez, A., Sedeño, L., García, A.M. (2017). *Neuroscience and Social Science: The Missing Link*. New York: Springer.

Kossowska, M., Czernatowicz-Kukuczka, A., Szumowska, E., & Czarna, A. (2016). Cortisol and moral decisions among young men: The moderating role of motivation toward closure. *Personality and Individual Differences*, *101*, 249–253.

Koster-Hale, J., Saxe, R., Dungan, J., & Young, L. L. (2013). Decoding moral judgments from neural representations of intentions. *Proceedings of the National Academy of Sciences*, *110*(14), 5648–5653.

Krueger, F., Parasuraman, R., Iyengar, V., Thornburg, M., Weel, J., Lin, M., Clarke, E., McCabe, K., & Lipsky, R. (2012). Oxytocin receptor genetic variation promotes human trust behavior. *Frontiers in Human Neuroscience*, *6*, 4.

Kvaran, T., & Sanfey, A. G. (2010). Toward an integrated neuroscience of morality: The contribution of neuroeconomics to moral cognition. *Topics in Cognitive Science*, *2*(3), 579–595.

Lotze, M., Heymans, U., Birbaumer, N., Veit, R., Erb, M., Flor, H., & Halsband, U. (2006). Differential cerebral activation during observation of expressive gestures and motor acts. *Neuropsychologia*, *44*(10), 1787–1795.

Marsh, A. A., & Cardinale, E. M. (2014). When psychopathy impairs moral judgments: Neural responses during judgments about causing fear. *Social Cognitive and Affective Neuroscience*, *9*(1), 3–11.

Marsh, A. A., Crowe, S. L., Henry, H. Y., Gorodetsky, E. K., Goldman, D., & Blair, R. J. R. (2011). Serotonin transporter genotype (5-HTTLPR) predicts utilitarian moral judgments. *PLoS One*, *6*(10), e25148.

Martínez, R. M., Chen, C.-Y., Liao, T.-T., Cheng, Y., Fan, Y.-T., Chou, S.-H., & Chen, C. (2020). The multifaceted effects of serotonin transporter polymorphism (5-HTTLPR) on anxiety, implicit moral attitudes, and harmful behaviors. *Frontiers in Psychology*, *11*, 1521.

Moll, J., de Oliveira-Souza, R., & Eslinger, P. J. (2003). Morals and the human brain: A working model. *Neuroreport*, *14*(3), 299–305.

Moll, J., De Oliveira-Souza, R., & Zahn, R. (2008). The neural basis of moral cognition: Sentiments, concepts, and values. *Annals of the New York Academy of Sciences*, 1124, 161–180.

Moll, J., & Schulkin, J. (2009). Social attachment and aversion in human moral cognition. *Neuroscience & Biobehavioral Reviews*, *33*(3), 456–465.

Moll, J., Zahn, R., de Oliveira-Souza, R., Krueger, F., & Grafman, J. (2005). The neural basis of human moral cognition. *Nature Reviews Neuroscience*, *6*(10), 799–809.

Northoff, G., & Bermpohl, F. (2004). Cortical midline structures and the self. *Trends in Cognitive Sciences*, *8*(3), 102–107.

O'Doherty, J. P. (2007). Lights, camembert, action! The role of human orbitofrontal cortex in encoding stimuli, rewards, and choices. *Annals of the New York Academy of Sciences*, *1121*(1), 254–272.

Palumbo, S., Mariotti, V., Anastasio, T., Rota, G., Lucchi, L., Manfrinati, A., Rumiati, R., Lotto, L., Sarlo, M., & Pietrini, P. (2020). A genetic profile of oxytocin receptor improves moral acceptability of outcome-maximizing harm in male insurance brokers. *Behavioural Brain Research*, 112681.

Paolucci, C. (2012). Social cognition between theories, simulations and narratives: The narrative practice semiotic hypothesis. *Intellectica. Revue de l'Association Pour la Recherche Cognitive*, *58*, 173–195.

Pascual, L., Gallardo-Pujol, D., & Rodrigues, P. (2013). How does morality work in the brain? A functional and structural perspective of moral behavior. *Frontiers in Integrative Neuroscience*, *12*. doi.org/10.3389/fnint.2013.00065

Peirce, C. S., & Buchler, J. (1955). *Philosophical Writings of Peirce*. New York: Dover.

Pellegrini, S., Palumbo, S., Iofrida, C., Melissari, E., Rota, G., Mariotti, V., Anastasio, T., Manfrinati, A., Rumiati, R., & Lotto, L. (2017). Genetically driven enhancement of dopaminergic transmission affects moral acceptability in females but not in males: A pilot study. *Frontiers in Behavioral Neuroscience*, *11*, 156.

Phelps, E. A. (2006). Emotion and cognition: Insights from studies of the human amygdala. *Annual Revision of Psychology*, *57*, 27–53.

Preckel, K., Scheele, D., Eckstein, M., Maier, W., & Hurlemann, R. (2015). The influence of oxytocin on volitional and emotional ambivalence. *Social Cognitive and Affective Neuroscience*, *10*(7), 987–993.

Roelofs, K., Minelli, A., Mars, R. B., Van Peer, J., & Toni, I. (2009). On the neural control of social emotional behavior. *Social Cognitive and Affective Neuroscience*, *4*(1), 50–58.

Ru, W., Fang, P., Wang, B., Yang, X., Zhu, X., Xue, M., Shen, G., Gao, X., & Gong, P. (2017). The impacts of Val158Met in Catechol-O-methyltransferase (COMT) gene on moral permissibility and empathic concern. *Personality and Individual Differences*, *106*, 52–56.

Saussure, F. de. (2011). *Course in General Linguistics*. New York: Columbia University Press.

Saxe, R., & Kanwisher, N. (2003). People thinking about thinking people. The role of the temporo-parietal junction in «theory of mind». *NeuroImage*, *19*(4), 1835–1842.

Scheele, D., Striepens, N., Kendrick, K. M., Schwering, C., Noelle, J., Wille, A., Schläpfer, T. E., Maier, W., & Hurlemann, R. (2014). Opposing effects of oxytocin on moral judgment in males and females. *Human brain mapping*, *35*(12), 6067–6076.

Schilbach, L., Wohlschlaeger, A. M., Kraemer, N. C., Newen, A., Shah, N. J., Fink, G. R., & Vogeley, K. (2006). Being with virtual others: Neural correlates of social interaction. *Neuropsychologia*, *44*(5), 718–730.

Sellaro, R., Güroğlu, B., Nitsche, M. A., van den Wildenberg, W. P. M., Massaro, V., Durieux, J., Hommel, B., & Colzato, L. S. (2015). Increasing the role of belief information in moral judgments by stimulating the right temporoparietal junction. *Neuropsychologia*, 77, 400–408.

Shenhav, A., & Greene, J. D. (2014). Integrative moral judgment: Dissociating the roles of the amygdala and ventromedial prefrontal cortex. *Journal of Neuroscience*, *34*(13), 4741–4749.

Singer, N., Sommer, M., Döhnel, K., Zänkert, S., Wüst, S., & Kudielka, B. M. (2017). Acute psychosocial stress and everyday moral decision-making in young healthy men: The impact of cortisol. *Hormones and Behavior*, *93*, 72–81.

Skitka, L. J. (2002). Do the means always justify the ends, or do the ends sometimes justify the means? A value model of justice reasoning. *Personality and Social Psychology Bulletin*, *28*(5), 588–597.

Starcke, K., Polzer, C., Wolf, O. T., & Brand, M. (2011). Does stress alter everyday moral decision-making? *Psychoneuroendocrinology*, *36*(2), 210–219.

Tappan, M. (1997). Language, culture, and moral development: A Vygotskian perspective. *Developmental Review*, *17*(1), 78–100.

Tappan, M. (2006). Moral functioning as mediated action. *Journal of Moral Education*, *35*, 1–18.

Treadway, M. T., Buckholtz, J. W., Martin, J. W., Jan, K., Asplund, C. L., Ginther, M. R., Jones, O. D., & Marois, R. (2014). Corticolimbic gating of emotion-driven punishment. *Nature Neuroscience*, *17*(9), 1270–1275.

Turiel, E. (2008). Thought about actions in social domains: Morality, social conventions, and social interactions. *Cognitive Development*, *23*(1), 136–154.

Vygotsky, L. (1978). *Mind and society*. Cambridge, MA: Harvard University Press.

Walter, N. T., Montag, C., Markett, S., Felten, A., Voigt, G., & Reuter, M. (2012). Ignorance is no excuse: Moral judgments are influenced by a genetic variation on the oxytocin receptor gene. *Brain and Cognition*, *78*(3), 268–273.

Wertsch, J. V., del Río, P., & Alvarez, A. (Eds.). (1995). *Sociocultural Studies of Mind*. Cambridge: Cambridge University Press.

Wolf, D., Mittelberg, I., Rekittke, L.-M., Bhavsar, S., Zvyagintsev, M., Haeck, A., Cong, F., Klasen, M., & Mathiak, K. (2018). Interpretation of social interactions: Functional imaging of cognitive-semiotic categories during naturalistic viewing. *Frontiers in Human Neuroscience*, *12*. doi: 10.3389/fnhum.2018.00296

Young, L., Bechara, A., Tranel, D., Damasio, H., Hauser, M., & Damasio, A. (2010). Damage to ventromedial prefrontal cortex impairs judgment of harmful intent. *Neuron*, *65*(6), 845–851.

Young, L., & Saxe, R. (2008). The neural basis of belief encoding and integration in moral judgment. *NeuroImage*, *40*(4), 1912–1920.

Young, L., & Saxe, R. (2009a). Innocent intentions: A correlation between forgiveness for accidental harm and neural activity. *Neuropsychologia*, *47*(10), 2065–2072.

Young, L., & Saxe, R. (2009b). An FMRI investigation of spontaneous mental state inference for moral judgment. *Journal of Cognitive Neuroscience*, *21*(7), 1396–1405.

Zeki, S., Goodenough, O. R., Zeki, S., & Goodenough, O. (2004). Law and the brain: Introduction. *Philosophical Transactions of the Royal Society of London. Series B: Biological Sciences*, *359*(1451), 1661–1665.

Zhang, L., Kong, M., Li, Z., Zhao, X., & Gao, L. (2018). Chronic stress and moral decision-making: An exploration with the CNI model. *Frontiers in Psychology*, *9*, 1702.

Zhang, J., Zhou, C., & Yu, R. (2020). Oxytocin amplifies the influence of good intentions on social judgments. *Hormones and Behavior*, *117*, 104589.

16

THE NEUROSEMIOTICS OF SOCIAL INTERACTION

Insights from second-person neuroscience

Leonhard Schilbach

Introduction: From semiotics to neurosemiotics

Semiotics traditionally has focused on the study of signs and their use during human communication. According to Eco (1979: 16), a sign is "*everything* that, on the grounds of a previously established social convention, can be taken as *something standing for something else*." In other words, social interactions help to introduce the use of words, expressive gestures, and so forth that represent something in the minds of the interaction partners. More recent approaches in the field of experimental semiotics have taken an empirical approach to address varied forms of communication, which people develop when they cannot access and use pre-established communication systems (Galantucci & Garrod, 2011). Here, an important assumption is that both individual cognition and the complex processes of social interaction need to be studied in order to understand how they are related and to help humans to make sense of the world and each other.

In particular, *experimental semiotics* focuses on social interaction from three different perspectives: while the first perspective focuses on different types of dyadic interactions, the second perspective focuses on the social diffusion of novel communication, and the third perspective investigates the effects that in-group and out-group dynamics have on the development on novel linguistic conventions (Galantucci & Garrod, 2011). All these approaches capitalize on the idea that observing the emergence of communication offers new opportunities for its scientific study. Furthermore, Galantucci & Garrod (2011) suggest that future work in experimental semiotics could fruitfully link up with the field of cognitive neuroscience to investigate the underlying neural bases of the emergence of new forms of communication. This approach can be seen as being aimed at the development of a field of neurosemiotics, an area of research that previously had been defined as referring to the "investigation of the neurophysiological substrata of semiotic behavior" (Bouissac, 1985: 223). In addition, I propose that the burgeoning and by now well-established field of social neuroscience is also relevant because it focuses on the neurobiology of interacting minds (Frith & Frith, 1999). While social neuroscience does not always explicitly refer to the semiotic tradition, and often focuses on nonverbal communication, it certainly does investigate highly relevant phenomena such as social cognition, mental state inference, and social interaction – all of which contribute to human beings' impressive communicative abilities. In particular, the recent development within social neuroscience of focusing on the dynamics of social interaction and how they relate to brain

DOI: 10.4324/9781003051817-20

function and the developmental establishment of higher order cognitive functions – a trend that has been described as aiming for a *second-person neuroscience* – might be of particular relevance for neurosemiotics. In other words, a truly social second-person neuroscience might be in a particularly promising position to gain insights into how patterns of social interaction and communication lead to distributed patterns of neural activity.

Importantly, human beings are never passive observers, but are always ready to continuously engage with the environment. Nevertheless, in its early phases, social neuroscience has often studied human social cognition as if humans primarily adopted an observational stance and did not interact or act collectively. Consequently, research in this field has often relied on methods that measure neural responses as if the brain's primary function were not to control behavior and adaptive responses, but to merely observe what goes on in the social world. More importantly, it seems that characteristics and limitations of the methodologies may also have affected the theories that are used to think about and explain social behavior. While social neuroscience started out with the great ambition to study the neurobiology of "interacting minds" (Frith & Frith, 1999), much of the research initially conducted clearly missed this mark and focused on the neural correlates of social observation – that is, what happens in the brain of a human observer when they see another human being performing some action that is not related to the observer. These shortcomings have led to the suggestion that the neurobiology of social *interaction* (rather than social *observation*) in fact constitutes the "dark matter" of social neuroscience (Schilbach et al., 2013). Against this background, another line of research has more recently been proposed, which takes social interaction seriously and focuses on the behavioral and neural mechanisms of real-life social interactions both within and across interacting brains (Redcay & Schilbach, 2019). This approach has been described as a *second-person neuroscience* because it rests on the assumption that social cognition from an interactor's point of view – characterized by emotional engagement and the reciprocity of the social interaction – is fundamentally different from a detached observational stance according to which we merely observe others (Schilbach et al., 2013).

In this chapter, I review studies that have taken an "interactive turn" to focus on the behavioral and neural mechanisms of social interaction and inform us about how human beings communicate and share their experiences in such situations. I start out by focusing on studies that have investigated how a social context – albeit minimal – changes the neural correlates of action control and how motoric responses to others can also be brought about automatically, as evidenced in the case of facial mimicry and other forms of behavioral contagion. I then move on to studies that have used full-body motion tracking to investigate interpersonal coordination and the exchange of gaze cues during social interaction and its underlying neurobiology. Finally, we discuss how second-person neuroscience might link up in fruitful and productive ways with neurosemiotics, opening important avenues for interdisciplinary research on the neurobiology of intersubjectivity. In the end, I turn towards the clinical relevance of second-person approaches and the discussion of social (communicative) impairments across many, if not all, psychiatric disorders, which have consequently been described as "disorders of social interaction" (Schilbach, 2016). A focus on interaction-based processes in particular appears to be crucial for improving our understanding of the behavioral and neurobiological mechanisms of psychiatric disorders in clinically beneficial ways.

Smile with me

Successful interpersonal communication depends to a large extent on the exchange of nonverbal information. The face is known to be of particular importance in this context, as facial expressions convey information about the emotional state of others but may also reflect their appraisal of a given situation (Erickson & Schulkin, 2003; Frijda & Tcherkassof, 1997; Kaiser & Wehrle, 2001). Interestingly, perceivers across the human lifespan spontaneously imitate the facial gestures of others (e.g., Meltzoff & Moore, 1977). This automatic phenomenon has been described as *facial mimicry*, a form of "physiological linkage" between individuals (Dimberg, 1982; Dimberg et al., 2000) that allows us to inhabit someone else's facial expressions (Merleau-Ponty, 1964), thus promoting interpersonal communication (Niedenthal et al., 2005). Mimicry reflects an internal simulation of a perceived emotion and could thereby facilitate understanding others' mental states (Niedenthal et al., 2010; Oberman et al., 2007). Conceptually, these findings have often been associated with the so-called simulationist accounts of social cognition, which describe how we use our own mental states to obtain a "*first-person* grasp" of the motor goals and intentions of other individuals (Rizzolatti & Sinigaglia, 2010: 264). In contrast to this view, which emphasizes similarities in self- and other-related processes, an interactionist or second-person view of social cognition construes interpersonally coordinated and responsive behavior as constituting "knowledge" or practical know-how of other minds (Schilbach et al., 2013).

To investigate the behavioral and neural correlates of facial mimicry, we performed a sequence of studies (Mojzisch et al., 2006; Schilbach et al., 2008; Schilbach et al., 2006) in which participants viewed short video sequences depicting an anthropomorphic virtual character that exhibited socially relevant facial expressions or arbitrary facial movements. Furthermore, it was varied whether or not the virtual character looked directly at the participant or towards the right or left in the direction of someone else. Behavioral results indicated that participants did not have difficulties in differentiating socially relevant from arbitrary mimic behavior. In spite of the explicit instruction to "put themselves into the shoes of the other," participants demonstrated a bias towards giving socially relevant facial expressions a higher rating of communicative relevance when they were self-directed rather than other-directed. In parallel, neuroimaging results showed that the perception of socially relevant nonverbal cues from an observer's viewpoint recruits brain regions that have been related to visuospatial processing, while the perception of identical, self-directed stimuli activates regions subserving emotional and evaluative processing, such as the amygdala and medial prefrontal cortex (Schilbach et al., 2006). Interestingly, the neuroimaging data also showed that the perception of arbitrary facial movements activated the so-called mirror neuron system (Rizzolatti & Sinigaglia, 2010). This suggests that "mirror" responses do not just occur when actions are highly familiar (Brass et al., 2007), but also when they are unpredicted and may constitute a form of prediction error signal (Heerey & Crossley, 2013).

In a follow-up experiment, the same paradigm was used while recording eye movements, pupil size, and facial electromyography (EMG). Attention allocation, as assessed by fixation duration, was specifically related to the perception of self-directed stimuli. EMG measurements showed that facial activity was influenced by the perception of socially relevant facial expressions, as reflected in spontaneous, involuntary facial responses (Mojzisch et al., 2006). Using the temporal information from the EMG study, we then re-analyzed the fMRI data. The findings showed that the occurrence of facial mimicry is associated with a differential increase of neural activity in the face motor area. This region is active during voluntary facial movements and during the perception of emotional vocalizations (e.g., laughter), thereby potentially preparing facial movements in response to the stimuli (Warren et al., 2006). This form of interaction readiness might promote behavioral synchrony across individuals.

Social context matters

While automatic behavioral responses may be important to link individuals and create rapport, human beings can also act voluntarily and suppress action tendencies. In order to investigate this capability and how it manifests in a minimal social context, we conducted another series of studies. Here, an action control paradigm was used, which required that participants performed spatially congruent or incongruent button presses to respond to an unpredictable change in a visual stimulus. Furthermore, the stimulus type was systematically varied to include both social (face) and non-social (geometric shape) stimuli. The results demonstrate that the so-called incongruency costs (i.e., longer reaction times needed to generate a spatially incongruent as compared to a congruent response) were significantly smaller for the social than for the non-social stimulus in healthy controls (Schilbach et al., 2011). This was surprising, because face stimuli and the gaze shifts shown in this task were thought to guide attentional resources much more than non-social stimuli, so that incongruent actions should become more difficult and time consuming. When considering, however, that the use of a face that looks directly at the study participant may have introduced a joint or we-centric reference frame, one could speculate that such a "division of labor" in a social setting could have helped to decrease the effort needed. In a follow-up neuroimaging study, we showed that the modulatory effect of social context on action control involved increased activity in subcortical structures subserving action execution and monitoring as well as social cognition (Schilbach et al., 2011). In other words, acting in the presence of someone else (or at least a face looking at us) significantly changes the neural networks relevant for action control, such that the brain may rely more on habitual social behavior while ramping up action monitoring to generate the fast behavioral adaptations that many human beings exhibit in the presence of others.

Joint orienting, shared attention, and reality

While the studies described above provide important insights into automatic processes of social understanding, they clearly do not capture the reciprocity of real-life social interactions. In other words, while a participant may exhibit a mimicry response or even an overt smile, this response will not have an impact on the agent whose facial expression has brought about the response. In order to close the loop between interaction partners, systematically manipulate, and measure the dynamics of social interaction, other methodological approaches are necessary. While many behavioral studies have shown effects of interpersonal synchrony and the related concept of mimicry, these phenomena may not be observable in all conditions (Hale & Hamilton, 2016). Dynamic coupling of individuals may also arise without direct synchrony of behavior (Hasson & Frith, 2016) and strict synchrony of movements may even be detrimental to the attainment of shared goals (Wallot et al., 2016). This suggests that additional mechanisms may be relevant, especially in naturalistic situations during which interaction partners may take different roles and mutually coordinate their behavior in complementary ways. Proxemic measures, such as distancing and orienting behaviors, could also be more sensitive than interpersonal synchrony at reflecting positive (and negative) attitudes toward other people in some social situations. In order to quantitatively measure social behavior during dyadic, real-world social interactions in unobtrusive manner, we have developed an infrared-based motion tracking system (Lahnakoski et al., 2020). This setup enables a detailed analysis of behavior both at the individual and at the interpersonal level. In other words, we can extract measures of interpersonal coordination, such as interpersonal distance, but also windowed cross-correlations of behavior, which can be informative about how much interaction partners mutually influence each other. The novel setup was validated in comparison to conventionally used wearable sensors. To study behavior during natural social interactions, we applied the system to track the body and head movements of participants sitting at a table engaged in conversations on pre-defined topics and while playing the game "Keep it steady," where participants pick out wooden sticks from an unstable bundle played alternately in either a cooperative or a competitive manner. After the task, participants evaluated their social interaction experience by answering a self-report questionnaire. During data analysis, we assessed interpersonal synchrony of movement as well as dyadic measures of proxemic behavior, such as joint orienting behavior and interpersonal distance. Our results demonstrate that patterns of proxemic behaviors, rather than more widely used measures of interpersonal synchrony, best predicted the subjective quality of the social interactions. Increased distance between participants predicted lower enjoyment, while increased joint orienting toward each other during cooperation correlated with increased effort reported by the participants. Importantly, the interpersonal distance was most informative of the quality of interaction when task demands and experimental control were minimal. In our study, we went on to train the so-called classifiers to automatically detect gaze behaviors during the interactions. While all behaviors were recognized above chance level, joint attention and eye contact/mutual gaze were particularly well recognized. Moreover, the prevalence of the automatically detected gaze behaviors were highly correlated with the manually annotated amounts for them, which again demonstrates that an automatic classification procedure can recognize these highly important phenomena during dyadic social interaction.

Importantly, eye contact and mutual gaze have profound psychophysiological effects on a human observer (Bateson et al., 2006; Kleinke, 1986). In fact, the ability to discriminate between direct and averted gaze exists across different species and may have evolved because direct gaze can signal that a predator is attending (Emery, 2000). Many animals therefore respond to direct gaze with displays of fear, aggression, or submission (Schwab & Huber, 2006). In humans, initial eye contact – in particular when combined with the so-called "eyebrow flash" (Grammer et al., 1988) – is transculturally recognized as an approach signal, and humans may expect that said gaze is directed towards them (Mareschal et al., 2013), whereas prolonged eye contact can be perceived as a threat signal (Nichols & Champness, 1971). Yet any gaze-based social interaction really only starts with two individuals looking at each other. An initial look towards someone increases the probability of an ensuing conversation and decreases the incidence of no talking (Carey, 1978). A model by Senju and Johnson (2009) suggests that the "eye contact effect" comes about through a subcortical route via the amygdala and low-level visual areas including the superior colliculus and the pulvinar. This subcortical mechanism is thought to modulate activity in brain areas involved in the detection of gaze direction, such as the superior temporal sulcus, as well as areas relevant for higher-order social cognition, such as the medial prefrontal cortex. Next to a tendency to establish eye contact, humans also have a tendency to follow others' gaze, because looking where others are looking can be useful at times. Also, gaze-following is one way to engage in joint attention, while the other consists in directing someone else's gaze towards an object or an aspect of the environment. This interactively constituted phenomenon of joint attention has been defined as attending to something "together with" someone and being aware that "we both" are attending (Schilbach et al., 2010). The importance of this phenomenon can hardly be overestimated because it creates a perceptual common ground for the interaction partners that would have to appear fundamental for any theory of semiotics, which typically assume a so-called semiotic triangle or quadrangle when including the human agent and have also been implied in theories of cultural evolution (Clark & Brennan, 1991). This quadrangle describes the relationship of a human agent, the sign itself, the term used, and the object in the world that is denoted. In terms of social interaction, this conception suggests that interaction partners are both part of semiotic quadrangles and that for the two to understand each other, the content that the quadrangles represent must fit or be aligned in a sufficient manner. Here, joint attention appears to be particularly relevant as data from human development indicates, for instance, that the occurrence and frequency with which children engage in joint attention events predicts language acquisition and vocabulary (Carpenter & Tomasello, 2000). Furthermore, a recent study has demonstrated that eye contact is positively correlated with synchrony across conversation partners as well as ratings of dyadic engagement (Wohltjen & Wheatley, 2021). Interestingly, it was shown that eye contact commences when interpersonal synchrony peaks, and predicts its subsequent decline. This pattern has been taken to suggest that eye contact is indicative of joint (or shared) attention but may also help to reduce synchrony when independent contributions to a conversation are called for.

In order to investigate the neural correlates of joint attention, we have devised an experimental setup that uses eye-tracking to systematically manipulate the gaze behavior of a face with whom study participants can engage in a gaze-based interaction while believing that the face belongs to/is controlled by another person (Brandi et al., 2020; Pfeiffer et al., 2014; Schilbach et al., 2010). Joint attention events can then be generated systematically while participants undergo neuroimaging scanning. Results demonstrate differences in the neural correlates of self- or other-initiated joint attention: directing someone else's gaze towards an object oneself differentially activated the ventral striatum, a part of the functional neuroanatomy of reward processing, and the degree of activity change in this region correlated with ratings of subjective experience, which indicated that participants enjoyed looking at objects more "together with" the virtual other than by themselves. Furthermore, our findings demonstrated that the so-called mentalizing network is robustly activated by the participation in gaze-based social interaction, even though the task did not ask for mental state attribution. This raises the interesting question of how such networks are shaped during development and whether social interactions might be a primary driving force for this before children develop the ability to explicitly attribute mental states to someone. Such a view appears consistent with a Vygotskian view of development, which suggests that, for example, the development of pretense is closely related to semiotic abilities and proceeds primarily in social contexts (Rakoczy, 2006).

In a follow-up study, we investigated whether joint attention is experienced as pleasant and motivating because it constitutes a form of cooperative behavior that relies on shared intentions or because it is an activity that is performed for the sake of mutual enjoyment (Pfeiffer et al., 2014). During the task, participants were asked to assess whether a virtual agent was either controlled by another human or by a computer, while in fact the agent was always controlled by a computer. In a between-subject design, the available information about the alleged other player was varied such that one group of participants was led to believe that the other group was helping to solve this task, whereas the other group thought the other players were naive to their task. On the behavioral level, this difference in instructions resulted in marked differences in the evaluation of the agent's gaze behavior. On the neural level, it was shown that even in the absence of a shared goal, a gaze-based interaction leads to a differential recruitment of reward-related brain regions.

Next to interaction-based single-brain studies, such as the joint attention study described above, recent years have also seen an increasing number of studies that use two-/dual-brain neuroimaging to gain new insights into how information is transferred between social partners and how they may build up shared representations – for a review, see Redcay and Schilbach (2019). These studies examine how activation within one brain can predict brain activation of one's social partner during dialogue, gestural communication, and emotion processing. Furthermore, conversational alignment across interaction partners is reflected by similarity at the neural level between partners. For example, greater similarity is seen at the neural level while viewing a movie clip when participants adopt a shared perspective (Lahnakoski et al., 2014; Yeshurun et al., 2017) or a similar emotional state (Nummenmaa et al., 2012). Other recent studies that are in line with the call for a second-person neuroscience have investigated how mutual engagement impacts the neural networks recruited during social interaction. Here, it has been shown that the mentalizing network is consistently sensitive to real-time interaction with a perceived or real social partner, regardless of task demands (Redcay et al., 2010; Rice & Redcay, 2016). From the conceptual side, it also appears important to ask whether mental state attributions that have been linked to activity change in the mentalizing network may also differ in situations of social interaction as compared to social observation. While a social interaction may immediately include a need to coordinate with the plans (and other mental states) of the other person, no such joint action plans might be necessary when I am only observing others. Here it would be important to differentiate how such a high-level alignment across persons may come about in a bottom-up rather than a top-down fashion (Clarke et al., 2019).

Returning to the topic of facial expressions in the context of social interactions, we conducted a study to investigate whether the occurrence of spontaneous facial mimicry is modulated by joint attention – that is, whether the person whose facial expression may be mimicked establishes eye contact and joint attention before (Neufeld et al., 2016). We again used EMG to assess spontaneous facial mimicry. Results showed that the occurrence of joint attention indeed augments spontaneous facial mimicry, but only in individuals with low compared to individuals with high autistic traits. These findings are in line with reports of reduced impact of joint attention on action imitation in individuals with autism spectrum disorder. Moreover, our findings suggest that it is important to investigate the interactions between empathic processes rather than testing these processes individually.

Second-person neuroscience meets neurosemiotics

Finally, we return to the question of the link between social neuroscience and neurosemiotics. As introduced above, neurosemiotics is interested in the neurobiological bases of semiotic behaviors. As these behaviors tend to be embedded in the context of social interactions (Galantucci & Garrod, 2011), we suggest that the newly forming field of *second-person neuroscience*, with its emphasis on (dyadic, but also multiperson) social interactions (Redcay & Schilbach, 2019), might link up particularly well with neurosemiotics and can offer important new avenues for interdisciplinary future research. An interesting line of research, for instance, could be concerned with the idea of how patterns of social interaction may influence patterns of brain activity by means of embodiment and internalization. One preliminary example of this can be found in neuroimaging studies showing that social interactive gaze behaviors recruit the so-called mentalizing network in the absence of instructions to explicitly attribute mental states to someone (Redcay & Schilbach, 2019). This has led to the suggestion that social interaction modulates activity in brain networks, which will later be reused to perform more abstract social cognitive and communicative functions. In other words, second-person neuroscience could help to investigate a gradient from more implicit to more explicit forms of communication and their underlying neurophysiology, as also suggested by neurosemiotics. In addition, semiotic typologies have been used to inform neuroimaging studies of social interaction (Wolf et al., 2018), constituting yet another point of contact. Such advancements are likely to be informative both on a theoretical and empirical level, but could also yield links to interactive and communicative impairments in clinical psychiatry. It is to the discussion of this topic that I now turn in the final section.

Second-person neuropsychiatry

Apart from its relevance for social neuroscience, the second-person approach of taking social interaction seriously also appears highly relevant for our understanding of psychiatric disorders. These disorders are ubiquitously characterized by social interaction difficulties and in terms of the practice of psychopathology – can only be defined by referring to intersubjectively shared conventions, which are captured in the relevant classification manuals. Because of those reasons, it has been suggested that psychiatric disorders can be thought of as "disorders of social interaction" (Schilbach, 2016). Consequently, a strong focus on social and communicative processes and determinants of mental illness appears to be crucial for improving our understanding of the behavioral and neural mechanisms of psychiatric disorders in a way that maximally benefits the patients (Schilbach, 2019). In this context, points of contact between semiotic traditions and psychopathology may also be worth exploring (Andersch, 2015).

Taking the notion of social interaction as a constituent element of the human condition seriously, we have recently suggested that the conception of psychiatric disorders as disorders of social interaction may allow to broaden the scope of scientific inquiry. Rather than focusing exclusively on individuals affected by mental illness and the disruptions of their interaction with healthy persons, we can also investigate what happens when two patients interact with one another. Here, social impairments sometimes appear to be less pronounced when, for example, two persons with autism interact compared with a situation where one autistic person and one non-autistic person interact, which has been described as a social interaction mismatch (Bolis et al., 2017; Schilbach, 2016) (see Figure 16.1). In line with this view, recent findings have indicated that real-life social network size is indeed related to interaction-based measures of neural activity (Preller et al., 2014), and that a psychiatric condition such as borderline personality disorder is characterized by state-dependent differences in neural activity that can only be detected across two people's brains (Bilek et al., 2017).

Conceptually, the notion of misalignment (or misattunement) may also be helpful to further analyze the levels on which social interaction and communication may fail. Combined with the

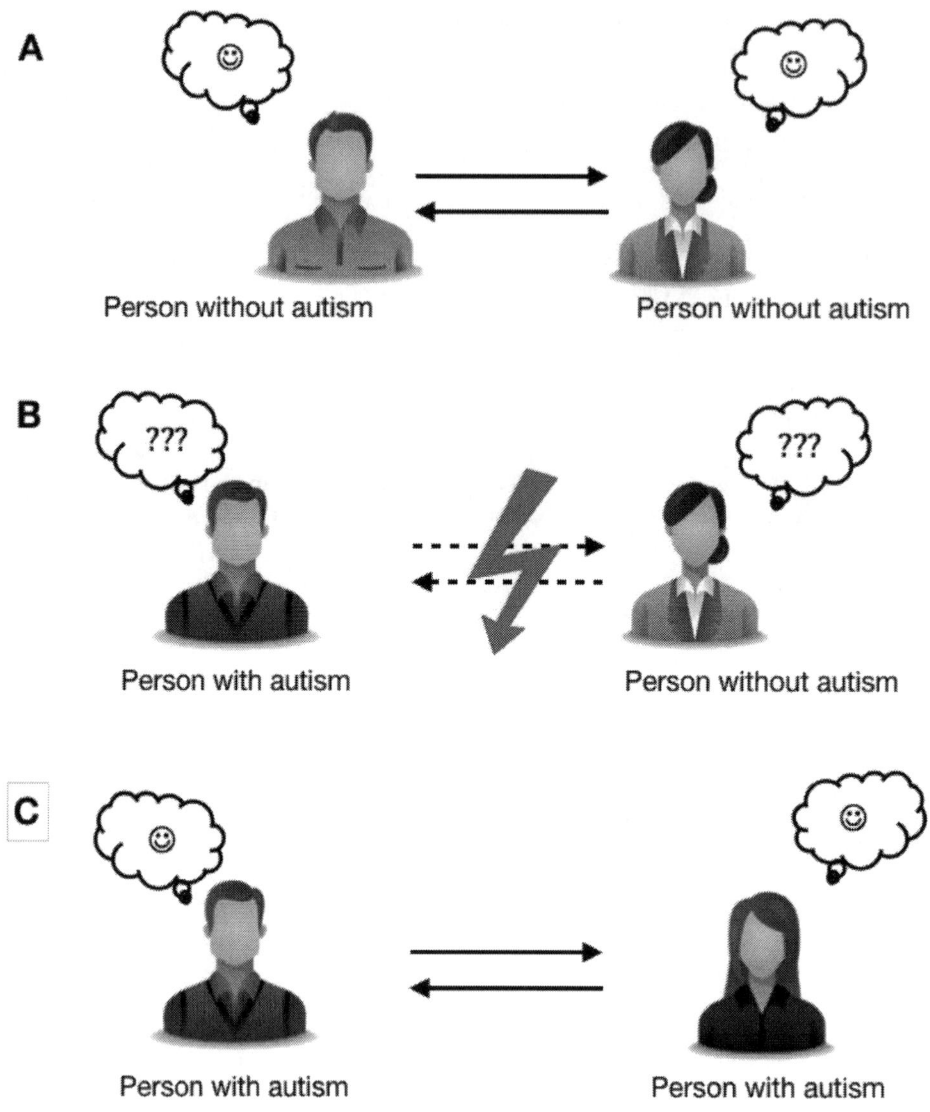

Figure 16.1 Schematic depiction of social interaction mismatch

A. Due to a relatively high level of interpersonal similarity in a dyad consisting of two persons without autism, the reciprocity of the social interaction is intact. B. Due to low interpersonal similarity in a dyad consisting of one person with autism and one person without autism, the reciprocity of the social interaction is reduced or breaks down. C. Due to a relatively high level of interpersonal similarity in a dyad consisting of two persons with autism, the reciprocity of the social interaction is intact. See e-book for a full-color version of this figure.

relevant empirical work in social neuroscience and psychiatry, such an integrative and biopsychosocial approach could also be linked to current endeavors in computational modeling, which attempt to mechanistically explain the cognitive and neural mechanisms of social (and other types of) behavior. Here, the so-called predictive coding framework has gained considerable attention in recent years. This framework assumes that the "Bayesian brain" generates a model of the world to predict what aspects of the environment may have caused incoming sensory information. This approach can also be applied to mechanistically investigate how people make social decisions and how they weigh social as compared with non-social information (Henco et al., 2020; Sevgi et al., 2020). Furthermore, the predictive coding framework also helps to understand how the brain generates expectations about what will happen next, given a certain input to the system and what the differential contributions of prior experience and current sensory experience may be (von der Lühe et al., 2016). This information can also be used to adapt behavior and allow perception and action to be based on these expectations (Bach & Schenke, 2017). With regard to social interaction and breakdowns or disorders thereof as part of psychiatric disorders, we have argued that the predictive coding framework can be extended from individual brains to two-person situations, where it might help to mathematically capture (mis-)alignment and social interaction (mis-)match and provide a Bayesian account of intersubjectivity (Bolis et al., 2017; Henco & Schilbach, 2021).

Conclusion

This chapter has reviewed recent developments in the burgeoning field of social neuroscience, which investigates the neurobiology of the human capacity for social interaction and communication and how it could be seen as contributing to the development of neurosemiotics. Since its inception, the field has seen tremendous progress, but has taken some time to warm up to the challenge of addressing social processes where they matter most – that is, during real-life social interactions. In line with the call for a *second-person neuroscience*, this development towards higher degrees of ecological validity has resulted in striking new insights into the workings of the so-called "social brain" and how different brain networks play key roles and interact to help us engage in and make sense of social encounters. Moving beyond the investigation of brains in isolation, *second-person neuroscience* also focuses on interacting persons (and brains) and on how social behavior is realized at an interpersonal level. This development appears highly relevant and important for the success of the field of neurosemiotics, which is naturally attracted to social interactions and how they function as common ground for a wide range of semiotic processes. Here, the constitutive role of social interactions for how meaning and significance emerges could be an important point of convergence. In other words, second-person neuroscience might link up in a particularly fruitful and productive way with neurosemiotics and can offer important new avenues for interdisciplinary research on the neurobiology of intersubjectivity. Finally, investigating the neurobiology of how human beings navigate and communicate during social interactions can also help to explain when and how communication works and when it breaks down. Taking an integrative and multimodal approach that includes a comprehensive characterization of interaction-based phenotypes in the clinic, second-person neuropsychiatry promises to shed new light on the mechanisms of social impairments and on the kinds of social interactions that may promote health or support therapeutic interventions (Lahnakoski et al. 2021).

References

Andersch, N. (2015). Symbolic form and mental illness: Ernst Cassirer's contribution to a new concept of psychopathology. In J. T. Friedman, & S. Luft (Eds.), *The Philosophy of Ernst Cassirer* (pp. 163–198). Berlin: De Gruyter.

Bach, P., & Schenke, K. C. (2017). Predictive social perception: Towards a unifying framework from action observation to person knowledge. *Social and Personality Psychology Compass, 11*(7), Article e12312. doi: 10.1111/spc3.12312

Bateson, M., Nettle, D., & Roberts, G. (2006). Cues of being watched enhance cooperation in a real-world setting. *Biology Letters, 2*(3), 412–414. doi: 10.1098/rsbl.2006.0509

Bilek, E., Stößel, G., Schäfer, A., Clement, L., Ruf, M., Robnik, L., Neukel, C., Tost, H., Kirsch, P., & Meyer-Lindenberg, A. (2017). State-dependent cross-brain information flow in borderline personality disorder. *JAMA Psychiatry, 74*(9), 949–957. doi: 10.1001/jamapsychiatry.2017.1682

Bolis, D., Balsters, J., Wenderoth, N., Becchio, C., & Schilbach, L. (2017). Beyond autism: Introducing the dialectical misattunement hypothesis and a Bayesian account of intersubjectivity. *Psychopathology*, *50*(6), 355–372. doi: 10.1159/000484353

Bouissac, P. (1985). Neurosemiotics, a definition. *Semiotic Inquiry*, 5, 223–224.

Brandi, M.L., Kaifel, D., Lahnakoski, J.M., & Schilbach, L. (2020) A naturalistic paradigm simulating gaze-based social interactions for the investigation of social agency. *Behavior Research Methods*, *52*, 1044–1055. doi: 10.3758/s13428-019-01299-x

Brass, M., Schmitt, R. M., Spengler, S., & Gergely, G. (2007). Investigating action understanding: Inferential processes versus action simulation. *Current Biology*, *17*(24), 2117–2121. doi: 10.1016/j.cub.2007.11.057

Carey, M.S. (1978). The role of gaze in the initiation of conversation. *Social Psychology*, *41*, 269.

Carpenter, M., & Tomasello, M. (2000). Joint attention, cultural learning, and language acquisition: Implications for children with autism. In A. M. Wetherby, & B. M. Prizant (Eds.), *Communication and Language Issues in Autism and Pervasive Developmental Disorder: A Transactional Developmental Perspective* (pp. 31–54). Baltimore, MD: Brookes.

Clark, H. H., & Brennan, S. E. (1991). Grounding in communication. In L. B. Resnick, J. M. Levine, & S. D. Teasley (Eds.), *Perspectives on Socially Shared Cognition* (pp. 127–149). Washington, DC: American Psychological Association. doi: 10.1037/10096-006

Clarke, S., McEllin, L., Francová, A., Székely, M., Buterfill, S.A., & Michael, J. (2019). Joint action goals reduce visuomotor interference effects from a partner's incongruent actions. *Scientific Reports*, *9*(1), 15414. doi: 10.1038/s41598-019-52124-6

Dimberg, U. (1982). Facial reactions to facial expressions. *Psychophysiology*, *19*(6), 643–647. doi: 10.1111/j.1469-8986.1982.tb02516.x

Dimberg, U., Thunberg, M., & Elmehed, K. (2000). Unconscious facial reactions to emotional facial expressions. *Psychological Science*, *11*(1), 86–89. doi: 10.1111/1467-9280.00221

Eco, U. (1979). *A Theory of Semiotics*. Indianapolis, IN: Indiana University Press.

Emery, N. J. (2000). The eyes have it: The neuroethology, function and evolution of social gaze. *Neuroscience and Biobehavioral Reviews*, *24*(6), 581–604. doi: 10.1016/s0149-7634(00)00025-7

Erickson, K., & Schulkin, J. (2003). Facial expressions of emotion: A cognitive neuroscience perspective. *Brain and Cognition*, *52*(1), 52–60. doi: 10.1016/s0278-2626(03)00008-3

Frijda, N. H., & Tcherkassof, A. (1997). Facial expressions as modes of action readiness. In J. A. Russell & J. M. Fernández-Dols (Eds.), *The Psychology of Facial Expression* (pp. 78–102). Cambridge: Cambridge University Press.

Frith, C. D., & Frith, U. (1999). Interacting minds: A biological basis. *Science*, *286*(5445), 1692–1695. doi: 10.1126/science.286.5445.1692

Galantucci, B., & Garrod, S. (2011). Experimental semiotics: A review. *Frontiers in Human Neuroscience*, *5*, 11. doi: 10.3389/fnhum.2011.00011

Grammer, K., Schiefenhövel, W., Schleidt, M., Lorenz, B., & Eibl-Eibesfeldt, I., (1988). Patterns on the face: The eyebrow flash in crosscultural comparison. *Ethology*, 77, 279–288. doi: 10.1111/j.1439-0310.1988.tb00211.x

Hale, J., & Hamilton, A. F. (2016). Cognitive mechanisms for responding to mimicry from others. *Neuroscience and Biobehavioral Reviews*, *63*, 106–123. doi: 10.1016/j.neubiorev.2016.02.006

Hasson, U., & Frith, C. D. (2016). Mirroring and beyond: Coupled dynamics as a generalized framework for modelling social interactions. *Philosophical Transactions of the Royal Society of London. Series B, Biological Sciences*, *371*(1693), 20150366. doi: 10.1098/rstb.2015.0366

Heerey, E. A., & Crossley, H. M. (2013). Predictive and reactive mechanisms in smile reciprocity. *Psychological Science*, *24*(8), 1446–1455. doi: 10.1177/0956797612472203

Henco, L., Brandi, M. L., Lahnakoski, J. M., Diaconescu, A. O., Mathys, C., & Schilbach, L. (2020). Bayesian modelling captures inter-individual differences in social belief computations in the putamen and insula. *Cortex*, *131*, 221–236. doi: 10.1016/j.cortex.2020.02.024

Henco, L., & Schilbach, L. (2021). Studying social inferences in and across social brains. *Biological Psychiatry. Cognitive Neuroscience and Neuroimaging*, *6*(8), 760–761. doi: 10.1016/j.bpsc.2021.04.008

Kaiser, S., & Wehrle, T. (2001). Facial expressions as indicators of appraisal processes. In K. R. Scherer (Ed.), *Appraisal Processes in Emotions: Theory, Methods, Research* (pp. 285–300) New York: Oxford University Press.

Kleinke, C. L. (1986). Gaze and eye contact: A research review. *Psychological Bulletin*, *100*(1), 78–100. doi: 10.1037/0033-2909.100.1.78

Lahnakoski, J. M., Eickhoff, S. B., Dukart, J., & Schilbach, L. (2021). Naturalizing psychopathology: Towards a quantitative real-world psychiatry. *Molecular Psychiatry*, doi: 10.1038/s41380-021-01322-8

Lahnakoski, J. M., Forbes, P., McCall, C., & Schilbach, L. (2020). Unobtrusive tracking of interpersonal orienting and distance predicts the subjective quality of social interactions. *Royal Society Open Science*, 7(8), 191815. doi: 10.1098/rsos.191815

Lahnakoski, J. M., Glerean, E., Jääskeläinen, I. P., Hyönä, J., Hari, R., Sams, M., & Nummenmaa, L. (2014). Synchronous brain activity across individuals underlies shared psychological perspectives. *NeuroImage, 100*(100), 316–324. doi: 10.1016/j.neuroimage.2014.06.022

Mareschal, I., Calder, A. J., & Clifford, C. W. (2013). Humans have an expectation that gaze is directed toward them. *Current Biology, 23*(8), 717–721. doi: 10.1016/j.cub.2013.03.030

Meltzoff, A. N., & Moore, M. K. (1977). Imitation of facial and manual gestures by human neonates. *Science, 198*(4312), 74–78. doi: 10.1126/science.897687

Merleau-Ponty, M. (1964). *The primacy of perception.* Evanston, IL: Northwestern University Press.

Mojzisch, A., Schilbach, L., Helmert, J. R., Pannasch, S., Velichkovsky, B. M., & Vogeley, K. (2006). The effects of self-involvement on attention, arousal, and facial expression during social interaction with virtual others: A psychophysiological study. *Social Neuroscience, 1*(3–4), 184–195. doi: 10.1080/174709106 00985621

Neufeld, J., Ioannou, C., Korb, S., Schilbach, L., & Chakrabarti, B. (2016). Spontaneous facial mimicry is modulated by joint attention and autistic traits. *Autism Research, 9*(7), 781–789. doi: 10.1002/aur.1573

Nichols, K. A., & Champness, B. G., (1971). Eye gaze and the GSR. *Journal of Experimental Social Psychology*, 7(6), 623–626.

Niedenthal, P. M., Barsalou, L. W., Winkielman, P., Krauth-Gruber, S., & Ric, F. (2005). Embodiment in attitudes, social perception, and emotion. *Personality and Social Psychology Review, 9*(3), 184–211. doi: 10.1207/ s15327957pspr0903_1

Niedenthal, P. M., Mermillod, M., Maringer, M., & Hess, U. (2010). The simulation of smiles (SIMS) model: Embodied simulation and the meaning of facial expression. *The Behavioral and Brain Sciences, 33(6)*, 417–480. doi: 10.1017/S0140525X10000865

Nummenmaa, L., Glerean, E., Viinikainen, M., Jääskeläinen, I. P., Hari, R., & Sams, M. (2012). Emotions promote social interaction by synchronizing brain activity across individuals. *Proceedings of the National Academy of Sciences of the United States of America, 109*(24), 9599–9604. doi: 10.1073/pnas.1206095109

Oberman, L. M., Winkielman, P., & Ramachandran, V. S. (2007). Face to face: Blocking facial mimicry can selectively impair recognition of emotional expressions. *Social Neuroscience, 2*(3–4), 167–178. doi: 10.1080/ 17470910701391943

Pfeiffer, U. J., Schilbach, L., Timmermans, B., Kuzmanovic, B., Georgescu, A. L., Bente, G., & Vogeley, K. (2014). Why we interact: On the functional role of the striatum in the subjective experience of social interaction. *NeuroImage, 101*, 124–137. doi: 10.1016/j.neuroimage.2014.06.061

Preller, K. H., Herdener, M., Schilbach, L., Stämpfli, P., Hulka, L. M., Vonmoos, M., Ingold, N., Vogeley, K., Tobler, P. N., Seifritz, E., & Quednow, B. B. (2014). Functional changes of the reward system underlie blunted response to social gaze in cocaine users. *Proceedings of the National Academy of Sciences of the United States of America, 111*(7), 2842–2847. doi: 10.1073/pnas.1317090111

Rakoczy, H. (2006). Pretend play and the development of collective intentionality. *Cognitive Systems Research*, 7(2–3), 113–127. doi: 10.1016/j.cogsys.2005.11.008

Redcay, E., Dodell-Feder, D., Pearrow, M. J., Mavros, P. L., Kleiner, M., Gabrieli, J. D., & Saxe, R. (2010). Live face-to-face interaction during fMRI: A new tool for social cognitive neuroscience. *NeuroImage, 50*(4), 1639–1647. doi: 10.1016/j.neuroimage.2010.01.052

Redcay, E., & Schilbach, L. (2019). Using second-person neuroscience to elucidate the mechanisms of social interaction. Nature Reviews *Neuroscience, 20*(8), 495–505. doi: 10.1038/s41583-019-0179-4

Rice, K., & Redcay, E. (2016). Interaction matters: A perceived social partner alters the neural processing of human speech. *NeuroImage, 129*, 480–488. doi: 10.1016/j.neuroimage.2015.11.041

Rizzolatti, G., & Sinigaglia, C. (2010). The functional role of the parieto-frontal mirror circuit: Interpretations and misinterpretations. *Nature Reviews Neuroscience, 11*(4), 264–274. doi: 10.1038/nrn2805

Schilbach L. (2016). Towards a second-person neuropsychiatry. *Philosophical Transactions of the Royal Society of London. Series B, Biological Sciences, 371*(1686), 20150081. doi: 10.1098/rstb.2015.0081

Schilbach, L (2019). Using interaction-based phenotyping to assess the behavioral and neural mechanisms of transdiagnostic social impairments in psychiatry. *European Archives of Psychiatry & Clinical Neuroscience, 269*, 273–274. doi: 10.1007/s00406-019-00998-y

Schilbach, L., Eickhoff, S. B., Mojzisch, A., & Vogeley, K. (2008). What's in a smile? Neural correlates of facial embodiment during social interaction. *Social Neuroscience, 3*(1), 37–50. doi: 10.1080/17470910701563228

Schilbach, L., Wilms, M., Eickhoff, S. B., Romanzetti, S., Tepest, R., Bente, G., Shah, N. J., Fink, G. R., & Vogeley, K. (2010). Minds made for sharing: Initiating joint attention recruits reward-related neurocircuitry. *Journal of Cognitive Neuroscience, 22*(12), 2702–2715. doi: 10.1162/jocn.2009.21401

Schilbach, L., Eickhoff, S. B., Cieslik, E., Shah, N. J., Fink, G. R., & Vogeley, K. (2011). Eyes on me: An fMRI study of the effects of social gaze on action control. *Social Cognitive and Affective Neuroscience, 6*(4), 393–403. doi: 10.1093/scan/nsq067

Schilbach, L., Timmermans, B., Reddy, V., Costall, A., Bente, G., Schlicht, T., & Vogeley, K. (2013). Toward a second-person neuroscience. *The Behavioral and Brain Sciences*, *36*(4), 393–414. doi: 10.1017/S0140525X12000660

Schilbach, L., Wohlschlaeger, A. M., Kraemer, N. C., Newen, A., Shah, N. J., Fink, G. R., & Vogeley, K. (2006). Being with virtual others: Neural correlates of social interaction. *Neuropsychologia*, *44*(5), 718–730. doi: 10.1016/j.neuropsychologia.2005.07.017

Schwab, C., & Huber, L. (2006). Obey or not obey? Dogs (*Canis familiaris*) behave differently in response to attentional states of their owners. *Journal of Comparative Psychology*, *120*(3), 169–175. doi: 10.1037/0735-7036.120.3.169

Senju, A., & Johnson, M. H. (2009). The eye contact effect: Mechanisms and development. *Trends in Cognitive Sciences*, *13*(3), 127–134. doi: 10.1016/j.tics.2008.11.009

Sevgi, M., Diaconescu, A. O., Henco, L., Tittgemeyer, M., & Schilbach, L. (2020). Social Bayes: Using Bayesian modeling to study autistic trait-related differences in social cognition. *Biological Psychiatry*, *87*(2), 185–193. doi: 10.1016/j.biopsych.2019.09.032

von der Lühe, T., Manera, V., Barisic, I., Becchio, C., Vogeley, K., & Schilbach, L. (2016). Interpersonal predictive coding, not action perception, is impaired in autism. *Philosophical Transactions of the Royal Society of London. Series B, Biological Sciences*, *371*(1693), 20150373. doi: 10.1098/rstb.2015.0373

Wallot, S., Mitkidis, P., McGraw, J. J., & Roepstorff, A. (2016). Beyond synchrony: Joint action in a complex production task reveals beneficial effects of decreased interpersonal synchrony. *PLoS One*, *11*(12), e0168306. doi: 10.1371/journal.pone.0168306

Warren, J. E., Sauter, D. A., Eisner, F., Wiland, J., Dresner, M. A., Wise, S. R., & Scott, S. K. (2006). Positive emotions preferentially engage an auditory-motor "mirror" system. *Journal of Neuroscience*, *26*(50), 13067–13075.

Wohltjen, S., & Wheatley, T. (2021). Eye contact marks the rise and fall of shared attention in conversation. *Proceedings of the National Academy of Sciences of the United States of America*, *118*(37), e2106645118. doi: 10.1073/pnas.2106645118

Wolf, D., Mittelberg, I., Rekittke, L.-M., Bhavsar, S., Zvyagintsev, M., Haeck, A., Cong, F., Klasen, M., & Mathiak, K. (2018). Interpretation of social interactions: Functional imaging of cognitive-semiotic categories during naturalistic viewing. *Frontiers in Human Neuroscience*, *12*, Article 296. doi: 10.3389/fnhum.2018.00296

Yeshurun, Y., Swanson, S., Simony, E., Chen, J., Lazaridi, C., Honey, C. J., & Hasson, U. (2017). Same story, different story. *Psychological Science*, *28*(3), 307–319. doi: 10.1177/0956797616682029

17

JOINT EPISTEMIC ENGINEERING

The neglected process in human communication

Arjen Stolk, Jana Bašňáková, and Ivan Toni

"There is not much dependence to be placed upon these Constructions that we put upon Signs and Words, which we understand but very little of, & at best can only give a probable Guess at their Meaning"

David Samwell, ship surgeon on James Cook's HMS Discovery, Hawaii, 1779

Introduction

There is virtually no limit to what human minds can conceive beyond the physical world. Those mental activities might appear inconsequential or delusional. Yet, when people collectively agree on mental constructs, those cultural innovations can change reality, as when we attribute value to intrinsically worthless banknotes. Ultimately, those cultural innovations are rooted in our communicative abilities (Levinson, 2006; Misyak et al., 2014). How human minds communicate and converge on mental constructs, however, remains a largely open question. By focusing on both cognitive and neurobiological mechanisms of meaning construal during interactive communication, neurosemiotics offers a promising approach to tackle this hard question (García et al., 2020). More precisely, this chapter adopts a neurosemiotic focus on the mechanistic unfolding of the processes that create relations between signs and referents.

A core assumption in language and communication research holds that interlocutors understand one another because they have approximated the same conceptual structures through lifelong exposure to publicly available signals and a common mental lexicon storing information regarding their meanings (Gaskell, 2007). On this assumption, human communication is largely understood when we know how conventional signals, such as words, gestures, and facial expressions, are encoded and decoded by individuals. However, that traditional view ignores two key features of human communication. First, as repeatedly emphasized by semioticians, there are many-to-many mappings between a signal's form and meaning (Kull, 2020). Given that no two people share the same experience and expertise, interlocutors rarely, if ever, share the same default set of candidate meanings when interpreting a signal (Clark & Marshall, 1981; Lewis, 1969). Second, the meaning of any signal is negotiable and ultimately depends on the contingently unfolding interaction between interlocutors (Brennan et al., 2010; Tomasello et al., 2005). This is seen in how everyday interaction consists of ambiguous words and behaviors that can only be discerned by individuals who know their context of use in an ongoing interaction. Notwithstanding helpful regularities in word order and dialogic turns (subject–verb–object structures, question–answer relationships, social scripts, and other stereotyped dependencies), everyday interaction is also astonishing in its flexibility. An utterance

DOI: 10.4324/9781003051817-21

can constitute a response to another verbal or non-verbal utterance that occurred at any point in time along the interaction's trajectory, thus irrespective of word order, turn sequence, or even communication modality. These fleeting conceptual dependencies between utterances cannot easily be analyzed outside the communicative contexts in which they are embedded, as state-of-the-art artificial agents – such as Alexa or Siri – try to do.

Building on previous suggestions (Clark, 1996; Grice, 1957; Peirce, 1931), we argue that a common language and its statistics do not explain how people in dialogue overcome fundamental communicative obstacles. The reason is that signals do not have stereotyped and publicly invariant consequences. The real challenge is to specify how people define a context rich enough to afford a signal a fair chance at being interpreted in the way it is intended at the moment of delivery, yet flexible enough to be continuously adjusted to the goals and needs of the conversation. We review recent work in neurosemiotics that has begun to shift focus from the context-free coding and decoding of signals to the construal of meaning within genuinely interactive contexts. Extending early observations of a shared conceptual space underlying human communication (Stolk et al., 2016; Toni & Stolk, 2019), here we introduce "joint epistemic engineering," an account of how interlocutors can understand each other in everyday conversation as well as in situations when meaning needs to be construed from scratch.

The basic insight is that a large portion of a signal's context of use is constructed on the fly by members of the interaction. In what follows, we illustrate how interlocutors use multilayered communicative signals as a tool to simultaneously probe, align, and shape their conceptual structures during social interaction, providing a shared and situated source of interpretational constraints. By embedding signals in the conceptual space generated through this engineering process, interlocutors rapidly zoom in on relevant features of a signal and coordinate both current and new reference points in their frame of reference of the interaction.

From pre-Darwinian types to contingently shared tokens

By way of analogy, considering human communication as a signal coding–decoding problem is a fallacy reminiscent of the focus that pre-Darwinian natural sciences had on biological types. In that pre-Darwinian view, time-invariant species were the fundamental units of biological organization, worthy of investigation because of their presumed immutability and optimality (Mayr, 1999). Arguably, one of Darwin's main conceptual innovations was to shift the focus of inquiry from biological types to tokens; from ideal species to individual organisms that might or might not pass through the filter of natural selection. In Darwin's framework, each accident of history became informative, showing how a biological replicator adapts to the current environmental circumstances in light of past adaptations. In contrast, the focus of linguistics has largely remained anchored on signal types – as seen, for instance, in the academic space devoted to investigating regularities in word order and turn-taking patterns (Gaskell, 2007; Sacks et al., 1974). Deviations from those regularities, frequent in real-life dialogue (Stivers, 2010), have largely been ignored as stochastic phenomena, rather than accidents of interactional history showing how interlocutors create and adapt to the current communicative circumstances.

Linguistic types are thought to offer optimal solutions to the problem of linking a set of signals to their meanings, with a pre-defined syntax combining signals compositionally to form a larger meaning (Gibson et al., 2019). Those solutions are optimal insofar as human communication is framed as an information-theoretic problem – that is, the problem of reducing uncertainty over the identity of a signal given the set of possible signals and referents (Shannon, 1948). Information-theoretic frameworks assume that linguistic signals have meanings shared with other members of our linguistic community, up to the point where those meanings are properties of those signals. However, while there are obvious surface regularities in the signals we use, they do not map reliably onto regularities in the content of the signals – for example, the sound /dɔg/ onto its possible referents. Those referents are high-dimensional concepts (e.g., an individual pet, a zoological category, a human villain), which require similar contextual constraints to afford similar interpretations across communicators. As a painter needs to decide which hue to contrive from her palette for achieving a fair chance the viewer will perceive a red apple in the context of that particular canvas (Conway, 2012), so a communicator needs to decide how to contrive a signal that will be interpreted as intended in the current communicative context, even when the signal might seem highly conventional.

Building on these considerations, this chapter raises two main conceptual issues, in line with a large body of work on experimental semiotics and pragmatics (Galantucci & Garrod, 2011; Noveck & Reboul, 2008). First, we advocate a shift from pre-Darwinian type-centered thinking, where signals have stereotyped and publicly invariant consequences, toward studying the actual tokens used during communicative interactions. Type-centered frameworks have been instrumental in extracting linguistic regularities from idealized material, like individual agents processing isolated sentences. Here we argue that, when signals are considered in their natural embedding of contingently unfolding social interaction, then human communication should be thought of as joint control of a shared conceptual space, rather than signal coding-decoding. Second, we emphasize that interlocutors' overlaps in signal-referent mappings and communicative contexts are a product of communication, not a default background. We explore a way in which these interpersonal disparities can be resolved on the fly, namely the suggestion that a communicative signal contains a multiplicity of semiotic functions. The basic insight is that a communicative token, besides being deployed to reduce uncertainty over the identity of its referent – a Shannon-signal (Shannon, 1948) – is also meant to ostensively mark its own communicative value – a Grice-signal (Grice, 1957) – and to offer cues for aligning the space of possible interpretations across interlocutors – a Peirce-signal (Peirce, 1931).

What is in a signal?

Shannon-signals

In the original transmission-capacity view of communication (Shannon, 1948), there is no mechanism for assigning meaning to a signal. A signal conveys information to a receiver when it reduces the receiver's uncertainty over the identity of that signal, given the set of possible signals and referents. It is assumed that both sender and receiver share a pre-existing set of signal-referent mappings, like two telegraph operators sharing the Morse code. Natural and simulated selection have led to numerous situations where conspecifics can rely on shared signal-referent mappings (Danchin et al., 2004; Kirby et al., 2014). In those situations, a communicator can generate Shannon-signals, since the set of possible signals and the set of signal-referent mappings are already fully shared by senders and receivers. Alarm calls of vervet monkeys, bees' dances, and human behavioral contagion are just a few examples of Shannon-signals. However, this communicative scheme requires repeated rounds of natural selection under consistent pressures to arise. Accordingly, it is not clear how it can account for the referential flexibility of human communication, as seen in the moment-to-moment variability in signal use across and within conversations. It is also not obvious how referential flexibility can be accounted for by ignoring signal-referent mappings altogether – for example, explanatory frameworks where signal use is determined exclusively by an iterated process of reciprocal influence and resistance between individuals, devoid of any reference (Dawkins & Krebs, 1978; Rendall & Owren, 2013).

Grice-signals

Addressing referential flexibility, Grice initiated an influential perspective on human communication, arguing that it requires interlocutors to have knowledge about one another's intentions and beliefs to disambiguate the intended meaning of a signal (Grice, 1957). A Grice-signal involves a sender producing a signal to: (1) induce functional changes in an interpreting receiver; (2) assess that the signal has been recognized as to induce those changes; and (3) ultimately give rise to functional changes that incorporate consequences of that recognition. As when a driver flashes their lights to an oncoming car, a signal is also meant to ostensively mark its own communicative value, signaling that we not only intend to influence the receiver (through the production of a stimulus), but also want them to recognize that we are acting with such intentions and, ultimately, respond on the basis of recognizing this (Sperber & Wilson, 1986). In this scheme, interlocutors can go beyond literal meaning as long as their respective speech acts adhere to the accepted purpose or direction of the conversation as well as universal principles of cooperation. As part of the latter, Grice indicates that each individual's contribution ought to be as relevant and informative as required, but not more than required for the current purpose of the exchange. He leaves unspecified, however, how interlocutors determine what quantity of information is appropriate for the current purposes. What is considered concise by one person could be pedantic to another.

Peirce-signals

Emphasizing interpretation, Peirce's triadic model highlighted a special role for meaning-making agents in the communication process, adding a third entity to dyadic models of communicative tokens and the mental concepts they kindled. A Peirce-signal (or, in Peircean terms, sign) is what it is interpreted to be, as when clouds signify rain to some, and ruins stand for ancient civilization to others. The triadic representation of a referent entails that a Peirce-signal can take any form, and that nothing is a communicative token unless it is interpreted as such (Peirce, 1931). Peirce further distinguished three primary signal types: icons, indices, and symbols. The former two bear a natural relationship with the object they represent, either through perceptual resemblance (icons – for example, two fingers up for the number *two*) or through physical or causal connection (indices – for example, two fingers for V for *victory*). For their part, symbols signify an object only via an arbitrary rule imposed by a community (for example, two fingers up conventionally standing for *peace*). The problem with this tripartite scheme, as is often the case with type-centered thinking, is that a closer look at everyday interactions frequently yields exceptions to the rule, in this instance that utterances can be composites of two or more signal types. For example, uttering "I caught a fish *this* long" while holding hands a certain distance apart both symbolizes and denotes the length of a caught fish (Clark, 1997). Peirce was aware of this obvious issue, considering the types not mutually exclusive. More generally, however, until we understand how people integrate or otherwise deal with different signal types, any type-centered framework of human communication remains fundamentally limited (Deacon, 2018). Or, as the ship's surgeon who sailed with James Cook noted in 1779, there is not much dependence to be placed on signal types: they only give a probable guess at a signal's meaning, raising the fundamental issue of understanding how people end up making similar guesses during communicative interactions.

Fixed-code fallacy

Overall, the multiplicity of functions and referents of a signal argue against the "fixed-code" view that has percolated into modern perspectives of language and communication (Harris, 1998). In these contemporary yet fundamentally pre-Darwinian perspectives, words have universal referents within a linguistic community and encode semantic constructs of thought. We argue that this fixed-code view of language use is an illusion. As we tend to think of language as being lawfully constituted by phonemes, words, and sentences, when in fact those elements are regularized and approximate low-dimensional projections from high-dimensional spoken utterances (Elman, 2004; Port, 2010), so we tend to think of communication as being constituted by signals exchanged between interlocutors, when in fact those signals are approximate low-dimensional behavioral projections from high-dimensional conceptual spaces in the interlocutors' minds. Put differently, communication requires a degree of conceptual overlap across interlocutors to afford comparable and contextually appropriate interpretations of a candidate behavior, inverting it into partially overlapping concepts (Veissière et al., 2019; Warglien & Gärdenfors, 2015). This situated inversion would allow those interlocutors to resolve the multiple ambiguities that permeate almost every human interaction, such as distinguishing between a reflexive and an embarrassed cough, or between /dɔg/ as a pet and /dɔg/ as a villain. These considerations on the context-dependency of a signal-referent trajectory beg the question of how interlocutors determine what counts as context, a fundamental yet largely overlooked issue to which we will turn next.

What counts as context?

Disambiguation

When context is brought into models of human communication, it is to arbitrate among the possible interpretations of a signal, as when adjudicating between the meanings of "financial institution" and "riverside" for the sound /bæŋk/. This view acknowledges the ambiguities intrinsic in many words. However, there are several problematic assumptions behind the notion that these ambiguities can be fully resolved through contextual factors biasing interpretation toward an intended referent. First, given that no two people share exactly the same experience and expertise, the fact that they are using the same expression does not guarantee perfect symmetry in their conceptual knowledge. When a mechanic talks about a car, they think in terms of "brake horsepower" and "electronic stability control," a representation only marginally overlapping with how their customer conceptualizes the same vehicle. Even if expertise in the moment of the conversation is broadly comparable, it seems unlikely that the condition of perfect symmetry between interlocutor can be a priori satisfied in the longer term, given how concepts can change over a lifetime, and even within the timespan of a conversation (Carpendale & Lewis, 2004). It is also unlikely that perfect symmetry is granted by community membership, as no community is sufficiently homogenous to provide full conceptual alignment across interlocutors (Clark & Marshall, 1981; Lewis, 1969). Second, even assuming perfect symmetry between interlocutors, context is not a clearly defined background, built bottom up from the sensory data. Signal-referent mappings are plagued by ambiguity; contexts are at least as ambiguous, and harder to define. We do not have sensory receptors for context – for example, a universal relevance detector (Sperber & Wilson, 1986). Calling upon context to achieve disambiguation ultimately moves the explanatory problem up a level, without delivering any actual explanation other than ad hoc heuristics with no generalization power.

Strategic reasoning

It could be argued that converging on a context is a problem that has already been solved in "game theory," the study of strategic coordination among rational agents. Moving beyond the standard practice of assuming full knowledge of goals and pay-off outcomes built into coordination games (cf. signal-referent mappings), Schelling asked how people could tacitly coordinate given minimal cues (Schelling, 1960). For instance, study participants are given hypothetical problems such as meeting with a stranger in New York City on a set date, requiring choosing a time and place. Participants tend to converge on a small set of solutions, a popular answer being noon at Grand Central Station in this particular task. The emergence of these "focal points" has largely been attributed to strategic reasoning, either in the form of modeling and choosing the best response of other players or of an imaginary group leader wanting to maximize group interest. These strategies would arguably afford sufficient flexibility to arrive at a different focal point (e.g., the Statue of Liberty), given another relatively well-defined situation (e.g., the stranger is a tourist). However, strategic reasoning presupposes rather than explains how rational agents come to operate on identical levels of granularity in their "New York" representation. For instance, it is unclear whether strategic reasoning would generate effective focal points across agents that do not know whether the coordination challenge is about New York City or New York State. Everyday interlocutors operating in open-ended situations cannot presume overlapping granularity in their contextual representations absent any mutual coordination.

Mutual coordination

It should follow from the above that "context" is as ambiguous and cognitively construed as the signal being disambiguated. We argue here that it is through the production and interpretation of the Peirce-signals embedded in their communicative history that interlocutors generate a shared context for constraining the possible interpretations of a signal. Besides exchanging signals, communicators jointly determine the detectability and interpretability of those signals. For instance, a communicator could furnish the sound /bæŋk/ with a pointed gaze towards the cupboard where both interlocutors know fishing equipment is stored. The mutually known knowledge about the cupboard's contents, and the physical presence of that piece of furniture, offer a situated source of interpretational constraints for the /bæŋk/ sound. The production of an additional Grice-signal (the pointed gaze) poses an interpretational request at the addressee's door, aimed at aligning the interpretational frames of /bæŋk/ across the two interlocutors. The addressee might get at the intended referent if she zooms into the focal point provided by the conjunction of the cupboard and her pre-existing shared knowledge with the speaker (the fishing equipment). This trivial example of a daily interaction illustrates the inadequacy of fixed-code approaches to human communication, and the hard inferential labor required to produce and interpret a multilayered signal.

Needless to say, the Peirce-signal generated when combining the gaze, the cupboard, and the presumed mutually known knowledge might fail to evoke in the addressee the intended context for the /bæŋk/ sound. Under those circumstances, repair operations, including asking for clarification, could prove important for achieving successful communication (Dingemanse et al., 2015). However, repair cannot be the main mechanism supporting successful communication. Calling upon repair to achieve disambiguation ultimately moves the explanatory problem into a secondary channel at least as complex as the original dialogue. In fact, repair procedures seem likely to be computationally more demanding, since the problem of figuring out what is being requested (or what to request) is compounded by the problem of providing a solution to the original ambiguities, and both are rapidly aggravated as time elapses in the turn-taking dynamics. Accordingly, interlocutors often tolerate possible misunderstandings to avoid interrupting a dialogue (Galantucci et al., 2020; Jefferson, 1988).

This tolerance towards possible misunderstanding might not be linked specifically to disagreements, but is a core feature of the communication process since interlocutors need to constantly juggle multiple possible interpretational frameworks. In the example above, the addressee might try to embed /bæŋk/ into different contexts – for example, a financial institution, a geographical feature, or a meteorological phenomenon as in a bank of clouds. The addressee might tentatively choose the financial option, but then pivot toward the geographical framework as that initially un-chosen option proves more consistent with the evidence provided by the interlocutor. Tolerance toward potential misunderstanding might result in enhanced dialogue functionality, but the driving factor of that tolerance might be the need to maintain epistemic flexibility in the face of signal-referent volatility. In the next section, we illustrate how interlocutors mutually develop shared conceptual spaces, epistemic systems that adapt at the same scale as the goals and needs of the interaction and afford a certain tolerance for local ambiguity and misunderstanding.

What do interlocutors construct?

Joint epistemic engineering

An explanatory framework of human communication needs to clarify how inherently asymmetric individuals rapidly arrive at mutually understood mental constructs from ambiguous signals that are referentially contingent on the current communicative circumstances. Existing frameworks tend to minimize those fundamental communicative obstacles – for example, signal ambiguity (Hasson et al., 2012; Rizzolatti & Arbib, 1998), interpersonal asymmetry (Pickering & Garrod, 2013), or type inadequacy (Gibson et al., 2019). We have recently argued, supported by neural evidence, that people overcome those obstacles because they solve, at each and every dialogue turn, a conceptual alignment challenge (Stolk et al., 2016). This alignment challenge entails that interlocutors continuously evaluate their conceptual structures for consistency with what is implied by the other in light of the ongoing interaction, just as a reader needs to find and maintain consistent relationships between concepts conveyed in this contribution (e.g., links between Peirce, /bæŋk/, and asymmetry). Here we zoom in on this epistemic engineering process, illustrating how interlocutors construct multilayered communicative signals to probe and give shape to their continually changing conceptual spaces. Using two conversational settings, one verbal and one non-verbal, we show that a signal can operate across different levels: to offer cues for aligning the space of possible interpretations across interlocutors (a Peirce-signal), while asking to be recognized as communicative (a Grice-signal); and reducing uncertainty over the identity of its referent (a Shannon-signal if the Peirce- and Grice-signals evoke the intended interpretational context).

Furthermore, we show how those multilayered signals are not processed in serial isolation. The contextual constraints suggested by the production of each Grice-signal and Peirce-signal accumulate and change as the interaction proceeds. By way of analogy, production of each signal can be thought of as a stroboscopic flash, designed by the communicator to transiently illuminate her own rapidly shifting conceptual landscape for the benefit of the interlocutor. Across multiple turn-taking cycles, the interlocutors flash those strobes to offer a glimpse of each other's conceptual landscapes, so they can be meshed together. The spectral qualities of the stroboscopic light can change over time, resolving finer details of the interlocutors' contextual framework as the interaction progresses successfully, or zooming back to a coarser granularity if a new dialogue is started. The integration window over multiple signals can also change as a function of interaction status, as when we open a dialogue confidently assuming mutual knowledge of an earlier conversation with the same interlocutor, or tentatively explore a newcomer with a pleasantry. Joint epistemic engineering is meant to emphasize that interlocutors are focused on controlling the shared conceptual landscape, rather than the consistency of signals or signal-referent mappings. By embedding signals in the shared conceptual space generated through the engineering process, interlocutors rapidly zoom in on relevant features of those signals, coordinate current reference points, and prepare the ground for anchoring new reference points.

Engineering a bar conversation

It is easy to overlook how joint epistemic engineering underpins everyday interaction. Consider the bar conversation shown in Figure 17.1.

The flow and apparent straightforward understanding between customer and bartender might mask the interpretational constraints necessary to make sense of a dialogue laced with semantic incoherence and ambiguity. Even before voicing "A cup of Joe," the customer would need to build a scaffold of conceptual information that approximates the scaffold presumably used by the bartender to interpret his utterance (black graph structures in Figure 17.2A). The customer needs to select background knowledge that coffee can be ordered from bars; that bartenders may be familiar with slang words for coffee; and so on (blue background structure in Figure 17.2A).

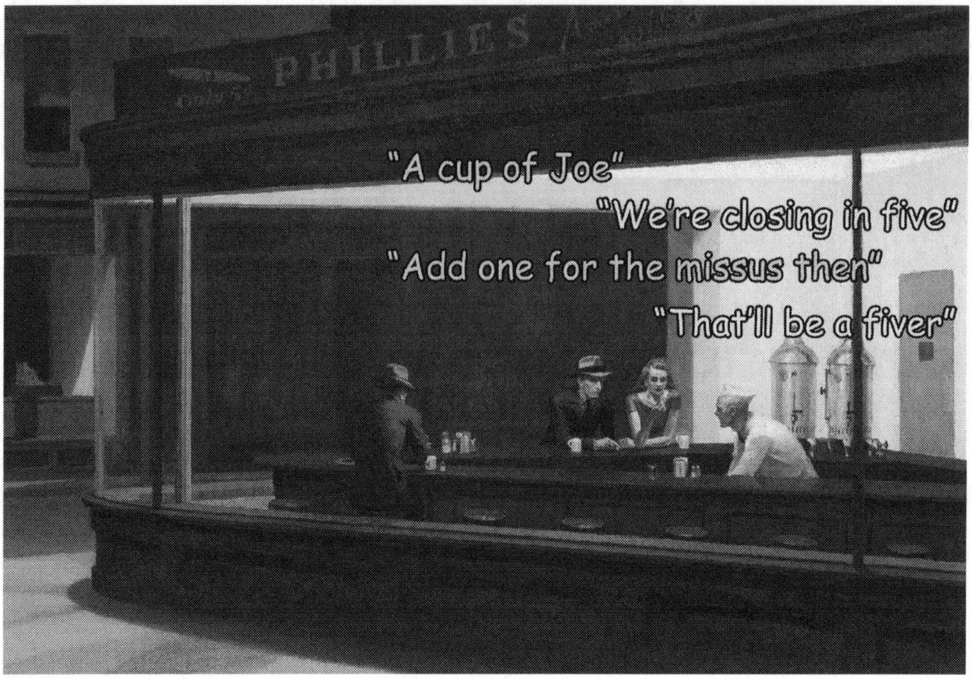

Figure 17.1 A prototypical (semantically incoherent but semiotically fluent) human interaction
Artwork courtesy of the Art Institute of Chicago. See e-book for a full-color version of this figure.

In fact, several possible-world scenarios might need to be prepared: the presumed bartender is a cleaner; the bar is already closed; etcetera. Accordingly, besides placing an order (a Shannon-signal), the customer's opening statement doubles as a tacit request to probe the conceptual scaffold shared with his interlocutor (a Peirce-signal), and to be recognized as such (a Grice-signal). The bartender's reply, "We're closing in five," despite bearing no semantic resemblance to the customer's opening utterance, suffices to address the customer's multilayered request. He confirms his ability and willingness to process the order (addition of coffee to the conceptual space, Figure 17.2B) as well as to engage in the joint engineering process. Besides conveying recognition of communicative intent (a Grice-signal) and additional details about the bar (a Shannon-signal), the bartender's disclosure of the approaching closing time also operates as a tacit invitation to negotiate the customer's current request (e.g., "I'm not serving," or "I'm serving but drink fast") or make another (e.g., a drink for his female companion) – that is, a Peirce-signal. This multiplicity of functions illustrates how interlocutors use signals to simultaneously coordinate current and anchor new reference points in their conceptual frame, effectively coordinating a situated source of interpretational constraints for each other's intrinsically ambiguous signals.

This bar conversation also illustrates how joint epistemic engineering offers the possibility to fluidly reference pockets of readily shareable background knowledge (blue and orange graph structures in Figure 17.2), amalgamating potentially unrelated conceptual structures into a space of meanings and relationships between those structures. For instance, the customer's specification of "the missus" in his reply, "Add one for the missus then," offers the bartender with an unsolicited set of cues to the identity of his female companion, ground he could have expanded on in a subsequent exchange. Perhaps the innovation within the bartender's response, "That'll be a fiver," hints at an alignment on the level of nonchalance still, consistent with the customer's slang use. But on its own, the bartender's response references a separate pocket of background knowledge (concept of payment, orange structure in

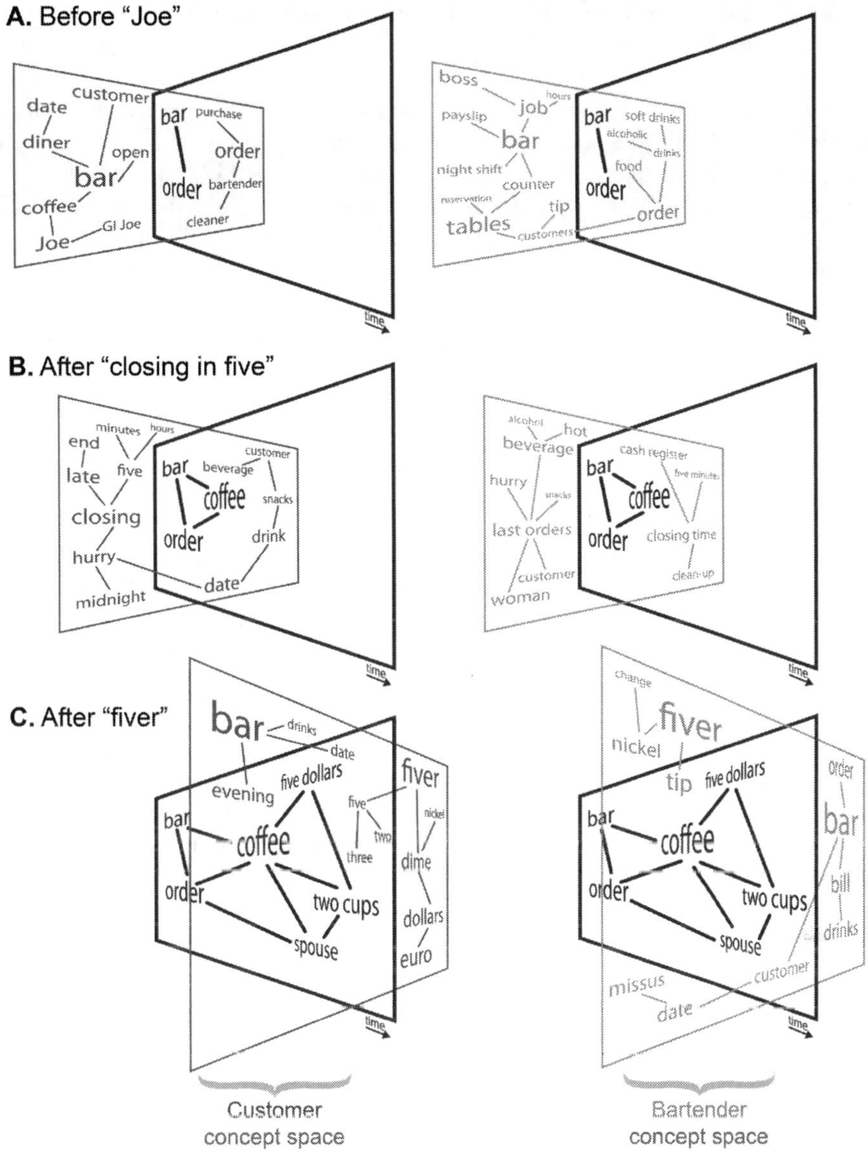

Figure 17.2 Epistemic dissections of three moments in a conversation

The situation corresponds to the bar conversation shown in Figure 17.1, illustrating how dialogue requires people to continually build a scaffold of conceptual information that approximates the scaffold used by the other (forming a shared conceptual space, black graph structures). This joint engineering process kicks in even before the first signal is produced and draws on individual background knowledge where possible (blue/orange graph structures). For instance, before voicing "A cup of Joe," the customer needs to select background knowledge that coffee can be ordered from bars or that bartenders might be familiar with slang words for coffee, while also preparing alternative scenarios (blue background structure, A). Though semantically incoherent with the customer's opening statement, the bartender's reply, "We're closing in five," suffices to address the customer's request that he can and is willing to process the order (addition of coffee to the conceptual space, B). As interaction unfolds, the interlocutors construct their multilayered signals to probe and give shape to their expanding conceptual spaces, keeping those spaces aligned with one another to provide a situated source of interpretational constraints (black structures, C). See e-book for a full-color version of this figure.

Figure 17.2C), knowledge he expects his interlocutor to also consider when hearing his response in the context of their current conceptual frame. Needless to say, that reference would have been out of place in other moments of the exchange (e.g., before the customer's order). Moreover, by exploiting the conceptual space they have jointly assembled and streamlined over their four utterances (black structures in Figure 17.2C), the interlocutors can rapidly generate plausible hypotheses about even novel signals, as when a customer would hear "fiver" for the first time. That epistemic inference would widely miss its target when working from the sensory data using context-free statistical regularities abstracted from speech/text corpora, as AI-based language processors do. Lacking a cognitive architecture for joint epistemic engineering, those artificial agents would fail to interpret "fiver" in the context of the customer's opening statement, instead limiting the search for relevant context to semantically, temporally, or arithmetically closer signals in the turn-taking sequence (e.g., "in five," "Add one").

Engineering a communication system

It could be argued that the previous example, while plausible, remains an armchair argument with no empirical evidence. In fact, even if the utterances had been recorded from a real diner, the conversational commentary would be purely speculative and rather descriptive. Fortunately, some researchers have managed to gather experimentally controlled observations on human communication, without losing sight of its core interactive features. The rationale of the approach is that when shared assumptions on what counts as a context and a signal are experimentally removed, then the production and interpretation of Grice-signals and Peirce-signals will become more apparent, revealing the mechanisms of joint epistemic engineering in the process. Although the approach might seem to rely on experimentally contrived situations (see Figure 17.3 for an example, discussed in more detail below), similar challenges are common when communication cannot count on a shared idiom.

Take the situation experienced by the Hawaiian people when Hawaii was visited by James Cook in 1779. As in many other "first encounters" between different groups (Leahy, 1936), people found ways to communicate reliably, and the British sailors spent a peaceful month on the island. Yet, shortly afterward, James Cook lost his life in a confrontation – apparently a consequence of miscommunications arising from a change of context, obvious to the Hawaiian people (the shift from the season of peace to the season of war) but completely opaque to the Western visitors. It is hardly surprising that during that episode, one of the crew members became sensitive to the fixed-code fallacy in Signs and Words (see Samwell's opening quote to this chapter).

Several groups have recently started to recreate first encounters in the lab (without most of the risks) as a way to gain experimental access to core generative processes supporting human communicative abilities (de Ruiter et al., 2010; Galantucci, 2005; Scott-Phillips et al., 2009; Selten & Warglien, 2007). This research program, under the general banner of "experimental semiotics" (Galantucci & Garrod, 2011; Toni & Stolk, 2019), has created various communication games where human participants interact using signals lacking a pre-existing conventional use (e.g., artificial words, scribbly drawings). Importantly, while signal and context accessibility are experimentally controlled, great care is usually taken to preserve the minimal condition for studying human communication – that is, the presence of two or more people in interaction. In our work, we have frequently used the "tacit communication game," in which two players converse on a three-by-three digital grid using the movements of a geometric shape (de Ruiter et al., 2010). In each round of the game, the two players have to jointly reproduce a target configuration of two shapes, one for each player (a circle, rectangle, or triangle). Crucially, however, the target configuration is shown to one of the players only, the sender, see Figure 17.3. Given that the other player, the receiver, cannot see this configuration, the sender needs to communicate the receiver's target position to the receiver while also ensuring that the final location and orientation of their own shape is as specified by the target configuration. The only means available to the sender for communicating with the receiver is by moving the sender's

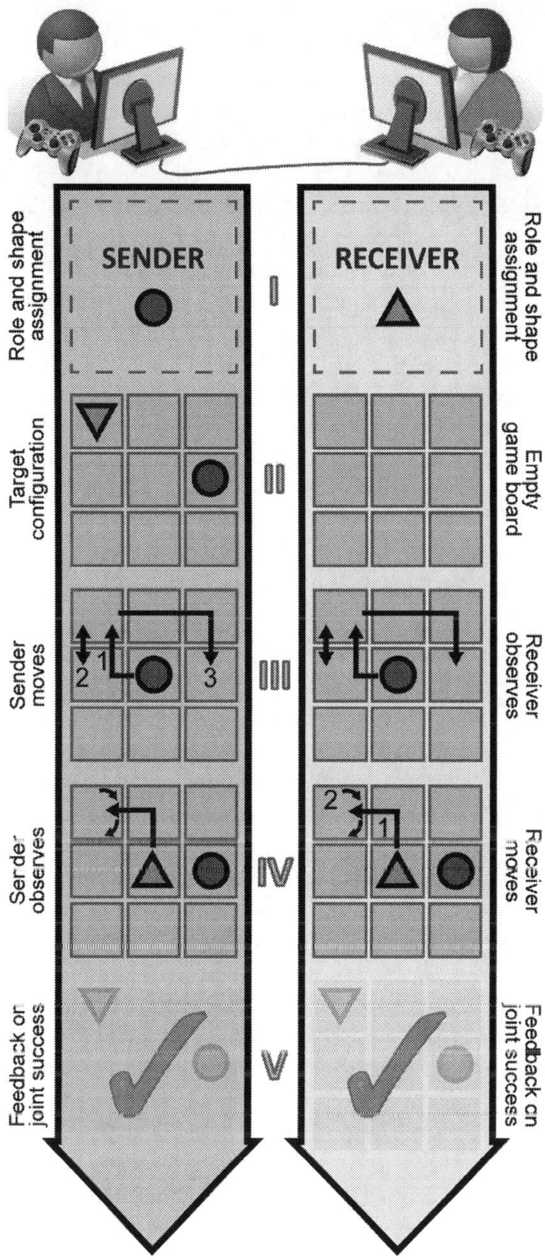

Figure 17.3 Tacit communication game

The joint goal of sender (left) and receiver (right) is to reproduce a target configuration of their two given shapes on a digital game board. This target configuration is shown to the sender only (event II). Given that the receiver cannot see the target configuration, a successful interaction requires the sender and receiver to construct and comprehend how the behavior of the sender's shape indicates the location and orientation of the receiver's shape (event III). Feedback is presented to both players with a green checkmark or red cross indicating joint success or failure (event V). A benefit of the novel communicative setting is that the shape behaviors lack conventional meaning, providing reliable access to the core process of how two humans converge on a shared meaning for a signal. An online version of the game can be found at www.MutualUnderstanding.nl. See e-book for a full-color version of this figure.

own shape around the grid using horizontal and vertical translations, and 90° clockwise rotations controlled by button presses on a handheld game controller. The only means available to the receiver for completing the configuration is by inferring the target location and orientation of their own shape based on the movements of the sender and positioning it accordingly using a second handheld game controller. As the receiver cannot ask for clarification, the only indication of whether her interpretation of the sender's signals was correct is feedback on the token's position received at the end of each trial. The sender not only has to monitor whether the receiver got the target location, but also whether they are adhering to the tacitly agreed-upon communicative strategy or making any changes in the way communicative signals have been used so far.

There are no a priori correct communication strategies in the tacit communication game, nor can the receiver solve the task by simply reproducing the movements of the sender's shape. Analogous to everyday multimodal communication involving ambiguous signals, the receiver needs to rapidly zoom in on relevant features of the sender's movements and infer a possible referent (a shape configuration) on the basis of those features. Example features include brief movement "pauses" on the receiver's target location, distinguishing it from other locations visited on the grid, as well as rotational movements, directional movements, and repeated stepping in and out from the receiver's target location ("wiggling"), with the latter three movement types typically used to indicate target orientation. A type-centered framework might assign those movement features to signals' referents as if they constitute optimal solutions to (parts of) a problem, but this would miss the local principles that govern their interpretations (Garrod & Anderson, 1987). For instance, it cannot be determined from a wiggling behavior alone whether it is intended to emphatically indicate the direction in which the receiver's shape needs to point, or whether the number of wiggles corresponds to the number of clockwise rotations the receiver needs to make to reach the target orientation, with some pairs using both strategies during a single game. These observations indicate how in this game, as in the bar conversation, the trajectory from a signal to its referent is contingent on the communicative context people develop together.

To illustrate how joint epistemic engineering could support rapidly understood new signal-referent trajectories, even when a different trajectory exists for a signal, we here turn to the case of the "missing wiggle." Before doing so, it should be mentioned that to drive interlocutors to continuously develop and coordinate their shared conceptual spaces, the tacit communication game increases the task difficulty across successive interactions. This is achieved by introducing deliberate mismatches between the geometric characteristics of the pairs' shapes, including situations where a receiver's target orientation is incompatible with the pair's current strategy. For instance, if a sender were able to successfully communicate the target orientation of the receiver's shape by rotating their own shape, this strategy would be negated when the sender's shape changed to a circle and the receiver's to a triangle. The sender would then have to find a new way to indicate the target orientation of the receiver's shape because rotations of a circle are not visible. A further level of difficulty is introduced by maintaining the same circle-triangle shape combination but having the receiver's triangle point outside the grid. If the sender had previously used a signal that involved repeatedly stepping in and out of the receiver's target location in the direction of the target orientation ("wiggling," number 2 double-headed arrow in Figure 17.3), an interaction where the receiver's triangle pointed outside of the grid would be impossible to solve using that signal.

Returning to our case, several pairs started to use a "pause" strategy to indicate that the triangle needed to point outside of the grid. Those pairs had previously converged on using movement pauses on receiver target locations to selectively indicate the communicative relevance of those grid locations, thus with no obvious role for pauses in conveying target orientation other than the default orientation. Hence, through a lens of associative learning, the use of a pause strategy would unambiguously mean that a triangle needed to be positioned in its default upward position, rather than outward-facing. How, then, could pairs have rapidly converged on a new use for an existing signal in the absence of any failures? A closer look at a pair's recent communicative history hints at a conceptual shift as to what movement features the pair mutually considered relevant in their communication. Specifically, the pair had recently converged on using a wiggle strategy to indicate the direction in which a triangle needed to point (as in Figure 17.3), applying this strategy even in cases where a triangle needed to point upward and previously a pause would have sufficed. In doing so, wiggling had not only become the prevalent feature for indicating target orientation in this pair, but the conceptual shift in feature relevance had implicitly relaxed the relationship between pauses and default orientations. Consequently, pauses could be introduced by the sender to signify orientation in situations where he could safely assume that the receiver would infer wiggles could not (i.e., a missing wiggle, see dashed lines in Figure 17.4), such as with outward-facing triangles. This epistemic inference illustrates how a shift in conceptual space can cause a signal to acquire a different meaning in (apparently) a single instance, as when a pause becomes a missing wiggle.

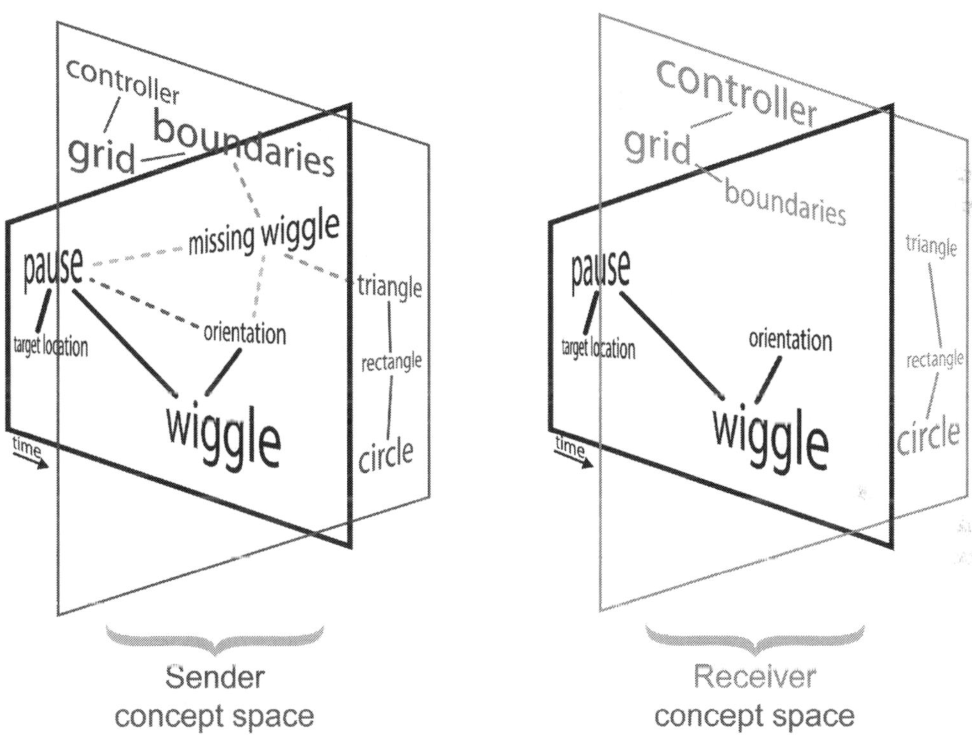

Figure 17.4 Epistemic dissection capturing the moment a signal acquires new meaning

The situation corresponds to the tacit communication game. The figure on the left captures the moment the sender used a pause, previously used exclusively to signal target location (solid black connection), to additionally signal orientation (dashed grey connection), a function previously reserved for wiggles (solid black connection). To understand this new use for behaviorally identical pauses (pause as a "missing wiggle"), the receiver would need to infer the implied change in their conceptual space driving that proposal. For instance, he would need to infer that the sender faced a situation in which wiggles could no longer be used to signal orientation, such as with an outward-facing triangle at the grid's boundary. He would also need to consider conceptual shifts supporting that new wiggle-less orientation-signaling strategy (dashed connections radiating out from "missing wiggle," left figure). If he then manages to convey agreement about that epistemic inference to the sender, the players can strengthen or add connections in their conceptual space supporting the sender's proposal (dashed grey connections on the left becoming solid in both left and right figures). See e-book for a full-color version of this figure.

What does the brain care about?

The previous sections provide prima facie evidence for moving beyond views of human communication as a signal coding–decoding problem. Whether during ordinary conversations or during "first encounters" deprived of a common language (Figures 17.2 and 17.4), interlocutors need to construct their signals to probe and give shape to their conceptual frame of reference, keeping it aligned with the current situation and with one another. By embedding signals in the shared conceptual space generated through this engineering process, interlocutors rapidly resolve the multiple ambiguities in every signal. Here we discuss recent work that has begun to empirically interrogate these theoretical issues at the implementation level by combining neuroscientific techniques with controlled studies of live social interaction – that is, the tacit communication game outlined above. To date, there are three major insights.

First, both production and comprehension of communicative signals are supported by a right-lateralized frontotemporal network, shown in Figure 17.5 A (Stolk et al., 2013). This network has been shown to contribute to pragmatic and mental state inferences when communicating with linguistic means, suggesting a role for right frontotemporal cortex in embedding utterances in their conversational context (Bašnáková et al., 2014; Beeman, 1993; Sabbagh, 1999).

Second, neural activity in this right-lateralized network predates in time the production and comprehension of communicative signals, i.e., before the initial dashed lines in Figure 17.5 A. This observation fits with the notion that communicative behaviors are selected and interpreted within the conceptual frame of reference people in dialogue develop together. Interference studies of anterior frontal and posterior temporal nodes of the network confirm and qualify the contribution of those cortical regions. Ventromedial prefrontal lesion patients, known for their social conduct deficits (Beer et al., 2006), were found to lack the specific ability to constrain their ongoing communication with knowledge implied by the current communicative circumstances, including the presumed abilities of an interlocutor (Stolk et al., 2015). Transient disruption of neural function in the right posterior superior temporal sulcus diminishes the ability to constrain the interpretation of communicative behaviors using knowledge abstracted from the recent communicative history (Stolk, Noordzij, Volman, et al., 2014). These causal observations emphasize the constraining role of contingently updated conceptual knowledge in social interaction.

Third, activity in one subregion of the right-lateralized frontotemporal network, the superior temporal gyrus (STG), becomes synchronized across interlocutors due to the accumulation of shared conceptual knowledge (Stolk, Noordzij, Verhagen, et al., 2014). This neural synchronization occurred only when interlocutors developed shared communicative solutions, and at a temporal scale closer to communicative episodes than the behaviors themselves, see Figure 17.5B. Conversely, neural synchronization was reduced over communicative episodes that did not require interlocutors to coordinate shared knowledge. These observations define a neural basis for the notion that interlocutors mutually coordinate their conceptual knowledge updates during social interaction.

The picture that emerges from these brain observations is one in which the meaning of a communicative signal is not a property of the signal, or of the individuals interpreting that signal. Rather, meaning is a property of conceptual knowledge inferred from prior beliefs and interactive behaviors embedded in the recent communicative history and kept aligned with the unfolding interaction to constrain communication. What neurophysiological mechanism allows a sustained yet adjustable influence of conceptual knowledge on transient signal production and comprehension? A clue is provided by the right-hemispheric frontotemporal structures found to support communication. Densely spaced neuronal populations with overlapping dendritic fields and thin axonal myelination endow those frontotemporal association areas with a relatively large-world architecture compared to their left hemisphere homologs (Hutsler & Galuske, 2003; Jung-Beeman, 2005). Highly interconnected populations of neurons might confer conceptual processing at varying levels of abstraction, offering a neuroanatomical infrastructure to flexibly scaffold and search for relevant context in communication.

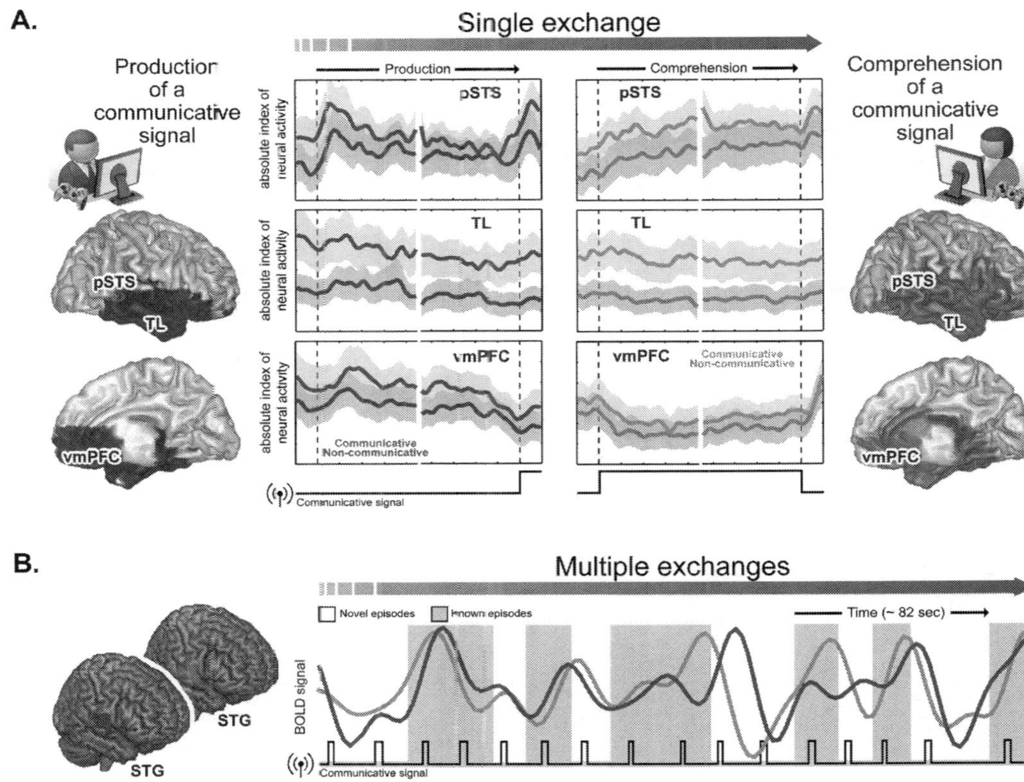

Figure 17.5 Neural dynamics of sharing conceptual spaces within communicative exchanges

The figure shows the dynamics within a single communicative exchange (A) and over multiple exchanges (B). Brain regions of a right-lateralized frontotemporal network supporting both production and comprehension of communicative signals (blue and orange, respectively) are already upregulated before a communicative signal is produced or comprehended (before the initial dashed in lines in A). Activity in one subregion, the superior temporal gyrus (STG, shown in B), tracked communicative success throughout the experiment (not shown) and was coherent across interlocutors at a temporal scale independent from individual communicative signals (blue and orange traces). Adapted from Stolk et al. (2016). See e-book for a full-color version of this figure.

Another clue is provided by the spectrotemporal nature of neural activity observed over the frontotemporal cortex. Temporally, frontotemporal regions are tonically upregulated during communicative interactions, showing strikingly similar phasic neural dynamics during the production and comprehension of both communicative and non-communicative events (blue/orange vs. grey traces in Figure 17.5A). This observation is consistent with an increasing body of evidence showing that contextual demands can modulate ongoing neural activity yet retain responsiveness to event-related neural processing (Abitbol et al., 2015). Indeed, tonic upregulation had measurable behavioral consequences on communicative performance (Stolk et al., 2013). Spectrally, the neural upregulation over the frontotemporal cortex had an extremely broad profile (not shown in Figure 17.5). Broadband shifts of neural activity are thought to reflect changes in the mean firing rates of neuronal populations, and their antecedence to observable events might be instrumental to integrate driving afferences with contextual information. Specifically, ongoing contextual inputs can temporarily hold selective neurons in an excitable state, increasing the probability of those neurons propagating event-related inputs, effectively integrating information associated with the input streams (Smith et al., 2013). This neuronal mechanism, based on upregulated broadband neural activity in the right frontotemporal cortex, might provide a neural marker of the conceptual frame of reference people build together in communication (Stolk et al., 2013).

What could possibly go wrong?

The theoretical and empirical observations presented in this chapter might be seen as exceptional situations that do not generalize to the daily interactions of a linguistic community. On the contrary, joint epistemic engineering might be relevant to understand communicative alterations despite a relatively intact command of language. For instance, individuals with damage to the right hemisphere may respond appropriately to clearly structured questions requiring specific answers – for example, "Where do you live?" Yet they produce irrelevant and verbose answers (in a Gricean sense) to open-ended questions such as "What did you do yesterday?" Patients seem unable to assemble their utterances into a coherent narrative, instead wending their way through a maze of disassociated detail, without answering the question (Myers, 1979). Comparable deficits have been noted in patients suffering frontotemporal dementia, where coherent conversations, as well as intrinsically motivated social relationships, are affected when the frontal lobe and right temporal pole degenerate (Mates et al., 2013). These clinical observations converge with the brain observations detailed above in linking a right-lateralized frontotemporal network to the processing of conceptual knowledge of the communicative context.

Ultimately, it will be important to make systematic pathophysiological comparisons between patient groups with communicative alterations, potentially isolating cognitive phenotypes that unify apparently disparate disorders – for example, schizophrenia, autism spectrum disorder, frontotemporal dementia (Ibáñez et al., 2018). For instance, it might emerge that patients with either of those disorders have problems creating and maintaining a shared conceptual space with an interlocutor. Recent evidence from our group suggests that this alteration is present in cognitively able adults on the autism spectrum (Wadge et al., 2019). Despite otherwise indistinguishable performance from neurotypical pairs, autistic pairs had lower communicative success in the tacit communication game. This communicative impairment was not simply a consequence of reduced cognitive flexibility or social motivation, as autistic individuals showed a similar propensity to change their signals following a misunderstanding with their partner. However, they struggled to assign meanings to signals based on the unique communicative context established through past interaction with their partner, showing more individual exploration when constructing those signals. As seen in the largely segregated interaction spaces between autistic individuals in Figure 17.6 (blue versus orange clusters), neurotypical pairs navigate open-ended communicative situations by continuously considering and aligning to the frame of reference defined by signals embedded in their communicative history (in a Peircean sense). These observations explain, for instance, why autistic individuals experience difficulties in everyday

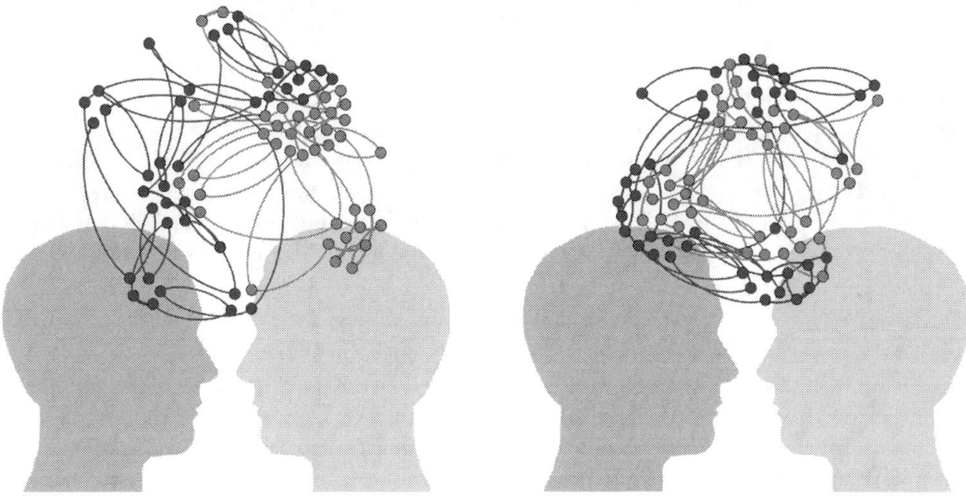

Figure 17.6 Pairwise interaction trajectories by an autistic pair and a neurotypical pair

Network visualizations of an autistic (left) and a neurotypical pair (right). The nodes represent communicative signals constructed by two individuals during a series of interactions in the tacit communication game. The nodes are clustered to show signals that were used repeatedly. The colored edges connect each individual's consecutively produced signals throughout the interaction (blue for one individual, orange for the other). It can be seen that autistic individuals showed more individual exploration when constructing signals, as indicated by relatively large clusters of individually used signals and small clusters of jointly used signals. By contrast, the neurotypical pair navigated the interaction space by continuously considering and aligning to recent signals from their partner, embedding those signals in a strongly interconnected space of meaning and relationships between one another's signals. ASD: autism spectrum disorder. Adapted from Wadge et al. (2019). See e-book for a full-color version of this figure.

context-dependent situations such as ironic or sarcastic conversation, but succeed in tests where they can capitalize on stereotyped cues to resolve linguistic ambiguities (Hahn et al., 2015).

Investigating the role of communicative context in language development is another research direction that, in our opinion, will provide important insights into the interplay between stereotyped and fleeting conceptual structures in epistemic engineering. For instance, while language processing is largely left-lateralized throughout life, necessary contributions from the right hemisphere may be seen early in life, gradually decreasing through childhood. Moreover, the right hemisphere may support basic language skills when the left hemisphere is compromised (Olulade et al., 2020). To date, there is no evidence for the opposite, with the left hemisphere seemingly not able to compensate for lost conversational abilities after early right hemisphere damage. As noted elsewhere (Sabbagh, 1999), this pattern of recovery is reminiscent of the pattern of linguistic and communicative development in autism. Vocabulary development is delayed but occurs in autistic children, yet communicative deficits persist through adulthood, as they would in right-hemisphere patients. We infer from its comparably small-world architecture that the left hemisphere is less able to cope with the flexibility demands of everyday interaction. Widely spaced neuron populations with few overlapping dendritic fields and greater levels of myelination endow the left hemisphere with functional stability and efficiency in terms of perturbation-resistant network hubs and shorter path lengths. Accordingly, the left hemisphere might be better equipped to generalize recurrent patterns of association when scaffolded by the conceptually flexible right hemisphere. These stereotyped dependencies, in turn, help communication by providing access to semantic structures and cues to a meaning (blue and orange background structures of Figure 17.2).

Conclusion

We have introduced joint epistemic engineering, a neurosemiotic account of how inherently asymmetric interlocutors can communicate effectively despite using signals that are referentially contingent on the current communicative circumstances. The basic insight is that interlocutors use multilayered communicative signals as a tool to organize and align their conceptual structures during social interaction. Besides reducing uncertainty over the identity of a referent in the interlocutors' minds (a Shannon-signal), a multilayered signal asks interlocutors to manage that declaration of communicative intent (a Grice-signal) and to coordinate the space of possible interpretations across interlocutors (a Peirce-signal). Accordingly, joint epistemic engineering offers the possibility to establish a communicative context in the presence of highly ambiguous signals, as well as to fluidly contextualize background knowledge relevant to the current situation, amalgamating potentially unrelated conceptual structures into a space of meanings and relationships between those structures. The hypothesized dependencies between those semiotic relations open the way to precisely characterize neural mechanisms that can implement the construal of meaning during interactive human communication. Future work should aim to understand how the elusive conceptual space generated during communication is instantiated in our brains, how its neural implementation is altered in disorders of human communication, and how joint epistemic engineering can bootstrap communication when infants learn to use linguistic signals in their daily interactions.

References

Abitbol, R., Lebreton, M., Hollard, G., Richmond, B. J., Bouret, S., & Pessiglione, M. (2015). Neural mechanisms underlying contextual dependency of subjective values: Converging evidence from monkeys and humans. *Journal of Neuroscience*, *35*(5), 2308–2320.

Bašnáková, J., Weber, K., Petersson, K. M., van Berkum, J., & Hagoort, P. (2014). Beyond the language given: The neural correlates of inferring speaker meaning. *Cerebral Cortex*, *24*(10), 2572–2578.

Beeman, M. (1993). Semantic processing in the right hemisphere may contribute to drawing inferences from discourse. *Brain and Language*, *44*(1), 80–120.

Beer, J. S., John, O. P., Scabini, D., & Knight, R. T. (2006). Orbitofrontal cortex and social behavior: Integrating self-monitoring and emotion-cognition interactions. *Journal of Cognitive Neuroscience*, *18*(6), 871–879.

Brennan, S. E., Galati, A., & Kuhlen, A. K. (2010). Two minds, one dialog: Coordinating speaking and understanding. In B. H. Ross (Ed.), *The Psychology of Learning and Motivation: Advances in Research and Theory* (pp. 301–344). Cambridge: Elsevier.

Carpendale, J. I. M., & Lewis, C. (2004). Constructing an understanding of mind: The development of children's social understanding within social interaction. *The Behavioral and Brain Sciences*, *27*(1), 79–96.

Clark, H. H. (1996). Using language. Cambridge: Cambridge University Press.

Clark, H. H. (1997). Dogmas of understanding. *Discourse Processes, 23*(3), 567–598.

Clark, H., & Marshall, C. (1981). Elements of discourse understanding. In Aravind K. Joshi, Bonnie L. Webber, & Ivan A. Sag (Eds.), *Definite Knowledge and Mutual Knowledge*, (pp. 10–63). Cambridge: Cambridge University Press.

Conway, B. R. (2012). Color consilience: Color through the lens of art practice, history, philosophy, and neuroscience. *Annals of the New York Academy of Sciences*, *1251*, 77–94.

Danchin, E., Giraldeau, L. A., Valone, T. J., & Wagner, R. H. (2004). Public information: From nosy neighbors to cultural evolution. *Science*, *305*(5683), 487–491.

Dawkins, R., & Krebs, J. R. (1978). Animal signals: Information or manipulation. In J. R. Krebs & N. B., & Davies (Eds.), *Behavioural Ecology: An Evolutionary Approach* (pp. 282–309). Oxford: Blackwell.

Deacon, T. W. (2018). Beneath symbols: Convention as a semiotic phenomenon. In S. C. Hayes & D. S. Wilson (Eds.), *Evolution & Contextual Behavioral Science: A Reunification*. (pp. 1–15). Los Angeles: New Harbinger.

de Ruiter, J. P., Noordzij, M. L., Newman-Norlund, S., Newman-Norlund, R., Hagoort, P., Levinson, S. C., & Toni, I. (2010). Exploring the cognitive infrastructure of communication. *Interaction Studies*, 11(1), 51–77.

Dingemanse, M., Roberts, S. G., Baranova, J., Blythe, J., Drew, P., Floyd, S., Gisladottir, R. S., Kendrick, K. H., Levinson, S. C., Manrique, E., Rossi, G., & Enfield, N. J. (2015). Universal principles in the repair of communication problems. *PloS One*, *10*(9), e0136100.

Elman, J. L. (2004). An alternative view of the mental lexicon. *Trends in Cognitive Sciences*, *8*(7), 301–306.

Galantucci, B. (2005). An experimental study of the emergence of human communication systems. *Cognitive Science, 29*(5), 737–767.

Galantucci, B., & Garrod, S. (2011). Experimental semiotics: A review. *Frontiers in Human Neuroscience, 5*. doi: 10.3389/fnhum.2011.00011

Galantucci, B., Langstein, B., Spivack, E., & Paley, N. (2020). Repair Avoidance: When faithful informational exchanges don't matter that much. *Cognitive Science, 44*(10), e12882. doi: 10.1111/cogs.12882

García, A. M., Franco-O'Byrne, D., & Ibáñez, A. (2020). Neurosemiotics: Blurbing a field beyond the "two cultures divide." In L'. Lacková, C. J. Rodríguez H., & K. Kull (Eds.), *Gatherings in Biosemiotics XX* (pp. 92–97). Tartu: University of Tartu Press.

Garrod, S., & Anderson, A. (1987). Saying what you mean in dialogue: A study in conceptual and semantic co-ordination. *Cognition, 27*(2), 181–218.

Gaskell, G. M. (2007). *The Oxford Handbook of Psycholinguistics*. Oxford: Oxford University Press.

Gibson, E., Futrell, R., Piantadosi, S. T., Dautriche, I., Mahowald, K., Bergen, L., & Levy, R. (2019). How efficiency shapes human language. *Trends in Cognitive Sciences, 23*(12), 1087.

Grice, H. P. (1957). Meaning. *The Philosophical Review, 66*(3), 377–388.

Hahn, N., Snedeker, J., & Rabagliati, H. (2015). Rapid linguistic ambiguity resolution in young children with autism spectrum disorder: Eye tracking evidence for the limits of weak central coherence. *Autism Research: Official Journal of the International Society for Autism Research, 8*(6), 717–726.

Harris, R. (1998). *Introduction to Integrational Linguistics*. Oxford: Pergamon Press.

Hasson, U., Ghazanfar, A. A., Galantucci, B., Garrod, S., & Keysers, C. (2012). Brain-to-brain coupling: A mechanism for creating and sharing a social world. *Trends in Cognitive Sciences, 16*(2), 114–121.

Hutsler, J., & Galuske, R. A. W. (2003). Hemispheric asymmetries in cerebral cortical networks. *Trends in Neurosciences, 26*(8), 429–435.

Ibáñez, A., García, A. M., Esteves, S., Yoris, A., Muñoz, E., Reynaldo, L., Pietto, M. L., Adolfi, F., & Manes, F. (2018). Social neuroscience: Undoing the schism between neurology and psychiatry. *Social Neuroscience, 13*(1), 1–39.

Jefferson, G. (1988). On the sequential organization of troubles-talk in ordinary conversation. *Social Problems, 35*(4), 418–441.

Jung-Beeman, M. (2005). Bilateral brain processes for comprehending natural language. *Trends in Cognitive Sciences, 9*(11), 512–518.

Kirby, S., Griffiths, T., & Smith, K. (2014). Iterated learning and the evolution of language. *Current Opinion in Neurobiology, 28*, 108–114.

Kull, K. (2020). Codes: Necessary, but not sufficient for meaning making. Constructivist Foundations. *Constructivist Foundations, 15*(2), 137–139.

Leahy, M. (1936). The Central Highlands of New Guinea. *The Geographical Journal, 87*(3), 229.

Levinson, S. (2006). On the human interactional engine. In N. Enfield & S. Levinson (Eds.), *Roots of Human Sociality*. (pp. 39–69). Oxford: Berg.

Lewis, D. K. (1969). *Convention: A Philosophical Study*. Princeton, NJ: Blackwell.

Mates, A. W., Mikesell, L., & Smith, M. S. (2013). *Language, Interaction, and Frontotemporal Dementia: Reverse Engineering the Social Mind*. Sheffield: Equinox.

Mayr, E. (1999). *Systematics and the Origin of Species, from the Viewpoint of a Zoologist*. Cambridge, MA: Harvard University Press.

Misyak, J. B., Melkonyan, T., Zeitoun, H., & Chater, N. (2014). Unwritten rules: Virtual bargaining underpins social interaction, culture, and society. *Trends in Cognitive Sciences, 18*(10), 512–519.

Myers, P. S. (1979). Profiles of communication deficits in patients with right cerebral hemisphere damage: Implications for diagnosis and treatment. *Clinical Aphasiology: Proceedings of the Conference 1979*, 38–46. http://aphasiology.pitt.edu/373/1/09-05.pdf

Noveck, I. A., & Reboul, A. (2008). Experimental pragmatics: A Gricean turn in the study of language. *Trends in Cognitive Sciences, 12*(11), 425–431.

Olulade, O. A., Seydell-Greenwald, A., Chambers, C. E., Turkeltaub, P. E., Dromerick, A. W., Berl, M. M., Gaillard, W. D., & Newport, E. L. (2020). The neural basis of language development: Changes in lateralization over age. *Proceedings of the National Academy of Sciences*, 201905590. doi: 10.1073/pnas.1905590117

Peirce, C. S. (1931). In Hartshorne, Charles Weiss, Paul Burks, Arthur W. (Eds.), *Collected Papers of Charles Sanders Peirce*. New York: Thoemmes Continuum.

Pickering, M. J., & Garrod, S. (2013). An integrated theory of language production and comprehension. *The Behavioral and Brain Sciences, 36*(4), 329–347.

Port, R. F. (2010). Language as a social institution: Why phonemes and words do not live in the brain. *Ecological Psychology, 22*(4), 304–326.

Rendall, D., & Owren, M. J. (2013). Communication without meaning or information: Abandoning language-based and informational constructs in animal communication theory. In U. E. Stegmann (Ed.), *Animal Communication Theory*, (pp. 151–188). Cambridge: Cambridge University Press.

Rizzolatti, G., & Arbib, M. A. (1998). Language within our grasp. *Trends in Neurosciences*, *21*(5), 188–194.
Sabbagh, M. A. (1999). Communicative intentions and language: Evidence from right-hemisphere damage and autism. *Brain and Language*, *70*(1), 29–69.
Sacks, H., Schegloff, E. A., & Jefferson, G. (1974). A simplest systematics for the organization of turn-taking for conversation. *Language*, *50*(4), 696.
Schelling, T. C. (1960). *The Strategy of Conflict*. Cambridge, MA: Harvard University Press.
Scott-Phillips, T. C., Kirby, S., & Ritchie, G. R. S. (2009). Signalling signalhood and the emergence of communication. *Cognition*, *113*(2), 226–233.
Selten, R., & Warglien, M. (2007). The emergence of simple languages in an experimental coordination game. *Proceedings of the National Academy of Sciences of the United States of America*, *104*(18), 7361–7366.
Shannon, C. E. (1948). A mathematical theory of communication. *Bell System Technical Journal*, *27*(3), 379–423.
Smith, S. L., Smith, I. T., Branco, T., & Häusser, M. (2013). Dendritic spikes enhance stimulus selectivity in cortical neurons in vivo. *Nature*, *503*(7474), 115–120.
Sperber, D., & Wilson, D. (1986). *Relevance: Communication and Cognition*. Hoboken, NJ: Blackwell.
Stivers, T. (2010). An overview of the question–response system in American English conversation. *Journal of Pragmatics*, *42*(10), 2772–2781.
Stolk, A., D'Imperio, D., di Pellegrino, G., & Toni, I. (2015). Altered communicative decisions following ventromedial prefrontal lesions. *Current Biology: CB*, *25*(11), 1469–1474.
Stolk, A., Noordzij, M. L., Verhagen, L., Volman, I., Schoffelen, J. M., Oostenveld, R., Hagoort, P., & Toni, I. (2014). Cerebral coherence between communicators marks the emergence of meaning. *Proceedings of the National Academy of Sciences*, *111*(51), 18183–18188.
Stolk, A., Noordzij, M. L., Volman, I., Verhagen, L., Overeem, S., van Elswijk, G., Bloem, B., Hagoort, P., & Toni, I. (2014). Understanding communicative actions: A repetitive TMS study. *Cortex*, *51*, 25–34.
Stolk, A., Verhagen, L., Schoffelen, J. M., Oostenveld, R., Blokpoel, M., Hagoort, P., van Rooij, I., & Toni, I. (2013). Neural mechanisms of communicative innovation. *Proceedings of the National Academy of Sciences of the United States of America*, *110*(36), 14574–14579.
Stolk, A., Verhagen, L., & Toni, I. (2016). Conceptual alignment: How brains achieve mutual understanding. *Trends in Cognitive Sciences*, *20*(3), 180–191.
Tomasello, M., Carpenter, M., Call, J., Behne, T., & Moll, H. (2005). Understanding and sharing intentions: The origins of cultural cognition. *The Behavioral and Brain Sciences*, *28*(5), 675–691.
Toni, I., & Stolk, A. (2019). Conceptual alignment as a neurocognitive mechanism for human communicative interactions. In P. Hagoort (Ed.), *Human language: From genes and brains to behavior, 249*. Cambridge, MA: MIT Press.
Veissière, S. P. L., Constant, A., Ramstead, M. J. D., Friston, K. J., & Kirmayer, L. J. (2019). Thinking through other minds: A variational approach to cognition and culture. *The Behavioral and Brain Sciences*, *43*, e90.
Wadge, H., Brewer, R., Bird, G., Toni, I., & Stolk, A. (2019). Communicative misalignment in autism spectrum disorder. *Cortex; a Journal Devoted to the Study of the Nervous System and Behavior*, *115*, 15–26.
Warglien, M., & Gärdenfors, P. (2015). Meaning negotiation. In F. Zenker, & P. Gärdenfors (Eds.), *Applications of Conceptual* Spaces: *The Case for Geometric Knowledge Representation* (pp. 79–94). New York: Springer.

18

TOWARDS A NEUROSEMIOTICS OF FRIENDSHIP

Claus Emmeche

Introduction: Why friendship?

The aim of this chapter is to get a sense of what a neurosemiotics of friendship might look like, investigating the difference between a semiotics of friendship and a neurosemiotics of friendship based upon neuroscientific research. The key premise has been lucidly articulated by Jorna (2009: 2831), who wrote: "Humans, whether they are conceived of as information processing systems or as neurological systems, are signals, signs and symbols using systems themselves. Therefore, neurosemiotics, largely, is also about ourselves." Insofar as friendship molds much of our lives, across ages and scenarios, then its study should not escape the purview of this nascent field.

Still, why use friendship as a case? What *is* friendship? Is it a real relation in the social world (like relations of family, class, or institutional roles)? Is it a human phenomenon involving subjective experience? Or is it a "construct" used in fields such as network research and social cognitive neuroscience, where such constructs are seen either as a hypothesized cause for certain patterns of behavior, or as a way to operationalize abstract notions, like friendship? These three characterizations are not disjunctive and they may all be adequate, depending upon context. Indeed, there are even more ways of characterizing friendship, drawing on insights from anthropology, history, philosophy, social psychology, and ethology, to name just some fields.

Friendship, in its everyday sense, designates a special social bond between two or more persons. Such a link has essentially relational and semiosic characteristics that are (neuro)biologically grounded and embedded in cultural and social matrices of norms, ideals, habits, ways of living, and ways of thinking and communicating. This richness foregrounds a broad variety of approaches relevant for illustrating the epistemic benefits of neurosemiotics. Although the term "friendship" has multiple meanings – a common one being *a voluntary relationship of mutual liking, trust, and support between the agents involved* – and is studied by many disciplines, it is fruitful to use the social relationship of friendship as a lens to better understand the social and semiotic nature of the self, thus emphasizing an important aspect of all social and psychic phenomena – namely, that they can be understood as mutually constituting each other (there can be no normal psyche without a social structuring environment and vice versa) within a set of neurobiological constraints and enablements. There is a subjective phenomenology particular to the human psyche, but it is embedded and enculturated within a social matrix that also needs to be accounted for (indicating the existence of a sociocultural phenomenology transcending the purely subjective, such as social norms, organizational habits, and institutions).

DOI: 10.4324/9781003051817-22

Similarly, the psyche is embodied in a human organism where (measurable and unmeasurable) brain processes are only a part of its total material biology. If it is true that neurosemiotics is largely about ourselves (as Jorna states in the opening quote), to understand ourselves is also to understand how we are placed in a sociosemiotic grid of "other selves," interacting with semiosic fluxes through our bodies (including our brains), in a cultural matrix codetermining who we are. If a friend can be seen as another social self (Aristotle's famous suggestion),[1] friendship is a good place to investigate social cognition and its neurosemiotics.

It is not purely coincidental that a seminal paper on neurosemiotics (Favareau, 2001) analyzed the then newly discovered mirror neurons and their role in empathy and the general emergence of intersubjectivity. What applies in general for the neurosemiotics of intersubjectivity is particularly crucial for the interplay between self and other in friendship. Favareau (2001: 86–87) argued that

> to equate the "self" as coterminous with biological proprioception, with the first-person perspective, or with a node in a social matrix is to impoverish the conception of "self" by several significant orders – for the self to *be* a self must be all of these recursively at once and more. The full "self" as we understand it in our daily lives is a dynamically determined self at every moment and the relations of which it is inextricably a part (itself, other, language) are likewise dynamically and perpetually co-construed. It is therefore as much a product of social interaction as of neurotransmission, for both the interpersonal and extrapersonal aspects of this self are deeply rooted in a massively non-linear, re-entrant ecology of signs.

As we will see below, the contemporary neuroscience of friendship lends itself, when interpreted neurosemiotically, to add a new dimension to Aristotle's notion of the friend as another self.

The theoretical framework for the following analysis, apart from Peircean semiotics (Peirce, 1931–1958; Stjernfelt, 2014), is a perspectival realist (Giere, 1999) philosophy of interdisciplinarity that acknowledges the irreducible complexity of the models and perspectives offered by the natural, human, and social sciences upon friendship phenomena in their evolutionary, biological, historical, psychological, social, political, and philosophical (including ethical) aspects (Caine, 2009; Hruschka, 2010; Digeser, 2016). There is not yet any single integrative theory of friendship, but many attempts have been made to trace friendship's evolutionary prehistory and culture-dependent universality, as well as the plurality of ways in which it can be enacted. Neurosemiotics is an important part of this territory of investigative attempts to map friendship phenomena in the real world.

Neuroscience needs semiotics

The meaning of "a semiotics of *X*" is exemplified by "a semiotics of ideology" – that is, the use of concepts, theories, and perspectives from semiotics to understand ideology as a real-world phenomenon. It comprises: (1) *the academic collective* as a social-institutional network of researchers gathering around the study of ideology; (2) *the epistemic object*, namely, ideology as constituted specifically through a semiotic perspective being applied to investigate it; and (3) *the real object* – for instance, the various political and religious ideologies existing throughout the history of human societies. To become a subject matter of investigation, a real object must be mediated to constitute an epistemic object, and this can happen in various ways through the application of different theoretical and methodological perspectives from different disciplines (Køppe, 2012). Thus, the epistemic object of ideology as a semiotic phenomenon is not identical to (but may share similarities with) the epistemic object of ideology as seen through the perspectives of sociology, political science, or anthropology, among other fields. The similarity between dimensions (1), (2), and (3), and the Peircean distinction between interpretants, representamens, and dynamical objects, will not escape the attention of a semiotically sensitive reader.[2] Thus, a semiotics of *X* involves *X* as a real dynamic object studied through the tools of semiotics, thereby constituting *X* as a semiotic phenomenon allowing investigators to ask specific questions and pursue their inquiry. If *X* is living processes as investigated within biology, a semiotics of *X* is the field of biosemiotics (Favareau, 2010a). This field is dependent upon research already done within standard biology, but biosemiotic approaches help by putting the material mechanisms of living systems as discovered by biologists into a broader perspective of signs, meaning, and communicative function, and also help to explain why biology has long been perfused with information and signal metaphors (Emmeche & Hoffmeyer, 1991) by actually taking these metaphors seriously and developing them into genuine biosemiotic concepts. In this sense, biosemiotics helps us to expand biology to better grasp communication in nature. Similarly, neurosemiotics helps us to expand the understanding achieved by the neurosciences.

But what is it that neurosemiotics (Leewen et al., 1992; Ivanov, 1993; Nöth, 2000; Jorna, 2009; Favareau, 2001, 2010a, 2010b) can offer specifically?[3] As we will see with the case of friendship, it can offer two things, both needed for better interpretations of the findings of neuroscience. First, neurosemiotics uses the tools of semiotics to study the forms of sign action underlying neurobiological processes and mechanisms as a basis for the emergence of cognitive, volitional, and emotional behavior as well as intentionality, functioning as an interdisciplinary bridge between semiotics and neuroscience in general. It emulates: (1) an academic interfield connecting semiotics with cognitive neuroscience; and (2) a special approach constituting an epistemic object of neurosemiosic processes; pointing to (3) real existing but hitherto undiscovered or unexplained phenomena that are thus brought under scrutiny. Second, it also offers a critical subjecting of neuroscientific findings to semiotic analysis: A scientific neuroscience research paper (a sign of knowledge) is a complex proposition with a predicate and a subject, stating true (or probably true, or false) claims about the properties of something – for example, "friendship has a neural correlate," (Güroğlu et al., 2008). Seen as such (namely, as a dicisign[4] or an argument), a research report can be analyzed semiotically by analyzing how this complex dicisign refers, what subsigns it consists of, the role of models and diagrams in it, its inferential structure, what (scientific, philosophical, cultural) discursive universes it involves, and the role of errors and uncertainties in its empirical grounding, among several other aspects. In this second sense, neurosemiotics parallels the philosophy of (neuro)science, but uses semiotic instead of philosophical methods.

A semiotics of friendship

Because a semiotics of *X* must take *X*'s potentials for and enactments of sign exchanges and interpretation as a focal point of analysis, a semiotics of friendship must analyze such a relation from the perspective of *semiosis* – that is, sign generation, representation, sign action and interpretation, and their processual roles in the interactive relations of two or more friends as they are located in a social web. If we focus on friendship between humans – knowing that some non-human animals can also relate in ways that best can be described as friendship (Denworth, 2020) – this situatedness in a social web involves markers or identity indices like age, gender, class, ethnicity, race, culture, and language. Being triadic relational structures in the Peircean sense, semiosic processes (where some signs stand for something to somebody or just some third instance) involve the mediation of qualities, existants, and general thoughts (or feelings, reactions, and concepts). It seems obvious that friendship – when seen as a communicative relationship between two or more human beings knowing each other well, having a reciprocal trust in each other, and a positive affective preference for each other for reasons that may be clear or obscure (or both) to those involved – is a social semiotic relation that by hypostatic abstraction (Peirce, 1958) has become a potential object of reflection for the agents involved, and a source of change of and by themselves. It is not a simple rule-based and purely instrumental relation (like my relation to my greengrocer when I buy broccoli); rather, it is a mutually valued, shared, and personal relation beyond mere economic, nutritional or other survival-related necessities. Friendship is similar to semiosis, as it is communicational, embodied, and depends upon a register of biolinguistic capacities that need to be in action and working before we can see it unfolding. One can even give a definition of friendship (Emmeche, 2014), emphasizing its relational triadicity as it is governed not just by the two friends but also by social norms.[5]

All these aspects need not involve the perspective of neuroscience, even though friendship is unfolding (psychologically, socially, culturally) within a set of neurobiological constraints and enablements, which is why a neurodegenerative disease can have the sad effect of ultimately ending a friendship (Rorty, 1993). One can analyze classic and modern conceptions of friendship from a semiotic perspective, give a semiotic definition of the relationship, and investigate the sign actions of its dynamisms (in formation, maintenance, and termination) quite independently of any focus on its neurobiological mechanisms, constraints or enablements. However, a neurosemiotics of friendship will have to draw upon insights about its neurobiology on some dimensional scale. Let us turn to our main example.

A neurosemiotics of friendship

There have been few, albeit quite remarkable, examples of research on friendship in the neurosciences (Brent et al., 2014; Chavez & Wagner, 2020; Denworth, 2020; Güroğlu et al., 2008; Wang et al., 2016; Woods et al., 2020). Recasting this work in a semiotic perspective may help shape our ideas of neurosemiotics as a nascent field of research.

We will focus upon an excellent study within cognitive social neuroscience by Carolyn Parkinson, Adam M. Kleinbaum, and Thalia Wheatley, which seems to indicate that friends often have some similarities at the neural level. First, let's remind ourselves about the social science notion of *homophily*, introduced by Paul Lazersfeld in the 1950s. This term denotes the tendency for people to have (non-negative) ties with people who are similar to themselves in socially significant ways. Much social science research has indicated that similarity seems to breed connection, and this pattern influences network ties of many types, including marriage, friendship, work, advice, support, information transfer, exchange, co-membership, and other types of relationship. The result is that people's personal networks are homogeneous with regard to many sociodemographic, behavioral, and intrapersonal characteristics (McPherson et al., 2001). The hypothesis investigated by Parkinson and Wheatley (from neuroscience) and Kleinbaum (from social network research) was that homophily – especially when manifested as friendship, but also more generally as closeness in a social network – can be detected at the neural level among people; that it might be shown that friends actually "click"' even at the neural level, not just on a social and emotional level. So if friends might be said to have an instant rapport with each other (in the sense of a close and harmonious relationship in which they understand each other's feelings or ideas and communicate well), this form of relatedness has a neural signature. Operationalizing friendship (to be discussed below) so as to be a measurable construct, seen as a relation in a social network, and using the scanning technique of functional magnetic resonance imaging (fMRI) on a concrete population of university students, the three researchers found that "[s]imilar neural responses predict friendship," to quote the title of their paper (Parkinson et al., 2018: 1). From a neurosemiotic perspective, the study is especially interesting both for what it reveals and for what it leaves unanswered, as we shall see. Their abstract, quoted here, will serve as our point of departure:

> Human social networks are overwhelmingly homophilous: individuals tend to befriend others who are similar to them in terms of a range of physical attributes (e.g., age, gender). Do similarities among friends reflect deeper similarities in how we perceive, interpret, and respond to the world? To test whether friendship, and more generally, social network proximity, is associated with increased similarity of real-time mental responding, we used functional magnetic resonance imaging to scan subjects' brains during free viewing of naturalistic movies. Here we show evidence for neural homophily: neural responses when viewing audiovisual movies are exceptionally similar among friends, and that similarity

> decreases with increasing distance in a real-world social network. These results suggest that we are exceptionally similar to our friends in how we perceive and respond to the world around us, which has implications for interpersonal influence and attraction.
>
> *(Parkinson et al., 2018: 1)*

So Parkinson et al. (2018) claim to have revealed a new aspect of friendship (and homophily more generally) called *neural homophily*, meaning that some neurological phenomena are more similar between friends than between nonrelated persons. It concerns the activity patterns of different brain regions when persons are exposed to (i.e., perceive and interpret) some meaningful stimuli. In the study these were 14 video clips covering a range of topics and genres such as comedy clips, documentaries, and debates. The clips were selected so that they would likely be unfamiliar to the subjects, effectively constraining the subjects' thoughts and attention to minimize mind wandering, and to evoke meaningful variability in responses, because different subjects attend to different aspects and have different cognitive as well as emotional reactions to them (i.e., they interpret content differently).

The subjects used for the first part of the study were a cohort of 279 first-year university students in a graduate program at Dartmouth's Tuck School of Business. All participants filled out a survey (administered in November of the students' first academic year) to characterize their internal social network. Forty-two students, who were interested in participating in the subsequent neuroimaging part of the study, did so in February.[6] A survey question read:

> Consider the people with whom you like to spend your free time. Since you arrived at [institution name], who are the classmates you have been with most often for informal social activities, such as going out to lunch, dinner, drinks, films, visiting one another's homes, and so on?

Classmates' names were supplied as listed in columns, with one column corresponding to each section of students in the graduate program. The subjects could indicate any number of social ties, and had no time limit for responding to this question. The survey only inquired about students' interactions with other members of their academic cohort, not individuals outside their group of classmates. Thus, a social network analysis could be made, mapping the nodes (students) and the edges (their ties) of the network. Friendship was operationalized as a mutually reported tie – that is, having two students both indicating a positive response to the abovementioned question (basically a checked box for the name in the survey's column of classmate's names). In network terms, an undirected edge would connect two actors only if both nominated the other "as a friend," as the scientists say, which may be friends but could also be just those with whom you will have spent some free time.[7] The protocol also allowed mapping social distance, operationalized as the smallest number of intermediaries or mutual social ties required to connect two individuals in the network. Demographic data about each subject's gender, ethnic identity, and country of citizenship were obtained from the school's register to control for mere demographic similarities.

In the subsequent fMRI study, the 42 students viewed the same series of video clips on various topics (music, politics, food, sport, science, comedy, satire) ranging in length from 88 seconds to more than five minutes and chosen, as mentioned, to evoke a range of different emotions. As participants watched the clips, the scanner recorded the responses of what in the analysis would be compartmentalized into 80 separate regions of their brains (for each hemisphere, 34 cortical areas and six subcortical structures). Then the researchers compared the responses of each student with the responses of every other student. The 42 students paired up in $42 \cdot 41/2 = 861$ distinct ways, and some of these dyads would classify as friends [social distance = 1] (because of mutual nomination in the survey), others as friends of friends [distance = 2], and so on, up to a category of distance 4 or more.

The results were quite remarkable. The neural responses of friend pairs were significantly more alike than those of non-friend pairs in terms of the calculated inter-subject time series correlations. For each of the 861 unique dyads, the Pearson correlation between the time series of fMRI responses (Figure 18.1) was computed for each of the 80 brain regions. The neural response similarity within each student dyad was summarized as a single variable; so for each dyad, a weighted average of normalized neural response similarities was computed, with the contribution of each brain region weighted by its average volume in the sample of fMRI subjects. It was shown that, overall, the more similar their neural responses, the shorter the distance between them in the social network. In statistical terms, for each one-unit increase in overall neural similarity, the odds that two people were friends increased by 47 percent. Even when the researchers controlled for the demographic (non-neural) similarities of people in each of the 861 pairs (features such as age, gender, and nationality), the correlation between neural response and position in the social network remained. Thus, neural similarity provided additional predictive power, above and beyond similarity in terms of the observed demographic variables, as seen when the "full model" was compared with a model that did not include neural similarity.

The authors further examined whether certain brain regions were driving the observed relationship. Broad regions of the ventral and dorsal striatum were thus detected, including the right nucleus accumbens, the bilateral caudate nucleus, the left putamen, the right amygdala, the right superior parietal lobule, and the left inferior parietal cortex (Parkinson et al., 2018: 1–14).[8] These are not delimited to the regions known to process social information, as Wheatly commented to a science journalist: "It was all over the brain, sensory regions, memory, language … You couldn't say here's the social brain network that is responsible for friendship. It was that friends' brains are remarkably similar across huge swathes of areas" (Denworth, 2020: 292). Yet the correlation was especially strong in areas related to shared perspective-taking, visual and auditory attention, and affective processing. Wheatly commented:

> Friends are literally seeing and hearing the world more similarly than people who are friends of friends and friends of friends of friends. It's coming down to the level of how you're processing sights and sounds. Given a music video, if you and I find some parts of the melody or some part of the visuals particularly engaging, then we're going to tune our eyes and ears to those parts.
>
> *(Denworth, 2020: 292)*[9]

The researchers also tested whether it was possible to predict friendship status based on similarity of the fMRI response time series across brain regions. The use of the word "prediction" here (and in the paper's title) should, of course, be taken with caution. When a journalist phrased the findings thus: "Parkinson and her colleagues also found that the brain responses alone could do a pretty good job of predicting whether two people were friends, mere acquaintances or total strangers" (Kaplan, 2018), "predicting" in this statistical sense used by the researchers means first training a machine learning algorithm to recognize patterns of neural similarities associated with four social distance categories (1, 2, 3, and 4+) from a subset of the total dataset from the dyads, and then to check whether this classifier program can "guess better" in the sense of deviating significantly from classifying completely randomly when exposed to data outside the training set. As mentioned, the 861 dyads were divided into four categories of social distance: "friends" defines a distance of 1 ($N = 63$); "a friend of a friend" implies a distance of 2 ($N = 286$); "a friend of a friend of a friend" entails a distance of 3 ($N = 412$); and the last category was dyads with a distance of 4 or more ($N = 100$). If the algorithm was making random guesses about a dyad's social distance, it would guess right 25 percent of the time.[10] But the classifier trained on the brain responses correctly identified friends 48 percent of the time (meaning there was close to a 50–50 chance of hitting a right answer if asked whether those in a particular dyad were friends – so much for statistical "prediction").[11] It also correctly classified

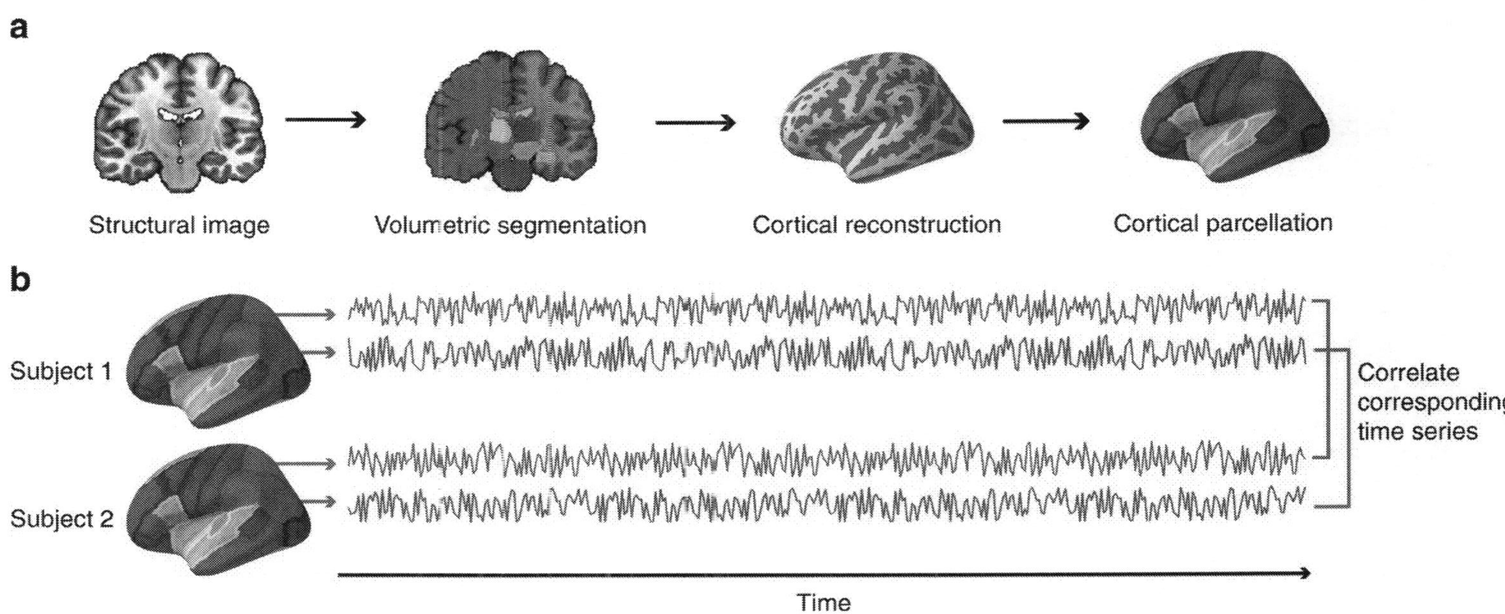

Figure 18.1 Computing inter-subject time series correlations

A. 80 anatomical regions of interest (ROIs) were derived for each individual; segmentation of cerebral cortex, subcortical white matter, and deep gray matter volumetric structures (signified by color in the image) was performed on the high-resolution scan of each individual's brain volume. Next, a cortical surface model was reconstructed and parcellated into anatomical units, here signified by different colors in the cortical parcellation scheme on the far right. B. For each individual, the average response time series within each ROI was extracted during video viewing. The correlation between time series extracted from each pair of corresponding ROIs was computed for each unique pair of subjects. For details see Parkinson et al. (2018). Credit: Creative Commons Attribution 4.0 International License. See e-book for a full-color version of this figure.

distance 2 relationships 39 percent of the time, distance 3 relationships 31 percent of the time, and distance 4 relationships 47 percent of the time, according to the study (Figure 18.2). When the algorithm guessed wrong, it was usually only off by one category.[12]

Disregarding our reservations about the meaning of "prediction," it is indeed remarkable that one can use time series correlations between any two brains perceiving the same material to indicate the likelihood that the persons involved are friends – or *could be* friends, as there was no deeper understanding involved about the actual nature of these mutually sympathetic nominations (liking to spend free time with another person).[13] If this study should be expanded (from being about potential friendship to become a neurosemiotics of realized friendship), more focus on the specific nature of the involved relationships would be needed. Standard analyses of social distance would not suffice and must be supplied with investigations of the qualitative sociology and psychology of the actual relationships. An interesting procedure would then be to first investigate the nature of the relationships involved and how they might be differentiated, eventually inspired by the classic trichotomy between friends of utility, friends of pleasure, and very good or best friends – which is empirically feasible (cf. Anderson & Fowers, 2020) – and then perform a similar analysis to see where "neural homophily" would be most salient. A hypothesis would be that there is no special neural homophily or similarity among friends of utility, but that there is so for friends of pleasure, while for very good friends the degree of similarity is more difficult, if not impossible, to guess (this group may also cover more distinct types of relationships) but it might take an intermediate position. A similar conjecture could be posed for the trichotomy of social, familiar, and communicating friendships (Little, 1993).

But what about the causality behind the correlation between social distance and brain patterns? "Do we become friends with people who respond to the environment similarly, or do we come to respond to the world similarly to our friends?" asked the researchers, and immediately admitted that "we cannot ascertain, based on these results alone, whether neural response similarity is a cause or consequence of friendship" (Parkinson et al., 2018: 1–14).[14] They plan to continue their research with follow-up studies in a longitudinal setting, to monitor whether, for instance, a group of students naturally gravitate towards those who see the world the same way as they do or if they become neurally more similar once they share experiences with their friends (Denworth, 2020). Another study has shown that neural similarity also correlated with social proximity for brains in the absence of external stimuli.[15]

A way to interpret a high degree of neural similarity in the time series of two persons' brains is to see this as an example of neural synchrony (Hasson, 2012). As cognitive neuroscientist Mathew Lieberman phrased it, the study is "one of only a handful of neural synchrony studies to use machine learning algorithms, such that neural synchrony is actually being used to predict something about the people whose brains are synchronized," the only difference being that while other studies predicted experiences and memories, Parkinson et al. (2018) "predicted aspects of the social structure of a large novel group from the similarity of their neural responses" (Lieberman, 2018: 371–372).

The neurosemiotics of opacity in data-intensive brain research

While using the term "predict" with care, however, a neurosemiotics of friendship should also ask: Who is doing the predicting? Is it the researchers or the algorithm trained on the data set? What kind of knowledge is achieved through this laborious exercise? Can we imagine the possibility of unpacking the classifier algorithm (which in this and many similar studies via machine learning becomes almost blackboxed)[16] and from its structure extract an understandable lesson or some explicit knowledge that would help us, as humans, not only to classify dyads to social distance categories more or less successfully (if we have a big and reliable dataset and good machine learning tools), but actually *know* in the explanatory sense about the detailed workings of neural homophily, and gain some sort of deeper understanding of the neurosemiotic mechanisms involved?

Compare such a statement as "I know a friendship when I see one but cannot tell you how I know this" when uttered by (a) a layperson, (b) a psychotherapist, and (c) a research group with a classifier algorithm à la Parkinson et al. (2018). We would only think of (a) and (b)'s utterances as scientific if their knowing how to identify friendship were accompanied by some general explanatory principles related to how they got this skill and what friendship is within some theoretical perspective; but we tend to think that (c)'s utterance is more scientific when it is based upon elaborate empirical research, including semi-automated inductive reasoning on brain scan data, including pattern recognition by machine learning. Yet, in all three cases, it may be more accurate to say that something is distinguished (or "predicted") and in this sense is "known," rather than seeing the knowledge attained as explanatory. The classifier algorithm used by Parkinson offers in itself no explanation of its skills of distinguishing social distance categories.

Of course, the neuroscientists cannot just look at the unprocessed fMRI scanning outputs and point out the locations where two persons' curves (indicating blood flow peaks) are similar enough in time response to count for something that can "predict" anything like friendship. The prediction is highly mediated by algorithms that achieve a form of tacit knowledge, akin to the skill a trained physician has in distinguishing freckles from skin cancer spots. The doctor has learned to do this by training and observing hundreds of cases, and receiving guidance from a skilled expert. Such a tacit knowledge is not explicit, but a cognitive capacity we have when we somehow "know more than we can tell" (Polanyi, 1983: 4). Polanyi's examples of this kind of knowledge include not just technicians' and doctors' ability to correctly diagnose diseases based upon perceptual clues, but also everyday skills such as face recognition – "we usually cannot tell how we recognize a face we know" (Polanyi, 1983: 4). In general, there exist many tasks whose execution we can understand intuitively, even though we cannot verbalize the rules or procedures behind them, and even if we can get machines to learn these tasks, we still do not posit an adequate theory of the social and cognitive processes.

Can the neuroscientist acquire the same kind of skill as the classifier algorithm? Here, a neurosemiotics of friendship involves a semiotics of pattern recognition and statistical prediction via artificial intelligence. The physician may do a good job distinguishing freckles from potentially dangerous spots, but dermatology cannot be just an intuitive skill in classifying skin. It is a science including an explicit biological understanding of the differences between normal and dangerous skin change processes. Likewise, social cognitive neuroscience needs more than pattern recognition of unexplained similarities between people's brains. It needs a transparent theory (not opaque models) of the mechanisms of neural homophily, and this theory may need to couple several levels of description, one for the perceptions of friendship among the agents involved, one about the social structure within which the friendship unfolds, and one about the neural mechanisms "underlying" social cognition and emotion (where a better metaphor than "underlie" may be to see the neural mechanisms as just forming one component of the total brain–psyche–culture system).[17]

Polanyi's appraisal of the role of tacit knowledge in science went along with his insistence on a personal aspect of scientific knowledge and understanding that in no way questioned the authority of a scientist's expertise. Yet who is the authoritative epistemic agent regarding the finding of neural homophily in Parkinson et al. (2018) if parts of the justification of this discovery (the data and their analysis) are epistemically opaque? Humphreys (2009) analyzed the *essential epistemic opacity* of a computational process (leading from an abstract model underlying a simulation to the output) relative to a researcher X. He defined such a process as being "essentially epistemically opaque to X if and only if it is impossible, given the nature of X, for X to know all of the epistemically relevant elements of the process" (Humphreys, 2009: 618). He later expanded the analysis to include *representational opacity* related to machine learning tools like deep neural networks, which perform successfully but whose underlying predictive principles are not fully understood (Humphreys, 2020). The numerical functions between the input values and a probability distribution over the classification types are so complex that interpreting and understanding these functions can be beyond the reach of humans.

A representation is opaque when it is non-transparent, and a *transparent* one presumes that the state of the system is represented "in a way that is open to explicit scrutiny, analysis, interpretation, and understanding by humans and transitions between those states are represented by rules that have similar transparent properties" (Humphreys, 2020: 19). No clear rules of how to come from a degree of neural similarity to friendship status could be offered by Parkinson's group. The central representation in their paper – summing up the data analysis (including the computed time series similarities of the 68880 dyad brain regions recorded) – is a confusion matrix (Figure 18.2), indicating the capacity of the constructed machine learning model to predict social distance based on neural similarities. It summarizes the results of the classifier algorithm (a support-vector network) after being trained on the dataset, but it can hardly be called transparent in the sense just stated.

So, while the epistemic authority is with the person in the case of tacit knowledge of a skilled expert in skin disease diagnosis, in the case of predictive classification of social distance in epistemic opaque computer assisted research, the authority of that "knowledge" is not personal, but technosocially distributed – that is, bound to wider communities of expertise and their computational technologies.

Related to the causality question is a question about what video contents were particularly significant in bringing friends' brains into synchrony or neural similarity? A reviewer of the paper suggested that some movies might be more diagnostic of dyad friendship than others, and asked "to see the overall model performance, prediction accuracy, or rank for individual movies." In their answer, Parkinson's group analyzed the data corresponding to each video clip separately and published these as a supplement. As seen in their Supplementary Table 3, only four of the 14 clips (two comedic videos, one soccer match clip, and a clip called "An Astronaut's View of Earth") provoked a separate neural similarity measure that was statistically significant (either at $p < .05$, $p < .01$, or $p < .001$), while this applied to all the 14 clips compared for both gender and nationality and to none of the

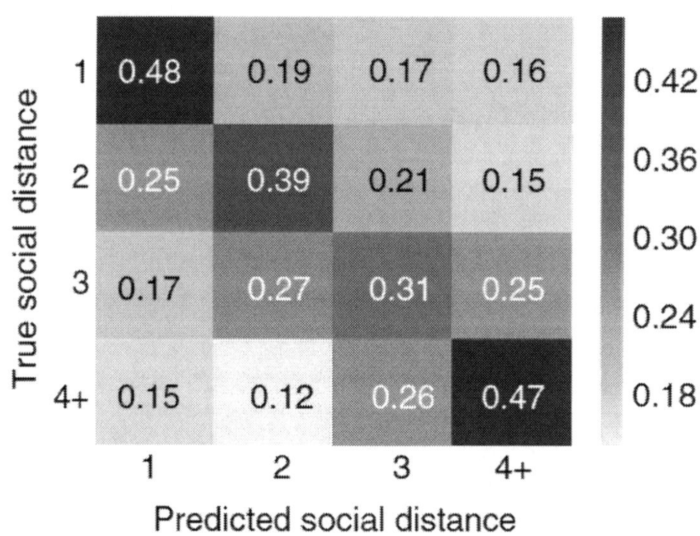

Figure 18.2 Prediction accuracy of classifiers able to predict friendship

Confusion matrix summarizing prediction accuracy of four-way classifiers trained to predict friendship or further distance between members of dyads in their social network based on patterns of neural similarity. Numbers and grey tones indicate how often the classifier predicted that dyads belonged to each social distance category (from Parkinson, et al., 2018; see their 'Methods' for further details). See e-book for a full-color version of this figure.

clips for ethnicity, handedness, or age. These results are difficult to interpret and received no further comments by the group.

However, their research is ongoing and Parkinson's group is determined to shed more light on the causality question. Neurosemiotics can help interpret the results of such lines of research and frame them as forms of knowledge that at once widens the epistemic authority to collective agency (interdisciplinary teams of experts) and make explicit the epistemic costs related to such styles of inquiry in the form of new kinds of scientific uncertainty and epistemic and representational opacity.

Concluding remarks on a friendly critique of common neurosense

To summarize the open questions of the study, substantial additional knowledge (about the way specific areas of the brain process visual and auditory stimuli and bind them together with the subject's previous individual or shared experience to a coherent interpretive response) is needed before we can begin to glimpse the fragments of a neurosemiotic theory of neural homophily that would provide us with explicit and transparent knowledge about the workings of friendship and its *sunaisthesis*, its seeing-together (Flakne, 2005).

Neurosemiotics helped us raise questions concerning the truth status of the research paper as a dicisign predicating neural similarity (and its predicting power) about a subject ("friendship" and, more general, "distance in a social network"). As a complex dicisign, the meaning of the research paper is not reducible to its title and the total argument it communicates helps to contextualize and moderate the simple proposition that "similar neural responses predict friendship." A neurosemiotic analysis contributes to make clear that the title could as well have been the less fancy but more accurate proposition "machine learning algorithms found associations between neural response similarity and preferences for socializing together among a set of first year university students." This clarification may seem commonsensical to the scientists involved, but would impact the way their message is understood by science communicators and the wider public. It may be needed to bring common sense in line with a popular "neurosense" to prevent its interpretation from degrading into nonsense claims. Why did the scientists not choose a more accurate heading? Perhaps this can be explained at the level of some overall social semiotic mechanisms of contemporary science, how it is funded, and the competition for publicity.

Finally, let us not forget the ethical aspect of neurosemiotics. Susan Petrilli and Augusto Ponzio (2010) maintain that human beings, endowed with a capacity of care for semiosis, are also "semioethic animals," with an obligation to reflect upon the conditions for responsible living in open societies. If, in the future, the propositional dicisign "similar neural responses predict friendship" can be proven to be true with more accuracy, several uses and misuses of this knowledge can be imagined, because such a dicisign is tied to instrumental techniques that not only can measure similarity of neural responses, but also could be deployed to control subjects based upon neural profiling information. So if there is reality behind Lieberman's suggestion that perhaps "companies will one day put together teams for projects based on getting the right balance of neural similarity and dissimilarity to optimize team performance and satisfaction" (Lieberman, 2018: 371–372), such a future may look scary from a wider political perspective and make it urgent, when developing a neurosemiotic perspective on the social realm of human beings, to also raise concerns about the ethical challenges to open and friendly societies raised by this brave new world.

Acknowledgements

Thanks to the editors Adolfo M. García and Agustín Ibáñez and an anonymous reviewer for helpful comments. Thanks goes also to Carolyn Parkinson and Paul Humphreys for personal communication.

Notes

1 In Aristotle's *Nicomachean Ethics* and his other writings on virtues and the art of living well, friendship played a major role. While he may have understood the notions of self and other quite differently from modern conceptions and contemporary individualistic psychology (Fowers & Anderson, 2018; Stern-Gillet, 1995: Chs 1 and 2), his take on friendship still inspires present-day research.

2 However, to spell out in detail a theory of science (and the dynamics of researchers, their ways of representing and intervening, and the nature so investigated) based on Peirce's semiotics is beyond the scope of this chapter.

3 For this question, an analogy to general fields like biology or linguistics may help. Also in them we find hyphenated or combined designations of specialized research areas – for example, neurobiology and evolutionary biology, neurolinguistics and historical linguistics. They both signify: (1) more or less well-defined institutional subdisciplines (often with their own journals, congresses, associations, research departments, and so on); (2) the specific topics dealt with (e.g., evolutionary or historical change, and neurological or linguistic mechanisms); and (3) the real-world phenomena that are highlighted by these approaches. Such hyphenated fields of research can have a more or less interdisciplinary character. The existence of neurobiology as a subfield does not sever it from the rest of biology or the general study of biological principles and mechanisms. A subfield like neurolinguistics, studying structures and processes in the human brain that underlie grammar and language communication, connects the two broad fields of biology and linguistics.

4 Peirce stated that, "In regard to its relation to its signified interpretant, a sign is either a Rheme, a Dicent, or an Argument. This corresponds to the old division Term, Proposition, & Argument, modified so as to be applicable to signs generally." (*Letters to Lady Welby*, MS [R] L463); Stjernfelt (2014); www.commens.org/dictionary/term/dicisign.

5 Thus, what Peirce observed about a person's thoughts – that "a person is not absolutely an individual. His thoughts are what he is 'saying to himself', that is, is saying to that other self that is just coming into life in the flow of time" ("What Pragmatism is," Peirce, 1958: Vol. 5, para. 421) – becomes even more accentuated considering the thinking of friends (Emmeche, 2017), and the dialogic aspect of science and philosophy.

6 The information given in this section is both from Parkinson et al. (2018) and brief interviews with the researchers given in Kaplan (2018), Knapton (2018), and especially Denworth (2020).

7 Note that the very notion of a friend differs from its operationalization in the social network survey. A mutual nomination here is not necessarily the same as a realized tie of friendship – that is, some of the dyads could be friends only potentially, in the sense of classmates one has been with most often for lunch, for example.

8 Compare the findings of Güroğlu et al. (2008: 903–910), whose results "revealed, among others, three regions of particular interest as selectively more strongly activated when subjects interacted with their friends than with other peers and celebrities: the amygdala and hippocampus, the nucleus accumbens, and the ventromedial prefrontal cortex."

9 Such findings add new meaning to Aristotle's notion of shared perception, *sunaisthesis*, and his comment that "a man also ought [*dei*] to share-his-friend's-consciousness of his existence [*sunaisthanesthai hoti estin*]" (Flakne, 2005: 37–63).

10 Given that the data were imbalanced across social distance categories, "data resampling and folding procedures were used to create a series of balanced data folds such that all dyads were included in the analyses" (Parkinson et al., 2018).

11 Parkinson et al. (2018) stated that "the classifier tended to predict the correct social distances for dyads in all distance categories at rates above the accuracy level that would be expected based on chance alone (i.e., 25% correct), with an overall classification accuracy of 41.25%." However, one can question whether "percentage of correct answers" is a good criterion for quality when the distribution of the four classes is so unequal: If you guess with the same probability distribution as the data, the percentage of correct guesses is given by: $(63^2 + 286^2 + 412^2 + 100^2) / 861^2 = 35.8\%$, and if you consequently guess "distance 3" (the most frequent category) you will get $412/861 = 47.9$ percent correct classifications. Seen in this light, 41 percent is not very convincing. I thank Henrik Nielsen for his helpful comments on this.

12 A part of the neurosemiotics (in sense no. 2 indicated above) would be occupied with correcting misinterpretations of neuroscience in social and popular media that easily appear when news reporters try to make sense of scientists' findings. Thus, a news feature about Parkinson et al. (2018) stated that: "The team also found that MRI response similarities could be used to predict not only if a pair were friends but also the social distance between the two" (Knapton, 2018); this phrasing suggests that the researchers could predict the degree of closeness between real (not just potential) "friends" (rather than predicting the dyad's belonging to one of the four social distance categories), thus alluding to the possibility of distinguishing by these methods between different kinds of friendship – an aspect that was clearly not involved here. Sometimes journalists might just have seen a press release about a study (for this study: see Dartmouth College, 2018) or spoken a few words with the scientists, so misunderstandings are not surprising, but in this case the quoted phrasing is

taken directly from the press release itself (where a better phrasing could have been "predict not only if a pair were friends but also the social distance between the any non-friend pair").

13 The researchers did not access the specific character of the 63 "friendship" (social distance 1) relations within the subgroup of 42 students who mutually reported that they spend time together, and thus cannot say anything beyond that definition of friendship. I thank Carolyn Parkinson (pers. communication) for pointing out that looking at gradations of interpersonal closeness among the dyads identified as "friends" based on that survey would likely require a much bigger sample size in order to have sufficient statistical power. Hopefully further research will allow them to be able to say more in the future.

14 Their paper acknowledges that a large body of research demonstrates that people in our immediate environment influence how we think, feel, and behave, but does not cite work specifically relevant for friendship. There are several relevant philosophical accounts of friendship – friends as mirroring their selves; or having a receptivity to being drawn by the friend and by her understanding of this, or being a plural agent with joint cares, a joint evaluative perspective, a pattern of interpersonally connected emotions, desires, judgments, and shared actions – see Helm (2017) for an overview. Friendship and its various processes, including collaboration between scientists or artists, is relevant for understanding embodied and embedded aspects of cognition (Emmeche, 2017).

15 Studying a group of people in a remote Korean village, Parkinson's team showed that neural similarity in individuals' resting-state brain activity could also predict proximity in their social network, even when controlling for demographic characteristics and self-reported personality traits (Hyon et al. 2020). They suggested that such patterns of brain activity during rest encode latent similarities of how people think and behave associated with friendship. However, a similar study on girls from a day and boarding school in the United Kingdom showed no evidence of a similar correlation (McNapp et al., 2020).

16 As Varoquaux and Thirion (2014) comment, "for progress in neuroscience, black-box prediction engines do not suffice as the key to understanding brain function lies in the properties of the signal used for prediction." Addressing another set of learning algorithms Tanaka et al. (2019) asked: "Are we simply replacing one complex system (a biological circuit) with another (a deep network), without understanding either?" These challenges are also neurosemiotic – that is, they connect a better multi-scale understanding of the brain's neural mechanisms (conceptualized computationally or semiotically) with the higher-order patterns of functional action. Similar questions are also raised in other fields of biology (Baker et al., 2018).

17 It is difficult to tell how to get to such a theory based on the kinds of data in study by Parkinson et al. (2018), but it may not be altogether impossible – cf. the patent by Li M. Fu (1991).

References

Anderson, A. R. & Fowers, B. J. (2020): An exploratory study of friendship characteristics and their relations with hedonic and eudaimonic well-being. *Journal of Social and Personal Relationships*, *37*(1), 260–280. doi: 10.1177%2F0265407519861152

Baker, R. E., Jose-Maria, P., Jayaratnam, J. & Antoine, J. (2018). Mechanistic models versus machine learning: A fight worth fighting for the biological community? *Biology Letters*, *14*(5), 20170660 doi: 10.1098/rsbl.2017.0660

Brent, L. J. N., Chang, S. W. C., Gariépy, J.-F. & Platt, M. L. (2014). The neuroethology of friendship. *Annals of the New York Academy of Sciences*, *1316*, 1–17. doi: 10.1111/nyas.12315

Caine, B. (Ed.) (2009). *Friendship: A History*. London: Equinox.

Chavez, R. S., & Wagner, D. D. (2020). The neural representation of self is recapitulated in the brains of friends: A round-robin fMRI study. *Journal of Personality and Social Psychology*, *118*(3): 407–416. doi: 10.1037/pspa0000178

Dartmouth College (2018). Your brain reveals who your friends are: Study illustrates how similar neural responses predict friendships. *ScienceDaily*, 30 January. www.sciencedaily.com/releases/2018/01/180130123643.htm

Denworth, L. (2020). *Friendship. The Evolution, Biology and Extraordinary Power of Life's Fundamental Bond*. London: Bloomsbury.

Digeser, P.E. (2016). *Friendship Reconsidered: What It Means and How It Matters to Politics*. New York: Columbia University Press.

Emmeche, C. (2014). Robot friendship: Can a robot be a friend? *International Journal of Signs and Semiotic Systems*, *3*(2), 26–42. doi: 10.4018/IJSSS.2014070103

Emmeche, C. (2017). Thinking with friends: Embodied cognition and relational attention in friendship. In F. Adams, O. Pessoa Jr., & J. E. Kogler Jr. (Eds), *Cognitive Science: Recent Advances and Recurring Problems* (pp. 47–58). Delaware, MD: Vernon Press.

Emmeche, C. & Hoffmeyer, J. (1991). From language to nature – the semiotic metaphor in biology. *Semiotica*, *84*(1/2), 1–42. doi: 10.1515/semi.1991.84.1-2.1

Favareau, D. (2001). Beyond self and other: The neurosemiotic emergence of intersubjectivity. *Sign Systems Studies*, *30*(1), 57–101.

Favareau, D. (2010a). Introduction: An evolutionary history of biosemiotics. In D. Favareau (Ed.), *Essential Readings in Biosemiotics* (pp. 1–77). Dordrecht: Springer.
Favareau, D. (2010b). Neurosemiotics. In P. Cobley (Ed.), *The Routledge Companion to Semiotics* (pp. 275–275). London: Routledge.
Flakne, A. (2005). Embodied and embedded: Friendship and the sunaisthetic self. *Epoché 10*(1), 37–63.
Fowers, B. J. & Anderson, A. R. (2018). Aristotelian *philia*, contemporary friendship, and some resources for studying close relationships. In T. Harrison & D. I. Walker (Eds.), *The Theory and Practice of Virtue Education* (pp. 184–196). London: Routledge.
Fu, L. M. (1991). Translation of a neural network into a rule-based expert system. *IJCNN-91-Seattle International Joint Conference on Neural Networks, Vol. 2,* p. 947. doi: 10.1109/IJCNN.1991.155551
Giere, R.N. (1999). *Science Without Laws*. Chicago: University of Chicago Press.
Güroğlu, B., Haselager, G. J. T., van Lieshout, C. F. M, Takashima, A., Rijpkema, M. & Fernández, G. (2008). Why are friends special? Implementing a social interaction simulation task to probe the neural correlates of friendship. *NeuroImage 39*, 903–910. doi: 10.1016/j.neuroimage.2007.09.007
Hasson, U., Ghazanfar, A. A., Galantucci, B., Garrod, S., & Keysers, C. (2012). Brain-to-brain coupling: A mechanism for creating and sharing a social world. *Trends in Cognitive Sciences, 16*, 114–121. doi: 10.1016/j.tics.2011.12.007
Helm, B. (2017). Friendship. In E. N. Zalta (Ed.), *The Stanford Encyclopedia of Philosophy*, https://plato.stanford.edu/archives/fall2017/entries/friendship
Hruschka, D.J. (2010). *Friendship: Development, Ecology, and Evolution of a Relationship*. Berkeley, CA: University of California Press.
Humphreys, P. (2009). The philosophical novelty of computer simulation methods. *Synthese, 169,* 615–626. doi: 10.1007/s11229-008-9435-2
Humphreys, P. (2020). Why automated science should be cautiously welcomed. In M. Bertolaso & F. Sterpetti (Eds.), *A Critical Reflection on Automated Science: Will Science Remain Human?* (pp. 11–26). Cham: Springer.
Hyon, R., Youmb, Y., Kimb, J., Cheyc, J., Kwakd, S., and Parkinson, C. (2020). Similarity in functional brain connectivity at rest predicts interpersonal closeness in the social network of an entire village. *Proceedings of the National Academy of Sciences, 117* (52), 33149–33160.
Ivanov, V.V. (1993). Neurosemiotics and neurobiology. *Semiotica, 94*(1–2), 103–121.
Jorna, R. J. (2009). Neurosemiotics. In M. D. Binder, N. Hirokawa, & U. Windhorst (Eds.), *Encyclopedia of Neuroscience* (pp. 2830–2833). Berlin: Springer.
Kaplan, K. (2018). Brain scans reveal that friends really are on the same wavelength. *Los Angeles Times*, January 30. www.latimes.com/science/sciencenow/la-sci-sn-friends-brains-same-20180130-story.html
Knapton, S. (2018). Friends really are on same wavelength, brain scans show. *The Telegraph*, January 30. www.telegraph.co.uk/science/2018/01/30/friends-really-wavelength-brain-scans-show
Køppe, S. (2012). A moderate eclecticism: Ontological and epistemological issues. *Integrative Psychology and Behavior, 46,* 1–19. doi: 10.1007/s12124-011-9175-6
Leeuwen, E. van, Dillmann, R., & Broekman, J. (1992). Neurosemiotics – the loss of reference. In M. Balat & J. Deledalle-Rhodes (Eds.), *Signs of Humanity: Proceedings of the IVth International Congress, International Association for Semiotic Studies. Barcelona, March 30–April 6, 1989* (pp. 969–980). Berlin: Mouton de Gruyter.
Lieberman, M. D. (2018): Birds of a feather synchronize together. *Trends in Cognitive Sciences, 22*(5), 371–372.
Little, G. (1993). *Friendship: Being Ourselves with Others*. Melbourne: Scribe.
McNabb, C.B., Burgess, L.G., Fancourt, F., Mulligan, N., FitzGibbon, L., Riddell, P., & Murayama, K. (2020). No evidence for a relationship between social closeness and similarity in resting-state functional brain connectivity in schoolchildren. *Scientific Reports, 10,* 10710. doi: 10.1038/s41598-020-67718-8
McPherson, M., Smith-Lovin, L., & Cook, J. M. (2001). Birds of a feather: Homophily in social networks. *Annual Review of Sociology, 27*, 415–444. doi: 10.1146/annurev.soc.27.1.415
Nöth, W. (2000). *Handbuch der Semiotik. 2. Auflage.* Stuttgart Weimar: Verlag J. B. Metzler.
Parkinson, C., Kleinbaum, A. M., & Wheatley, T. (2018). Similar neural responses predict friendship. *Nature Communications, 9*(1), 332. doi: 10.1038/s41467-017-02722-7
Peirce, C. S. (1931–1958). *Collected Papers of Charles Sanders Peirce, Vol. 1–6*, (C. Hartshorne & P. Weiss, Eds.), *Vols.* 7–8, A. W. Burks (Ed.). Cambridge, MA: Harvard University Press. [References: CP, followed by vol., and paragraph number].
Petrilli, S. & Ponzio, A. (2010). Semioethics. In P. Cobley (Ed.), *The Routledge Companion to Semiotics* (pp. 150–162). London: Routledge.
Polanyi, M. (1983 [1966]). *The Tacit Dimension*. Gloucester, MA: Peter Smith.
Rorty, A. O. (1993). The historicity of psychological attitudes: Love is not love which alters not when it alteration finds. In: N. K. Badhwar (Ed.), *Friendship: A Philosophical Reader* (pp. 73–88). Ithaca, NY: Cornell University Press.

Stern-Gillet, S. (1995). *Aristotle's Philosophy of Friendship.* Albany, NY: State University of New York Press.

Stjernfelt, F. (2014). *Natural Propositions. The Actuality of Peirce's Doctrine of Dicisigns.* Boston: Docent Press.

Tanaka, H., Nayebi, A., Maheswaranathan, N., McIntosh, L., Baccus, S. A., & Ganguli, S. (2019). From deep learning to mechanistic understanding in neuroscience: the structure of retinal prediction. https://ganguli-gang.stanford.edu/pdf/19.DeepRetinaUnderstanding.pdf

Varoquaux, G. & Thirion, B. (2014). How machine learning is shaping cognitive neuroimaging. *GigaSci*, 3, 28. doi: 10.1186/2047-217X-3-28

Wang, Y., Song, J., Guo, F., Zhang, Z., Yuan, S. & Cacioppo, S. (2016). Spatiotemporal brain dynamics of empathy for pain and happiness in friendship. *Frontiers in Behavorial Neuroscience*, *10*, 45. doi: 10.3389/fnbeh.2016.00045

Woods, B. K., Forbes, E. E., Sheeber, L. B., Allen, N. B., Silk, J. S., Jones, N. P., & Morgan, J. K. (2020). Positive affect between close friends: Brain–behavior associations during adolescence. *Social Neuroscience*, 15(2), 128–139. doi: 10.1080/17470919.2019.1662840

19

NEUROSEMIOTICS AND IDEOLOGY

A linguistic view

Annabelle Lukin and David Butt

Introduction

Despite distinct sociocultural origins, the study of ideological phenomena has much to offer the emerging field of neurosemiotics. Ideology – the human potential to construe one's experiences of some happening or state of affairs in a variety of ways – has traditionally been a central concept for the social and political sciences. But its "unrelenting pertinence" (Žižek, 1994: 1) has seen it break into fields as diverse as psychiatry (Wexler, 2006) as well as cognitive neuroscience and neuropsychology (Zmigrod & Tsakiris, 2021). In this much newer research environment, ideology has moved into the laboratory, and brains identified as home to specific ideological positions – for example, "liberals" vs. "conservatives" (Ahn et al., 2014; Kaplan et al., 2016; Leong et al., 2020; Nam et al., 2021; Rabin, 2020) and pro-Brexiteers (Zmigrod et al., 2018) – have been recruited in attempts to investigate "the neural basis of political cognition" (Leong et al., 2020: 27731), to elucidate "neural predictors" of political orientation as part of a search for "tools for ideology's biological measurement" (Ahn et al., 2014: 2697), to develop "a cognitive anatomy of ideologies" (Zmigrod et al., 2021: 11), and to challenge the orthodoxy that ideological variation is essentially a function of external factors (culture, society, environment) without some foundation in biology (Claessens et al., 2020).

Under this gaze, ideology has been reconsidered within established methods and discourse for the study of bio-semio-social behavior. In this process, the considerable literature on ideology in the social and political sciences, which has a history going back more than 200 years (McLellan, 1986), has been bypassed. Ideology in the laboratory is a narrow phenomenon, often defined in partisan terms despite party-based politics being a relatively recent historical development (Weber, 2004), or as dogmatic or doctrinally defensive behavior, embedded in cognitive or personality traits or categories, then measurable via a variety of psychological testing products. The enormous technological and statistical infrastructure of the cognitive and psychological sciences has been part of this enterprise, providing a basis for claims that micro-neuro phenomena can explain macro-ideological patterns of behavior. While the complex problem of causality in the relations of brain and ideology is acknowledged (Zmigrod et al., 2021), the thrust of this research is a search for neural and psychological/cognitive factors or mechanisms which "underlie," "predict," or "determine" ideological positions and behavior. Even genes have been linked to ideological stances (Alford et al., 2005; Claessens et al., 2020). Such studies typically avoid the use of the naturalistic texts that are the everyday vehicles of ideology (Leong et al., 2020), and they eschew discussion of the considerable structural and historically unique

DOI: 10.4324/9781003051817-23

innovations of modernity favorable to the spread of ideologies – printing, mass literacy, mass/social media, universal suffrage, the rise of standard languages, and the nation-state as the only viable political entity (Anderson, 1983; Gellner, 1983; Malešević, 2019). Since it has been argued that, under the conditions of modernity, ideology has become a deeper, more powerful force in communities than in previous epochs (Malešević, 2010, 2019), the impact of such forces on the collective shaping of minds cannot be overlooked.

Yet, clearly brain structure and processes are an integral part of the production and reproduction of ideological formations. Indeed, given the pervasiveness and power of ideology – consider, for instance, its central role in legitimating the brutal inter-state violence that was a hallmark of the twentieth century and that resulted in 110 million deaths directly caused by war (Malešević, 2010) – it seems likely that the brain is not only a generative site of ideology, but that the brain's properties facilitate the endless ideological creativity of humans. We will argue that this ideological creativity is a function both of properties of language and properties of the brain. We deal first with the ideological nature of language. We consider how ideology arises in language by looking through an evolutionary lens. We explain the ideological power of language as a function of the emergent complexity of language as humans left proto-language behind and created a semiotic system of many dimensions. Considering language as a crucial element in the evolutionary story of the human brain (Deacon, 1997; Edelman, 1992), the second part of the chapter presents key motifs in modern neuroscientific thinking that resonate with the ideological nature of language. The decision to consider first language and ideology and then the brain is not, however, intended to suggest priority.

While all semiotic systems are involved in shaping the environments of meaning in which young brains grow and mature, we focus on language because it is the "engine-room" of ideology (Lukin, 2019), being central to the creation and maintenance of ideologies. Language has a reach across all domains of our lives, and of all the semiotic modalities "at once defies time, is capable of being reflexive, classifies reality, construes communicable human experience and articulates the many voices of a culture with equal facility" (Hasan, 2005: 134). But ideology is also characteristic of language, deriving from the complexity and indeterminacy of language. As argued by leading neuroscientists, such as Deacon (1997) and Edelman (1992), this complexity of language is essential to the evolution of modern humans, shaping the nature and structure of their brains. It follows, therefore, that the human capacity for ideology is part of the human evolutionary story.

To explore the mutual commonalities of these research fields, we begin by examining the distinct origins of the terms "ideology" and "neurosemiotics," and present three key reasons for why neurosemiotics should engage with ideology. We then consider the concept of ideology with respect to two major uses of the term – what is referred to as the "particular" and the "total" view of ideology (Mannheim, 1936). We will argue, following Halliday, for the "total" view – that is, that language is inescapably ideological, precisely because ideological innovation is itself part of the internal organization of language. We will present Halliday's model of the rise of language out of an earlier proto-linguistic semiotic (encompassing and extending Saussure's model of the sign), through which language comes to have the essential properties of an apparently unlimited, "semogenic" (meaning-generating) system (Butt, 2001, 2015; Halliday, 2003a, 2003b). These properties are the "multistratal" complexity of language (i.e., its ordering of various levels of phonetics/phonology, lexicogrammar, and semantics), the metafunctional complexity of language (the three simultaneous functions of language, which all lexicogrammatical structures are in the service of), and the realizational complexity of language (the combination of both the arbitrary relation between lexicogrammar and expression, and a natural relation between lexicogrammar and semantics). As Deacon (1997: 69) notes in a chapter with the title "Symbols Aren't Simple," in fact the ideological potential of language is part of language's emergent complexity – a complexity that Halliday argues "defines the brain of homo sapiens" and is "what constitutes it as specifically human" (Halliday, 2003c: 390). From our discussion of the emergent complexity of language, with ideology as a feature of this complexity, we then draw out connections to some key themes in neuroscience. Our discussion includes topics such as the size, extent, complexity, and metastability of the brain; the non-computational nature of the brain; the hierarchical organizations of brain structure and processes; and Edelman's concept of "degeneracy" (Edelman & Gally, 2001).

Why ideology and neurosemiotics

Coined in the late eighteenth century, the concept of ideology is now over 200 years old. The rise of the concept of an "ism" – attested as early as the mid-seventeenth century[1] – suggests that the general idea of ideology had been in the ether for some time prior to the formal use of the term "ideology" by French Enlightenment philosopher Destutt de Tracy, in the foment of the French Revolution (Kennedy, 1979). By contrast, the term "neurosemiotics" is hyper-modern, associated with recent decades as the twentieth century became the century of brain sciences. Although early lexical combinations with the morpheme "neuro" are attested to from the eighteenth century, the term "neuroanatomy" is in evidence only by 1900,[2] while "neuroscience" is attested in the *Oxford English Dictionary* from just the early 1960s.[3] The term "neurosemiotics," originating in the late 1970s (Bouissac, 1998), is – like the earlier term "biosemiotics", coined in 1962 according to Barbieri (2009) – a call to interdisciplinarity. These intellectual innovations attest to an intellectual drive to explain how the human organism "transcend[s] the brute indexicality of physically present, coextensive and discrete relata ... to participate *interactively* across its own organizational levels – levels which include the intrinsically dynamic elements of neuron, body, sign and world" (Favareau, 2002: 5).

With the focus in this handbook on new synergies, it is timely, for a number of reasons, to bring the concept of ideology into direct contact with that of neurosemiotics. First, as we enter the third decade of the twentieth century, even more than in previous eras, ideological phenomena are setting the terms of human ways of living (Malešević, 2010). As every nation on Earth is currently living through a devastating pandemic, ideologies about the role of government, the delivery of and access to health services, corporate rights to intellectual property, and individual freedoms and responsibilities have an extended reach technologically, and are deeper in their consequences: a "battleground" of beliefs is leaving a growing body count. At the same time, one of the greatest existential challenges faced by humans, climate change due to global warming, is at the mercy of the ease with which public awareness and opinion can be shaped by those with vested interests in the burning of polluting fossil fuels. These are but two of many ideological domains that could be cited: the habits of mind/meaning that we call, for example, "racism," "sexism," "homophobia," "nationalism," "militarism" are real and powerful forces in the ways communities live and organize their resources (Weber, 2004).

Second, ideology presents the ultimate challenge for interrelating the scale of phenomena that the discipline of "neurosemiotics" must traverse. Part of the value of "ideology" to neurosemiotics is that it is an integrating principle: it can provide a counterweight to the tendencies in the cognitive sciences towards a focus on "fragments of analytically decomposed units," such as "bodiless faces," "language-free actions," or "situation-independent words" (Ibáñez & García, 2018: 56). Ideologies are shared, large-scale, supra-individual, multi-modal, historically, and socially variable phenomena: they depend on the intricate structure and potential of the human brain in reciprocal engagement with the intricate structure and potential of human language. Without having to be entirely consistent or coherent, ideologies provide principles of unity and continuity in the interpretation of human experience (Thompson, 1984). They are, arguably, a means of maintaining homeostasis (Damasio, 2012: p.47ff). As such, a reconciliation of the terms "ideology" and "neurosemiotics" invites and requires a scholarly gaze, which can encompass the large scale vistas of human behaviors in their socio-cultural contexts with the features and characteristics of human brains that enable the production and reproduction of ideologies.

Third, as neurosemiotics debates its conceptual foundations, it must test different theories of the central phenomena of the field. Different scientific theories of brain and mind, or of sign and meaning, as well as theories of the interaction of these phenomena, can be thought of as having their own distinct ideologies. In addition, since the progress of neurosemiotics is dependent on language, and language is (as we will argue) ideologically saturated (Vološinov, 1973), then attention to ideology is important for the field to be self-reflective and self-aware. Every category or principle in neurosemiotics is formed out of the ideologically rich resource of language. As much as a grounding in scientific method is important for the field, neurosemiotics – like all science – is shaped by the ideologies of its era and its progenitors. For neurosemiotics to deliver on the promise of its grand title, it must be able to interrogate its own ideological biases. For example, the "classical" definition of neurosemiotics – an "epistemological domain which includes the scientific investigation of the neurological processes *underlying* communicative behavior in all its forms" (Bouissac, 1986: 204, emphasis added) – reflects what we might call a "neuro-first" bias, part of an ideology which has been described as "neurofetishism" (Cornejo & Valsiner, 2018: 5). When neurological processes are described as "underlying" ideology, they are in some sense construed as having primacy, either in phenomenal or in explanatory terms, or both. If the emerging field of neurosemiotics continues to speak in terms of the biological or neurological "basis" of phenomena, it will contribute to maintaining the assumptions it is seeking to challenge.

Given the force of ideology in all our lives, private and professional, then a field encapsulated by a term like "neurosemiotics" ought to turn its attention to the concept of ideology.

Defining ideology

"Ideology" as a self-conscious concept has had over 200 years of discussion, debate, and disagreement within philosophy, sociology, and political science. If there was a prize for the most contested concept, "ideology would very nearly rank first" (Giddens, 1983: 18). Despite these definitional difficulties, emphasis on ideological debate has persisted through a plethora of academic fashions (Malešević & MacKenzie, 2002), and "ideology" has been pursued further under a variety of analogues and partial synonyms. These include, for example, "worldview," "subjectivity," "discursive formation," "*zeitgeist*," "*habitus*," "frames," and "*umwelt*."

"Ideology" has been used with two principal meanings, described as the "particular" view and the "total" view of ideology (Mannheim, 1936). In the "particular" view, ideology is reduced to particular sets of ideas/beliefs considered to be misguided or distorted with reference to some set of conditions. The partial view suggests that while some minds can be fooled into a misrecognition of the way things are, other minds can experience reality directly without the mediation of false conceptions. Two large historical figures – Napoleon and Marx – played key roles in the construction of this narrow, pejorative view of ideology. Napoleon used the concept to criticize his enemies, whom he called "ideologues" (McLellan, 1986), while for Marx ideologies were connected to the unequal distribution of power and resources, as in his famous dictum "the ideas of the ruling class are in every epoch the ruling ideas" (Marx & Engels, 1985: 64). For Marx, ideology was understood within the terms of the classic bifurcation of "materialism" and "idealism," between "real, active men … on the basis of their real life-process" and "the phantoms formed in the human brain" (Marx & Engels, 1985: 47).

In the second and "total" conception of the term, ideology is pervasive and inescapable, denoting the "ideology of an age or of a concrete historico-social group," and referring to "the characteristics and composition of the total structure of the mind of this epoch or of this group" (Mannheim, 1936: 56). From this perspective, the concept connects to traditions in philosophies of epistemology and the sociology of knowledge, in which human thinking arises and operates "not in a social vacuum but in a definite social milieu" (Mannheim, 1936: 80). Where the partial view of ideology is synonymous with "false consciousness," in the total view ideology is akin to patterns of consciousness *per se*. All thinking is marked by the socially, historically, and culturally based experience of thinkers. Indeed, as Mannheim argued, thought "is a particularly sensitive index of social and cultural change" (Mannheim, 1936: 83) and is therefore "inherently" ideological (Mannheim, 1936: 53). From this perspective, even science cannot escape the influence of ideology, an intellectual conundrum referred to as "Mannheim's paradox" (Geertz, 1973: 194): if ideology is inescapable, then all attempts to analyze ideology are also ideological acts. This does not discount the value of any particular scholarly project: it can still be judged on its efficacy in explaining its object of study.

The total view of ideology is closer to the original concept of ideology when it was coined at the end of the eighteenth century. Then it referred to the study of the "history of our means of knowledge," in order to lay out "the first principles of all other branches of our knowledge" (Destutt de Tracy, 1817: ix). Ideology no longer holds this meaning, but in the context of this handbook, we note that the original meaning grew out of an inquiry that, had the study been current, would have been described as "neurosemiotic." When invoking the term, Destutt de Tracy took inspiration from the philosophical work of Étienne Bonnot de Condillac (1714–1780), whose *Essay on the Origin of Human Knowledge*, published in 1746, was striving to balance humans' biological and cognitive endowments with the role of experience, including in particular the role of signs in the emergence of knowledge and reasoning (Condillac, 2001). Condillac argued that words were "like bonds that prevent [ideas] from coming apart," adding that "you will admit that you cannot take a single step without finding yourself in a state of chaos, if you do not have signs to determine the number of simple ideas you have collected together" (Condillac, 2001: 81). The original concept of ideology, therefore, derives from a philosophical reflection on the interaction between the biological inheritance of humans in interaction with signs as organizing principles for interpreting human experience. This seems to us to be a key to the resonance between ideology and neurosemiotics.

We argue that the plasticity of language and of the brain favors the total view of ideology. Yet, whether in its "partial" or "total" view, the concept, by virtue of its claims to explain the malleability of the human mind, touches on issues that are already at the center of neurosemiotics, namely, the need to see the brain/mind complex in relation to humans' socio-historically located meaning-making practices. While, in relation to epistemological inquiry, the study of ideology appears to be an outsider to the experimental fields of neuroscience, the more recent vectors of neuroscientific theory from Vygotsky to Edelman have all emphasized the status of semiotic behavior as the *sine non qua* of the evolution of higher order consciousness. Ideology is a concept, then, that merits a place in the interdisciplinarity of sciences of human experience. In fact, ideology has the potential to open up new questions – especially in relation to meaning and motivations in context – and to contribute to the genuine interdisciplinarity demanded by the binomial neurosemiotics.[4]

The ideological potential of language

In this section, we explain the origins of ideology in the evolution of language. Though ideology is a manifestation of the complementarity of the brain and language, we focus here on the profound interconnection between language and ideology, which reaches right back into the evolution of language. The intersection of language and ideology has received less attention in linguistics than it deserves, and linguistic theories have offered very different accounts of ideology – see Lukin (2019). Some linguists have had little or nothing to say about the role of language in ideological innovation. Chomsky, for instance, despite coauthoring a classic work in the field of propaganda studies (Herman & Chomsky, 2002), rejects any role for linguistics in the study of power and politics (Lukin, 2019: p10–11). Others, in fields as diverse as cognitive linguistics (e.g., Lakoff), critical discourse analysis (e.g., Fairclough), and pragmatics (e.g., Verscheuren), argue that language is often, but not always, ideological (Lukin, 2019). Linguists such as Vološinov, Halliday, and Hasan have argued that language is inescapably ideological (with Vološinov making this claim in the late 1920s, presenting the first semiotic account of ideology). To truly recognize the pervasiveness and power of ideology, linguistic theories must be able to explain how language, in consort with our brains, enables our astonishing potential for ideological creativity. As Hasan argues, linguistic theories ought to be tested against their potential to explain the ideological power of language (Hasan, 2009).

The linguistic claim from Chomsky that language has no ideological power worthy of serious consideration (Otero, 2004) can be dismissed as simply observationally inadequate: it relies on seeing language as a completely inert medium through which pre-existing cognitive content can be expressed. Further, to argue that language is only sometimes ideological, and that therefore it can be used in non-ideological ways, is also untenable. This position requires that language be, simultaneously, two completely distinct substances: on the one hand, an agent in the process of construing meaning when it is ideological; and on the other, a mere mirror of experience when it is functioning without ideological parameters. Those who propose this position have not explained how language could be both of these things at the same time. When linguistic theories are tested in the crucible of ideology, those that survive embrace ideology as a fundamental property of language.

To explain ideological creativity in language, we need to look into the deep history of language, in particular the extended moment in the evolution of language in which humans moved from proto-language (a type of semiotic system shared with many other species) to the complex, uniquely human semiotic of modern language. In the evolutionary history of language, and in its ontogenetic development in individuals, meaning is a function of what Halliday and others have called "proto-language." For Halliday, proto-language is a bistratal semiotic system, along the lines of the *signifié/signifiant* of the Saussurean sign. Proto-language, Halliday (2002: 353) argues, "probably evolved out of the contradiction between the two primary modes of experience, the material and conscious." Halliday reminds us that proto-language is not a collection or aggregate of individual signs, but rather a "two-dimensional semiotic space constituting a sign system" (Halliday, 2002: 353). Human proto-linguistic sign systems, according to Halliday, exhibit a microfunctional organization in which two forms of consciousness – action and reflection – intersect with two domains of experience, the dyadic dynamic of "you and me" versus that of "the rest." In this intersection, proto-languages generate four distinct "microfunctions": the regulatory, the instrumental, the interactional, and the personal (Halliday, 2002: 353) (see Figure 19.1).

Despite proto-language in this phase of human evolution and development being considerably simpler than what comes after, proto-language exhibits key qualities that are important for a neurosemiotic approach to ideology. First, proto linguistic sign systems grow out of functional pressures grounded in human sociality. Second, the proto-linguistic sign, even prior to the rise of the more intricate organization of language, is a complex reconciliation of meaning and matter. It constructs an interface between the phenomena of human experience and the meanings through which such phenomena are brought into a shared interactive space – the principle Saussure called the "signified." The sign requires a second interface (Saussure's "signifier") since "there can be no meaning without expression" (Halliday, 2002: 354). At this interface, meaning is turned towards the material body of the meaning-making subject as articulation or gesture. The process is no less than "the transduction of the phenomenal back into the phenomenal via these two interfaces of content and expression" (Halliday, 2002: 355). The formation of proto-linguistic signs, as such, dissolves the

Form of consciousness / Domain of experience	Action	Reflection
1st/2nd person	Regulatory	Interactional
3rd person	Instrumental	Personal

Figure 19.1 The proto-language *microfunctions*
Taken from Halliday (2002: 353).

"material" versus "ideal" binary on which Cartesian philosophy has rested for hundreds of years (Butt, 2015).

In these fundamental properties of the sign, two key characteristics of language are evident: the dependency of meaning on expression means that meaning-making is an embodied and intersubjective activity (Halliday, 2002: 354). Being grounded in the human body and human interaction, sign systems therefore depend on and realize human sociality. They grow by virtue of human connections, by humans who are always located in some particular geographical, historical, and cultural space and time. At the same time, the interface of the signifier with phenomena of human experience is a process of transforming experience into shared meanings. This process is not a passive reflection or encoding of already determined content, but an active construal of experience via a process of "reciprocal delimitation," the mysterious means by which the *signifié* and *signifiant* carve out the mutuality of their fused conceptual domains in the brain – note, crucially, that *both* sides of Saussure's sign are conceptual.

Since all languages depend on this conjunction of two fundamentally distinct substances, Hasan has proposed that this "conjunction of two dissimilars" binds "the signal and its meaning into a unity," and, as such, forms part of the "biogenetic capital that the baby has inherited as a member of the human species" (Hasan, 2016a: 103). Babies must navigate the conjunction of two dissimilars well before they are capable of being taught this principle. The generative power of this biogenetic capital can only be realized if there is "validation and reciprocity": a system of values, salience, and motivations must emerge, inherent in the sign process. Without an already acculturated (*viz.,* already ideologized) caregiver to engage in joint semiosis, this biogenetic capital goes without activation (Hasan, 2016a). Not only does this caregiving have to happen in the ecology of social and cultural contexts – as this is simply how humans live – but the contexts provide the motivating environments in which this biogenetic capital can express itself (Hasan, 2016b).

As powerful as this simple sign principle is, the evolution of language shows that human cultures had to move beyond proto-linguistic-based communication. In a critical move in our evolution, human cultures collectively generate the semiotic force that splits the sign apart – a moment described in Lukin (2019: 18) as the "semiotic big bang." In this process, a wholly abstract level of structural organization, lexicogrammar, becomes interpolated between the content and expression planes of the sign. Figure 19.2 represents Halliday's comparison of the multistratal organization of language (Figure 19.2b), compared with proto-language (Figure 19.2a). Figure 19.2b shows lexicogrammar as an internal level of language, with an interface to meaning and the ecosocial environment, and to phonetics and the human body. Lexicogrammar, created by "the collective human consciousness," provides humans with "a semiotic space which is truly elastic, in that it can expand in any number of directions" (Halliday, 2002: 356). Through this process, meaning in human language becomes "grammaticalized" – that is, linguistic meanings come to be realized in patterns of grammatical configurations, with the consequence that the symbolic organization of language becomes "freed from direct dependence on the phenomenal, and can develop a structure of its own" (Halliday, 2002: 356). Lexicogrammar, the primary innovation that transforms proto-languages into adult human language, provides the essential semiotic machinery for language to be ideological. Indeed, Halliday has described grammar as "the ideological interpretant that is built into language itself" (Halliday, 2003d: 135). Humans are "ideological creatures that search for meaning" (Malešević, 2019: 61), and the emergence of lexicogrammar is the socio-historical or collective product of this search.

In its shift to becoming a stratally more complex semiotic system, language has gained additional properties of organization. It retains its arbitrary relation between content and expression, indicated in Figure 19.2b by double dotted lines. Yet, in becoming more stratally complex, language has also become realizationally complex, adding to the arbitrary mode of realization a new principle of realization that relates lexicogrammar and semantics, and that amplifies the power of the arbitrariness of the sign. Thus, Halliday argues, the relation between these strata is "natural," not arbitrary. This means that the systems of grammar in a language – using English as the example, systems such as polarity,

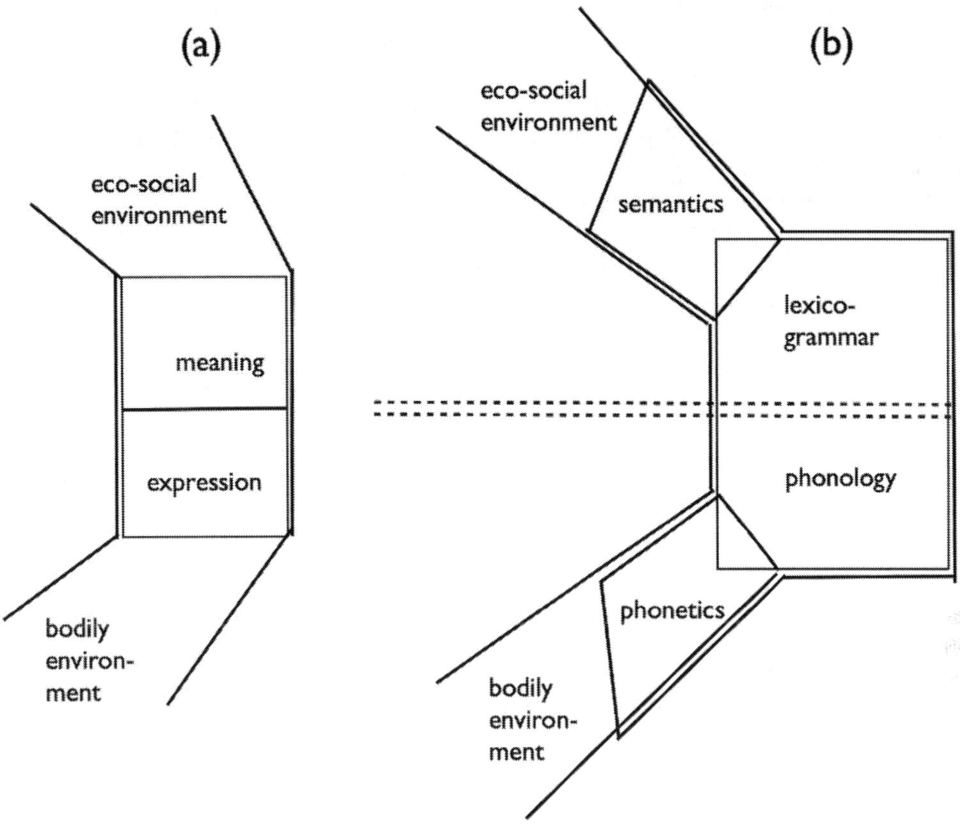

Figure 19.2 The stratal organization of proto-language and language
Taken from Halliday (2003b).

number, person, tense/aspect, and mood – give us back as linguistic systems aspects of our experience of and interactions with our ecosocial environment. It also means that every shift on one stratum demands a change on the other: a different choice in the lexicogrammar will have a semantic consequence, however nuanced. Combining now two principles of realization – the arbitrary and the natural – language becomes an expanding, ideologically plastic, semogenic potential, limited only by "human articulatory and auditory capabilities and the capacity of the human brain" (Halliday, 2003d: 75).

The natural relation of lexicogrammar to semantics – as the nature of grammatical systems in languages shows – ensures that ideologies are patterns of meanings that stay close to human experience. Grammatical systems, while they vary across the diversity of human languages, are not arbitrary: they are indexical of cultural preoccupations about phenomena such as time, cause, agency, thingness, process, relevance, interactive roles, and so on. These grammatical systems are a reflection of a further principle in the organization of language, also opened up by the stratificational complexity of language. The interpolation of the wholly abstract stratum of lexicogrammar, combined with the arbitrary nature of the sign, enables linguistic structure to be "metafunctional." Humans, through their collective socio-semiotic pressure on language, generate meaning-making systems that allow them – indeed, require them – to combine meanings that are at the same time interpersonal, ideational, and textual. The metafunctional character of language means that it is simultaneously a system for acting and thinking, as well as for building text and relevance to context. Language itself has been shaped by the two modes of being – acting and thinking – and their manifestation in meaning (Halliday, 2013). For Halliday, acting, or "enacting," means "ongoingly manag[ing] our interactions with other people, from the small-scale encounters of daily life to the pronouncements with which we maintain our social networks and our own identities within them" (Halliday, 2003d: 74). Interpersonally, grammar is a "form of praxis, and the key evolutionary step for this was dialogue" (Halliday, 2003d: 74). By the process of thinking, or "construing," Halliday means "that we are all the time rehearsing and reinforcing our sense of reality, recognizing and naming categories of phenomena such as processes and entities, and the complex relationships among them" (Halliday, 2003d: 74). Here, Halliday argues, grammar functions as a theory – "a well-tried theory of human experience, no less." The key evolutionary development for this mode of experience was reference (Halliday, 2003d: 74).

Because language users combine meanings of three distinct kinds, built into the linguistic system is a principle of organization that ensures there is no neutral mode of representation. The construing of experience has to be done with regard to some addressee, ranging from a known specific individual, to a mass virtual audience, and is always a product of culture. Language does not prioritize one of these metafunctions over another: the modes of meaning – the ideational and the interpersonal – co-evolved. Speakers choose from the various systems that constitute the ideational and the interpersonal metafunctions, but this freedom to combine options from these two metafunctions is limited by the need for meaning-making to be coherent with respect to some context of situation. Halliday's "textual function" provides the resources by which speakers organize the flow of discourse to create coherent text responsive to the pressure of social context. In bringing these two different meaning types into single structures, language creates a "parallel universe of its own: a world that is made of meaning, and hence instantiated in the semiotic process" (Halliday, 2003a: 276). Halliday (2003a) argues that it is in the "interstices" between the experiential and the interpersonal function that bias comes into the text – in other words, that simply by creating text, ideological principles come into play.

In addition, the complexity of language means the act of making meaning has to be a largely unconscious affair. Halliday shows, for example, that a single lexical verb can be formulated into at least 40,000 distinct options, taking into account the grammatical systems of tense, polarity, modality, finiteness, voice, and aspect, among others (Halliday, 2003b). Language could not function if humans were consciously choosing all elements of wording and structure, even in the production of simple text. This complexity, combined with the narrowing of options under the force of context, provides impetus for prior patterns of choice to become "least effort" options, creating habitual "fashions of speaking" (viz., ideologies), carved out from the endless potential of language.

Halliday has argued that this "explosion into grammar" as humans collectively create the multilevel semiotic system of language (Halliday, 2002: 355) enabled for us nothing less than the move from primary consciousness – the "tyranny of the extended present," in the words of Edelman – to higher-order consciousness, a state that Edelman has argued is language-dependent (Edelman, 1992: 395). In its new form, language achieves "a massive reconciliation of conflicting principles of order – this being the only way of 'semioticizing' our complex ecosocial environment in a way that is favorable to our survival" (Halliday, 2003b: 29). In heralding the arrival of the potential for language to construe alternative, even contradictory versions of experience, the development that enables the emergence of "higher-order consciousness" also brings with it the ideological potential of language.

The ideological brain

We have argued that ideologies are facilitated by the organization of language. Yet there must also be a congruence between the organization of language and the organization of neuronal dynamics that realize ideological productivity. In short, brains become "ideologized," so we must ask: What is it in the structure, properties, and especially the functions of human brains that make them so ideologically creative? In response to this question, we turn to an ensemble of specialist research which marks a significantly dramatic revision of the popular, deterministic ideas that ruled over human sciences, from psychology and cognitive sciences, and evolutionary theory in the early to the mid twentieth century – for critiques of determinism see, for example, Edelman & Tononi (2000: 37–50) on neural Darwinism, and Shapiro (2011: 145–147) on evolution viewed from the science of the twenty-first century. These revisions emphasize certain significant properties and principles concerning the growth and dynamics of neuronal formation in human brains. These properties include the evolutionary benefit of the combination of variability and metastability in the vectors of change in the brain; the numerical size or "population" character of neurons; that neuronal organization has no computer-like central processor (viz., the brain is organic, not algorithmic); that the brain involves layers or strata, which enable levels of activation and inhibition for arriving at a threshold or "choice"; and that the brain and language are paradigmatic cases of a positive feature, "degeneracy" (an architecture that finds more than one route to realize a goal or function). In considering these changes of outlook for the development of neurosemiotics, we arrive at a fresh vision of how the potential for investigating ideologies from biological and neuroscientific perspectives has joined closely with the novel social sciences and population thinking that gave the topic of "ideology" its burst of relevance from the eighteenth to the twentieth centuries.

Size, extent, complexity, and metastability of the brain

A starting point for our discussion is the enormous congruence between the semiotic potential of a linguistic system and the seemingly unlimited circuitry available in the brain. Halliday emphasizes the infinite potential of the stratified system of a language – recall the earlier discussion of the number of possible structural forms for a single lexical verb being at least 40,000 (Halliday, 2003b). Like language, the brain is capable of an astounding degree of innovation, having, according to Edelman, ten followed by a million noughts of alternative circuits, more than all the atoms in the cosmos, the latter being only ten with 79 zeros (Edelman & Tononi, 2000: 38). Language and brain, therefore, display architectures that appear unlimited. Size and extent are indexical of complexity in the phenomena. The increasing complexity in language, of which ideological variability is a realization, is both enabled by and enabling of the development of the complexity of the human brain. Deacon (1997: 344), in his co-evolution thesis, argues that "a robust and persistent trend in brain structure evolution reflects forces of natural selection acting on major brain functions [and that this] correlate[s] with the development of a unique human facility for symbols." This echoes our discussion on the human biogenetic capacity to unite two "dissimilars," which is the foundation of the sign. Drawing on Edelman, Halliday (2003c: 395) argues that "the brain has evolved in coping with ever more complex environments; what is significant is not just the complexity of the organism but the complexity of its relationship with its environment."

As in language, the extent and complexity of neuronal populations and circuitry in the brain in fact assist in maintaining equilibrium in the system, or metastability. In a system of systems (like the central nervous system, or language, or social patterns), change is less likely to be chaotic since it needs to be realized across a layered and hierarchical architecture. To come about at all, change has to come about on a number of levels. Dehaene (2014: 167) reminds us of an idea suggested by William James, namely that consciousness looks like "an organ added for the sake of steering a nervous system grown too complex to regulate itself." Metastability in the brain is an echo of our discussions earlier of "fashions of speaking": habitual patterns favor the creation and iteration of ideologies.

The brain is not like a computer

The brain, again as emphasized by Edelman, is not computer-like: it is selectional, not instructional, and it carries out "categorizations on value" (Edelman 1992: 227). The brain is crucially *inexact* – that is, non-determinative in any absolute sense (Edelman & Tononi, 2000: 47). There is, then, an enormity of potential for dealing with the probabilistic dynamism of the lived conditions of a total organism. The "ideological brain" is also based on the potential for variation, for the extravagant realizations that semiotic systems offer. These extravagant realizations are the foundations of neuronal adaptation, now accentuated in the popularized metaphor of "plasticity." As noted by Dehaene (2014) as well as Edelman and Tononi (2000) at various points in their work, a crucial fact about the brain is that in it you see an architecture that defies central command and fixed determinations while eschewing categorial "instruction." It uses "selection," with its Darwinian meaning, as in the transfer of Edelman's concepts from his study of immunology over to populations of neurons: "Neural Darwinism." Dehaene's use of the metaphor of a "workspace" has some characteristics of what might be called a "neuronal parliament," where values are passed up from ensembles or coordinations of action *and* inhibition in the circuits. As with ideological creativity, it is the multiplicity of possible responses to living, the abundance of construals of experiences, that supports innovative adaptations to experience. These possibilities become the potential for widely "broadcasted" messages through the central nervous system (broadcasting being for Dehaene another key metaphor characterizing the signatures of consciousness).

Hierarchy, stratification, value, and re-entry: The modeling of brain structure and function

Ideologies are the outcome of values (realized as significant differences), which "decide" the global response of the organism. The neuronal ensemble, across hierarchies of organization, realizes ideology – that is, the ensemble embodies it. The hierarchical organization of the evolved human brain can be illustrated by a range of factors. Every reference to levels (or to the strata of different kinds of organization) constitutes a statement of hierarchy. Both long-standing and emerging neuroscientific discussion of the interplay of hierarchy of levels in the brain and central nervous systems are analogical with respect to the multistratal organization of human semiotic behavior. In the mid-nineteenth century, Hughlings Jackson propounded a theory of the brain's hierarchical evolution – see extended discussions by Meares (1999, 2012) and reference in Arbib (2012: 153). Jackson emphasized levels of higher complexity that could be subject to disaggregation or disinhibition due to physical damage or trauma, resulting in a regress to responses from more "primitive" systems – for instance, of fear and flight. Feinberg and Mallatt (2016: 26ff) write in terms of "complex neuronal hierarchies" as they set out a detailed account of the stages of evolutionary development of "experience" over the 520 million years of vertebrate evolution. The significance of neuronal hierarchies can also be illustrated by a discussion of bottom-up/top-down messaging in the brain. An example comes from Dehaene (2014) in his application of Granger causality analysis to the complexity of connections in the "Brain Web." Although there has to be ascending messages which "climb up to increasingly abstract representations," another question arises from the "tangled relations." Dehaene (2014: 139) asks why "top-down projections often outnumber ascending ones." In testing for signatures of consciousness – that is, those that reach the 300 millisecond threshold of conscious "ignition" – he suggests that "anterior regions were desperately interrogating sensory areas" and that their failure to respond "resulted in the absence of conscious perception" (Dehaene, 2014: 140).

"Value" may seem to be a concept of a very different kind, but it is linked to hierarchy, and it is a term that appears at the core of theories of the neuronal selection and consciousness – *viz.*, in the reciprocation in the dynamic core hypothesis of Edelman; in the relevance "router" of the global neuronal workspace of Dehaene and Baars (Dehaene, 2014: 140); and in the discussion of biological value, biological "idioms," and "leitmotif of life regulation" (Damasio, 2012: 59). To pass messages across strata or different levels in a system, the selectional process of a message is regarded as a "value." Therefore, a value is a difference with consequences. The dominant traffic of messages within the brain suggests exchanges between distinct regions and circuits – for instance, between perception and behavior. Such exchanges must then build and/or confirm values across levels which count as "decisions." The interdependence of the terms of the sub-heading (hierarchy, stratification, value, re-entry) becomes apparent since the last term, *re-entrant* neurons, enables the traffic of *values* in *hierarchies* of neuronal reciprocation between brain regions. Edelman and Tononi explain "re-entry" as follows:

> Re-entry depends on the possibility of cycles of signaling in the thalamocortical meshwork and other networks mentioned earlier. It is the ongoing, recursive interchange of parallel signals between *reciprocally connected areas* [emphasis added] of the brain, an interchange that continually coordinates the activities of these area's maps to each other in space and time … reentry allows for a unity of perception and behavior that would be otherwise impossible given the absence in the brain of a unique, computerlike central processor with detailed instructions or of algorithmic calculations for the coordination of functionally segregated areas.
>
> *(Edelman & Tononi, 2000: 48–49)*

The analogy between neuronal and biological systems of selection on the one hand, and semiotic/ideological factors on the other, is extremely direct in the thinking of Damasio. The connection appears to be homological, rather than just analogy:

> Consciousness enabled humans to repeat the leitmotif of life regulation by means of a collection of cultural instruments – economic exchange, religious beliefs, ethical rules, laws, arts, science, technology. Still, the survival intention of the eukaryotic cell and the survival intention implicit in human consciousness are one and the same.
>
> *(Damasio, 2012: 59)*

Degeneracy

Edelman and colleagues emphasize the capacity of a system to reconfigure itself in order to reach a potential outcome (goal) by an alternative structural arrangement (Edelman & Gally, 2001). They offer a list of 22 systems that illustrate this active potential. Language is listed among these biological phenomena. We suggest that ideological thinking could be added as an index of the generative output of brains with regard to selectional principles, anticipating the demands on the basis of experience. Such output could be viewed negatively, as over-generative, much in the way that some theorists evaluate consciousness as a maladaptive aspect of humans – see a discussion of examples in Dehaene (2014: 89–114). The partial view of ideology is a similar case of emphasizing the negative consequences of a human potential. While the degree of openness of an unconstrained system promotes the probability of novel responses to experience, it may also thereby increase the chance of complex and maladaptive choice. Yet "degeneracy" is the systemic character central to behavioral and semiotic innovation.

Concluding remarks: Integrating ideology into neurosemiotics

The semiotic brain emerges as an organ which has evolved with an anticipation of – or a readiness to accept – guidance as to how it can circumvent its own structural limitations. The properties of and perspectives on the brain, as outlined in the four subsections above are, we believe, representative of an already established platform of research in which neuro- and socio-contextual perspectives can and must be integrated and refined through critique and interdisciplinary dialogue. We have argued that the origins of ideology lie in an inquiry that in our modern idiom would be considered "neurosemiotic" in orientation, suggesting both a deeper history for neurosemiotics, as well as a natural link to the problem of ideology. Modern developments in neuroscience, both technological – for example, the imaging of Posner and Raichle (1994) – and conceptual – for example, the population-based neural Darwinism of Edelman (1992) – provide new opportunities for the kind of bio-semio-social explanation of mind that Condillac initiated in the mid eighteenth century. In linguistics, while the emphatic Cartesianism and Platonism of some proponents of idealized universals overshadowed much of the latter part of the twentieth century, key technological developments – for example, the rise of corpus linguistics (McEnery & Hardie, 2013) – and conceptual advances – for example, the recognition of ideology as a feature of the complexity and indeterminacy of language, discussed above – also open up new possibilities for understanding the power and reach of ideology. The combination of these technological and conceptual developments enables linguists to bring out the unconscious, collective ideological patterning in discourse that human communities produce and are shaped by.

The problem of ideology has increased urgency, since the conditions of modernity allow for a wider and deeper reach of ideologies, including that our models of reality are increasingly distant from direct local experience. The neurosemiotic agenda must therefore embrace the problem of ideology, and consider how it might contribute to a deeper understanding of the processes by which brains become minds in their encounters with meaning. That brains become ideologized is a reality about which none of us can be in doubt: all of us deal in our face-to-face and digitally-mediated interactions with individuals shaped by the ideologies of their communities. If brains are ideologized it is because they are "ideologizable." We have argued that this is a natural extension of the co-evolution of the brain and language (Deacon, 1997) and the co-evolution of language and ideology (discussed above).

We have offered some discussion of the properties of the brain that might explain its role in human ideological creativity, and we have emphasized some principles which are necessary to accommodate the problem of ideology in a neurosemiotic context. While there will always be experimental research seeking to explain human ideological behavior with reference to neural or genetic determinism, these positions are in contradiction to the principles of brain organization that appear to be the basis of a gathering and dramatically different consensus. One career-long investigation characterizes the exciting prospects of future research about claims of human nature. Feldman Barrett (2017: 166–169) argues against the fixed topological mapping of brain regions, noting, for example, the paucity and contradictory character of evidence over Broca's region as the language area directly related to Broca's aphasia (Feldman Barrett, 2017). Given the role Broca's claims have played in assumptions in linguistics and psychology, there is much at stake here. Feldman Barrett notes that lesions in that area are neither a necessary nor a sufficient condition for Broca's aphasia; and that recent consensus is that the "region" is not language-specific at all, but "part of several intrinsic networks, including the interoceptive and control networks". She emphasizes: "Where language is concerned, the control network helps your brain choose between conflicting options" (Feldman Barrett, 2017: 167). This is very much like the kind of network that would be congruent with Halliday's ideas about language as a dynamic open system, a system best represented by networks of options – that is, in paradigms.

Feldman Barrett's emphatic rejection of Broca's claim for language to be "located" in the brain is part of her overall rejection of classical "brain blob" theories – the idea that "the brain evolved as a bunch of blobs with distinct, dedicated functions" (Feldman Barrett, 2017: 167). Her specific focus is on understanding the brain in relation to "how emotions are made" (the title of her 2017 book). Emotions, she argues, are neurally distributed and language-dependent. Each instance of an emotion is a "whole brain state" and gets unity through a conceptual/linguistic category, like the word *fear*. Such a unit results, then, from the properties of the brain and the language-mediated process of socialization. She argues that nature endowed our brains with "the raw materials to wire itself with a conceptual system" (Feldman Barrett, 2017: 103). Feelings like fear are the conjunction of this natural endowment with the "input from a chorus of helpful adults who spoke emotion words to you in a deliberate and intentional way" (Feldman Barrett, 2017: 103). If something such as the feeling of fear needs to be semiotically constructed, how much more so the complex semiotic structures and patterns that we know as ideologies. When a notion as fundamental – that is, seemingly natural – as our feeling of fear needs to be reconstrued through the languages and personal contexts of humans, our proclivity for the complex semiotic ensembles we describe as "ideologies" merits novel interdisciplinary efforts.

As we pursue a more multidimensional – neurosemiotic – explanation of ideology, the question is not where ideologies are found in brains, but how brains help create and reproduce ideological phenomena, and why. The next steps towards an answer to these questions will require neurosemiotic innovation: a new openness to understanding ideology, brain, and social priorities as realized in the specifics of our languages.

Notes

1 "ism, n." OED Online. Oxford University Press, December 2021.
2 "neuroanatomy, n.-" OED Online. March 2021. Oxford University Press. www.oed.com/view/Entry/235294?redirectedFrom=neuroanatomy
3 "neuroscience, n.-" OED Online. March 2021. Oxford University Press. www.oed.com/view/Entry/235290?redirectedFrom=neuroscience
4 This presentation of ideology is necessarily brief: a useful summary of the literature can be found in McLellan (1986).

References

Ahn, W., Kishida, K. T., Gu, X., Lohrenz, T., Harvey, A., Hibbing, J. R., Dayan, P., & Montague, R. R. (2014). Nonpolitical images evoke neural predictors of political ideology. *Current Biology, 24*, 2693–2699. doi: 10.1016/j.cub.2014.09.050

Alford, J. R., Funk, C. L., & Hibbing, J. R. (2005). Are political orientations genetically transmitted? *American Political Science Review, 99*, 153–167. doi: 10.1017/S0003055405051579

Anderson, B. (1983). *Imagined Communities: Reflections on the Origin and Spread of Nationalism*. New York: Verso.

Arbib, M. A. (2012). *How the Brain Got Language: The Mirror System Hypothesis*. Oxford: Oxford University Press.

Barbieri, M. (2009). A short history of biosemiotics. *Biosemiotics, 2*, 221–245. doi: 10.1007/s12304-009-9042-8

Bouissac, P. (1986). Semiotics in Canada. In P. Bouissac (Ed.), *The Semiotic Web* (pp. 191–252). Berlin: Mouton de Gruyter.

Bouissac, P. (Ed.). (1998). *Encyclopedia of Semiotics*. Oxford: Oxford University Press.

Butt, D. G. (2001). Firth, Halliday and the development of systemic functional theory. In S. Auroux, E. F. K. Koerner, H. Niederehe, & K. Versteegh (Eds.), *History of the Language Sciences: An International Handbook on the Evolution of the Study of Language from the Beginnings to the Present*, Vol. 2 (pp. 1806–1838). Berlin: Walter de Gruyter.

Butt, D. G. (2015). The "history of ideas" and Halliday's natural science of meaning. In J. J. Webster (Ed.), *The Bloomsbury Companion to M. A. K. Halliday* (pp. 17–61). London: Bloomsbury.

Claessens, S., Fischer, K., Chaudhuri, A., Sibley, C. G., & Atkinson, Q. D. (2020). The dual evolutionary foundations of political ideology. *Perspective, 4*, 336–345. doi: 10.1038/s41562-020-0850-9

Condillac, E. B. D. (2001). *Essay on the Origin of Human Knowledge* (H. Aarsleff, Trans.). Cambridge: Cambridge University Press.

Cornejo, C., & Valsiner, J. (2018). Neurosciences in psychology: What stays after the "decade of the brain" has passed? In A. Ibáñez and A, M. García, *Contextual Cognition: The Sensus Communis of a Situated Mind* (pp. v–ix). Heidelberg: Springer.

Damasio, A. (2012). *Self Comes to Mind: Constructing the Conscious Brain*. New York: Vintage.

Deacon, T. (1997). *The Symbolic Species: The Co-evolution of Language and the Human Brain*. New York: Penguin.

Dehaene, S. (2014). *Consciousness and the Brain: Deciphering How the Brain Codes our Thoughts*. New York: Penguin.

Destutt de Tracy, A. (1817). *A Treatise of Political Economy: Elements of Ideology* (T. Jefferson, Trans.). Georgetown, VA: Joseph Milligan.

Edelman, G. (1992). *Bright Air, Brilliant Fire: On the Matter of the Mind*. New York: Penguin.

Edelman, G., & Gally, J. A. (2001). Degeneracy and complexity in biological systems. *Proceedings of the National Academy of Sciences of the United States of America, 98*(24), 13763–13768. doi: 10.1073/pnas.231499798

Edelman, G., & Tononi, G. (2000). *A Universe of Consciousness: How Matter Becomes Imagination*. New York: Basic Books.

Favareau, D. (2002). Constructing representema: on the neurosemiotics of self and vision. *Semiotics, Evolution, Energy and Development Journal, 2(4)*, 3–24.

Feinberg, T. E., & Mallatt, J. M. (2016). *The Ancient Origins of Consciousness: How the Brain Created Experience*. Cambridge, MA: MIT Press.

Feldman Barrett, L. (2017). *How Emotions are Made: The Secret Life of the Brain*. Boston: Houghton Mifflin Harcourt.

Geertz, C. (1973). *The Interpretation of Cultures*. London: Basic Books.

Gellner, E. (1983). *Nations and Nationalism*. New York: Cornell University Press.

Giddens, A. (1983). Four theses on ideology. *Canadian Journal of Political and Social Theory/Revue canadienne de théorie politique et sociale, 7(1–2)*, 18–21.

Halliday, M. A. K. (2002). How do you mean? In J. J. Webster (Ed.), *On Grammar. Volume 1 in the Collected Works of M. A. K. Halliday* (pp. 352–368). London: Continuum.

Halliday, M. A. K. (2003a). Is the grammar neutral? Is the grammarian neutral? In J. J. Webster (Ed.), *On Language and Linguistics. Volume 3 in the Collected Works of M. A. K. Halliday* (pp. 271–292). London: Continuum.

Halliday, M. A. K. (2003b). On the architecture of human language. In J. J. Webster (Ed.), *On Language and Linguistics. Volume 3 in the Collected Works of M. A. K. Halliday* (pp. 1–29). London: Continuum.

Halliday, M. A. K. (2003c). On language in relation to the evolution of human consciousness. In J. J. Webster (Ed.), *On Language and Linguistics. Volume 3 in the Collected Works of M. A. K. Halliday* (pp. 390–432). London: Continuum.

Halliday, M. A. K. (2003d). Language and the order of nature. In J. J. Webster (Ed.), *On Language and Linguistics. Volume 3 in the Collected Works of M. A. K. Halliday* (pp. 116–138). London: Continuum.

Halliday, M. A. K. (2013). *Halliday in the 21st Century. Volume 11 in the Collected Works of M. A. K. Halliday*. Edited by J. J. Webster. London: Bloomsbury.

Hasan, R. (2005). Semiotic mediation and three exotropic theories: Vygotsky, Halliday and Bernstein. In J. J. Webster (Ed.), *Language, Society and Consciousness. Volume 1 in the Collected Works of Ruqaiya Hasan* (pp. 130–156). London: Equinox.

Hasan, R. (2009). Language in the processes of socialization. In J. J. Webster (Ed.), *Semantic Variation: Meaning in Society and Sociolinguistics. Volume 2 in the Collected Works of Ruqaiya Hasan* (pp. 119–179). London: Equinox.

Hasan, R. (2016a). *Context in the System and Process of Language. Volume 4 in the Collected Works of Ruqaiya Hasan*. Edited by J. J. Webster. London: Equinox.

Hasan, R. (2016b). Wherefore context? The ontogenesis of meaning exchange. In J. J. Webster (Ed.), *Context in the System and Process of Language. Volume 4 in the Collected Works of Ruqaiya Hasan* (pp. 95–126). London: Equinox.

Herman, E., & Chomsky, N. (2002). *Manufacturing Consent: The Political Economy of the Mass Media*. London: Pantheon Books.

Ibáñez, A., & Garcia, A. M. (2018). *Contextual Cognition: The Sensus Communis of a Situated Mind*. Heidelberg: Springer.

Kaplan, J. T., Gimbel, S. I., & Harris, S. (2016). Neural correlates of maintaining one's political beliefs in the face of counterevidence. *Scientific Reports*, 6, 39589.

Kennedy, E. (1979). "Ideology" from Destutt de Tracy to Marx. *Journal of the History of Ideas, 40(3)*, 353–368. doi: 10.2307/2709242

Leong, Y. C., Chen, J., Willer, R., & Zaki, J. (2020). Conservative and liberal attitudes drive polarized neural responses to political content. *Proceedings of the National Academy of Sciences, 117(44)*, 27731–27739. doi: 10.1073/pnas.2008530117

Lukin, A. (2019). *War and Its Ideologies: A Social-semiotic Theory and Description*. Heidelberg: Springer.

Malešević, S., & MacKenzie, I. (Eds.). (2002). *Ideology after Poststructuralism*. London: Pluto Press.

Malešević, S. (2010). *The Sociology of War and Violence*. Cambridge: Cambridge University Press.

Malešević, S. (2019). *Grounded Nationalisms*. Cambridge: Cambridge University Press.

Mannheim, K. (1936). *Ideology and Utopia: An Introduction to the Sociology of Knowledge* (L. Wirth & E. Shils, Trans.). London: Harcourt, Brace & Co.

Marx, K., & Engels, F. (1985). *The German Ideology*. London: Lawrence and Wishart.

McEnery, T., & Hardie, A. (2013). The history of corpus linguistics. In K. Allan (Ed.), *The Oxford Handbook of the History of Linguistics* (pp. 727–745). Oxford: Oxford University Press.

McLellan, D. (1986). *Ideology*. Oxford: Oxford University Press.

Meares, R. (1999). The contribution of Hughlings Jackson to an understanding of dissociation. *American Journal of Psychiatry, 156(12)*, 1850–1855. doi: 10.1176/ajp.156.12.1850

Meares, R. (2012). *Borderline Personality Disorder and the Conversational Model: A Clinician's Manual*. New York: W.W. Norton.

Nam, H. H., Jost, J. T., Meager, M. R., & Van Bavel, J. J. (2021). Toward a neuropsychology of political orientation: Exploring ideology in patients with frontal and midbrain lesions. *Philosophical Transactions of the Royal Society B*, 376 20200137, 1–9. doi: 10.1098/rstb.2020.0137

Otero, C. P. (2004). *Noam Chomsky: Language and Politics*. New York: A.K. Press.

Posner, M. I., & Raichle, M. E. (1994). *Images of Mind.* New York: Scientific American Library.
Rabin, J. S. (2020). Blue brain, red brain: The biopsychology of political beliefs and behavior. In J. D. Sinnott & J. S. Rabin (Eds.), *The Psychology of Political Behavior in a Time of Change* (pp. 15–53). Heidelberg: Springer.
Shapiro, J. A. (2011). *Evolution: A View from the 21st Century.* London: FT Press Science.
Thompson, J. B. (1984). *Studies in the Theory of Ideology.* New York: Polity Press.
Vološinov, V. (1973). *Marxism and the Philosophy of Language* (L. Matejka & I. R. Titunik, Trans.). London: Seminar Press.
Weber, M. (2004). *The Vocation Lectures.* London: Hackett.
Wexler, B. E. (2006). *Brain and Culture: Neurobiology, Ideology, and Social Change.* Cambridge, MA: MIT Press.
Žižek, S. (1994). Introduction: The spectre of ideology. In S. Žižek (Ed.), *Mapping Ideology* (pp. 1–33). Verso.
Zmigrod, L., Eisenberg, I. W., Bissett: G., Robbins, T. W., & Poldrack, R. A. (2021). The cognitive and perceptual correlates of ideological attitudes: A data-driven approach. *Philosophical Transactions of the Royal Society B, 376*, 20200424, 1–14. doi: 10.1098/rstb.2020.0424
Zmigrod, L., Rentfrow, J., & Robbins, T. W. (2018). Cognitive underpinnings of nationalistic ideology in the context of Brexit. *Proceedings of the National Academy of Sciences, 115(19)*, E4532–E4540. doi: 10.1073/pnas.1708960115
Zmigrod, L., & Tsakiris, M. (2021). Computational and neurocognitive approaches to the political brain: Key insights and future avenues for political neuroscience. *Philosophical Transactions of the Royal Society B, 376*, 20200130, 1–6. doi: 10.1098/rstb.2020.0130

20

THE INTERPLAY OF CULTURE, RELIGION, AND BIOLOGY

Joni Y. Sasaki and Hannah I. Pearson

Introduction

The human mind craves meaning. An admirer of a sculpture muses on the artist's intention. Seeing a friend's furrowed brow elicits concern. In the wake of widespread suffering from natural disasters or disease, many are left wondering *why*? A shared human experience is that we are able to perceive various events and stimuli, and then represent them in our minds to interpret their meaning. Notably, these meanings can vary systematically and predict different psychological outcomes across individuals and societies. In order to explain how these different outcomes may arise, the field of cultural neuroscience has focused on the interaction of culture and biology. Not only are "nature" and "nurture" both necessary for understanding human cognition and behavior, but biological and cultural factors work together in complex ways to predict important outcomes. Similarly, the field of neurosemiotics aims to understand communicative behavior by integrating the external world – including the physical environment and human social interactions – with internal, underlying biological processes (Bouissac, 1986).

In this chapter, we first provide a brief historical context for cultural neuroscience focused on cultural psychology, which traditionally deals with ethnic or national forms of culture. Next, we argue that a full interpretation of the interplays of culture, brain, and genes requires considering how different cultural groups construe meaning to understand the world around them. This is followed by specific examples from religion as a central form of human culture (Cohen, 2009). We then build upon these findings with research and theory in neurosemiotics, tying together culture, meaning, and neurosemiotics. Finally, we propose future research avenues that may capitalize on meaning to integrate culture and biology, and we discuss the unique challenges of doing so.

Meaning in cultural psychology

Meaning is inherently social and, as such, it is inherently cultural. As Bruner (1990: 67) notes, "one of the crowning achievements of human development" comes from the way people not only communicate but also constantly negotiate divergent meanings via cultural narratives and traditions, and by using cognitive capacities such as theory of mind or the ability to represent mental states of the self and others. While the particular meaning of stimuli can be subjective, the "point" of construing meaning is often to share it with others. A person seeing a row of tulips in a garden, for instance, may

DOI: 10.4324/9781003051817-24

interpret them as intentionally planted. She can then express that meaning publicly and negotiate others' interpretations of what they see. In this way, her interpretation of the tulips becomes *social*, or shared. That shared sense of meaning can be passed on to others and refined over time so that the meaning maintained takes on a slightly different form from her original, individualized sense of meaning. This process of sharing, changing, and maintaining meaning over time is *cultural*. Thus, it may come as no surprise that meaning is central to the study of human psychology, given that we are social and cultural beings.

A central tenet in cultural psychology is that culture and the mind "make each other up" (Shweder, 1995: 41). The human mind is equipped to adopt meanings from its socio-cultural environment, and likewise, the socio-cultural environment itself is created and shaped by the individuals who overlay their own interpretations and shared meanings across time. Cultural psychology has demonstrated how culture shapes numerous aspects of an individual. While many of these aspects – particularly cognition – may previously have been studied as if they were universal, cross-cultural research suggests otherwise.

For example, Nisbett et al. (2001) found that East Asians tended to hold bigger picture, more holistic cognitive tendencies whereas Westerners tended to think more analytically about objects and their categorizations. For their part, Markus and Kitayama (1991) discuss how individuals think about themselves in connection to others around them and theorize that East Asian individuals tend to view the self as more connected to or interdependent with others compared with Western individuals, who view themselves as more independent or separate from others (Markus & Kitayama, 1991). Additionally, interdependent and independent construals of the self, as well as other cultural beliefs, can impact other aspects of an individual, such as their emotion (Mesquita & Frijda, 1992), motivation (Heine et al., 2001), development (Greenfield et al., 2003), and morality (Haidt et al., 1993).

In this sense, Heine et al. (2001) reported differing motivations between Japanese and North American participants. They found that despite sharing the goal of wanting to do their best, Japanese participants held more critical views of the self and had self-improvement motivations compared with North Americans, who focused more on their own strengths, holding a self-enhancement motivation style. In another example, Haidt et al. (1993) found that morality varies across not only different countries, but also different socioeconomic statuses. In particular, participants varied in how they reacted to scenarios involving moral violations (e.g., flag burning, breaking promises, eating a dead pet dog).

Across both basic and complex psychological processes, evidence from cultural psychology as a whole suggests that meanings shared in different cultures can vary systematically and, crucially, shape the way people think and behave. In what follows, we will touch on not only cross-cultural viewpoints, but also other aspects of culture such as religion, as we bridge these fields with the chapter's main focus of neurosemiotics.

Meaning in cultural neuroscience and genetics

Cultural neuroscience is a relatively new field combining theories and methods from cultural psychology and neuroscience. Research in this area focuses on the interaction of cultural and biological factors in predicting psychological outcomes (Chiao & Ambady, 2007), and the general framework of cultural neuroscience connects findings across different levels of analysis, including the broader *societal level* operating within evolutionary processes; the *person-level* through interactions of cultural, genetic, and situational factors; and the *physiological level* via neural, cardiovascular, endocrine, immune, and other responses (Kim & Sasaki, 2014). Importantly, culture permeates every level of analysis, from individual processes "under the skin" (Kitayama & Salvador, 2017) to shared group processes "outside the head" (Morling & Lamoreax, 2008). Being influenced by all these levels, our meaning-making capacities are central to the field of cultural neuroscience.

Cultural neuroscience research relies on cultural meanings

In cultural neuroscience, empirical evidence becomes difficult, if not impossible, to interpret without integrating appropriate cultural meanings. Illuminating work has found that people in different cultures can show disparate brain activation patterns while engaging in the same behavioral task. For instance, Gutchess et al. (2010) used functional magnetic resonance imagining (fMRI) techniques to examine East Asians' and Americans' neural activity as they categorized the meaning of various objects. When participants experienced a conflict in the semantic task, they seemed to use different strategies to resolve it. East Asians showed neural activation indicating top-down controlled processes that were mediated by frontal-parietal networks, while Americans' activation patterns indicated greater reliance on semantic information via temporal lobes, alongside conflict detection and monitoring demands via the cingulate gyrus. This evidence suggests that culture shapes the neural activity underlying semantic processing. One possibility is that, at a psychological level, people may interpret different meanings as they try to categorize concepts and also use different strategies to resolve conflicts in meaning. However, additional tasks and experimentation are needed to interpret divergent neural activation patterns for different cultural groups.

In another fMRI study relevant to cultural meaning, Tang et al. (2006) examined cultural differences in neural activity during arithmetic processing among English and Chinese speakers. The study involved simple addition or numerical quantity comparisons. Although there were no behavioral between-group differences, meaningful differences emerged in neural activation patterns. When thinking about arithmetic calculations, native English speakers primarily tended to engage perisylvian areas associated with language processing, including Broca and Wernicke, while native Chinese speakers tended to engage premotor association areas linked to visuo-spatial processing. Put simply, when asked whether "5 plus 3 equals 8," for example, both English and Chinese speakers may correctly respond behaviorally in the affirmative with the appropriate button-press. However, their underlying neural activation pattern seems to vary as they provide this behavioral response. Although these two cultural groups arrive at the same answer, English speakers may compute the problem more verbally by "asking" themselves whether "5 plus 3 equals 8." Chinese speakers may instead tend to work through the problem by visualizing five objects next to three objects spatially and then considering abstractly whether they "see" eight objects in total. While there are many fMRI studies that document neural activation associated with specific behaviors, the importance of Tang et al.'s (2006) findings is that different meanings between cultures potentially arise at the level of neural activity, but not in behavior. This cultural difference is consistent with earlier behavioral research. For example, using articulatory suppression techniques, Kim (2002) demonstrated that European Americans may think more linguistically, and East Asians more abstractly, during a reasoning task. Though a definitive link between brain activations and behavioral output can be difficult to establish, the fMRI study from Tang et al. (2006) also illuminates a useful benefit of bringing neuroscience into more traditional psychological studies of culture and meaning: neural measures can at times address the issue of awareness and reportability of different meanings beyond outward behavior.

Meaning is necessary to interpret findings in cultural neuroscience. At the same time, neuroscience provides crucial insights that can deepen our understanding of how culture shapes the mind. This same principle can be applied in other integrative fields. Some researchers argue that we may never capture the full picture without integrative areas such as biosemiotics, because culture and natural sciences would continue to be studied separately (Cobley, 2016). The aim of biosemiotics, and presumably its subfield of neurosemiotics, is not to have one topic take over the other, but to combine them into a well-rounded explanation of how we find meaning in the world around us (Cobley, 2016).

Benefits of integrating neuroscience into cultural psychology

Neuroscience utilizes techniques and perspectives that were unavailable to scientists a generation ago, injecting undeniable excitement into many fields. There are unique benefits of integrating neuroscience into the study of meaning in areas as broad as psychology, culture, and semiotics. In this section, we discuss some of the benefits of integrating neuroscience into the study of meaning, particularly the ability to address implicit versus explicit processes.

Meanings are often studied explicitly, using self-report or face-valid behavioral measures. Yet meanings are not always explicit. Indeed, people often interpret the meaning of stimuli, situations, and behaviors in an implicit fashion, below the threshold of awareness. What people say about their intentions may not always correspond to what they do because they may have implicit reasons for their behaviors that they are unable to explicitly report (Nisbett & Wilson, 1977). This presents a challenge for more traditional investigations of meaning, including works in cultural psychology and semiotics, because investigators may often focus on meanings that participants can explicitly acknowledge and accurately report.

By integrating neuroscientific perspectives, as has been done in cultural neuroscience and neurosemiotics, research has uncovered important differences in semantic processing. For example, Hedden et al. (2008) used fMRI techniques to demonstrate that people from East Asian versus European American cultures may at times show a similar pattern of neural activation but in response to divergent stimuli due to distinct meanings of these stimuli across cultures. In this study, researchers examined cross-cultural differences in relative judgments, which depend on the context, versus absolute judgments, which are more independent of the context. For example, when judging the length of a line drawn within a box, participants can make a more context-*independent* judgment that ignores the size of the surrounding box, or a more context-*dependent* judgment that considers the length of the line in relation to the surrounding box. This study found that when making context-*independent* judgments (which are less preferred in East Asian cultural contexts), East Asian participants showed neural activation patterns indicating greater use of attentional control. However, Western European Americans showed a neural activation pattern indicating greater attentional control when making content-*dependent* judgments (which are less preferred in Western cultural contexts). These results demonstrate that the literal content of stimuli did not predict neural activation patterns consistently across cultures. Instead, specific cultural meanings of the stimuli may have been responsible for predicting people's neural responses, suggesting that interpreting these results in cultural neuroscience requires meaning.

Conversely, within neurosemiotics, some researchers have begun exploring how commonly seen stimuli, more specifically non-verbal behaviors such as gesturing with your palms facing up, may be deeply rooted in neural pathways. Givens (2016) argues that although gesturing with your hands up may convey many different meanings depending on the context of the situation, neural roots dating back to 500 million years ago help our brains determine when to use the gesture and how to interpret it when we see the gesture being used around us. For example, the palm-up gesture with a shrug may be a well-known symbol for asking a question or being confused. We may believe we are making a conscious decision to do this, but in reality the feelings associated with being confused (e.g., defensiveness) may trigger parts of our brain (e.g., the limbic system) to send signals through our brain and spinal cord, which causes us to make this gesture in response to confusion. After making that gesture, mirror neurons are triggered within the neural and limbic system to help decode the true meaning of the gesture and emotion behind it within the given context (Givens, 2016). Non-verbal gestures may not be the only sort of communication that can be interpreted cross-culturally. Ćwiek et al. (2021) found that many novel vocalizations of specific, widely understood concepts (e.g., sleep, eat, child, fire) can be understood cross-culturally, even by speakers of different languages. In these examples, interpreting the results requires understanding what a particular neural pattern means in connection to both the individual's behavior and their surrounding context.

Meaning in religion

Despite its contributions, research in cultural neuroscience often highlights a particular form of culture. Although "culture" in cultural neuroscience is most often studied as nationality or ethnicity, there are many other forms of culture, including social class, region, and religion (Cohen, 2009). Religion, in particular, may be at least partially understood through the lens of culture and, more broadly, can be considered a system of meaning, thus inviting neurosemiotic insights.

Overlaps and distinctions between religion and culture

Religion has key overlapping features with national or ethnic culture (Cohen & Hill, 2007), perhaps most importantly its reliance on socially shared meaning and symbols (Geertz, 1973). Yet, at the same time, religion often involves features that are unique from culture, including its emphasis on the supernatural, sacred, or "divine." Belief in supernatural powers and events that defy physical or natural explanation, as well as ritualistic behaviors linked to these beliefs, is a key component of religion (Atran & Norenzayan, 2004; James, 1963). In order to account for both overlapping and unique features of these two concepts, we thus construe religion as *partially overlapping* with culture. Though scholars tend to disagree on an exact definition of religion, for the purposes of this chapter we conceive of religion as a form of culture consisting of shared meanings and symbols centered on the supernatural, sacred, or divine. We aim to consider implications that not only apply broadly across both religion and culture as meaning systems, but also may be specific to each.

Historical examples of meaning in religion

Religion's unique emphasis on the sacred or supernatural may be particularly relevant for the study of meaning, as thinking about the supernatural and engaging in religious traditions require a cognitive understanding of representation and the ability to create symbolic artifacts and rituals, beyond literal objects or actions in the natural world. This unique emphasis on the sacred may have implications for integrating neuroscience perspectives into the study of religion, even though intuitively and historically religion has been understood as quite separate from the "natural," physical, and literal.

Though there is no consensus on the origin of religion, the world's first known temple, Göbekli Tepe, was said to be built in the Fertile Crescent 11,000 years ago, and archaeological records of basic religious beliefs, practices, and symbols are even older. The use of religious symbols in Blombos Cave in South Africa and deliberate burial rituals in the Qafzeh site in Israel, for instance, date back to about 100,000 years ago (Culotta, 2009). While there is some dispute over whether or not we can consider early findings of cave drawings and burial practices as definitive proof of "religion" *per se*, it seems clear that these are important precursors to meaning-making in connection to supernatural phenomena. Interestingly, cases of these symbols and rituals can be found all over the world, from small figurines discovered in Germany to religious hierarchies in ancient Egypt (Culotta, 2009). This evidence points to the early prevalence of religion and religious practice, which crucially revolved around meaning.

Historically, symbolic meaning has been heavily emphasized within religious groups and can vary greatly given that divergent meanings can be attributed to the same elements (Geertz, 1973). Take the Eucharist, for example. In a non-religious context, bread and wine in and of themselves are secular; you do not have to follow a particular religion in order to eat bread or drink wine. Conversely, within Christianity, this supernatural practice turns the same seemingly secular objects into religious, ritualistic symbols. Depending on the religio-cultural context, the meaning and behavior surrounding bread, wine, and many other symbols take on a completely different meaning. According to Paul Tillich (1955), symbols have a specific purpose: to point beyond themselves and participate in the meaning and power behind the thing that they symbolize. Tillich (1955: 191) goes on to say that symbols, particularly religious symbols, are necessary to "open up to a reality for which non-symbolic speaking is inadequate." The meaning that religious symbols provide extends beyond one's personal meaning in life and can shape how we think, perceive, and interact with the world around us.

Psychological research demonstrating meaning in religion

Some research within the cognitive science of religion suggests that, psychologically, these symbols may even work unconsciously. For example, Weisbuch-Remington and colleagues (2005) primed Christian participants with masked images of positive (e.g., Jesus and Mary) versus negative (e.g., Satan and Hell) Christian symbols and induced the threat of death versus a control (i.e., a trip to the dentist) to examine how exposure to religious symbols, even beneath awareness, may influence individuals' physiological and cognitive responses to threat. Participants who were exposed to the negative religious prime *and* were asked to speak about their own death were more likely than those in the other conditions (i.e., who viewed the positive images and/or spoke about the dentist) to show a cardiovascular pattern consistent with feeling threatened. Additionally, when conducted on both Christian and non-Christian participants and with non-Christian control images included, the initial pattern of results did not hold among non-Christian participants or for the control images. These findings suggest that the meaning behind symbols may be specific to both the context and the particular beliefs of the individuals viewing the symbols, even when the religious meaning is processed unconsciously.

These findings may also extend beyond the lab setting and carry real-world implications. In a field study conducted by Guéguen et al. (2015), they found that the presence of a cross necklace – an important religious symbol in many branches of Christianity – impacted prosocial behavior. More specifically, when passersby were approached by an individual handing out organ donation cards, which are used as consent to be an organ donor in France, they were more likely to accept the card when the individual handing the cards out was wearing a cross necklace versus not wearing a cross necklace. Results of this study suggest that religious primes, even in a real-world setting, impact behavior and can lead to more prosocial choices – see also Shariff et al. (2015). Religious priming effects demonstrate how people make decisions and find meaning in seemingly unrelated situations around them, even without awareness.

Utilizing theories and research techniques grounded in neurosemiotics when studying various forms of culture, including religion, can add depth to how we understand culture and the search for meaning. Within the broader study of biosemiotics, researchers from both biological sciences and the humanities have come together to discuss how combining the two helps uncover a more complete picture of the world (Favareau et al., 2017). With the help of modern takes on semiotics, such as biosemiotics and neurosemiotics, researchers are able to move beyond purely mechanical, biological, or humanities-based understandings within their own expertise and embrace a fuller scope of human experience (Favareau et al., 2017). Because meaning unites religion and culture, theories and evidence from neurosemiotics may be an important bridge to understanding recent advances in cultural neuroscience.

The unique utility of neuroscience in the study of religion

Integrating neuroscience into "classic" cultural investigations focusing on national or ethnic culture has proved fruitful. It may likewise be useful – perhaps especially so – to incorporate neuroscience into cultural investigations of religion. Neuroscience research on the cognitive underpinnings of religious belief, for instance, has demonstrated that religious priming, or leading people to think about the supernatural, can impact neurophysiological responses to errors. Specifically, when exposed to a religious prime, individuals who made an error showed reduced amplitude of the error-related negativity (ERN), a signal typically indicating defensive responses to making an error (Inzlicht & Tullett, 2010). This finding suggests that religion may lead believers to experience less distress in the face of their own errors and suggests one potential mechanism for the previously found link between religion and well-being (Powell, Shahabi, & Thoreson, 2003). Interestingly, these results hold only for people who believe in supernatural concepts, suggesting that religion can provide a system of meaning or explanation specifically for those who believe in or hold this meaning system. Thinking about the concepts of *spirit*, *divine*, and *sacred*, as is typically done in religious priming studies, while meaningful to believers, may not always have the same effects for non-believers – for a meta-analysis, see Shariff et al. (2015) – thus highlighting the centrality of meaning when studying religion through the use of neuroscientific techniques. These findings suggest that our conceptions of, and interactions with, the world rely on external stimuli and internal reactions.

Relatedly, Holbrook et al. (2020) investigated the commonly studied relationship between religiosity and ideological threat by limiting the contribution of a particular brain area through non-invasive transcranial magnetic stimulation (TMS). This replication of the research of Holbrook et al. (2016) sought to specifically examine the impact of downregulatory TMS on the posterior medial frontal cortex (pMFC), an area of the brain that seems to be associated with attending to various potential threats and discrepancies, versus an unrelated, control area of the brain. Results showed that when participants were reminded of their own death, receiving the TMS downregulation in the pMFC (versus control) led to *lower* endorsement of positive aspects of religion, such as the belief in an all-knowing and loving God. However, this same effect of TMS did not occur among participants in the control condition (i.e., writing about their morning routine). Researchers note that this finding could be suggestive of an "alarm effect" related to the preconceived associations between religion and death (e.g., Hell). It seems that when the part of the brain responsible for these alarms is downregulated, the meaning behind religiosity changes. More specifically, by downregulating one of the areas often associated with threats via TMS, the threat of one's own death seems to make participants less likely to view religion positively than when this area is able to sound the alarm as usual. In line with the goal of neurosemiotics, this finding suggests that integrating neuroscience into the study of religion can uncover crucial information that may aid in or even change previous findings to obtain a clearer picture of human thought and behavior.

The need for meaning in gene–environment interaction and religion research

Although fMRI and electroencephalography predominate in cultural neuroscience, other methods prove critical to derive neurosemiotic insights. Genetics is a case in point. Theoretical and empirical contributions from the gene–environment interaction (G × E) framework indicate that genetic influences can be moderated by environmental features (Caspi et al., 2002; 2003). This framework has been incorporated by cultural neuroscience research to examine the interplay between biological and cultural factors in gene–*culture* interactions (Kim & Sasaki, 2014). Such interactions have been found on a number of psychological outcomes, including cognitive tendencies (Kim et al., 2010a), emotion perception and suppression (Ishii et al., 2014; Kim et al., 2011), and social support use (Kim et al., 2010b). Moreover, genes in the dopamine system could be linked to acquiring cultural norms more broadly (Kitayama et al., 2016). Overall, this research demonstrates the complexity of the relationship between culture and biology, based on evidence of gene–culture coevolution occurring at the macro- and historical-level of analysis (Chiao & Blizinsky, 2010; Feldman & Laland, 1996) and gene–environment interactions occurring at the more micro and present-day level (Kim & Sasaki, 2014).

Yet interpreting these complex interactions across time and populations calls for semantic considerations. Culture and religion are meaningful forms of the environment that can be used to predict when gene–environment interactions may occur, and why (Sasaki & Kim, 2017). For example, people with certain variants (4-repeat allele carriers) of the dopamine receptor polymorphism *DRD4* are more likely to behave prosocially compared to those with "risky" variants (2- or 7-repeat allele carriers) (Bachner-Melman et al., 2005). However, Sasaki et al. (2013) found that this genetic pattern reversed when priming religious concepts. Results of their G × E investigation showed that people with 2-/7-repeat allele variants of *DRD4*, who should be more sensitive to reward, were actually *more* prosocial than those with 4-repeat allele variants when they were primed with religious concepts. In other words, for people who are motivated toward particular goals, such as the presence of reward and lack of punishment, thinking about religion may provide a meaningful motivation to behave prosocially. However, without religion or a comparable meaning system made salient, people with a genetic sensitivity to reward may lack sufficient motivation for prosocial behavior. These findings demonstrate how religion can provide the meaning necessary to motivate certain behaviors for people with specific genetic tendencies. Yet the religion–prosociality link occurred only for people with certain genotypes, suggesting that genes may illuminate one factor influencing "individual differences," while potentially explaining why religious belief and involvement can lead to quite different outcomes depending on the person.

Previous research on G × E interactions has examined how religiosity may play a role in these relationships as an environmental influence (Sasaki & Kim, 2020). Meyers et al. (2019), for instance, investigated how religious involvement may act as a moderator in the relationship between genetic factors and cannabis use/cannabis use disorders (CUD). This study used polygenic risk scores (PRS), which allow modeling of complex traits such as substance use and abuse through aggregating variations in genes and can help identify specific genetic risk markers for cannabis use. Results of this study showed that the link between PRS and self-reported cannabis use/CUD was moderated by frequency of religious service attendance such that this link was *weakened* for individuals who reported higher rates of religious service attendance. Incorporating genetics research into already established questions about the relationship between religiosity and real-world behaviors, including how church attendance may be related to taboo behaviors such as substance use, can provide new insights on how "nature" and "nurture" work together to predict the way people find meaning and make choices in the world around them.

In another example, Beaver et al. (2009) examined the impact that the interaction between religious belief and genetics, namely the dopamine D2 receptor gene (*DRD2*), may have on involvement in delinquent behaviors. Their results suggest that the A-1 allele of *DRD2* increased self-reported delinquent behavior specifically for males with a lack of religious beliefs and that higher religiosity in general seemed to act as a protective environmental factor against delinquency. These findings suggest it is the combination of genetic and environmental factors, such as religion, that help us to understand how and when to protect ourselves from potential challenges throughout our lives. While some may think that the connection between delinquency and religiosity is self-explanatory, researchers are able to more thoroughly piece together mechanisms for how the relationship works by utilizing genetic analyses.

Across these investigations, the integration of both environmental and genetic factors allowed researchers to understand how systems of meaning, including culture and religion, can act as critical modulating factors shaping biologically linked tendencies and behavioral outcomes (Figure 20.1). Specifically, culture and religion can be understood as partially overlapping systems of meaning that often interact. Systems of meaning can also shape the way biological factors, including genes, contribute to neurobiological processes and predict different psychological outcomes. At the same time, environmental factors including social situations can shape gene expression, as in gene-environment interactions.

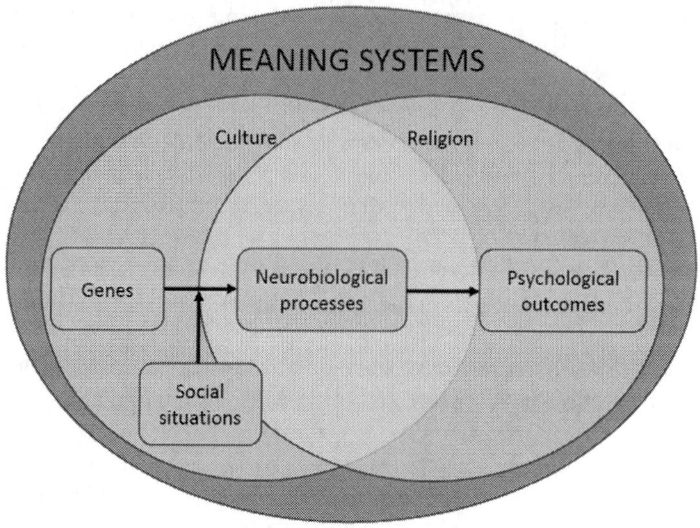

Figure 20.1 Culture and religion as meaning systems

Theoretical illustration of how culture and religion, as systems of meaning, shape the interrelationships among biological factors (including genes and neurobiological processes), social situations, and psychological outcomes. See e-book for a full-color version of this figure.

Future research and challenges in cultural neuroscience and religion

The focus on meaning is central to cultural neuroscience and religion, leading to great advances in these fields. Yet what are some current gaps in the literature, and what are the challenges that need to be addressed? As is the case in psychology as a whole, much of the research in cultural psychology and cultural neuroscience has focused on certain social groups, while neglecting others. In psychology, the vast majority of investigations tend to include Western, educated, industrialized, rich, democratic (WEIRD) societies (Heinrich et al., 2010), and in cultural psychology there is disproportionate representation of East–West ethno-cultural comparisons and a heavy focus on ethnic and national cultures rather than other forms of culture (Cohen, 2009). Thus, future research should prioritize sampling from non-Western regions of the world and especially from underrepresented ethno-cultural groups, such as Black and Indigenous people of color, and understudied religious groups, particularly non-Christians.

There are many opportunities to examine existing research in the area of cultural psychology, and in the study of religion in particular, through the lens of neuroscience. For instance, neuroscience may illuminate previous investigations that examine religion as a form of culture, including research on religio-cultural differences in psychological judgments of mental states between Judaism and Protestantism (Cohen & Rozin, 2001). Research from a more classic cultural psychological perspective on this topic finds that Protestants are more likely to moralize inappropriate mental states compared with Jewish individuals, and these judgments are evidenced by perceivers' explicit responses to statements about various targets' thoughts and behaviors (Cohen & Rozin, 2001). Incorporating perspectives from neuroscience may be useful for either corroborating these findings or revealing novel insights. For example, brain regions associated with detecting and monitoring semantic inconsistencies, such as the cingulate gyrus (as found in Gutchess et al., 2010), may be relevant for uncovering whether, consistent with self-reported beliefs, compared with Jewish individuals, Protestants show greater cingulate gyrus activation when presented with information that a target holds an inappropriate mental state and yet behaves appropriately (i.e., a thought-behavior mismatch). On the other hand, Jewish individuals may show similar cingulate gyrus activation to Protestants, suggesting that they cognitively detect a conflict between a target's thoughts and actions and are perhaps motivated to resolve this conflict in different ways than are Protestants. This pattern of results would raise the question of whether Jewish individuals might, via more implicit means, show some alternative form of negative behavioral reaction toward a target with inappropriate thoughts, or whether a detection of thought–behavior mismatch in this case does not meaningfully predict their behavior.

Incorporating neurosemiotic techniques into religion research specifically can be useful for theoretical reasons. Since a unique feature of religion is the component of the supernatural, sacredness, or "the divine," which is considered outside of physical or natural meaning systems, utilizing biological and neurological research can ground what may seem abstract to many in the physical world. Many religious stories and concepts rely on "eyewitness testimonials, narratives, symbols, and personal, experiential evidence" (Nieminen et al., 2020: 448), which are inherently imbued with meaning. Through the use of symbols, people are able to connect the supernatural, sacred, and divine to their own individual reality (Tillich, 1955). These symbols and the patterns we see in them are passed down through the generations and used as their own type of evidence rather than experimental proof (Nieminen et al., 2020). In fact, the unfalsifiability of certain religious beliefs may support human psychological motivations to flexibly maintain one's worldview or system of meaning (Friesen et al., 2015).

At the same time, an interesting implication of integrating neuroscience into the study of *religious meaning* in particular is that evidence for religious meaning at the level of neurophysiological or genetic explanation could, for some believers, be perceived as in conflict or irrelevant to their own interpretation of their religious beliefs. While neurosemiotic approaches may be useful to integrate with religion in theory, researchers must be aware of practical concerns when sharing research with religious communities including potential mistrust of certain methods and the reasons why that lack of trust exists. For many reasons, it may be challenging to use neuroscience and genetics research on religion to motivate real-world solutions, particularly for sensitive issues, such as interreligious conflict, religiously motivated violence, and faith-based decision-making more broadly.

Additionally, when studying religion and culture, it is important to consider individual differences within the groups themselves. A comparison of Christian and Jewish individuals may need to also consider potentially relevant differences between Orthodox and Reform Jewish individuals, depending on the outcome of interest. Even within the same overarching religious group, there are layers upon layers of nuance that need to be taken into account. The same religion can take on different meanings depending on the broader national or ethno-cultural context, leading to different psychological outcomes (Sasaki & Kim, 2011), suggesting that both ethno-cultural and religious differences – and importantly, the interaction of the two – may be crucial in future investigations. Besides any denominational and ethno-cultural differences, religion often comes with purposely picking specific beliefs and practices to follow, which can ultimately make the beliefs and practices of a religion highly individualized. Within the Western world, particularly the United States, there has been a focus on religious individualism and privatism (Greer & Roof, 1992). Bellah et al. (1985) even go so far as to speculate that with each individual coming up with their own belief system, it is not out of the question to think there may be just as many individual religions around us as there are individual people and cultures around the world. Incorporating neuroscience into these investigations may add a layer of common ground to connect individuals to each other, perhaps discovering more generalizable meanings about the groups we study.

Integrating culture, semiotics, and neuroscience

Research within cultural psychology, semiotics, and cultural neuroscience have all independently made important contributions to what we know about the world around us. Understanding how we find meaning could start from any or all of these pathways, but by integrating the fields, we may be able to gain a more complete understanding of semiotics. Neurosemiotics as a field has already inherently begun the process of integrating multiple research areas by combining the study of semiotics, more specifically biosemiotics, with neuroscience research (Favareau, 2002).

García et al. (2020: 93) bring these integrations one step further by advocating for neurosemiotics to be the way for research to "overcome the so called 'two cultures divide,'" referring to the current trend in separating what is considered "social" from "natural or physical." As one of the primary goals of neurosemiotics is to study how we communicate and interact with the environment from an integrated perspective (García et al., 2020), it seems only fitting that culture, an intuitively social concept concerning established symbolic beliefs and practices, would fit into that explicit goal. Cultural psychology and related fields that incorporate meaning, such as the psychology of religion, fit into various subfield components proposed by García et al. (2020), including how forms of communication are culturally transmitted, the way we communicate and interact socially, and variation in meanings across time and groups.

Integrating culture and religion research into neurosemiotics is not inherently different from current theoretical approaches in neurosemiotics. The clear connections between these fields provides an excellent opportunity to advance research in both cultural psychology and neurosemiotics. The core concepts underlying culture, religion, semiotics, and neuroscience research cannot be separated if we want to truly understand and interact with the world, so why separate them within the realm of research?

Conclusion

Cultural neuroscience is still relatively new, yet the centrality of meaning in this field is old. Cultural psychology, a precursor to cultural neuroscience, has focused on meaning as a defining component of what culture is and how it shapes the human mind (Shweder, 1995), and a key cognitive basis of religion is the human ability to represent meaning (Culotta, 2009). Similarly, neurosemiotics has emerged as a promising field through which researchers can integrate the study of meaning in the social world with theories and methods from neuroscience.

There are challenges in studying complex constructs, and "meaning" is no exception, but just as the human mind cannot help but construe meaning, fields as broad as cultural neuroscience, genetics, religion, and neurosemiotics cannot thrive without it.

References

Atran, S., & Norenzayan, A. (2004). Religion's evolutionary landscape: Counterintuition, commitment, compassion, communion. *Behavioral and Brain Sciences*, *27*, 713–770.

Bachner-Melman, R., Girsenko, I., Nemanov, L., Zohar, A. H., Dina, C., & Ebstein, R. P. (2005). Dopaminergic polymorphisms associated with self-report measures of human altruism: A fresh phenotype for the dopamine D4 receptor. *Molecular Psychiatry*, *10*, 333–335.

Beaver, K. M., Gibson, C. L., Jennings, W. G., & Ward, J. T. (2009). A gene × environment interaction between DRD2 and religiosity in the prediction of adolescent delinquent involvement in a sample of males. *Biodemography and Social Biology*, *55*, 71–81.

Bellah, R. M., Madsen, R., Sullivan W. M., Swidler, A., & Tipton, S. M. (1985). *Habits of the Heart*, 219–249. Berkeley, CA: University of California Press.

Bouissac, P. (1986). Semiotics in Canada I. In T. A. Sebeok & D. J. Umiker-Sebeok (Eds.), *The Semiotic Web*, 191–252. Berlin: Mouton de Gruyter.

Bruner, J. (1990). *Acts of Meaning*. Cambridge, MA: Harvard University Press.

Caspi, A., McClay, J., Moffitt, T. E., Mill, J., Martin, J., Craig, I. W., Taylor, A., & Poulton, R. (2002). Role of genotype in the cycle of violence in maltreated children. *Science*, *297*(5582), 851–854.

Caspi, A., Sugden, K., Moffitt, T. E., Taylor, A., Craig, I. W., Harrington, H., McClay, J., Mill, J., Martin, J., Braithwaite, A., & Poulton, R. (2003). Influence of life stress on depression: Moderation by a polymorphism in the 5-HTT gene. *Science*, *301*(5631), 386–389.

Chiao, J.Y., & Ambady, N. (2007). Cultural neuroscience: Parsing universality and diversity across levels of analysis. In S. Kitayama & D. Cohen (Eds.), *Handbook of Cultural Psychology*, (pp. 237–254). New York: Guilford Press.

Chiao, J.Y., & Blizinsky, K. D. (2010). Culture-gene coevolution of individualism-collectivism and the serotonin transporter gene. *Proceedings of the Royal Society B: Biological Sciences, 277*, 529–537.

Cobley, P. (2016). *Cultural Implications of Biosemiotics*. Dordrecht: Springer.

Cohen, A. (2009). Many forms of culture. *American Psychologist, 64*, 194–204.

Cohen, A.B., & Hill, P.C. (2007). Religion as culture: Religious individualism and collectivism among American Catholics, Jews, and Protestants. *Journal of Personality*, 75, 709–742.

Cohen, A. B., & Rozin, P. (2001). Religion and the morality of mentality. *Journal of Personality and Social Psychology, 81*, 697–710.

Culotta, E. (2009). On the origin of religion. *Science, 326*, 784–787.

Ćwiek, A., Fuchs, S., Draxler, C., ... Perlman, M. (2021). Novel vocalizations are understood across cultures. *Scientific Reports, 11*(1), 10108. doi: 10.1038/s41598-021-89445-4

Favareau, D. (2002). Constructing representema: On the neurosemiotics of self and vision. *Semiotics, Evolution, Energy, and Development Journal, 2*, 3–24.

Favareau, D., Kull, K., Ostdiek, G., Maran, T., Westling, L., Cobley, P., Stjernfelt, F., Anderson, M., Tønnessen, M., & Wheeler, W. (2017). How can the study of the humanities inform the study of biosemiotics? *Biosemiotics, 10*(1), 9–31.

Feldman, M. W., & Laland, K. N. (1996). Gene-culture coevolutionary theory. *Trends of Ecology & Evolution, 11*, 453–457.

Friesen, J. P., Campbell, T. H., & Kay, A. C. (2015). The psychological advantage of unfalsifiability: The appeal of untestable political and religious ideologies. *Journal of Personality and Social Psychology, 108*(3), 515–529.

García, A. M., Franco-O'Byrne, D., & Ibáñez, A. (2020). Neurosemiotics: Blurbing a field beyond the "two cultures divide". In L. Lacková, C. Rodríguez & K. Kull (Eds.), *Gatherings in Biosemiotics XX*, (pp. 92–97). Tartu: University of Tartu Press.

Geertz, C. (1973). *Interpretation of Cultures: Selected Essays by Clifford Geertz*. New York: Basic Books.

Givens, D. B. (2016). Reading palm-up signs: Neurosemiotic overview of a common hand gesture. *Semiotica, 210*, 235–250.

Greenfield, P., Keller, H., Fuligni, A., & Maynard, A. (2003). Cultural pathways through universal development. *Annual Review of Psychology, 54*, 461–490.

Greer, B. A., & Roof, W. C. (1992). "Desperately seeking sheila": Locating religious privatism in American society. *Journal for the Scientific Study of Religion, 31*, 346–352.

Guéguen, N., Bougeard-Delfosse, C., & Jacob, C. (2015). The positive effect of the mere presence of a religious symbol on compliance with an organ donation request. *Social Marketing Quarterly, 31*, 1203–1216.

Gutchess, A. H., Hedden, T., Ketay, S., Aron, A., & Gabrieli, J. D. E. (2010). Neural differences in the processing of semantic relationships across cultures. *Social Cognitive and Affective Neuroscience, 5*, 254–263.

Haidt, J., Koller, S. H., & Dias, M. G. (1993). Affect, culture, and morality, or is it wrong to eat your dog? *Journal of Personality and Social Psychology, 65*, 613–628.

Hedden, T., Ketay, S., Aron, A., Markus, H. R., & Gabrieli, J. D. E. (2008). Cultural influences on neural substrates of attentional control. *Psychological Science, 9*, 12–17.

Heine, S. J., Lehman, D. R., Ide, E., Leung, C., Kitayama, S., Takata, T., & Matsumoto, H. (2001). Divergent consequences of success and failure in Japan and North America: An investigation of self-improving motivations and malleable selves. *Journal of Personality and Social Psychology, 81*, 599–615.

Heinrich, J., Heine, S. J., & Norenzayan, A. (2010). Most people are not WEIRD. *Nature, 466*, 29.

Holbrook, C., Iacoboni, M., Gordon, C., Proksch, S., & Balasubramaniam, R. (2020). Posterior medial frontal cortex and threat-enhanced religious belief: A replication and extension. *Social Cognitive and Affective Neuroscience, 15*, 1361–1367.

Holbrook, C., Izuma, K., Deblieck, C., Fessler D. M. T., & Iacoboni, M. (2016). Neuromodulation of group prejudice and religious belief. *Social Cognitive and Affective Neuroscience, 11*, 387–394.

Inzlicht, M., & Tullett, A. M. (2010). Reflecting on God: Religious primes can reduce neurophysiological response to errors. *Psychological Science, 21*, 1184–1190.

Ishii, K., Kim, H. S., Sasaki, J.Y., Shinada, M., & Kusumi, I. (2014). Culture modulates sensitivity to the disappearance of facial expression associated with serotonin transporter polymorphism (5-HTTLPR). *Culture and Brain, 2*, 72–88.

James, W. (1963). *The Varieties of Religious Experience*. New Hyde Park, NY: University Books.

Kim, H. S. (2002). We talk therefore we think? A cultural analysis of the effect of talking on thinking, *Journal of Personality and Social Psychology, 83*, 828–842.

Kim, H., & Sasaki, J.Y. (2014). Cultural neuroscience: Biology of the mind in cultural contexts. *Annual Review of Psychology, 64*, 487–514.

Kim, H. S., Sherman, D. K., Mojaverian, T., Sasaki, J. Y., Park, J., Suh, E. M., & Taylor, S. E. (2011). Gene–culture interaction: Oxytocin receptor polymorphism (OXTR) and emotion regulation. *Social Psychological and Personality Science, 2*, 665–672.

Kim, H. S., Sherman, D. K., Sasaki, J.Y., Xu, J., Chu, T. Q., Ryu, C., Suh, E. M., Graham, K., & Taylor, S. E. (2010b). Culture, distress, and oxytocin receptor polymorphism (OXTR) interact to influence emotional support seeking. *Proceedings of the National Academy of Sciences of the United States of America, 107*(36), 15717–15721.

Kim, H. S, Sherman, D. K., Taylor, S. E., Sasaki, J. Y., Chu, T. Q., Ryu, C., & Xu, J. (2010a). Culture, the serotonin receptor polymorphism (5-HTR1A), and locus of attention. *Social Cognitive and Affective Neuroscience, 5*, 212–218.

Kitayama, S., King, A., Hsu, M., Liberzon, I., & Yoon, C. (2016). Dopamine-system genes and cultural acquisition: The norm sensitivity hypothesis. *Current Opinions in Psychology, 8*, 167–174.

Kitayama, S., & Salvador, C. E. (2017). Culture embrained: Going beyond the nature-nurture dichotomy. *Perspectives on Psychological Science, 12*, 841–854.

Markus, H. R., & Kitayama, S. (1991). Culture and the self: Implications for cognition, emotion, and motivation. *Psychological Review, 98*, 224–253.

Mesquita, B., & Frijda, N. H. (1992). Cultural variations in emotions: A review. *Psychological Bulletin, 112*, 179–204.

Meyers, J. L., Salvatore, J. E., Aliev, F., Johnson, E. C., McCutcheon, V. V., Su, J., Kuo, S. I., Lai, D., Wetherill, L., Wang, J. C., Chan, G., Hesselbrock, V., Foroud, T., Bucholz, K. K., Edenberg, H. J., Dick, D. M., Porjesz, B., & Agrawal, A. (2019). Psychosocial moderation of polygenic risk for cannabis involvement: The role of trauma exposure and frequency of religious service attendance. *Translational Psychiatry, 9*(1), 269. doi: 10.1038/s41398-019-0598-z

Morling, B., & Lamoreaux, M. (2008). Measuring culture outside the head: A meta-analysis of individualism-collectivism in cultural products. *Personality and Social Psychological Review, 12*, 199–221.

Nieminen P., Loikkanen J., Ryökäs E., & Mustonen A. (2020) Nature of evidence in religion and natural science. *Theology and Science, 18*, 448–474.

Nisbett, R., Peng, K., Choi, I., & Norenzayan, A. (2001). Culture and systems of thought: Holistic versus analytic cognition. *Psychological Review, 108*, 291–310.

Nisbett, R. E., Wilson, T. D., (1977). Telling more than we can know: Verbal reports on mental processes. *Psychological Review, 84*, 231–259.

Powell, L. H., Shahabi, L., Thoreson, C. E. (2003). Religion and spirituality: Linkages to physical health. *American Psychologist, 58*, 36–52

Sasaki, J. Y., & Kim, H. S. (2011). At the intersection of culture and religion: A cultural analysis of religion's implications for secondary control and social affiliation. *Journal of Personality and Social Psychology, 101*, 401–414.

Sasaki, J. Y., & Kim, H. S. (2017). Nature, nurture, and their interplay: A review of cultural neuroscience. *Journal of Cross-Cultural Psychology, 48*, 4–22.

Sasaki, J. Y., & Kim, H. S. (2020). The ego dampening influence of religion: Evidence from behavioral genetics and psychology. *Current Opinions in Psychology, 40*, 24–28.

Sasaki, J. Y., Kim, H. S., Mojaverian, T., Kelley, L. D., Park, I., & Janušonis, S. (2013). Religion priming differentially increases prosocial behavior among variants of dopamine D4 receptor (DRD4) gene. *Social Cognitive and Affective Neuroscience, 8*, 209–215.

Shariff, A. F., Willard, A. K., Andersen, T., & Norenzayan, A. (2015). Religious priming: A meta-analysis with a focus on prosociality. *Personality and Social Psychology Review, 20*, 27–48.

Shweder, R. (1995). Cultural psychology: What is it? In N. R. Goldberger & J. B. Veroff (Eds.), *The culture and psychology reader*, 41–86. New York: New York University Press.

Tang, Y., Zhang, W., Chen, K., & Feng, S. (2006). Arithmetic processing in the brain shaped by cultures. *Proceedings of the National Academy of Sciences, 103*, 10775–10780.

Tillich, P. (1955). Religious symbols and our knowledge of God. *The Christian Scholar, 38*, 189–197.

Weisbuch-Remington, M., Mendes, W. B., Seery, M. D., & Blascovich, J. (2005). The nonconscious influence of religious symbols in motivated performance situations. *Personality and Social Psychology Bulletin, 31*, 1203–1216.

PART IV

Further semiotic domains

21

WHAT MAKES US HUMAN? FACE IDENTITY RECOGNITION

Bruno Rossion

Introduction

The human brain is an organ weighing 1.2–1.5 kg that, together with the spinal cord, forms the central nervous system. It contributes to regulating body functions, processing sensory inputs of the environment, and controlling bodily actions. It is widely considered to be the most complex biological organ of the human body, consisting of about 86 billion nerve cells, or neurons, which present an astonishing level of morphological and functional variability. Each neuron is connected to other neurons by tens of thousands of synaptic connections, making this system extremely complex and difficult to understand. While the human brain is the product of a long biological evolution, it differs considerably from the brain of other animal species at multiple micro- and macroscopic levels of anatomo-functional organization (Bryant & Preuss, 2018; Gazzaniga, 2009; Herculano-Houzel, 2016; Kaas, 2019).

In its interaction with the environment, the brain can essentially be considered as a biological organ of recognition (Edelman, 2004): its primary function is to *discriminate* a myriad of sensory stimuli coming from a diverse, inherently ambiguous, and dynamic environment, and *to generalize* (or reproduce) these discriminative/selective responses across various instances of these stimuli based on their physical properties, as well as the brain's own biological constraints and past experience. For example, the adult human brain is able to recognize a wide range of stimuli as edible fruits, or different instances of insects as dangerous or harmless, and behave adaptively when facing them in daily life.

In psychology, the term "recognition" usually implies a judgment of previous occurrence (specifically "the ability to identify information as having been encountered before," according to the *APA Dictionary of Psychology*; see also Mandler, 1980). This is problematic if only because it confines recognition to experience, ruling out the contribution of phylogenetic memory. With such a restrictive semantic definition, *recognition* usually refers to a function different from *categorization* – two terms that are used preferentially by relatively independent scientific communities in psychology and cognitive (neuro)science (Palmeri & Gauthier, 2004). Here, I adopt a more general biological perspective, considering that recognition is essentially a categorization function that, in human adults, is largely automatic and associated with different levels of consciousness (Rossion & Retter, 2020). Without this recognition/categorization function (i.e., if each stimulus were treated as unique at every moment in time), we would be overwhelmed by the amount of sensory inputs received,

DOI: 10.4324/9781003051817-26

and lost in our interaction with the world. Hence, recognition/categorization is arguably the most important brain function, providing a key platform for learning, memory, attention, decision-making, language, and social communication, among other faculties (Murphy, 2002).

Inputs from the environment are dealt with by various sensory receptors in biological organisms, with vision being largely considered in the scientific community as the most elaborate sensory modality in humans (and primates in general). Visual stimuli vary substantially across time and space, with variations of luminance and wavelength providing extremely rich inputs. In humans and other primates, considerable brain portions deal mainly, or only, with visual inputs (Felleman & Van Essen, 1991) and the experimental studies in cognitive (neuro)science devoted to vision largely outnumber studies performed with stimuli suited to other sensory modalities (Hutmacher, 2019).

Among all sensory inputs to the human visual system, human faces constitute arguably the most important in our environment: they convey many cues for social communication and are frequently encountered, especially in modern societies and in the age of (social) media. Further, a face is a complex stimulus, containing multiple nameable parts (e.g., eyes, mouth, nose) and internal sources of physical variations interpreted in terms of shape, texture, and color. The face is thus extremely well suited for investigating the most refined mechanisms of recognition. In particular, often considered as the quintessential whole, or *Gestalt*, the face appears as the ideal stimulus to understand the complex relationships between wholes and parts in (visual) recognition (Rossion, 2013). For all these reasons, the human face undoubtedly holds a special place in scientific research, having become possibly the most widely studied stimulus in cognitive (neuro)science (Calder et al., 2011).

The key point of this chapter is that face recognition is specific to the human species in terms of expertise and neural mechanisms. This is not only because a human face is a powerful nonverbal stimulus communicating meaning, but more fundamentally because its recognition based on visual inputs only, in the adult human brain, originates from and is built upon multimodal (including verbal) associations. The recognition of identity from the face, face identity recognition (FIR), is used here as the primary example to illustrate this view. Since facial identity is not an objective conveyor of information to decode, but rather a sign to interpret based on semantic knowledge, understanding the biological bases of FIR is important for the agenda of neurosemiotics, and a neurosemiotic perspective can inspire future research on this topic.

Following this brief introduction, the chapter is divided into five further sections to first introduce the face as a stimulus, followed by insights on FIR, its development, and its fundamental difference between humans and other animal species. The next section will describe the human-specific neural circuitry subtending this function, highlighting key differences in cortical face networks with the best available animal model in cognitive neuroscience, the macaque brain. Following this analysis, an original model for the developmental origin and structuring of human cortical memories of face identities based on reentrant semantically driven identity representations will briefly be proposed before concluding remarks are made on this neurosemiotic perspective of human face (identity) recognition.

The human face as a powerful sign of social communication

Faces emerged through evolution in animal species over half a billion years ago as a biological interface between the central nervous system and the physical environment (McNeill, 2000). From a biophysical perspective, a face is a collection of sensory receptors – typically the eyes, nose, mouth, and ears – positioned together at the front of the body and in proximity to the brain. Importantly for an animal's survival, this arrangement enables information from the outside world to be reacted to appropriately and rapidly (Rossion & Retter, 2020). Many animal species have a face, with the sensory receptors organized in an overall quasi-symmetric configuration that often bears a striking resemblance to the human face (Bruce & Young, 1998). Despite this similarity, the human face has many characteristics that make it unique, even when compared with our closest cousin, the chimpanzee: a large head size relative to the body, a flat face due to the development of the prefrontal cortex, tooth size reduction, a prominent nose, a chin, less facial hair, thinner eyebrows, and a relatively small distance between the nose and the eyes.

Since populations of modern humans – *Homo Sapiens* – started to leave Africa around 100,000 years ago and settle on different continents, their body morphology, including the face, transformed in response to different natural selection pressures – that is, different physical and social environments (Ruff, 2002). Consequently, despite the extremely high genetic similarity between different modern human populations (Cavalli-Sforza & Cavalli-Sforza, 1995), there are important and markedly visible differences between their faces, both in terms of the bone structure and the reflectance of light on the skin (Bruce & Young, 1998). For instance, sub-Saharan Africans have darker skin and wider, more bulbous noses than Asians or Western Europeans, with the latter being characterized by thinner, pointier noses (Farkas, 1994; Zaidi et al., 2017).

In modern human populations, the face evolved to have primary importance for social functioning, conveying both quickly changeable cues to recognize/categorize emotion from the expression, the direction of attention from the position of the head and gaze, and the state of health from the skin tone – as well as relatively invariant cues to recognize/categorize age, sex, race, attractiveness, and personality traits such as dominance and trustworthiness (Bruce & Young, 1998; Todorov, 2017). The face is thus a multifaceted, ecologically valid construct with extreme importance for human social life. In this sense, the human face is an extremely powerful sign conveying meaning to the observer, and should be a primary object of study of (neuro)semiotics.

Face identity recognition: A human-specific expertise

The challenge and quality of human face identity recognition

Recognizing a face as belonging to a specific identity, or FIR, is particularly challenging in humans. This difficulty follows from two main factors. First, while individual faces certainly differ more in humans than in other animal species (Sheehan & Nachman, 2014), all human faces, particularly within a genetically homogenous group, share similar features and their overall configuration, so FIR requires fine-grained visual discrimination processes. Second, the same face identity can vary substantially under different viewing conditions (Figure 21.1), to the point where two views of the same identity may often differ physically more than two different facial identities (Burton et al., 2016).

A third factor, usually neglected, is that in most modern human societies, the number of different people encountered (in real life or through the media) is extremely large and variable over time. For this reason, the number of *categories* of human facial identities is, if not infinite, extremely large and undetermined. Hence, contrary to other face recognition functions (e.g., emotional expression, sex, age), for which there is a small and relatively stable number of categorizations to make, FIR is a wide-open flexible recognition function, making it extremely challenging. This challenge explains why there is so much natural interindividual variability in this ability in the normal population (Wilmer, 2017), and why this ability is easily lost in many neurological, neurodevelopmental and psychiatric disorders (Barton et al., 2021).

These three factors also explain why, despite major investments in technology and substantial progress over the past decades, artificial algorithms for FIR still struggle to come close to human performance and can be fooled relatively easily.[1] Since early 2020 and the COVID-19 pandemic, artificial FIR has also struggled to surmount the new challenges posed by face masks.[2]

Despite this challenge, in humans identity recognition is based primarily on the face, which among body parts carries by far the largest morphological and genetic diversity (Sheehan & Nachman, 2014). Young adults in modern societies are able to accurately identify thousands of faces on average (Jenkins et al., 2018), rapidly – that is, at a glance, and within a few hundreds of milliseconds of processing (Hsiao et al., 2008; Yan & Rossion, 2020) – and largely automatically (i.e., without volition). Thanks to these characteristics (accuracy, speed, automaticity, large and variable number of exemplars

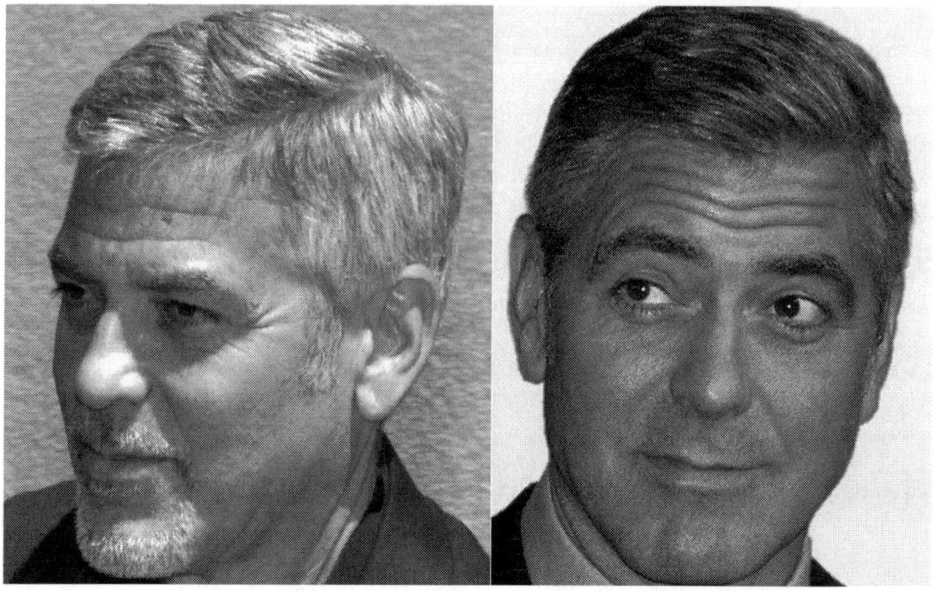

Figure 21.1 A face identity recognition (FIR) as categorization

FIR requires producing a **selective** response to a view of a face (e.g., George Clooney) compared with other (familiar or unfamiliar) face identities and to *generalize* this response across widely different signals – for example, very different views of George Clooney's face as in the display. Due to large changes in viewing conditions but also facial appearance during the lifetime, the objective physical difference can be much smaller between one view of a face identity and another facial identity (e.g., Clooney and a Clooney lookalike) than between two views of the same face identity. According to the neurosemiotic view advocated here, generalization across different views of a face identity is not based on invariant unimodal visual representations derived from an objective analysis of facial features, but is necessarily rooted in multimodal semantic memory. Pictures licensed under the Creative Commons Attribution – Share Alike 3.0 Unported. Attribution: Georges Biard. See e-book for a full-color version of this figure.

to recognize), neurotypical human adults can be considered genuine *experts* at FIR (Carey, 1992; Rossion, 2018a).

Expertise in FIR is thought to be based on the ability of the neurotypical adult brain to recognize a face identity holistically/configurally – that is, as a single unit rather than a collection of independent features (Tanaka & Farah, 1993). This recognition mode is well illustrated by visual phenomena such as the composite face illusion, in which identical top face halves aligned with differing bottom face halves, produce the vivid impression of different top face halves (Figure 21.2). This visual illusion provides compelling evidence that the recognition of the identity of a face part is mandatorily affected by the identity of the other parts (Rossion, 2013; Tanaka & Farah, 1993; Young et al., 1987) and that FIR goes well beyond the stimulus given. The importance of holistic face identity recognition is supported, among other observations (e.g., Van Belle et al., 2010), by the disruption of the composite face illusion following stimulus inversion (Rossion, 2013; Young et al., 1987; Figure 21.2) and in cases of prosopagnosia (Ramon et al., 2010), a sudden, massive, and category-selective impairment of FIR following brain damage (Bodamer, 1947; for a recent review, see Rossion, 2018b).

Development, genetics, and experience

To what extent is human FIR genetically predetermined and to what extent does it arise due to visual experience? On the one hand, developmental difficulties at FIR – most often called "developmental or congenital prosopagnosia" (Behrmann & Avidan, 2005), but more correctly "prosopdysgnosia"

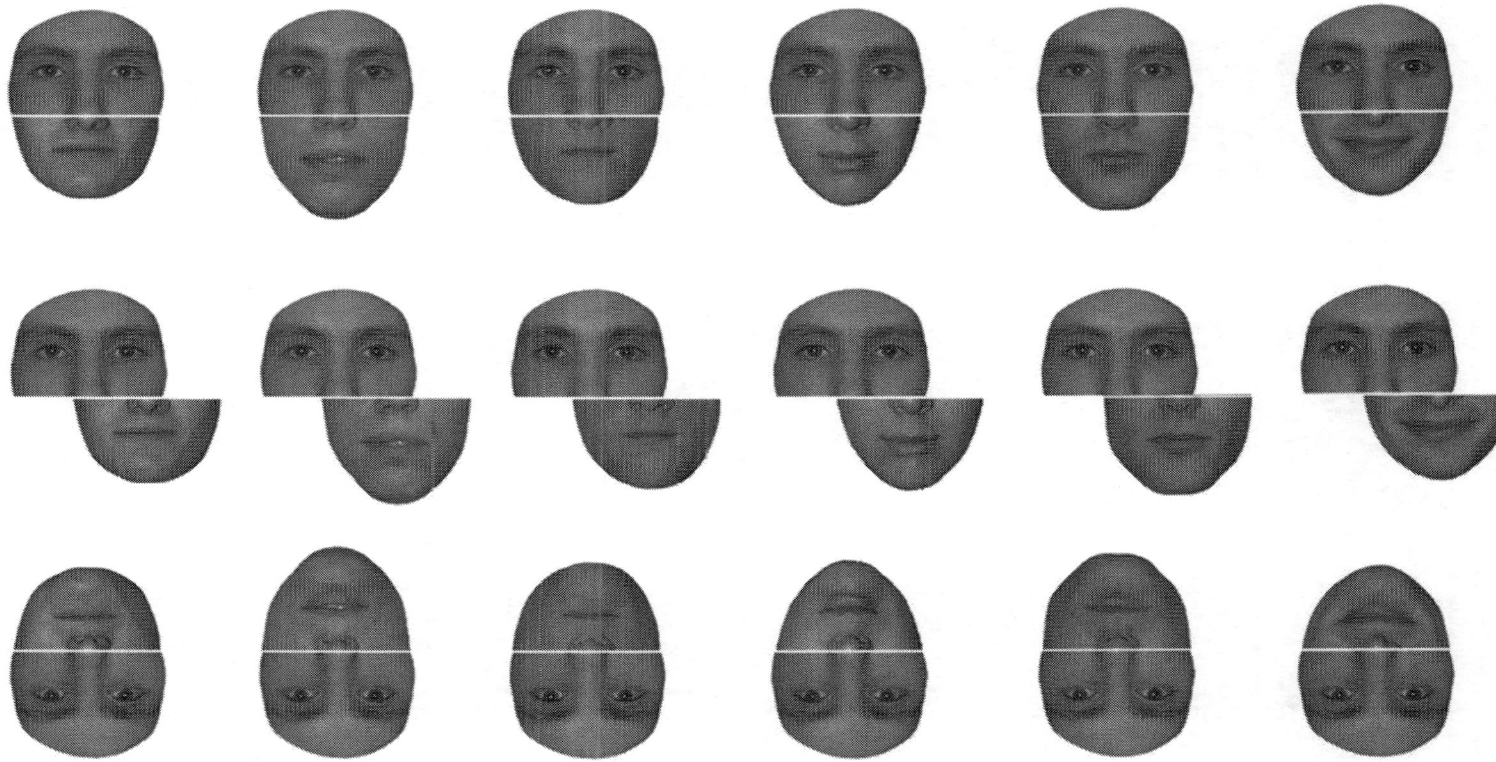

Figure 21.2 The composite face illusion

This powerful illusion shows that FIR goes beyond the stimulus given. A. All five top halves (above the thin line) are physically identical. Yet, when they are aligned with distinct bottom halves (all of different identities, neutral expression, taken under the same lighting conditions), they are perceived as being different. B. If the bottom halves differ but are spatially misaligned with the top halves, one has no difficulties in perceiving the top face halves as being indeed identical. C. The same as in A but the display has been vertically flipped, showing inverted faces. All 5 "top" halves (here at the bottom of the display below the thin line) are physically identical and one does not see them as being different. See e-book for a full-color version of this figure.

(see Rossion, 2018c) – may run in families (Susilo & Duchaine, 2013), and monozygotic twins' performance at FIR tasks are more strongly correlated than dizygotic twins' performance (Wilmer et al., 2010). These observations have led to claims that genetics largely determine FIR ability. On the other hand, early visual experience appears to be critical for the development of FIR based on holistic representations (Le Grand et al., 2004) and also leads to the fine-tuning of FIR ability; at nine months of age, infants show lower FIR performance for non-experienced than frequently experienced faces – for example, other-species faces (Pascalis et al., 2002) and other-race human faces (Kelly et al., 2007). Nevertheless, even after nine years of age a predominant exposure to other-race faces can reverse such an early bias in FIR (Sangrigoli & de Schonen, 2004). Thus, experience appears to be necessary and influential for FIR, which continues to improve during development until adulthood (Carey, 1992). While some authors consider that this long development is essentially explained by the maturation of general cognitive factors (Crookes & McKone, 2009), there is substantial behavioral and neural evidence for a progressive, specific improvement of FIR. For instance, the face inversion effect, measured as the difference in performance for recognizing the identity of upright versus inverted faces, emerges only at a few years of age and increases until adulthood (Hills & Lewis, 2018). Moreover, the spatial extent and degree of face-selectivity in the human ventral occipito-temporal cortex, as described in the next section, continues to develop past age seven into adulthood (Golarai et al., 2017).

Importantly, although the notion of expertise has been around for decades in the field of human face recognition (Diamond & Carey, 1986; Carey, 1992), it is generally conflated with the view that expertise necessarily arises from visual experience only, and that it could be developed in a similar way for virtually any kind of non-face stimuli learned during development or even in adulthood (Diamond & Carey, 1986; Gauthier & Tarr, 1997). In this vein, "acquired" domain-general expertise has often been radically opposed to "innate" domain-specific (i.e., only for faces) expertise (McKone et al., 2007). Instead, current evidence suggests that, despite a large amount of interindividual variability in FIR ability (Wilmer et al., 2010), neurotypical human adults possess a domain-specific expertise in FIR, which emerges both from genetic factors and experience. The level of expertise that humans reach in FIR appears particularly salient when compared with FIR performance of other animal species.

A human-specific expertise in FIR

Animal species other than humans undoubtedly rely on faces of conspecifics for social communication, with the face of non-human primates, in particular, conveying important cues for recognizing emotional expression and attention from gaze and head direction (e.g., Emery et al., 1997). Yet whether the face is used as a (primary) cue for identity recognition in non-human species is much more debatable. Behavioral studies have shown that many non-human species, such as sheep (Peirce et al., 2000), fish (Wang & Takeuchi, 2017), and even wasps (Sheehan & Tibbetts, 2011) can discriminate pictures of faces of different conspecifics, drawing parallels to human performance. However, FIR performance of non-human species often follows long operant-conditioning procedures and, despite the use of a small number of individual exemplars (with often the exact same images repeated extensively), remains relatively modest (Rossion & Taubert, 2019; Figure 21.3A). Moreover, successful performance on such tasks appears to be based on low-level image characteristics (with limited across-image generalization) and/or external traits of the face – for example, antennae for wasps or ears for sheep; see respective references above (Figure 21.3A).

Importantly, this limited ability also holds for the species often considered as offering the best available animal model for the human visual system (and even for complex visual object recognition – see DiCarlo et al., 2012): the macaque monkey. Interestingly, macaques are poor at behavioral FIR tasks, requiring hundreds of trials to reach acceptable levels of performance on simple image discrimination tasks, with little generalization over new images (Parr et al., 2008) (Figure 21.3B). This is also the case for other monkey species, such as Capuchin monkeys (Pokorny & de Waal, 2009; see

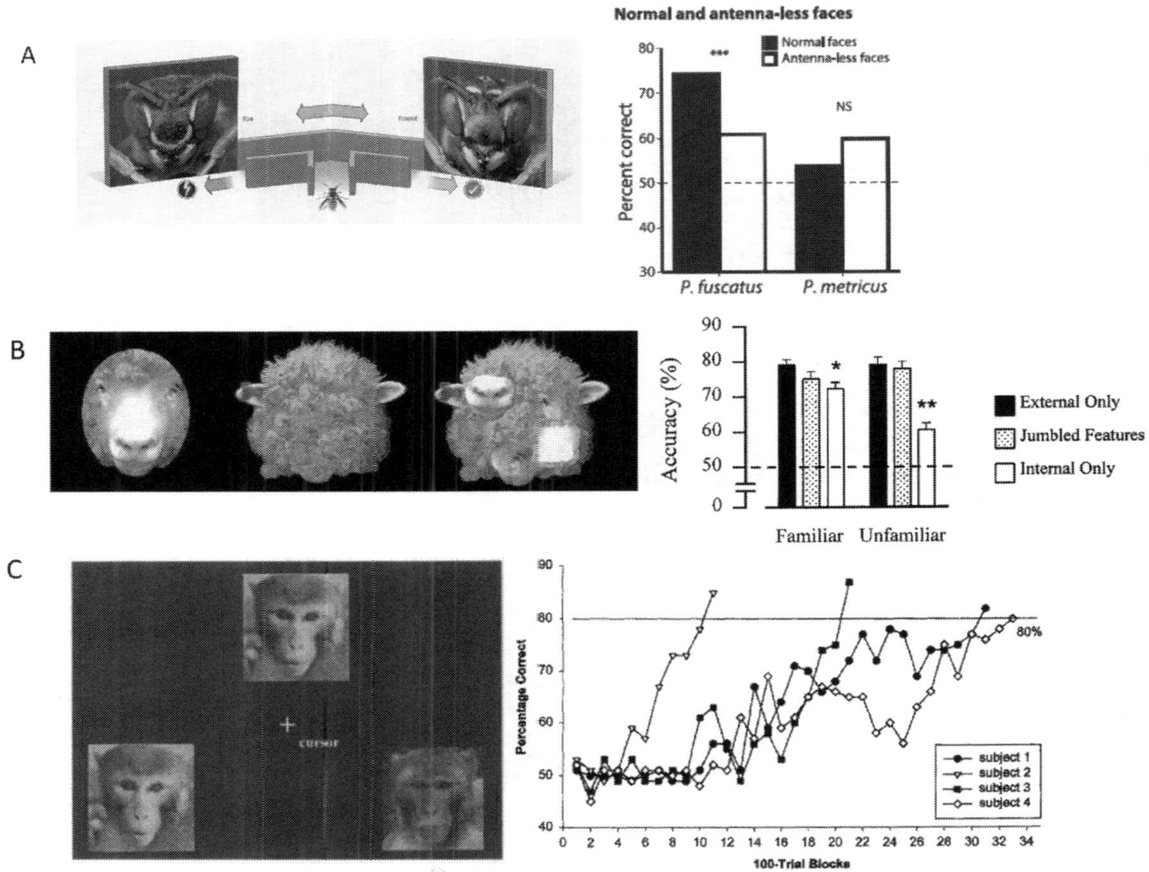

Figure 21.3 Many animal species can be trained to discriminate the identity of conspecifics from their faces

A. Polistes fuscatus wasps as shown in A, whose recognition performance depends heavily on the presence of the antenna (from Sheehan & Tibbetts, 2011; with permission). B. Similarly, sheep can be trained to discriminate images of conspecifics, but with a

Figure 21.3 (Continued)

limited performance that, unlike in humans, is based on piecemeal information, especially external features (from Peirce et al., 2000, with permission). C. Left. Example of a sequential 2 alternative forced-choice or match-to-sample task used in the studies of Parr and colleagues (Parr et al., 2000, 2008) in which a target face is presented on top, and disappears when the monkey contacts it with a cursor driven by a joystick. After the target face is contacted, it is cleared from the monitor, and the two comparison stimuli appear below. In some versions of the task, the target face remains on the screen. Note that the two images to match are strictly identical. Right. Results of the four macaques tested at this trivial task with blocks of 100 trials, showing that they need between 1100 and 3300 trials to reach criterion (>80% performance). Introducing a new image set after reaching criterion leads to a significant drop of performance, even though the task still requires a simple image comparison (from Parr et al., 2008, with permission under a PMC Creative Commons License). See e-book for a full-color version of this figure.

the extensive review of Rossion & Taubert, 2019). Importantly, since monkeys' performance drops after the introduction of new images, this modest performance is not due to difficulties at specific task acquisition. Moreover, monkeys do not rely on qualitatively similar processes to humans for FIR. That is, they rely primarily on external features (Parr et al., 2008), and generally fail to show a decrease of performance with stimulus (picture-plane) inversion (Bruce, 1982; Griffin, 2020; Rossion & Taubert, 2019), one of the most compelling effects in human studies (Rossion, 2008). Moreover, unlike humans (e.g., Bruce et al., 2001), they do not perform better for matching pictures of familiar than unfamiliar faces for their identity (Micheletta et al., 2015; Pokorny and de Waal, 2009).

Overall, these observations cast strong doubt as to the appropriateness of the (macaque) monkey as a model for understanding the neural basis of human FIR. Although behavioral studies suggest that chimpanzees, and perhaps other apes, are better than macaques at FIR and might rely on more qualitatively similar processes to humans (Taubert et al., 2012), humans may be the only animal species living in a large social group to naturally use the face as the primary source of information for FIR (as opposed to smell, vocalization, non-facial body cues and so on), reaching expertise levels that appear unparalleled in the animal world.

Face identity recognition: A human-specific neural circuitry

What are the neural mechanisms supporting human FIR? For the reasons presented above, answering this question would go a long way towards understanding recognition/categorization, arguably the most fundamental brain function. As we shall see below, the answer to this question is also important for the agenda of neurosemiotics, which should be concerned not only with how semantic knowledge about people's identity is associated with visual constructs in the human brain, but by how semantic knowledge constrains and even generates face recognition based on visual inputs.

A right-lateralized network of face-selective regions

The neural bases of human FIR were first hinted at in patients presenting prosopagnosia – that is, after lesions to the ventral occipito-temporal cortex (VOTC), in particular the right fusiform gyrus (Cohen et al., 2019; Meadows, 1974). Since the mid-1990s, functional magnetic resonance imaging (fMRI) studies have identified clusters of voxels (of a few cubic millimeters) responding significantly more to pictures of faces than nonface objects, especially along the VOTC (in particular, the lateral fusiform gyrus) and the superior temporal sulcus (STS) (Figure 21.4) – for reviews and models, see Duchaine & Yovel (2015), Grill-Spector et al. (2017), and Haxby et al. (2000). While the human VOTC network has been associated with the recognition of relatively stable aspects of a face, in particular its identity, the more dorsal STS network is thought to be involved in the recognition of rapidly changing (i.e., dynamic) aspects of faces, such as eye gaze direction, head orientation, and facial expression (Allison et al., 2000; Bernstein & Yovel, 2015).

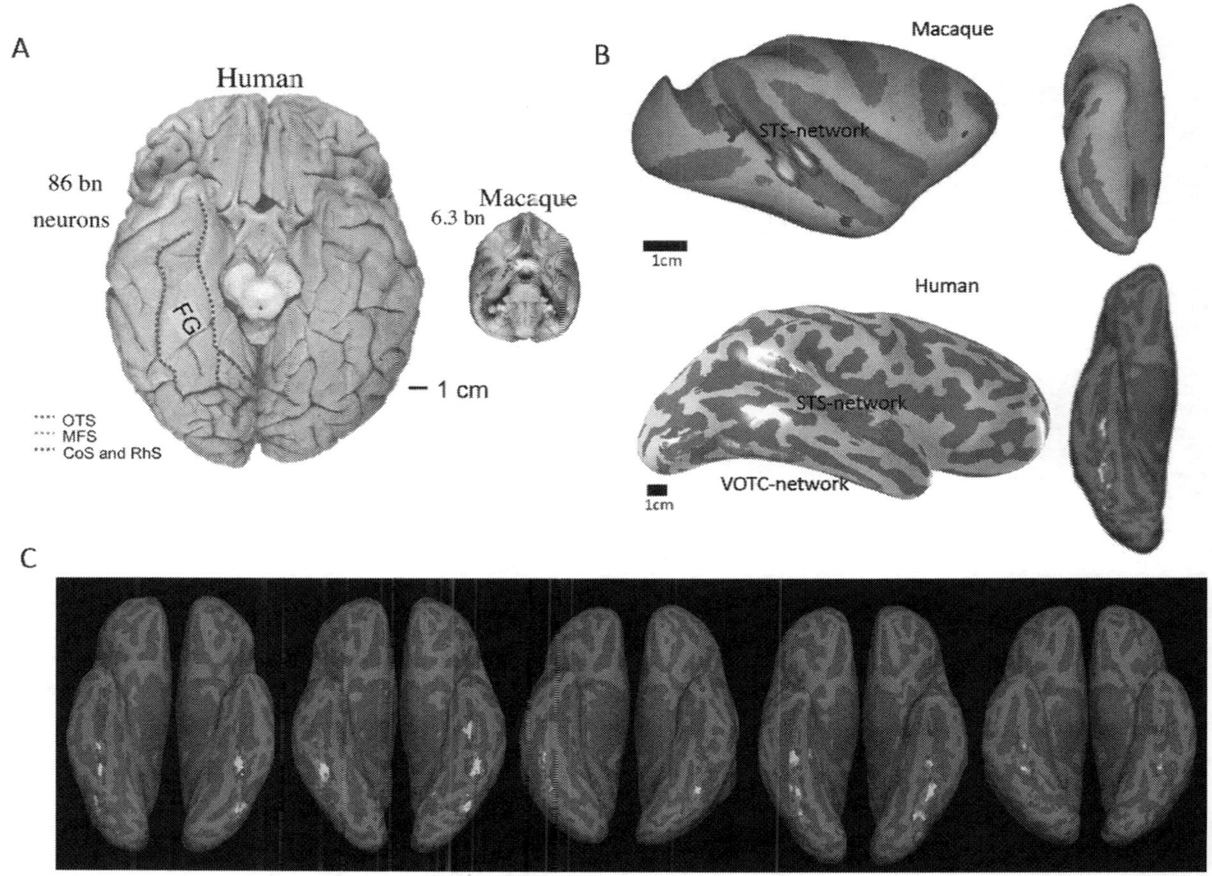

Figure 21.4 Human specificity of neural circuits for face identity recognition

A. Ventral view of a human and a macaque brain at relative sizes. The human brain contains approximately 86,000 million neurons, about 13.5 times more than a macaque brain (6376 million) (Herculano-Houzel, 2016). In humans, the key neural structures for face identity recognition run from

Figure 21.4 (Continued)

the lateral section of the inferior occipital gyrus (IOG) to the posterior (pFG), middle lateral (lFG) and anterior fusiform gyrus (aFG) up to the temporal pole. In comparison, the posterior ventral occipito-temporal cortex of the macaque brain is limited to one sulcus, with little gyrification, and no fusiform gyrus (Bryant & Preuss, 2018). B. Inflated segmented brains showing typical locations of posterior face-selective regions in macaques and humans (adapted from Weiner & Grill-Spector, 2015; with permission under a PMC Creative Commons License). In macaques, these regions are essentially found in the STS, whereas humans have regions in both the STS and the VOTC (1, 2, 3, 4 on the figure). C. Ventral surface of individual human brains, showing the wide variability across five individuals in terms of the number and size of face-selective responses (data unsmoothed, obtained here with a highly sensitive and specific fMRI face localizer, Gao et al., 2018). This ventral network of face-selective regions is found primarily in the lateral fusiform gyrus and does not exist in monkeys. See e-book for a full-color version of this figure.

Neurofunctional models of human face recognition have been generated, with modular roles attributed to clusters of voxels (usually referred to as face-selective areas) in the VOTC and STS (Duchaine & Yovel, 2015; Haxby et al., 2000) (see Figure 21.4). The face-selective cluster in the lateral middle fusiform gyrus, known as fusiform face area (FFA; Kanwisher et al., 1997) has been divided into several subclusters, such as the pFus-faces/FFA-1 and mFus-faces/FFA-2, which have been linked to cytoarchitectonically distinct regions (Grill-Spector et al., 2017).

In recent years, there has been a rise in fMRI studies using multivariate pattern analysis to "decode" the representations of (unfamiliar) individual faces in the cortical face network in order to localize and better define the neural bases of FIR. Unfortunately, these studies often report weak and inconsistent effects essentially driven by image-based cues (Nestor et al., 2011; see Rossion, 2014). In comparison, fMR-adaptation studies (Grill-Spector & Malach, 2001), which are based on reduced fMRI signal to repeated facial identities as compared with different stimuli, have reported more consistent effects in face-selective VOTC regions (Davies-Thompson et al., 2009; Gauthier et al., 2000).

However, such effects have not been reported in more anterior regions of the VOTC, which are affected by large magnetic susceptibility artifacts in fMRI (Rossion et al., 2018; Wandell, 2011). This drop in signal-to-noise ratio creates a "gap" between posterior VOTC regions and more anterior regions in the temporal pole (e.g., between regions 3 and 4 in Figure 21.4B), this latter region being linked to multimodal semantic associations, in particular knowledge about people (Collins et al., 2016; Gainotti, 2013; Lambon-Ralph et al., 2010). Interestingly, at the functional level, this gap caused by methodological factors corresponds to the advocated dissociation between "perception" and "semantic memory" for faces (Duchaine & Yovel, 2015; Haxby et al., 2000). However, lesion analyses of prosopagnosia (Cohen et al., 2019) as well as focal electrical intracerebral recordings (Jacques et al., 2020; Jonas et al., 2016) and direct stimulation (Jonas & Rossion, 2021), point to a key role of populations of neurons throughout the anterior ventral temporal cortex, rather suggesting a continuous cortical representation of faces along the whole VOTC.

The lack of a ventral face-selective network in macaque monkeys

Since there is no reason to expect, and no evidence whatsoever, that each facial identity would be uniquely associated with a specific brain region or even a neuronal population at the level of a single voxel in fMRI (containing millions of neurons; Logothetis, 2008), it is generally assumed that a full understanding of the neural mechanisms of human FIR requires complementary neural measures at finer spatial scales of brain organization, all the way down to the level of single neurons. This is where rhesus monkeys have served as a non-human primate model, potentially bridging what we learn from human lesion studies and neuroimaging to activity at the level of the single cell.

Single neurons responding selectively to faces were found in the macaque temporal cortex originally by Gross et al. (1972). Further single cell studies performed during the 1980s reported large numbers of these face-selective neurons, describing their response properties in detail (e.g., Perrett et al., 1982; see Desimone, 1991 for review). Since early studies reported variability in the firing rate of single neurons in response to images of different individual faces, this variability has been proposed as a mechanism for FIR (Rolls, 1992). Specifically, each face-selective neuron of a small population does not respond only to one face, but has a different relative response, in terms of the number of spikes/second, to each of the members of a set of facial identities. Thus, the firing rate across a population of such neurons can convey information about different individuals – that is, a distributed neural code (Rolls, 1992). Importantly, this information is thought to relate directly to physical properties of the stimuli: faces that are physically similar/different appear to be represented by similar/different distributed patterns of spike rates across the neuronal population – a "face space" (Leopold et al., 2006; Young & Yamane, 1992). In recent years, this seminal work has been extended to target, and compare, the coding of different facial identities in fMRI-defined face-selective regions of the macaque brain (Tsao et al., 2006). For instance, an influential study reported that the firing rates of approximately 200 neurons sampled from face-selective regions in two macaque brains could be used to decode visual similarity among 2000 humanoid pictures of faces and claimed to have finally cracked the neural code that allows the human brain to perform FIR (Chang & Tsao, 2017; see also Freiwald, 2020; Hesse & Tsao, 2020).

However, this claim is unsubstantiated (Rossion & Taubert, 2017), and the view that variable spike rates in a small population of neurons in the monkey brain offer a mechanistic account of human FIR is fatally flawed for several reasons. First, as described above, monkeys are poor at recognizing the identity of conspecifics from their faces only. Moreover, even if the animals tested in experiments are usually raised in captivity, there is no reason to expect that they would be better at identity recognition of *human* faces (as used in most of these studies). Second, when they succeed at learning to recognize a modest number of facial identities in photographs, monkeys rely on different cues and qualitatively different processes compared with humans, most likely using a part-based analysis of low-level visual characteristics rather than extracting a holistic, fine-grained representation to individuate the face at a glance. Third, there are major relevant differences at the neural level between humans and macaques (Figure 21.4), who last shared a common ancestor 25–30 million years ago (Kaas, 2019). For a start, the human brain contains about 13.5 times more neurons than the macaque brain (Herculano-Houzel, 2016) and this difference is not homogenous across regions. For instance, the primary visual cortex is relatively much larger in macaques than humans – 10 percent of the total cortical surface versus 3 percent, respectively (Van Essen, 2005). In contrast, the temporal lobe is much smaller and thinner in macaques than humans, even accounting for body size differences (Bryant & Preuss, 2018; Rilling & Seligman, 2002).

Beyond (relative) size, they are also major differences in gyrification between the brains of macaques and humans (Zilles et al., 2013). In humans, the VOTC is divided by two major sulci: the collateral sulcus (CS) more medially, and the occipito-temporal sulcus (OTS) more laterally, these two sulci defining the borders of *the fusiform gyrus*, the most important structure for human FIR, as noted above. In contrast, monkeys possess only one main ventral sulcus, labelled as the OTS, therefore lacking a fusiform gyrus – among other substantial neuroanatomical differences with the human VOTC (Figure 21.4A–B).

Given their lack of the hominoid-specific fusiform structure (Weiner & Zilles, 2016), it is not surprising that macaque monkeys do not hold a ventral face-selective cortical network (Bryant & Preuss, 2018). Rather, their face-selective regions are found more dorsally, mainly in the STS, where face-selective neurons have been recorded in this species since the earliest studies. Critically, bilateral removal of the entire STS in macaque monkeys has no or little effect on their learned ability to discriminate faces of conspecifics for their identity, but disrupts their sensitivity to gaze orientation (Heywood & Cowey, 1992). This latter observation supports the view that these face-selective STS regions in the monkey brain are involved in recognizing dynamic aspects of faces, such as eye gaze direction, head orientation, and facial expression, rather than identity (Allison et al., 2000; Bernstein & Yovel, 2015; Perrett et al., 1985; Taubert et al., 2020).

Finally, in humans, face-selective cortical regions are typically larger in size and level of activation in the right as compared to the left hemisphere (Rossion et al., 2012; Sergent et al., 1992). While the factors driving this right hemispheric lateralization remain largely unknown (Rossion & Lochy, 2022), regions of the right but not the left hemisphere appear critical for FIR (Cohen et al., 2019; Jonas & Rossion, 2021; Sergent & Signoret, 1992). This contrasts with the strictly bilateral cortical face network observed in monkeys (Tsao et al., 2008).

Overall, these anatomo-functional differences between species, together with the lack of human-like ability at FIR in macaque monkeys as reviewed in the previous section, support the exciting view that the ventral face-selective recognition system – which is mainly found all along the lateral fusiform gyrus and adjacent sulci (Figure 21.4) – emerged relatively recently in evolution, and may even have developed specifically in the human species.[3]

The key role of reentrant semantically driven identity representations

If the monkey brain offers only an inadequate model of human FIR, how can we clarify the neural mechanisms of this key function in our species? One answer is technical: neuroscientists should focus in the coming years on electrophysiological recording of neuronal populations and single neurons in the *human* cortical face-network. Human recordings of single neurons have been performed for decades with microelectrodes in patients with epilepsy refractory to medication (Fried et al., 2014). Yet this approach remains very rare and technically challenging. Moreover, for technical and clinical reasons, these studies focus on specific brain structures such as the medial temporal lobe (e.g., hippocampus, amygdala), where so-called concept cells (i.e., neurons responding to multimodal inputs defining a famous person, scene, or object) have been reported (Quian-Quiroga, 2020; Quian-Quiroga et al., 2005). Notwithstanding these limitations, recent studies have started to explore multi- and single-unit spiking activity in face-selective human VOTC regions (Khuvis et al., 2021), providing hope to make progress in our understanding of the neural basis of human FIR in the years to come. However, perhaps more fundamentally, another answer to the question above is conceptual: to make sense of future findings at this level, and integrate them with the large corpus of data collected at multiple levels of brain organization with various techniques of cognitive neuroscience, the prevalent theoretical framework in human face recognition research needs to be fundamentally reevaluated. This is where a neurosemiotic perspective, as advocated in this book and briefly discussed below, can be inspiring.

Human face recognition is generally considered a problem of vision, according to which we need to resolve how the analysis of physical features of a face stimulus impinging on the eye's retina leads to a hierarchical succession of visual representations in the cortex until an invariant visual representation of facial identity is extracted (DiCarlo et al., 2012; Freiwald, 2020; Hesse & Tsao, 2020). It is only *after* this invariant unimodal (visual) representation is built from objective features of the stimulus that it would be associated with semantic knowledge about that face (Bruce & Young, 1986; Jiang et al., 2006; Duchaine & Yovel, 2015). In fact, despite the use of various (and often confusing) terminologies, this dissociation goes well beyond face (identity) recognition and reflects a general conceptual gap that is made in human cognitive (neuro)science between "(visual) perception" and "(semantic) memory," or between "perceptual/visual categorization" (i.e., categorization thought to be based on the decoding of objective physical attributes of stimuli) and "conceptual/semantic categorization" (i.e., abstract categorizations based on our knowledge of the world).

Usually originating from a tradition of research that started with early stages of visual processing (Hubel & Wiesel, 1962), and the first influential computational approach of vision of Marr (1982), monkey neurophysiologists have adopted this hierarchical view of visual recognition, including face recognition, to the core. These researchers consider the visual recognition system as being essentially hierarchical, with increasingly complex visual representations progressively built from the computational analysis and (linear or nonlinear) combination of objective physical features of stimuli (DiCarlo et al., 2012; Freiwald, 2020; Hesse & Tsao, 2020). Since representations of facial identities are thought to be computationally extracted, independently of any previous encounter with these faces, and are based on physically objective features, the inputs (i.e., face images) can even be well-reconstructed from the pattern of neural activity at a specific stage in the system (Chang & Tsao, 2017). According to this hierarchical computational view, memory representations of familiar faces located in more anterior regions of the system, such as the anterior temporal lobe or the parahippocampal gyrus (Landi & Freiwald, 2017), are contacted only following computational extraction of invariant visual representations. The goal of this research program, based on this standard framework, is therefore to elucidate the nature (content) of visual representations at each of the stages of the system and the computations applied to these representations.

However, in our species at least, FIR goes well beyond vision and fully incorporates semantics, including verbal representations. Take the face stimuli of Figure 21.1, for instance: in many instances, physical similarity is much higher between one view of a face identity (George Clooney's face) and another (unfamiliar or familiar) face identity than between two views of George Clooney's face. This is even clearer when comparing veridical facial identities to their caricatures or their lookalikes. In this context, how could the visual recognition system build an invariant representation of all views of a face identity (e.g., George Clooney), independently of knowledge (semantic memory) about this person? And while there is probably no lookalike that we would seriously confuse with Donald Trump's inimitable face, how do we readily recognize him as a Parisian trash bin?[4] These examples serve to illustrate that conceptualizing FIR as a problem of vision only, with (semantic) memory representations intervening afterwards, is not tenable. This standard position in human face recognition research, according to which a series of perceptual stages precedes access to semantic knowledge, leads to fundamental incoherencies, such as the rejection of unfamiliar FIR to non-expert low-level visual processes (Megreya & Burton, 2006; Young & Burton, 2018), despite overwhelming evidence that such faces are processed holistically in high-level human visual cortical areas (Jacques et al., 2020; see Rossion, 2018b). Moreover, this standard position of a dissociation between perceptual processing stages and semantic memory makes it virtually impossible to understand how unfamiliar faces can (rapidly) become familiar.

To resolve these issues, an alternative view is proposed here according to which semantic representations – that is, the source of information we possess that enables us to bring meaning to words, objects, and all other nonverbal stimuli such as smell or sound (Lambon-Ralph et al., 2010) – in the ventral anterior temporal lobe developmentally *precede* and *build* unimodal (i.e., visual) face-selective representations of identity in the posterior VOTC, *constraining* these representations throughout lifetime via reentrant neuronal connections. That is, one learns that different views of a face belong to the same identity not only because they often occur in close temporal succession (Wallis & Bülthoff, 2001), but because they are associated with the same context, affects, auditory, and even olfactory inputs (Rekow et al., 2021), as well as abstract verbal cues – for example, names and all kinds of semantic associations (Dixon et al., 1998; Eick et al., 2020; Schwartz & Yovel, 2016). This is how two completely different views of an unknown George Clooney can become associated in our brain: thanks to their non-visual semantic commonalities, they both initially lead to the firing of a largely overlapping population of neurons in the ventral anterior temporal cortex because we encounter them in common multimodal contexts. And, contrary to the standard model of human face recognition, this multimodal person representation is not contacted *after* the extraction of view-invariant visual representations: to the contrary, it constitutes the earliest – in terms of developmental origin and learning – and (only fully) invariant representations of "facial" identity. In humans, these multimodal person representations are located in anterior regions of the VOTC – that is, the ventral anterior temporal lobe (Collins et al., 2016) – being heavily constrained by language-related inputs.

Through re-entry – that is, bidirectional rapid exchange of inputs along reciprocal axonal fibers (Edelman & Gally, 2013) – these selective populations of neurons synchronize their activity with populations of neurons located more posteriorly in the VOTC, down to non-retinotopic visual regions of the inferior occipital gyrus, posterior and midfusiform gyrus (Figure 21.5). If multimodal recognition in ventral anterior temporal regions is successful, this leads to strengthening of connections with selective populations of neurons in posterior VOTC regions – a process occurring through Hebbian associative learning mediated by the hippocampus (Squire et al., 2015). Since these posterior VOTC regions receive concurrent direct inputs from (retinotopic) low-level visual areas, there is a progressive selection of their neuronal populations receiving the patterns of low-level visual inputs associated with successful recognition. Through this associative process, in these posterior VOTC regions, facial identities become progressively distinguishable based on low-level visual inputs only. Thus, unimodal (i.e., visual) cortical memories (Fuster, 2009) are built "inside-out," from semantics to vision. In a mature system, these cortical visual memories are essential to immediately distinguish novel faces from one another, even in the absence of semantic associations, and facilitate learning – that is, transforming unfamiliar faces into familiar ones.

Importantly, this dynamic recurrent process leads to *distributed* cortical memories (of facial identities) all along the human VOTC (Figure 21.5). Rather than fixed hierarchical computational stages with an invariant, purely visual representation extracted from the input and subsequently associated with semantic memory, there is an antero-posterior *gradient* of selected semantic-visual feature representation (Figure 21.5). Hence, even "visual" posterior VOTC face-selective regions can be modulated in their early activity by multimodal inputs linked to faces and facial identities, such as human voices (Blank et al., 2015), identity-related names (Ambrus et al., 2019), semantic associations (e.g., "job title" – Eick et al., 2020) or even face-related words (García et al., 2020). Yet, in a fully

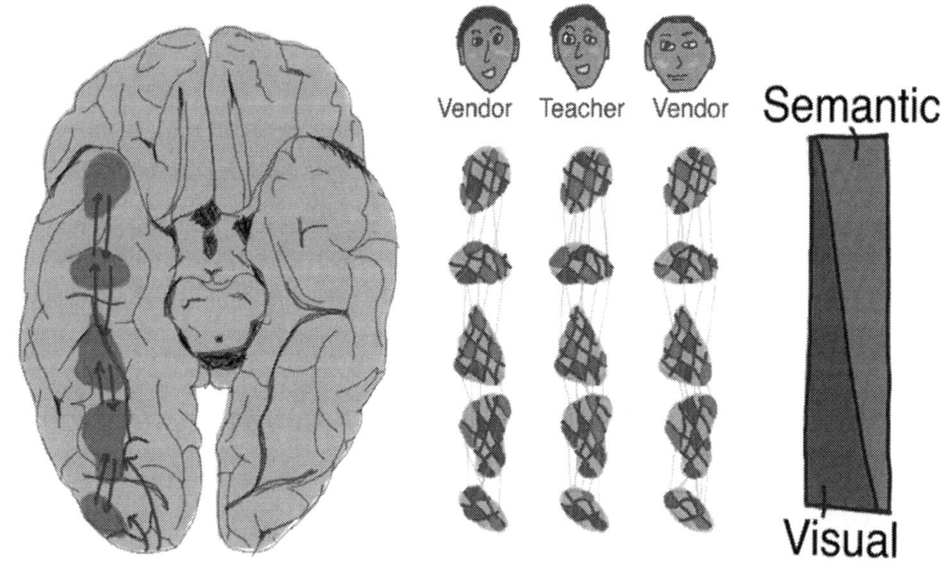

Figure 21.5 Face identity recognition in the human ventral occipito-temporal cortex

Different face-selective populations of neurons ("clusters") are linked by reentrant connections. Through a gradient of sensitivity from purely visual to semantic features along the VOTC, different facial identities could be represented by partly overlapping groups of neurons within these clusters, providing increased invariance across physical variations in the antero-posterior direction. Note that while five clusters of roughly similar sizes are represented here, their number and spatial extent vary across individual brains (Figure 21.4C). See e-book for a full-color version of this figure.

developed neurotypical adult brain, their main source of inputs to distinguish identities comes from low-level visual regions. This is the reason why, in a mature system, selective destruction of these posterior VOTC face-selective regions – such as the "FFA" in the right hemisphere – may cause prosopagnosia, a modality-specific memory impairment limited to face identity (Rossion, 2018a).

Finally, another implication of this visuo-semantic inverse gradient is that, although there are general anatomical constraints for these selective populations of neurons to end up roughly in the same cytoarchitectonic VOTC regions – for example, the lateral rather than the medial fusiform gyrus (Grill-Spector et al., 2017) – they also vary tremendously in terms of variability, size, spatial distribution, and number across individual brains (Figure 21.4C) (Gao et al., 2022), reflecting specific cultural and idiosyncratic visuo-semantic experiences with faces. Consequently, any scientific attempt to define general computational/representational stages at each level of a well-defined hierarchy of brain areas across all individual brains is bound to fail.

While a full elaboration of this original view goes beyond the scope of this chapter, if proved correct it would firmly place human face (identity) recognition beyond the realm of vision, as part of the larger field of neurosemiotics.

Conclusions: Towards a neurosemiotics of human face recognition?

A fundamental function of the central nervous system is to recognize stimuli of the environment in order to generate adaptive behavior. This function is not achieved by a series of computations applied to well-defined distinct representational stages but "merely" by associating specific populations of neurons to specific stimuli and being able to reproduce these selective responses across variable instances of the stimuli. At this very coarse level of description, there is no fundamental difference between the recognition of the identity of conspecifics from the face, FIR, across a number of animal species – for example, Polistes fuscatus wasps, sheep, macaque monkeys and humans. In humans, however, FIR requires a very fine-grained level of visual discrimination among many exemplars and, especially immense generalization abilities that go well beyond objective physical features. Thanks to extensive experience during development and the social pressure to rapidly and accurately recognize the identity of a large and variable number of face identities, this leads to an unparalleled level of expertise at FIR in neurotypical human adults, characterized by high accuracy levels, speed, automaticity and holistic recognition. This FIR expertise is supported by a distributed category-selective right-lateralized network in the VOTC, a network that is not found in macaque monkeys and that, across individual human brains, presents with a large amount of interindividual variability in size, localization, and number of cortical nodes (Gao et al., 2022). The VOTC face network originates as a semantic selective neural response in the ventral anterior temporal lobe, gradually generating and driving visual face-selectivity in posterior regions through re-entrant connections to support human-specific expertise at FIR (Figure 21.5).

According to this view, face (identity) recognition, even for unfamiliar faces, necessarily concerns meaning in the nervous system rather than a reactive information processing decoding, making it a semiotic process (Queiroz & El-Hani, 2006). That is, what determines the diagnosticity of low-level visual inputs (i.e., their "ability" to lead to successful recognition of a face or of a specific face identity) is not only their objective content (i.e., features to "decode"), but how these inputs are (and have been) successfully associated with semantic knowledge (in the past). Since it is not merely an object to decode visually, but a sign that is always interpreted based on past and present successful associations in the nervous system, this perspective puts the human face firmly in the field of neurosemiotics.

Acknowledgements

I thank Talia Retter for editing the manuscript and generating Figure 21.5, Jacques Jonas for contributing to Figure 21.4 and in-depth discussion of the comparative neuroanatomy of the human and macaque brain, Marie-Alphée Laurent and Benoit Cottereau for the macaque monkey activation maps in Figure 21.4, and Adolfo García and Agustin Ibáñez for their helpful comments on a previous version of this chapter.

Notes

1 www.theguardian.com/uk-news/2018/may/15/uk-police-use-of-facial-recognition-technology-failure
2 National Institute of Standards and Technology Interagency or Internal Report 8311.
3 Despite these obvious differences, a number of prominent scientists in the field consider that the monkey brain holds the exact same number of face-selective regions as the human brain (Tsao et al., 2008; Weiner & Grill-Spector, 2015) and that the STS cortical face network in the monkey brain should be divided into two parts: (1) a dorsal part, homologous to the face-selective STS network in humans; and (2) a ventral part, corresponding to the human face-selective VOTC network (Freiwald et al., 2016; Tsao et al., 2008; Weiner & Grill-Spector, 2015; Yovel & Freiwald, 2013) (Figure 21.4). According to this view, the putative ventral part of the monkey STS system would have been "pushed" onto the ventral cortical surface over the course of human evolution by the expansion of regions engaged in language and social cognition, in particular the temporal parietal junction. However, the hypothesis of a one-to-one homology of regions across the two species and of a ventral displacement of lower STS clusters through human evolution is far-fetched and contradicted by considerable anatomo-functional evidence (Gao et al., 2022; Rossion & Taubert, 2019), falling flat in comparison with the wealth of converging evidence supporting the view that the face-selective VOTC network is indeed specific to the human lineage.
4 www.boredpanda.com/funny-donald-trump-bin-photoshop-battle/?utm_source=google&utm_medium=organic&utm_campaign=organic

References

Allison, T., Puce, A., & McCarthy, G. (2000). Social perception from visual cues: Role of the STS region. *Trends in Cognitive Sciences*, *4*, 267–278. doi: 10.1016/s1364-6613(00)01501-1

Ambrus, G.G., Amado, C., Krohn, L., & Kovacs, G. (2019). TMS of the occipital face area modulates cross-domain identity priming. *Brain Structure and Function*, *224*, 149–157. doi: 10.1007/s00429-018-1768-0

Barton, J. J., Davies-Thompson, J., & Corrow, S. L. (2021). Prosopagnosia and disorders of face processing. In *Handbook of Clinical Neurology*, *Vol. 178* (pp. 175–193). New York: Elsevier.

Behrmann, M. & Avidan, G. (2005). Congenital prosopagnosia: Face-blind from birth. *Trends in Cognitive Sciences*, *9*, 180–187. doi: 10.1016/j.tics.2005.02.011

Bernstein, M. & Yovel, G. (2015). Two neural pathways of face processing: A critical evaluation of current models. *Neuroscience & Biobehavioral Reviews*, *55*, 536–546. doi: 10.1016/j.neubiorev.2015.06.010

Blank, H., Kiebel, S. J., & von Kriegstein, K. (2015). How the human brain exchanges information across sensory modalities to recognize other people. *Human Brain Mapping*, *36*, 324–39. doi: 10.1002/hbm.22631

Bodamer, J. (1947). Die Prosopagnosie. *Archiv fur Psychiatrie und Zeitschrift fur Neurologie*, *179*, 6–54. doi: 10.1007/BF00352849

Bruce, C. (1982). Face recognition by monkeys: Absence of an inversion effect. *Neuropsychologia*, *20*, 515–521. doi: 10.1016/0028-3932(82)90025-2

Bruce, V., Henderson, Z., Newman, C., & Burton, A. M. (2001). Matching identities of familiar and unfamiliar faces caught on CCTV images. *Journal of Experimental Psychology: Applied*, 7, 207–218. doi: 10.1037//1076-898X.7.3.207

Bruce, V., & Young, A. (1986). Understanding face recognition. *British Journal of Psychology*, 77, 305–327. doi: 10.1111/j.2044-8295.1986.tb02199.x

Bruce, V., & Young, A. (1998). *In the Eye of the Beholder: The Science of Face Perception*. New York: Oxford University Press.

Bryant, K. & Preuss, T. (2018). A comparative perspective on the human temporal lobe. In E. Bruner, N. Ogihara, & H. Tanabe (Eds.), *Digital Endocasts: From Skulls to Brains* (pp. 239–258). New York: Springer.

Burton, A. M., Kramer, R. S., Ritchie, K. L., & Jenkins, R. (2016). Identity from variation: Representations of faces derived from multiple instances. *Cognitive Science*, *40*, 202–223. doi: 10.1111/cogs.12231

Calder, A. J., Rhodes, G., Johnson, M. H., & Haxby, J. V. (Eds). (2011). *The Oxford Handbook of Face Perception*. Oxford: Oxford University Press.

Carey, S. (1992). Becoming a face expert. *Philosophical Transactions of the Royal Society of London. Series B, Biological Sciences*, *335*, 95–103. doi: 10.1098/rstb.1992.0012

Cavalli-Sforza, L. L. & Cavalli-Sforza, F. (1995). *The Great Human Diasporas: The History of Diversity and Evolution*. Massachusetts: Addison-Wesley.

Chang, L. & Tsao, D.Y. (2017). The code for facial identity in the primate brain. *Cell, 169*, 1013–1028. doi: 10.1016/j.cell.2017.05.011
Cohen, A. L., Soussand, L., Corrow, S. L., Martinaud, O., Barton, J. J. S., & Fox, M. D. (2019). Looking beyond the face area: Lesion network mapping of prosopagnosia. *Brain, 142*, 3975–3990. doi: 10.1093/brain/awz332
Collins, J. A., Koski, J. E., & Olson, I. R. (2016). More than meets the eye: The merging of perceptual and conceptual knowledge in the anterior temporal face area. *Frontiers in Human Neuroscience, 10*, 189. doi: 10.3389/fnhum.2016.00189
Crookes, K. & McKone, E. (2009). Early maturity of face recognition: No childhood development of holistic processing, novel face encoding, or face-space. *Cognition, 111*, 219–247. doi: 10.1016/j.cognition.2009.02.004
Davies-Thompson, J., Gouws, A., & Andrews, T. J. (2009). An image-dependent representation of familiar and unfamiliar faces in the human ventral stream. *Neuropsychologia, 47*, 1627–1635. doi: 10.1016/j.neuropsychologia.2009.01.017
Desimone, R. (1991). Face-selective cells in the temporal cortex of monkeys. *Journal of Cognitive Neuroscience, 3*, 1–8. doi: 10.1162/jocn.1991.3.1.1
Diamond, R. & Carey, S. (1986). Why faces are and are not special: An effect of expertise. *Journal of Experimental Psychology: General, 115*, 107–117. doi: 10.1037//0096-3445.115.2.107
DiCarlo, J. J., Zoccolan, D., & Rust, N. C. (2012). How does the brain solve visual object recognition? *Neuron, 73*, 415–34. doi: 10.1016/j.neuron.2012.01.010
Dixon, M. J., Bub, D. N, & Arguin, M. (1998). Semantic and visual determinants of face recognition in a prosopagnosic patient. *Journal of Cognitive Neuroscience, 10*, 362–376. doi: 10.1162/089892998562799
Duchaine, B. & Yovel, G. (2015). A revised neural framework for face processing. *Annual Review of Vision Science, 1*, 293–416. doi: 10.1146/annurev-vision-082114-035518
Edelman, G. M. (2004). Biochemistry and the sciences of recognition. *Journal of Biological Chemistry, 279*, 7361–7369. doi: 10.1074/jbc.X400001200
Edelman, G. M. & Gally, J. A. (2013). Reentry: A key mechanism for integration of brain function. *Frontiers in Integrative Neuroscience*, 7, 63. doi: 10.3389/fnint.2013.00063
Eick, C. M., Kovacs, G., Rostalski, S. M., Rohrig, L., & Ambrus, G. G. (2020). The occipital face area is causally involved in identity-related visual-semantic associations. *Brain Structure and Function, 225*, 1483–1493. doi: 10.1007/s00429-020-02068-9
Emery, N. J., Lorincz, E. N., Perrett, D. I., Oram, M. W., & Baker, C. I. (1997). Gaze following and joint attention in rhesus monkeys (Macaca mulatta). *Journal of Comparative Psychology, 111*, 286–93. doi: 10.1037/0735-7036.111.3.286
Farkas, L. G. (1994). *Anthropometry of the Head and Face*. New York: Raven Press.
Felleman, D. J. & van Essen, D. C. (1991). Distributed hierarchical processing in the primate cerebral cortex. *Cerebral Cortex, 1*, 11–47. doi: 10.1093/cercor/1.1.1-a
Freiwald, W. A. (2020). The neural mechanisms of face processing: Cells, areas, networks, and models. *Current Opinion in Neurobiology, 60*, 184–191. doi: 10.1016/j.conb.2019.12.007
Freiwald, W., Duchaine, B., & Yovel, G. (2016). Face processing systems: From neurons to real-world social perception. *Annual Review of Neuroscience, 39*, 325–346. doi: 10.1146/annurev-neuro-070815-013934
Fried, I., Rutishauser, U., Cerf, M., & Kreiman, G. (2014). In I. Fried, U. Rutishauser, M. Cerf, & G. Kreiman (Eds.), *Single Neuron Studies of the Human Brain: Probing Cognition*. Cambridge, MA: MIT Press.
Fuster, J. M. (2009). Cortex and memory: Emergence of a new paradigm. *Journal of Cognitive Neuroscience, 21*, 2047–2072. doi: 10.1162/jocn.2009.21280
Gainotti, G. (2013). Is the right anterior temporal variant of prosopagnosia a form of "associative prosopagnosia" or a form of "multimodal person recognition disorder"? *Neuropsychology Review, 23*, 99–110. doi: 10.1007/s11065-013-9232-7
Gao, X., Gentile, F., & Rossion, B. (2018). Fast periodic stimulation (FPS): A highly effective approach in fMRI brain mapping. *Brain Structure and Function, 223*, 2433–2454. doi: 10.1007/s00429-018-1630-4
Gao, X., Wen, M., Sun, M., & Rossion, B. (2022). A genuine interindividual variability in number and anatomical localization of face-selective regions in the human brain. *Cerebral Cortex*, bhab519. doi: 10.1093/cercor/bhab519
García, A. M., Hesse, E., Birba, A., Adolfi, F., Mikulan, E., Caro, M. M., Petroni, A., Bekinschtein, T. A., García, M. C., Silva, W., Ciraolo, C., Vaucheret, E., Sedeño, L., & Ibáñez, A. (2020). Time to face language: Embodied mechanisms underpin the inception of face-related meanings in the human brain. *Cerebral Cortex, 30*, 6051–6058. doi: 10.1093/cercor/bhaa178
Gauthier, I., & Tarr, M. J. (1997). Becoming a "Greeble" expert: Exploring mechanisms for face recognition. *Vision Research, 37*, 1673–1682. doi: 10.1016/S0042-6989(96)00286-6
Gauthier, I., Tarr, M. J., Moylan, J., Skudlarski, P., Gore, J. C., & Anderson, A. W. (2000). The FFA is part of a network that processes faces on an individual level. *Journal of Cognitive Neuroscience, 12*, 495–504. doi: 10.1162/089892900562165

Gazzaniga, M. S. (2009). *Human: The Science Behind What Makes Us Unique*. New York: Harper Perennial.

Golarai, G., Liberman, A., & Grill-Spector, K. (2017). Experience shapes the development of neural substrates of face processing in human ventral temporal cortex. *Cerebral Cortex, 27*, 1229–1244. doi: 10.1093/cercor/bhv314

Griffin, J. W. (2020). Quantifying the face inversion effect in nonhuman primates: A phylogenetic meta-analysis. *Animal Cognition, 23*, 237–249. doi: 10.1007/s10071-019-01340-8

Grill-Spector, K., & Malach, R. (2001). FMR-adaptation: A tool for studying the functional properties of human cortical neurons. *Acta Psychologica, 107*, 293–321. doi: 10.1016/s0001-6918(01)00019-1

Grill-Spector, K., Weiner, K. S., Kay, K., & Gomez, J. (2017). The functional neuroanatomy of human face perception. *Annual Review of Vision Science, 3*, 167–196. doi: 10.1146/annurev-vision-102016-061214

Gross, C. G., Rocha-Miranda, C. E., & Bender, D. B. (1972). Visual properties of neurons in the inferotemporal cortex of the macaque. *Journal of Neurophysiology, 35*, 96–111. doi: 10.1152/jn.1972.35.1.96

Haxby, J. V., Hoffman, E. A., & Gobbini, M. I. (2000). The distributed human neural system for face perception. *Trends in Cognitive Sciences, 4*, 223–233. doi: 10.1016/s1364-6613(00)01482-0

Herculano-Houzel, S. (2016). *The Human Advantage: A New Understanding of How Our Brain Became Remarkable*. Cambridge, MA: MIT Press.

Hesse, J. K. & Tsao, D.Y. (2020). The macaque face patch system: A turtle's underbelly for the brain. *Nature Reviews Neuroscience, 21*, 695–716. doi: 10.1038/s41583-020-00393-w

Heywood, C. A. & Cowey, A. (1992). The role of the "face-cell" area in the discrimination and recognition of faces by monkeys. *Philosophical Transactions of the Royal Society of London B, 335*, 31–37. doi: 10.1098/rstb.1992.0004

Hills, P. J. & Lewis, M. B. (2018). The development of face expertise: Evidence for a qualitative change in processing. *Cognitive Development, 48*, 1–18. doi: 10.1016/j.cogdev.2018.05.003

Hsiao, J. H. & Cottrell, G. W. (2008). Two fixations suffice in face recognition. *Psychological Science, 19*, 998–1006. doi: 10.1111/j.1467-9280.2008.02191.x

Hubel, D. H. & Wiesel, T. N. (1962). Receptive fields, binocular interaction and functional architecture in the cat visual cortex. *The Journal of Physiology, 160*, 106–154. doi: 10.1113/jphysiol.1962.sp006837

Hutmacher, F. (2019). Why is there so much more research on vision than on any other sensory modality? *Frontiers in Psychology, 10*, 2246. doi: 10.3389/fpsyg.2019.02246

Jacques, C., Rossion, B., Volfart, A., Brissart, H., Colnat-Coulbois, S., Maillard, L., Jonas, J. (2020). The neural basis of rapid unfamiliar face individuation with human intracerebral recordings. *NeuroImage*, 221, 117174. doi: 10.1016/j.neuroimage.2020.117174

Jenkins, R., Dowsett, A. J., & Burton, A. M. (2018). How many faces do people know? *Proceedings of the Royal Society B, Biological Sciences, 285*(1888). doi: 10.1098/rspb.2018.1319

Jiang, X., Rosen, E., Zeffiro, T., Vanmeter, J., Blanz V., & Riesenhuber, M. (2006). Evaluation of a shape-based model of human face discrimination using fMRI and behavioral techniques. *Neuron, 50*, 159–172. doi: 10.1016/j.neuron.2006.03.012

Jonas, J., Jacques, C., Liu-Shuang, J., Brissart, H., Colnat-Coulbois, S., Maillard, L., & Rossion, B. (2016). A face-selective ventral occipito-temporal map of the human brain with intracerebral potentials. *Proceedings of the National Academy of Sciences of the United States of America, 113*, E4088–E4097. doi: 10.1073/pnas.1522033113

Jonas, J., & Rossion, B. (2021). Intracerebral electrical stimulation to understand the neural basis of human face identity recognition. *European Journal of Neuroscience*, 54(1), 4197–4211. doi: 10.1111/ejn.15235

Kaas, J. H. (2019). The origin and evolution of neocortex: From early mammals to modern humans. *Progress in Brain Research, 250*, 61–81. doi: 10.1016/bs.pbr.2019.03.017

Kanwisher, N., McDermott, J., & Chun, M. (1997). The fusiform face area: A module in human extrastriate cortex specialized for face perception. *Journal of Neuroscience, 17*, 4302–4311. doi: 10.1523/JNEUROSCI.17-11-04302.1997

Kelly, D. J., Liu, S., Ge, L., Quinn, P. C., Salater, A. M., Lee, K., Liu, Q., & Pascalis, O. (2007). Cross-race preferences for same-race faces extend beyond the African versus Caucasian contrast in three-month-old infants. *Infancy, 11*, 87–95. doi: 10.1080/15250000709336871

Khuvis, S., Yeagle, E. M., Norman, Y., Grossman, S., Malach, R., & Mehta, A. (2021). Face-selective units in human ventral temporal cortex reactivate during free recall. *Journal of Neuroscience, 41*, 3386–3399. doi: 10.1523/JNEUROSCI.2918-19.2020

Lambon-Ralph M. A., Sage, K., Jones, R. W., & Mayberry, E. J. (2010). Coherent concepts are computed in the anterior temporal lobes. *Proceedings of the National Academy of Sciences of the United States of America, 107*(6), 2717–2722. doi: 10.1073/pnas.0907307107

Landi, S. M., & Freiwald, W. A. (2017). Two areas for familiar face recognition in the primate brain. *Science, 357*(6351), 591–595. doi: 10.1126/science.aan1139

Le Grand, R., Mondloch, C., Maurer, D., & Brent, H. (2004). Impairment in holistic face processing following early visual deprivation. *Psychological Science, 15*, 762–768. doi: 10.1111/j.0956-7976.2004.00753.x

Leopold, D. A., Bondar, I. V., & Giese, M.A. (2006). Norm-based face encoding by single neurons in monkey infero-temporal cortex. *Nature, 442*, 572–575. doi: 10.1038/nature04951

Logothetis, N. K. (2008). What we can do and what we cannot do with fMRI. *Nature, 453*, 869–878. doi: 10.1038/nature06976

Mandler, G. (1980). Recognizing: The judgment of previous occurrence. *Psychological Review, 87*, 252–271. doi: 10.1037/0033-295X.87.3.252

Marr, D. (1982). *Vision: A Computational Investigation into Human Representation and Processing of Visual Information*. San Francisco, CA: Freeman.

McKone, E., Kanwisher, N., & Duchaine, B. C. (2007). Can generic expertise explain special processing for faces? *Trends in Cognitive Sciences, 11*, 8–15. doi: 10.1016/j.tics.2006.11.002

McNeill, D. (2000). *The Face: A Natural History*. Boston: Little, Brown.

Meadows, J. C. (1974). The anatomical basis of prosopagnosia. *Journal of Neurology, Neurosurgery, and Psychiatry, 37*, 489–501. doi: 10.1136/jnnp.37.5.489

Megreya, A. M. & Burton, A. M. (2006). Unfamiliar faces are not faces: Evidence from a matching task. *Memory & Cognition, 34*, 865–876. doi: 10.3758/BF03193433

Micheletta, J., Whitehouse, J., Parr, L. A., Marshman, P., Engelhardt, A., & Waller, B. M. (2015). Familiar and unfamiliar face recognition in crested macaques (Macaca nigra). *Royal Society Open Science, 2*, 150109. doi: 10.1098/rsos.150109

Murphy, G. L. (2002). *The Big Book of Concepts*. Cambridge, MA: MIT Press.

Nestor, A., Plaut, D. C., & Behrmann, M. (2011). Unraveling the distributed neural code of facial identity through spatiotemporal pattern analysis. *Proceedings of the National Academy of Sciences of the United States of America, 108*(24), 9998–10003. doi: 10.1073/pnas.1102433108

Palmeri, T. J., & Gauthier, I. (2004). Visual object understanding. *Nature Reviews Neuroscience, 5*, 291–303. doi: 10.1038/nrn1364

Parr, L. A., Heintz, M., & Pradhan, G. (2008). Rhesus monkeys (Macaca mulatta) lack expertise in face processing. *Journal of Comparative Psychology, 122*, 390–402. doi: 10.1037/0735-7036.122.4.390

Pascalis, O., de Haan, M., & Nelson, C. A. (2002). Is face processing species-specific during the first year of life? *Science, 296*(5571), 1321–1323. doi: 10.1126/science.1070223

Peirce, J. W., Leigh, A. E., & Kendrick, K. M. (2000). Configurational coding, familiarity and the right hemisphere advantage for face recognition in sheep. *Neuropsychologia, 38*, 475–483. doi: 10.1016/s0028-3932(99)00088-3

Perrett, D. I., Rolls E. T., & Caan W. (1982). Visual neurones responsive to faces in the monkey temporal cortex. *Experimental Brain Research, 47*, 329–342. doi: 10.1007/BF00239352

Perrett, D. I., Smith, P. A. J., Potter, D. D., Mistlin, A. J., Head, A. S., Milner, A. D., & Jeeves, M. A. (1985). Visual cells in the temporal cortex sensitive to face view and gaze direction. *Proceedings of the Royal Society B*, 223, 293–317. doi: 10.1098/rspb.1985.0003

Pokorny, J. J., & de Waal, F. B. (2009). Face recognition in capuchin monkeys (Cebus apella). *Journal of Comparative Psychology, 123*, 151–160. doi: 10.1037/a0014073

Queiroz, J., & El-Hani, C. (2006). Towards a multi-level approach to the emergence of meaning processes in living systems. *Acta Biotheoretica, 54*, 179–206. doi: 10.1007/s10441-006-8177-0

Quian-Quiroga, R. (2020). No pattern separation in the human hippocampus. *Trends in Cognitive Sciences, 24*, 994–1007. doi: 10.1016/j.tics.2020.09.012

Quian-Quiroga, R., Reddy, L., Kreiman, G., Koch, C, & Fried, I. (2005). Invariant visual representation by single neurons in the human brain. *Nature, 435*, 1102–1107. doi: 10.1038/nature03687

Ramon, M., Busigny, T., & Rossion, B. (2010). Impaired holistic processing of unfamiliar individual faces in acquired prosopagnosia. *Neuropsychologia, 48*, 933–944. doi: 10.1016/j.neuropsychologia.2009.11.014

Rekow, D., Baudouin, J. Y., Poncet, F., Damon, F., Durand, K., Schaal, B., Rossion, B., & Leleu, A. (2021). Smells like real faces: Odor-driven face pareidolia in the infant brain. *Proceedings of the National Academy of Sciences of the United States of America, 118*(21), e2014979118. doi: 10.1073/pnas.2014979118

Rilling, J. K. & Seligman, R. A. (2002): A quantitative morphometric comparative analysis of the primate temporal lobe. *Journal of Human Evolution, 42*, 505–533. doi: 10.1006/jhev.2001.0537

Rolls, E. T. (1992). Neurophysiological mechanisms underlying face processing within and beyond the temporal cortical area. *Philosophical Transactions of the Royal Society of London B, 335*, 11–21. doi: 10.1098/rstb.1992.0002

Rossion, B. (2008). Picture-plane inversion leads to qualitative changes of face perception. *Acta Psychologica, 128*, 274–289. doi: 10.1016/j.actpsy.2008.02.003

Rossion, B. (2013). The composite face illusion: A window to our understanding of holistic face perception. *Visual Cognition, 121*, 139–253. doi: 10.1080/13506285.2013.772929

Rossion, B. (2014). Understanding face perception by means of prosopagnosia and neuroimaging. *Frontiers in Bioscience, 6*, 258–307. doi: 10.2741/E706

Rossion, B. (2018a). Humans are visual experts at unfamiliar face recognition. *Trends in Cognitive Sciences, 22*, 471–472. doi: 10.1016/j.tics.2018.03.002

Rossion, B. (2018b). Damasio's error – prosopagnosia with intact within-category object recognition. *Journal of Neuropsychology, 12*, 357–388. doi: 10.1111/jnp.12162

Rossion, B. (2018c). Prosopdysgnosia? What could it tell us about the neural organization of face and object recognition? *Cognitive Neuropsychology, 35*, 98–101. doi: 10.1080/02643294.2017.1414778

Rossion, B., Hanseeuw B, & Dricot, L. (2012). Defining face perception areas in the human brain: A large-scale factorial fMRI face localizer analysis. *Brain and Cognition, 79*, 138–157. doi: 10.1016/j.bandc.2012.01.001

Rossion, B., Jacques, C., & Jonas, J. (2018). Mapping face categorization in the human ventral occipito-temporal cortex with direct neural intracranial recordings. *Annals of the New York Academy of Science, 1426*, 5–24. doi: 10.1111/nyas.13596

Rossion, B., & Lochy, A. (2022). Is human face recognition lateralized to the right hemisphere due to neural competition with left lateralized visual word recognition? A critical review. *Brain Structure and Function*, 227(2), 599–629. doi: 10.1007/s00429-021-02370-0

Rossion, B., & Retter, T. L. (2020). Face perception. In D. Poeppel, M.S. Gazzaniga & G. Mangun (Eds). *The Cognitive Neurosciences* (6th edn, pp. 129–139). Cambridge, MA: MIT Press.

Rossion, B., & Taubert, J. (2017). Commentary: The code for facial identity in the primate brain. *Frontiers in Human Neuroscience, 11*, 550. doi: 10.3389/fnhum.2017.00550

Rossion, B., & Taubert, J. (2019). What can we learn about human individual face recognition from experimental studies in monkeys? *Vision Research, 157*, 142–158. doi: 10.1016/j.visres.2018.03.012

Ruff, C. (2002). Variation in human body size and shape. *Annual Review of Anthropology, 31*, 211–232. doi: 10.1146/annurev.anthro.31.040402.085407

Sangrigoli, S. & de Schonen, S. (2004). Effect of visual experience on face processing: A developmental study of inversion and non-native effects. *Developmental Science*, 7, 74–87. doi: 10.1111/j.1467-7687.2004.00324.x

Schwartz, L. & Yovel G. (2016). The roles of perceptual and conceptual information in face recognition. *Journal of Experimental Psychology: General, 145*, 1493–1511. doi: 10.1037/xge0000220

Sergent, J., Ohta, S., & Macdonald, B. (1992). Functional neuroanatomy of face and object processing: A positron emission tomography study. *Brain, 115*, 15–36. doi: 10.1093/brain/115.1.15

Sergent, J., & Signoret, J.-L. (1992). Varieties of functional deficits in prosopagnosia. *Cerebral Cortex, 2*, 375–388. doi: 10.1093/cercor/2.5.375

Sheehan, M. J., & Nachman, M. W. (2014). Morphological and population genomic evidence that human faces have evolved to signal individual identity. *Nature Communications, 5*(4800), 1–10. doi: 10.1038/ncomms5800

Sheehan, M. J., & Tibbetts, E. A. (2011). Specialized face learning is associated with individual recognition in paper wasps. *Science, 334*, 1272–1275. doi: 10.1126/science.1211334

Squire, L. R., Genzel L, Wixted, J.T., & Morris, R. G. (2015). Memory consolidation. *Cold Spring Harbor Perspectives in Biology*, 7(8), a021766. doi: 10.1101/cshperspect.a021766

Susilo, T., & Duchaine, B. (2013). Advances in developmental prosopagnosia research. *Current Opinion in Neurobiology, 23*(3), 423–429. doi: 10.1016/j.conb.2012.12.011

Tanaka, J. W., & Farah, M. J. (1993). Parts and wholes in face recognition. *Quarterly Journal of Experimental Psychology, 46A*, 225–245. doi: 10.1080/14640749308401045

Taubert, J., Aagten-Murphy, D., & Parr, L. A. (2012). A comparative study of face processing using scrambled faces. *Perception, 41*, 460–473. doi: 10.1068/p7151

Taubert, J., Japee, S., Murphy, A. P., Tardiff, C. T., Koele, E. A., Kumar, S, Leopold, D. A., & Ungerleider, L. G. (2020). Parallel processing of facial expression and head orientation in the macaque brain. *Journal of Neuroscience, 40*, 8119–8131. doi: 10.1523/JNEUROSCI.0524-20.2020

Taubert, J., Qureshi, A. A., & Parr, L. A. (2012). The composite face effect in chimpanzees (*Pan troglodytes*) and rhesus monkeys (*Macada mulatta*). *Journal of Comparative* Psychology, *126*, 339–46. doi: 10.1037/a0027287

Todorov, A. (2017). *Face Value: The Irresistible Influence of First Impressions*. Princeton, NJ: Princeton University Press.

Tsao, D. Y., Freiwald, W. A., Tootell, R. B., & Livingstone, M. S. (2006). A cortical region consisting entirely of face-selective cells. *Science, 311*, 670–674. doi: 10.1126/science.1119983

Tsao, D. Y., Moeller, S., & Freiwald, W. A. (2008). Comparing face patch systems in macaques and humans. *Proceedings of the National Academy of Sciences of the United States of America, 105*, 19514–19519. doi: 10.1073/pnas.0809662105

Van Belle, G., de Graef, P., Verfaillie, K., Busigny, T., & Rossion, B. (2010). Whole not hole: Expert face recognition requires holistic perception. *Neuropsychologia, 48*, 2609–2620. doi: 10.1016/j.neuropsychologia.2010.04.034

Van Essen, D. C. (2005) Surface-based comparisons of macaque and human cortical organization. In S. Dehaene (Ed.), *From Monkey to Brain: Proceedings of a Fyssen Foundation Colloquium* (3–20). Cambridge, MA: MIT Press.

Wallis, G., & Bülthoff, H. H. (2001). Effects of temporal association on recognition memory. *Proceedings of the National Academy of Sciences of the United States of America, 98*, 4800–4804. doi: 10.1073/pnas.071028598

Wandell B. A. (2011). The neurobiological basis of seeing words. *Annals of the New York Academy of Sciences, 1224*(1), 63–80. doi: 10.1111/j.1749-6632.2010.05954.x

Wang, M.Y., & Takeuchi, H. (2017). Individual recognition and the "face inversion effect" in medaka fish (Oryzias latipes). *eLife, 6*(e24728), 1–18. doi: 10.7554/eLife.24728

Weiner, K. S., & Grill-Spector, K. (2015). The evolution of face processing networks. *Trends in Cognitive Sciences, 19*, 240–241. doi: 10.1016/j.tics.2015.03.010

Weiner, K. S., & Zilles, K. (2016). The anatomical and functional specialization of the fusiform gyrus. *Neuropsychologia, 83*, 48–62. doi: 10.1016/j.neuropsychologia.2015.06.033

Wilmer, J. B. (2017). Individual differences in face recognition: A decade of discovery. *Current Directions in Psychological Science, 26*(3), 225–230. doi: 10.1177/0963721417710693

Wilmer, J. B., Germine, L., Chabris, C. F., Chatterjee, G., Williams, M., Loken, E., Nakayama, K., & Duchaine, B. (2010). Human face recognition ability is specific and highly heritable. *Proceedings of the National Academy of Sciences of the United States of America, 107*, 5238–5241. doi: 10.1073/pnas.0913053107

Yan, X., & Rossion, B. (2020). A robust neural familiar face recognition response in a dynamic (periodic) stream of unfamiliar faces. *Cortex, 132*, 281–295. doi: 10.1016/j.cortex.2020.08.016

Young, A. W., & Burton, M. (2018). Are we face experts? *Trends in Cognitive Sciences, 22*, 100–110. doi: 10.1016/j.tics.2017.11.007

Young, A. W., Hellawell, D., & Hay, D. C. (1987). Configural information in face perception. *Perception, 16*, 747–759. doi: 10.1068/p160747

Young, M.P., & Yamane, S. (1992). Sparse population coding of faces in the inferotemporal cortex. *Science, 29*, 1327–1331. doi: 10.1126/science.1598577

Yovel, G., & Freiwald, W. A. (2013). Face recognition systems in monkey and human: Are they the same thing? *F1000Prime Rep, 5*, 10. doi: 10.12703/P5-10

Zaidi, A. A., Mattern, B. C, Claes, P., McEvoy, B., Hughes, C., & Shriver, M. D. (2017). Investigating the case of human nose shape and climate adaptation. *PLOS Genetics*, (3), e1006616. doi: 10.1371/journal.pgen.1006616

Zilles, K., Palomero-Gallagher, N., & Amunts, K. (2013). Development of cortical folding during evolution and ontogeny. *Trends in Neurosciences, 36*, 275–284. doi: 10.1016/j.tins.2013.01.006

22

MUSICAL SIGNS AND THE HUMAN ORGANISM

Amy M. Belfi

Introduction

The field of neurosemiotics has been described as the "investigation of neurological processes underlying communicative behavior in all its forms," including "the perception of the environment as meaningful" (Bouissac, 1986: 204–206). This chapter will focus on music as one such form of "communicative behavior" – although it is debatable whether music should be considered a form of communication in the same way as language (Slevc & Patel, 2011) – and will review evidence of the neural systems underlying meaning in music. There are many questions one can ask about the capacity of music to convey meaning: Can music convey meaning at all? If so, what types of meaning are conveyed by music? How does music convey meaning (i.e., what musical features contribute to the generation of meaning)? Is musical meaning persistent across cultures? These questions have been posed and discussed by scholars in a variety of disciplines, spanning the sciences and humanities. However, the goal of this chapter is not to provide novel theoretical accounts of musical meaning or to definitively answer such questions; instead, it begins with the assumption that music does convey meaning and provides an overarching review of evidence to this extent. Given the focus of this volume (on *neuro*semiotics), I will provide a broad overview of both formative and recent scientific work investigating the neural correlates of musical meaning.

To connect this work with the semiological tradition, this chapter will also highlight how musical meaning may result from the various sign qualities of music. Sign qualities of the Peircean tradition are discussed, including how music can serve as a symbolic, indexical, and/or iconic sign to convey various types of meaning. While the concept of "meaning" in music seems to underlie many topics in the field of music cognition, the present chapter will focus primarily on two types of meaning in music: emotional associations and other semantic associations. Finally, we will consider studies on how quickly meaning emerges when listening to music, suggesting that music can convey both emotional and semantic associations on rapid timescales.

Neurocognitive components of music

Before discussing the capacity of music to convey meaning, I will briefly review key components of music and the neurological systems underlying their perception. Specifically, this section will

DOI: 10.4324/9781003051817-27

focus on pitch, tonality, and rhythm – for a more comprehensive review of these musical features and their neural correlates, see Loui & Przysinda (2019). First, the musical attribute of pitch ranges along a perceptual spectrum from low to high and is crucially related to the acoustic property of frequency: higher-frequency sounds tend to be perceived as higher-pitched; lower-frequency sounds tend to be perceived as lower-pitched. The neural regions underlying pitch perception are primarily those involved in auditory perception more generally, such as the primary auditory cortex (Bendor & Wang, 2005). Furthermore, damage to structures in the auditory pathway is associated with deficits in pitch perception, leading to one form of "amusia" (Särkämö et al., 2009).

Building off the perception of individual pitches, tonality describes the perceived relationship between pitches within a specific musical context. That is, within each musical key, notes are arranged in a hierarchical manner, with certain pitches occurring more frequently than others. Tonality influences the perception of both melody and harmony: melodies consist of pitches presented sequentially over time, while harmony is the simultaneous presentation of pitches. Even untrained listeners learn to anticipate the likelihood of certain melodic and harmonic musical events within a tonal context. For example, when given a musical context and asked to rate how well certain notes "fit," listeners accurately reproduce the expected tonal hierarchies (Krumhansl & Shepard, 1979).

One frequent approach to understanding the neural correlates of melodic and harmonic perception consists of investigating brain responses to violations of musical expectations. For example, when listeners hear musical chords that are unexpected within a tonal context, these evoke a specific electrophysiological response in the brain, termed the early right anterior negativity, or ERAN (Koelsch et al., 2000). The ERAN may be analogous to the early left anterior negativity (ELAN), which is found in response to violations of linguistic syntax (Fiveash et al., 2018). The ERAN has also been suggested as a neural marker of "intramusical" meaning, such that meaning emerges from references to itself, instead of references to concepts in the external world (Koelsch, 2011).

Finally, rhythm has been defined as a pattern of time intervals between stimuli (Grahn, 2012). Similarly, the musical "beat" is the perceived sense of pulse within a musical rhythm. "Meter" refers to the hierarchical organization of musical beats and designates which beats are accented. Neuroimaging studies of rhythm perception consistently implicate motor-related brain structures, such as the motor cortex, the cerebellum, and the basal ganglia (Chen et al., 2008; Gordon et al., 2018).

Emotional associations

Colloquially, the meaning of music often refers to its emotional properties. Indeed, one of the most frequently reported reasons for listening to music is that it evokes enjoyment and pleasure (Sanflippo et al., 2020). First, a distinction must be made between emotions *expressed* by music versus emotions *induced* by music. For example, when hearing the song "Walking on Sunshine," a listener (in particular, one familiar with Western music) would likely identify that the song expresses happiness (that is, it *sounds happy*). But the same listener may not actually experience feelings of happiness in response to the song. That is, "Walking on Sunshine" may *sound* happy, but may not actually induce feelings of happiness in a particular listener. Perhaps the listener feels sad when hearing the song because it evokes a gloomy past experience; that person may also feel annoyed because the song is played non-stop on the radio; and for some individuals the song may stir no feelings at all. While a fully comprehensive exploration of musical emotions is beyond the scope of this chapter, I will address foundational and recent evidence on the neural correlates of both emotions expressed and induced by music – for thorough reviews on the neural basis of musical emotions, see Koelsch (2014) and Omigie (2016); for discussions of how musical emotions fall into broader psychological theories of emotion, see Schiavio et al. (2017) and Warrenburg (2020).

Emotions expressed by music

Emotional expression in music has been suggested to arise from indexical sign qualities, such that the music is indexing a psychological state typically associated with human thoughts or emotions (Frit, 2013; Koelsch, 2011). This type of musical meaning has also been referred to as motivational-structural meaning, in reference to the relationship between motivational and/or affective characteristics of the listener and the structural features of the music (Cross, 2009). The capacity of music to express basic emotions has substantial empirical support (Dalla Bella et al., 2001; Heaton et al., 1999; Terwogt & Van Grinsven, 1988; Vieillard et al., 2008). Typically, four basic emotions are considered in this type of work: happiness, sadness, threat/fear, and peacefulness. These emotions can, to a certain degree, be delineated by specific musical features. For example, happy-sounding music often has a fast tempo and a major mode (i.e., is in a major key), while sad-sounding music has a slow tempo and a minor mode.

While the process of interpreting emotions conveyed by music is certainly more complex than simply identifying differences in tempo and mode, the interaction of these two features serves as an indexical sign for basic emotions in music. For example, others have stated that the emotional content in music is reflects its indexical sign qualities (Fritz et al., 2013; Koelsch, 2011), which suggests that the combination of a fast tempo and a major mode are indexing the expression of happiness. Some evidence suggests that these musical features correspond to basic emotions in vocal prosody. For example, the minor third is a musical interval frequently used to convey sadness, and analysis of speech patterns indicates that the minor third tends to be used in sad-sounding speech (Curtis & Bharucha, 2010). Interval size, therefore, seems to be one of many psychoacoustic features that are similar between the emotional meaning of music and vocal prosody in speech (Coutinho et al., 2013). Such musical features may be seen as indexical signs because the listener may interpret them as representing the emotional qualities of the composer, or of the piece of music itself (similar to identifying the emotions another person is feeling based on their vocal prosody). However, the relationship between musical features and emotion identification could also be symbolic in nature (i.e., that the musical features tied to specific emotions are arbitrary and culturally specific). Yet some evidence has indicated that even individuals with minimal exposure to Western music are able to accurately recognize such basic emotions in music (Fritz et al., 2009; Laukka et al., 2013), suggesting that emotion recognition in music might not be entirely culturally determined.

Several brain structures have been implicated in emotion identification in music. These include key structures within the limbic system, such as the amygdala, and regions involved in reward networks, such as the nucleus accumbens (NAcc) and the ventromedial prefrontal cortex (vmPFC), and other areas involved in affective processing at large. Neuropsychological work underscores the amygdala as a key region underlying the ability to perceive basic emotions in music – for a review, see Frühholz et al. (2014). For example, individuals with damage to the amygdala are selectively impaired at recognizing threat/fear in music (Gosselin et al., 2011; Gosselin et al., 2007; Gosselin et al., 2005), echoing their deficits in identifying fear from facial expressions (Adolphs et al., 1994; Adolphs et al., 1999). These findings are supported by neuroimaging evidence suggesting the role of the amygdala in identifying basic emotions, particularly fear, in music (Aubé et al., 2015).

Music can also communicate more complex emotions or intentions (Steinbeis & Koelsch, 2009). For example, both musically trained and untrained listeners are can identify complex intentions expressed by music, such as "domineering," "insolent," or "caring" (Aucouturier & Canonne, 2017). In one experiment (Downey et al., 2013), participants were asked to match a piece of music to either a mental state (e.g., dreading) or a non-mental state (e.g., raindrops). Patients with behavioral variant frontotemporal dementia, who have damage to the prefrontal cortex, performed poorly on the mental state condition, but not on the non-mental state condition. Further, performance on the mental state task was associated with the volume of the vmPFC, a core region for social and emotional processing, including interpreting the intentions of other human actors (Roy et al., 2012; Schneider & Koenigs,

2017). The vmPFC, then, may be a critical region for interpreting complex emotions in music, but not other semantic associations.

Beyond these core structures, emotion recognition in music likely requires a widespread network of regions interacting with one another. For example, individuals with left-hemisphere brain damage show deficits in recognizing basic emotions in music, while individuals with right hemisphere damage do not (Pralus et al., 2020). Therefore, widespread hemispheric damage, regardless of specific lesion location, can disrupt the process of emotion recognition in music. It is also likely that interactions between emotion-related regions (such as the amygdala and the vmPFC) and regions involved in auditory perception underlie the interpretation of emotional meaning in music. That is, neural regions responsible for decoding the structural features of music are also involved in the interpretation of its emotional content. Multivariate neuroimaging methods have been useful for identifying such interactions. For example, neural responses in the auditory cortex can accurately predict the emotional content of both music and voices (Paquette et al., 2018). Additionally, fMRI evidence indicates that the emotional content of music can be accurately classified based on neural responses in auditory cortical regions, including the superior temporal gyrus. Furthermore, this classification of musical emotions was shown to rely on rhythmic and timbral features of the music (Sachs et al., 2018). In sum, musical features seem capable of denoting particular emotions, and the perception of such emotions is associated with neural activity in systems important for both emotional processes and auditory perception.

Emotions experienced by the listener

The capacity for music to induce emotions in listeners has been referred to as "musicogenic meaning", such that meaning is construed by a listener interpreting "physical, emotional, and self-related" effects evoked by the music (Koelsch, 2011: 99). However, it is important to note that various types of musical meaning may overlap. For example, such musicogenic meaning (e.g., felt emotional responses to music) is likely the result of intramusical meaning (e.g., violations of expectations based on implicit knowledge of musical structure) and/or extramusical meaning (e.g., semantic or autobiographical associations evoked by the music). Of note, conveyed and felt emotions can be related – for example, through emotion contagion: "That song *sounds sad*, so it makes me *feel sad*." In fact, musical emotions can be evoked through this and many other routes (Juslin, 2013).

To briefly consider such interactions, we will first discuss the relationship between intramusical meaning and emotion evocation. Intramusical meaning has been defined as musical meaning in which the music references itself, or meaning in terms of understanding the musical structure and relations among musical elements (Koelsch, 2011; Koopman & Davies, 2001). It has long been suggested that music evokes emotions through systematic establishment, fulfilment, and violations of listeners' expectations (Huron, 2006; Meyer, 1956). Such musical expectations can be learned implicitly, and quickly, through repeated exposure to music with a consistent structure (Loui & Wessel, 2008; Loui et al., 2010; Rohrmeier & Rebuschat, 2012). Listeners are then able to form predictions about what comes next within a piece of music, which can then lead to either the fulfilment or violation of such predictions.

Abundant work indicates that musical predictions and expectations are part of the process by which music induces pleasure (or displeasure) – for a review, see Belfi & Loui (2020). In one recent study, participants listened to musical chord progressions and were given an arbitrary choice that led to either a consonant or dissonant chord ending. Participants were not explicitly made aware of which choices led to the consonant outcome, but over the course of the experiment they were more likely to make choices associated with consonant endings (Gold et al., 2019). The authors found that reward prediction errors (the difference between the decision outcome and the best expected outcome) significantly correlated with activity in the NAcc. This is one of many studies implicating the NAcc, and other regions in the reward system, in musical reward (Ferreri et al., 2019; Mas-Herrero et al., 2018; Salimpoor et al., 2011; Salimpoor et al., 2013). In this way, just as tempo and mode may serve as musical signs for expressing basic emotions, consonance/dissonance may denote the pleasantness of music – although consonance is not always rewarding, nor dissonance unpleasant (McDermott et al., 2016; Popescu et al., 2019).

In investigating the neural correlates of emotional responses to music, one fruitful approach has been to study individuals who do not experience pleasing emotional responses to music, which has been termed "musical anhedonia" (Mas-Herrero et al., 2013; Satoh et al., 2011). Musical anhedonia has been observed in individuals with focal brain damage (Belfi et al., 2017; Griffiths et al., 2004; Satoh et al., 2011, 2016) and in about 5 percent of healthy persons (Mas-Herrero et al., 2013). Neuropsychological and neuroimaging evidence indicates that musical anhedonia likely involves abnormal connectivity between auditory and reward regions in the brain (Loui et al., 2017; Martínez-Molina et al., 2016; Mas-Herrero et al., 2014). This suggests that music induces feelings of pleasure via connections between systems that generate expectations from acoustic input (intramusical meaning) and reward regions involved in processing the results of such predictions, such as the NAcc.

Interim summary

To summarize, previous work has indicated that music can convey emotional content, both by expressing and inducing emotions. Emotional responses to music may in part be tied to particular musical features (e.g., tempo and mode), and the violation and confirmation of expectations. The neural systems underlying the ability to both recognize and experience emotions from music include regions important for auditory perception, emotion, and reward. It is likely that the ability to perceive and experience emotions from music is the result of network-level interactions between these structures.

Other semantic associations

Of course, music can convey meanings beyond emotional ones. Semantic associations evoked by music have been frequently studied via event-related potentials (ERPs). The N400 is an ERP component that reflects semantic integration or contextual congruence and is larger in response to words that are semantically incongruent with a preceding context (Kellenbach et al., 2000). Not just found in response to language, the N400 has also been identified in other modalities such as action sequences (Reid & Striano, 2008) and mathematical equations (Jost et al., 2003). One foundational study on semantic associations in music sought to investigate whether a musical context could evoke a N400 response to subsequently presented words (Koelsch et al., 2004). Participants listened to either spoken language or music. Each context was followed by a semantically congruent or incongruent word. In both the language and music contexts, semantically incongruent words evoked large N400 responses, suggesting that the musical context did conjure semantic associations, and therefore primed the semantic processing of a subsequent word. This music-related N400 effect has been replicated in further studies (Daltrozzo & Schön, 2009a, 2009b).

Semantic concepts evoked by music

While the ERP results described above provide evidence that music can evoke semantic associations (and that the neural responses are similar to those evoked by semantic knowledge in other modalities), the question remains of *what* concepts music evokes. The associations between music and various semantic concepts may be both iconic and symbolic. In some cases, music serves as an iconic sign – that is, the musical sounds may resemble sounds or other properties of external objects. This may occur when listeners hear a piece of music that *sounds like* raindrops, or a bird, or an ascending sequence of notes that connotes the concept of a staircase. Music may have symbolic sign qualities when it conveys conventional or explicit extramusical associations that are understood in a culturally specific context (e.g., a national anthem). One particularly relevant example of music evoking semantic associations is the leitmotif, a recurring musical theme that references a particular person or situation – for example, in the operas of Wagner (Baker & Müllensiefen, 2017).

Along these lines, a recent study investigated whether listeners can perceive narratives in music (Margulis, 2017). Participants listened to excerpts of orchestral music and were asked whether they imagined a story or elements of a story (characters, events, or settings). Participants imagined a narrative 59 percent of the time while listening to music, suggesting that narrative experiences of music are fairly common. In terms of the content of these narratives, participants showed substantial agreement – for example, in response to a piece by Telemann, 88 percent of participants described a "grand affair" involving ballrooms, dancing, celebrations, weddings, and the like. This study suggests that music can evoke specific concepts, and that the precise content of that meaning is relatively consistent across listeners. It is likely that such associations were not due solely to the iconic sign quality of the music, but possibly due to its symbolic sign qualities (e.g., music evoked narrative involving a grand ball because listeners had experienced hearing such music during ball scenes in films).

This provides evidence that music can consistently evoke semantic associations, but does not indicate whether these music–concept links are due to musical features representing items in the real world (e.g., iconic meaning) or associations limited by culture and experience (e.g., symbolic meaning). To address this issue, one study investigated the "universal" nature of iconic meaning in music (Fritz et al., 2013). Participants consisted of German and Marfa listeners (the Marfa are a community of individuals entirely unfamiliar with Western music). Participants listened to excerpts of music that were selected to correspond with a particular concept, such as KING, CELEBRATION, or STORM, and were asked to choose which concept was associated with the excerpt. Within cultures, listeners tended to agree about which concepts mapped on to which pieces. There was minimal overlap between cultures, suggesting that iconic meaning in music is culturally specific. This suggests that music can serve as an iconic sign only for listeners experienced with the particular type of music (i.e., specific qualities of the music point to specific semantic concepts, but only for those familiar with the music). This is in contrast to other work indicating that the emotional associations of music could be accurately identified by the Marfa listeners (Fritz et al., 2009).

Whether music conveys certain semantic associations may change based on a listener's familiarity with the music. For unfamiliar music, music may denote particular concepts via symbolic sign qualities, based on prior experiences with similar types of music, or via iconic sign qualities, as the music mimics objects or events in the world. For highly familiar music, it is likely that music has semantic associations based on explicit connections between that particular music and certain contexts in which a listener has previously heard the music. For example, a listener may hear the melody for "Pomp and Circumstance" and know "this is the song played at graduation ceremonies" – in this case, the song is associated with the sematic concept of "graduations." Work in persons with focal brain damage suggests that the anterior temporal lobes play a critical role in the association between highly familiar music and particular concepts. One study found that individuals with damage to the left temporal pole due to primary progressive aphasia were able to recognize familiar melodies, but showed deficits in matching melodies with related semantic concepts. For example, individuals with left temporal polar damage had difficulties associating the "Wedding March" with the concept of "wedding" or accurately identifying a piece as a lullaby (Macoir et al., 2016).

Other cross-modal associations

Music can also evoke various types of visual imagery – for a review, see Taruffi & Küssner (2019). In a large sample of online participants ($n = 669$), researchers found that 77 percent of respondents reported experiencing visual imagery at some point during music listening (Küssner & Eerola, 2019). The most frequently reported music-evoked visual image was that of a nature scene or landscape. In addition to concrete visual images, abstract images (such as shapes, colors, or geometric objects) were frequently evoked in response to music.

One line of work that provides a potential explanatory mechanism for these music–imagery associations has identified consistent patterns of associations between music and color: faster musical pieces in a major mode tend to be associated with brighter and more saturated colors – for example, yellow – while slower pieces in a minor mode are associated with darker colors – for example, blue (Palmer et al., 2013; Whiteford et al., 2018). While the musical features of tempo and mode corresponded with certain colors, these music–color relationships were primarily mediated by emotional factors. That is, instead of serving as a direct reference for a color, the music was associated with an emotion that was similar to the emotion associated with a color. For example, a fast tempo/major mode song sounds happy and yellow looks happy. It may not be the case that the *felt* emotions, or the strength of emotional responses, to the music/colors are similar, but that the association between color and music is due to shared emotional properties. Therefore, yellow was associated with the song based on their shared emotional properties, rather than music being a direct referent to the color (Isbilen & Krumhansl, 2016).

Cross-modal associations have also been detected between music and other sensory concepts. One recent study (Guetta & Loui, 2017) indicated that listeners can consistently match music to tastes based on certain musical features. For example, lower-pitched and legato notes sound "bitter," while staccato notes sound "salty". Like the evidence from music–color associations above, the authors interpreted these findings to indicate that music evokes cross-modal associations via emotional connections, rather than directly evoking these concepts (Wang et al., 2015). This work suggests that while music may seem to serve as an iconic sign by evoking saltiness or yellowness, perhaps it is the indexical sign quality of music that mediates these effects: music induces a similar emotion to the color yellow, and these emotional characteristics are what cause the interpretation of music as denoting yellow.

Self-related meaning

Self-related meaning in music has been described as "meaning-for-the-subject" (Koopman & Davies, 2001), and as a type of musicogenic meaning (Koelsch, 2011). One particularly relevant way music conveys self-related meaning is through the evocation of personally significant autobiographical memories, which can be particularly vivid and emotional (Janata et al., 2007). When compared with other sensory stimuli, music appears to serve as a memory cue to evoke memories that have greater episodic richness than those evoked by images of persons (Belfi et al., 2020; Belfi et al., 2016). Other work has indicated that autobiographical memories evoked by music contain more sensorimotor details than memories evoked by verbal cues (Zator & Katz, 2017). This suggests that music may evoke a context in which a memory was encoded. Listening to music then triggers reminiscence and vivid reexperiencing of the original event.

Music-evoked autobiographical memories have been linked to the medial prefrontal cortex (Baird et al., 2020; Belfi et al., 2018; Ford et al., 2011; Janata, 2009). This region is engaged during music-evoked remembering and, when damaged, persons have fewer episodically rich memories in response to music. Note that the medial prefrontal cortex also plays a role in music-evoked emotions (as described earlier), suggesting that emotion may be an important component in the capacity for music to evoke episodically detailed autobiographical memories. Music even evokes vivid autobiographical remembering in individuals with certain types of dementia, and is perhaps more effective at doing so than other types of memory cues (Baird et al., 2018; Cuddy et al., 2017; El Haj et al., 2012). In this way, music may convey self-related meaning when other signs may lose their effectiveness, such as in Alzheimer's disease.

Interim summary

To summarize, music can evoke consistent semantic associations across listeners. These associations can range from narrative structures, to specific semantic concepts, to other cross-modal associations such as colors, shapes, tastes, and movement patterns. Additionally, music seems particularly capable of evoking self-related concepts, such as episodically-rich autobiographical memories.

Timecourse of meaning in music

Substantial prior research has sought to determine the point at which music becomes meaningful, and whether different types of meaning emerge on different timescales. For example, a listener may hear the first few notes of a highly familiar melody, such as "Pomp and Circumstance," but it may not yet evoke the concept of "graduations." Given a few more notes, this association may emerge. The music, therefore, did not convey this meaning until the listener had received sufficient musical information.

The emotional content of music can be inferred from very minimal information. When listening to 300- or 400-millisecond clips of popular music, listeners ratings of perceived emotion were highly consistent with ratings they made of longer (15-second) clips of the same pieces (Krumhansl, 2010). Similarly, listeners could accurately discriminate between emotionally moving and emotionally neutral music in as little as 250 milliseconds (Filipic et al., 2010). Additionally, listeners are able to identify the aesthetic appeal of a piece of music within 750 milliseconds (Belfi, Kasdan, et al., 2018). The ability to detect emotions from such brief excerpts suggests that certain features, such as timbre, may play a particularly important role in this initial or quick emotion detection (as many other musical components, such as melodic structure, may require a longer amount of time to detect). One paper specifically investigated the ability to identify emotions based on timbre, by investigating the affective meaning of individual instrument sounds (Eerola et al., 2012). Participants listened to one-second clips of a diverse set of instruments and rated them on emotional dimensions. Participants consistently rated certain instruments as conveying certain emotions, and these ratings mapped on to acoustic features. This suggests that even single notes can convey emotional meaning.

Not only do different instrumental timbres convey different emotions, but single instrument sounds can convey different emotions even when played on the same instrument. One study investigated ERP responses to deviant emotional tones played on the same instrument (Goydke et al., 2004). For example, participants heard a "sad violin" tone as a standard pitch, and a "happy violin" as a deviant, in addition to deviants with a different musical timbre (a flute). The deviant "happy violin" pitch evoked a mismatch negativity, suggesting that the brain was able to detect this subtle difference in emotional content. Interestingly, the mismatch negativity response of this emotional deviant was nearly identical to that of the timbral deviant, suggesting that emotion is processed on a similar timescale to that of other acoustic features, such as timbre.

Similar to the work on emotion identification, musical familiarity can be determined from very brief excerpts. Listeners can discriminate between familiar and unfamiliar excerpts within 500 milliseconds (Filipic et al., 2010), or about five to seven notes (Büdenbender & Kreutz, 2016; Dalla Bella et al., 2003). Additionally, participants can identify the musical artist and song title of 400-millisecond clips of popular music with above-chance accuracy (Krumhansl, 2010). Distinct neurophysiological responses have been observed for familiar versus unfamiliar melodies within 200–500 milliseconds after melody onset, such that there is a larger N400 response for familiar melodies (Daltrozzo et al., 2010). This suggests that familiar melodies "become familiar" within this window, and the heightened N400 represents the neural activation of conceptual associations with the melody.

Neuropsychological studies shed further light on the issue. One study investigated the role of the medial temporal lobes (MTLs) in identifying familiar melodies by studying patients with focal brain damage (Huijgen et al., 2015). Both healthy comparisons and individuals with right and left MTL lesions were able to distinguish between familiar and unfamiliar excerpts within 500 milliseconds. This suggests that MTL integrity is not necessary for recognizing famous musical melodies.

Interim summary

To summarize, listeners can infer meaning from music on a remarkably quick timescale. They are able to detect the familiarity, the emotional qualities, and even the aesthetic appeal of music within hundreds of milliseconds. This suggests that music can convey meaning even when minimal musical information is provided.

Conclusion

This chapter discussed various types of musical meaning, focusing on emotional and other semantic associations. To connect the evidence with the broader field of neurosemiotics, one can note that music does convey meaning, and these types of meaning are in some ways similar to other methods of communicating. That is, music can evoke emotions and specific concepts, and the neural correlates of such musical meanings are similar to those found in studies of language and other domains (e.g., the N400, ERAN versus ELAN). That said, music is certainly not entirely the same as language. For example, meanings evoked by music are often less specific than those denoted by language, and the intention behind music is not necessarily to communicate in the same sense as linguistic communication (Slevc, 2012; Slevc & Patel, 2011).

Note that the interpretation of meaning in music is not solely determined by musical sign qualities. Indeed, there are interactions between listeners' prior background and knowledge and the context in which the music is heard. Furthermore, there is not necessarily a one-to-one mapping between musical sign qualities and musical meaning – as discussed here, for example, emotional responses to music are likely the result of interactions between indexical, symbolic, and iconic musical signs, and may result from other sematic associations with the music. Pointing to the effects of these musical sign qualities is challenging, as they likely all influence a listener's interpretation of the music. Still, evidence suggests that music can both express and induce emotions, and convey specific concepts, all of which can be denoted in a relatively short timescale. Neural systems involved in auditory perception, emotional responses, and semantic and lexical retrieval, and the interactions among these networks, likely underlie the generation of such forms of musical meaning. Like other communicative and artistic phenomena, these multidimensional synergies are part and parcel of our daily neurosemiotic experiences.

References

Adolphs, R., Tranel, D., Damasio, H., & Damasio, A. (1994). Impaired recognition of emotion in facial expressions following bilateral damage to the human amygdala. *Nature*, *372*, 669–672. doi: 10.1038/372669a0

Adolphs, R., Tranel, D., Hamann, S., Young, A. W., Calder, A. J., Phelps, E. A., Anderson, A., Lee, G. P., & Damasio, A. R. (1999). Recognition of facial emotion in nine individuals with bilateral amygdala damage. *Neuropsychologia*, *37*(10), 1111–1117. doi: 10.1016/s0028-3932(99)00039-1

Aubé, W., Angulo-Perkins, A., Peretz, I., Concha, L., & Armony, J. L. (2015). Fear across the senses: Brain responses to music, vocalizations and facial expressions. *Social Cognitive and Affective Neuroscience*, *10*(3), 399–407. doi: 10.1093/scan/nsu067

Aucouturier, J.-J., & Canonne, C. (2017). Musical friends and foes: The social cognition of affiliation and control in improvised interactions. *Cognition*, *161*, 94–108. doi: 10.1016/j.cognition.2017.01.019

Baird, A., Brancatisano, O., Gelding, R., & Forde, W. (2018). Characterization of music and photograph evoked autobiographical memories in people with Alzheimer's disease. *Journal of Alzheimer's Disease*, *66*(2), 693–706. doi: 10.3233/JAD-180627

Baird, A., Brancatisano, O., Gelding, R., & Thompson, W. F. (2020). Music evoked autobiographical memories in people with behavioural variant frontotemporal dementia. *Memory*, *28*(3), 323–336. doi: 10.1080/09658211.2020.1713379

Baker, D. J., & Müllensiefen, D. (2017). Perception of leitmotives in Richard Wagner's *der ring des nibelungen*. *Frontiers in Psychology*, *8*, 662. doi: 10.3389/fpsyg.2017.00662

Belfi, A. M., Bai, E., & Stroud, A. (2020). Comparing methods for analyzing music-evoked autobiographical memories. *Music Perception*, *37*(5), 392–402. doi: 10.1525/mp.2020.37.5.392

Belfi, A. M., Evans, E., Heskje, J., Bruss, J., & Tranel, D. (2017). Musical anhedonia after focal brain damage. *Neuropsychologia*, *97*, 29–37. doi: 10.1016/j.neuropsychologia.2017.01.030

Belfi, A. M., Karlan, B., & Tranel, D. (2016). Music evokes vivid autobiographical memories. *Memory*, *24*(7), 979–989. doi: 10.1080/09658211.2015.1061012

Belfi, A. M., Karlan, B., & Tranel, D. (2018). Damage to the medial prefrontal cortex impairs music-evoked autobiographical memories. *Psychomusicology: Music, Mind, and Brain*, *28*(4), 201–208. doi: 10.1037/pmu0000222

Belfi, A. M., Kasdan, A., Rowland, J., Vessel, E. A., Starr, G. G., & Poeppel, D. (2018). Rapid timing of musical aesthetic judgments. *Journal of Experimental Psychology: General*, *147*(10), 1531–1543. doi: 10.1037/xge0000474

Belfi, A. M., & Loui, P. (2020). Musical anhedonia and rewards of music listening: current advances and a proposed model. *Annals of the New York Academy of Sciences*, *1464*(1), 1–16. doi: 10.1111/nyas.14241

Bendor, D., & Wang, X. (2005). The neuronal representation of pitch in primate auditory cortex. *Nature*, *436*(7054), 1161–1165. doi: 10.1038/nature03867

Bouissac, P. (1986). Semiotics in Canada I. In T. A. Sebeok & D. J. Umiker-Sebeok (Eds.), *The Semiotic Web* (pp. 191–252). Berlin: Mouton de Gruyter.

Büdenbender, N., & Kreutz, G. (2016). Long-term representations of melodies in Western listeners: Influences of familiarity, musical expertise, tempo and structure. *Psychology of Music*, *45*(5), 665–681. doi: 10.1177/0305735616671408

Chen, J. L., Penhune, V. B., & Zatorre, R. J. (2008). Listening to musical rhythms recruits motor regions of the brain. *Cerebral Cortex*, *18*(12), 2844–2854. doi: 10.1093/cercor/bhn042

Coutinho, E., Dibben, N., Coutinho, E., & Dibben, N. (2013). Psychoacoustic cues to emotion in speech prosody and music psychoacoustic cues to emotion in speech prosody and music. *Cognition and Emotion*, *27*, 658–684. doi: 10.1080/02699931.2012.732559

Cross, I. (2009). The evolutionary nature of musical meaning. *Musicae Scientiae*, *13*(2), 179–200. doi: 10.1177/1029864909013002091

Cuddy, L. L., Sikka, R., Silveira, K., Bai, S., & Vanstone, A. (2017). Music-evoked autobiographical memories (MEAMs) in Alzheimer's disease: Evidence for a positivity effect. *Cogent Psychology*, *4*(1), 1–20. doi: 10.1080/23311908.2016.1277578

Curtis, M. E., & Bharucha, J. J. (2010). The minor third communicates sadness in speech, mirroring its use in music. *Emotion*, *10*(3), 335–348. doi: 10.1037/a0017928

Dalla Bella, S., Peretz, I., & Aronoff, N. (2003). Time course of melody recognition: A gating paradigm study. *Perception & Psychophysics*, *65*, 1019–1028. doi: 10.3758/BF03194831

Dalla Bella, S., Peretz, I., Rousseau, L., & Gosselin, N. (2001). A developmental study of the affective value of tempo and mode in music. *Cognition*, *80*(3), B1–B10. doi: 10.1016/s0010-0277(00)00136-0

Daltrozzo, J., & Schön, D. (2009a). Is conceptual processing in music automatic? An electrophysiological approach. *Brain Research*, *1270*, 88–94. doi: 10.1016/j.brainres.2009.03.019

Daltrozzo, J., & Schön, D. (2009b). Conceptual processing in music as revealed by N400 effects on words and musical targets. *Journal of Cognitive Neuroscience*, *21*(10) 1882–1892. doi: 10.1162/jocn.2009.21113

Daltrozzo, J., Tillmann, B., Platel, H., & Schön, D. (2010). Temporal aspects of the feeling of familiarity for music and the emergence of conceptual processing. *Journal of Cognitive Neuroscience*, *22*(8), 1754–1769. doi: 10.1162/jocn.2009.21311

Downey, L. E., Blezat, A., Nicholas, J., Omar, R., Golden, H. L., Mahoney, C. J., Crutch, S. J., & Warren, J. D. (2013). Mentalising music in frontotemporal dementia. *Cortex*, *49*(7), 1844–1855. doi: 10.1016/j.cortex.2012.09.011

Eerola, T., Ferrer, R., & Alluri, V. (2012). Timbre and affect dimensions: Evidence from affect and similarity ratings and acoustic correlates of isolated instrument sounds. *Music Perception*, *30*(1), 49–70. doi: 10.1525/mp.2012.30.1.49

El Haj, M., Fasotti, L., & Allain, P. (2012). The involuntary nature of music-evoked autobiographical memories in Alzheimer's disease. *Consciousness and Cognition*, *21*(1), 238–246. doi: 10.1016/j.concog.2011.12.005

Ferreri, L., Mas-Herrero, E., Zatorre, R. J., Ripollés, P., Gomez-Andres, A., Alicart, H., Olivé, G., Marco-Pallarés, J., Antonijoan, R. M., Valle, M., Riba, J., & Rodriguez-Fornells, A. (2019). Dopamine modulates the reward experiences elicited by music. *Proceedings of the National Academy of Sciences of the United States of America*, *116*(9), 3793–3798. doi: 10.1073/pnas.1811878116

Filipic, S., Tillmann, B., & Bigand, E. (2010). Judging familiarity and emotion from very brief musical excerpts. *Psychonomic Bulletin & Review*, *17*, 335–341. doi: 10.3758/PBR.17.3.335

Fiveash, A., Thompson, W. F., Badcock, N. A., & McArthur, G. (2018). Syntactic processing in music and language: Effects of interrupting auditory streams with alternating timbres. *International Journal of Psychophysiology*, *129*, 31–40. doi: 10.1016/j.ijpsycho.2018.05.003

Ford, J. H., Addis, D. R., & Giovanello, K. S. (2011). Differential neural activity during search of specific and general autobiographical memories elicited by musical cues. *Neuropsychologia, 49*(9), 2514–2526. doi: 10.1016/j.neuropsychologia.2011.04.032

Fritz, T., Jentschke, S., Gosselin, N., Sammler, D., Peretz, I., Turner, R., Friederici, A. D., & Koelsch, S. (2009). Universal recognition of three basic emotions in music. *Current Biology, 19*(7), 573–576. doi: 10.1016/j.cub.2009.02.058

Fritz, T., Schmude, P., Jentschke, S., Friederici, A. D., & Koelsch, S. (2013). From understanding to appreciating music cross-culturally. *PLoS One, 8*(9), e72500. doi: 10.1371/journal.pone.0072500

Frühholz, S., Trost, W., & Grandjean, D. (2014). The role of the medial temporal limbic system in processing emotions in voice and music. *Progress in Neurobiology, 123*, 1–17. doi: 10.1016/j.pneurobio.2014.09.003

Gold, B. P., Mas-Herrero, E., Zeighami, Y., Benovoy, M., Dagher, A., & Zatorre, R. J. (2019). Musical reward prediction errors engage the nucleus accumbens and motivate learning. *Proceedings of the National Academy of Sciences of the United States of America, 116*(8), 3310–3315. doi: 10.1073/PNAS.1809855116

Gordon, C. L., Cobb, P. R., & Balasubramaniam, R. (2018). Recruitment of the motor system during music listening: An ALE meta-analysis of fMRI data. *PLoS One, 13*(11), e0207213. doi: 10.1371/journal.pone.0207213

Gosselin, N., Peretz, I., Hasboun, D., Baulac, M., & Samson, S. (2011). Impaired recognition of musical emotions and facial expressions following anteromedial temporal lobe excision. *Cortex, 47*(9), 1116–1125. doi: 10.1016/j.cortex.2011.05.012

Gosselin, N., Peretz, I., Johnsen, E., & Adolphs, R. (2007). Amygdala damage impairs emotion recognition from music. *Neuropsychologia, 45*(2), 236–244. doi: 10.1016/j.neuropsychologia.2006.07.012

Gosselin, N., Peretz, I., Noulhiane, M., Hasboun, D., Beckett, C., Baulac, M., & Samson, S. (2005). Impaired recognition of scary music following unilateral temporal lobe excision. *Brain, 128*(3), 628–640. doi: 10.1093/brain/awh420

Goydke, K. N., Altenmüller, E., Möller, J., & Münte, T. F. (2004). Changes in emotional tone and instrumental timbre are reflected by the mismatch negativity. *Cognitive Brain Research, 21*(3), 351–359. doi: 10.1016/j.cogbrainres.2004.06.009

Grahn, J. A. (2012). Neural mechanisms of rhythm perception: Current findings and future perspectives. *Topics in Cognitive Science, 4*(4), 585–606. doi: 10.1111/j.1756-8765.2012.01213.x

Griffiths, T. D., Warren, J. D., Dean, J. L., & Howard, D. (2004). "When the feeling's gone": A selective loss of musical emotion. *Journal of Neurology, Neurosurgery & Psychiatry, 75*(2), 341–345.

Guetta, R., & Loui, P. (2017). When music is salty: The crossmodal associations between sound and taste. *PLoS ONE, 12*(3), e0173366. doi: 10.1371/journal.pone.0173366

Heaton, P., Hermelin, B., & Pring, L. (1999). Can children with autistic spectrum disorders perceive affect in music? An experimental investigation. *Psychological Medicine, 29*(6), 1405–1410. doi: 10.1017/S0033291799001221

Huijgen, J., Dellacherie, D., Tillmann, B., Clément, S., Bigand, E., Dupont, S., & Samson, S. (2015). The feeling of familiarity for music in patients with a unilateral temporal lobe lesion: A gating study. *Neuropsychologia, 77*, 313–320. doi: 10.1016/j.neuropsychologia.2015.09.007

Huron, D. (2006). *Sweet Anticipation: Music and the Psychology of Expectation*. Cambridge, MA: MIT Press.

Isbilen, E. S., & Krumhansl, C. L. (2016). The color of music: Emotion-mediated associations to Bach's well-tempered clavier. *Psychomusicology: Music, Mind, and Brain, 26*(2), 149–161. doi: 10.1037/pmu0000147

Janata, P. (2009). The neural architecture of music-evoked autobiographical memories. *Cerebral Cortex, 19*(11), 2579–2594. doi: 10.1093/cercor/bhp008

Janata, P., Tomic, S. T., & Rakowski, S. K. (2007). Characterization of music-evoked autobiographical memories. *Memory, 15*(8), 845–860. doi: 10.1080/09658210701734593

Jost, K., Hennighausen, E., & Rösler, F. (2003). Comparing arithmetic and semantic fact retrieval: Effects of problem size and sentence constraint on event-related brain potentials. *Psychophysiology, 40*(6), 1000–1000. doi: 10.1111/1469-8986.00119

Juslin, P. N. (2013). From everyday emotions to aesthetic emotions: Towards a unified theory of musical emotions. *Physics of Life Reviews, 10*(3), 235–266. doi: 10.1016/j.plrev.2013.05.008

Kellenbach, M. L., Wijers, A. A., & Mulder, G. (2000). Visual semantic features are activated during the processing of concrete words: Event-related potential evidence for perceptual semantic priming. *Cognitive Research, 10*(1–2), 67–75. doi: 10.1016/S0926-6410(00)00023-9

Koelsch, S. (2011). Towards a neural basis of processing musical semantics. *Physics of Life Reviews, 8*(2), 89–105. doi: 10.1016/j.plrev.2011.04.004

Koelsch, S. (2014). Brain correlates of music-evoked emotions. *Nature Reviews Neuroscience, 15*, 170–180. doi: 10.1038/nrn3666

Koelsch, S., Gunter, T., Friederici, a D., & Schröger, E. (2000). Brain indices of music processing: "Nonmusicians" are musical. *Journal of Cognitive Neuroscience, 12*(3), 520–541. doi: 10.1162/089892900562183

Koelsch, S., Kasper, E., Sammler, D., Schulze, K., Gunter, T., & Friederici, A. D. (2004). Music, language and meaning: Brain signatures of semantic processing. *Nature Neuroscience*, 7, 302–307. doi: 10.1038/nn1197

Koopman, C., & Davies, S. (2001). Musical meaning in a broader perspective. *Journal of Aesthetics and Art Criticism*, *59*(3), 261–273. doi: 10.1111/1540-6245.00024

Krumhansl, C. L. (2010). Plink: "thin slices" of music. *Music Perception*, *27*(5), 337–354. doi: 10.1525/mp.2010.27.5.337

Krumhansl, C. L., & Shepard, R. N. (1979). Quantification of the hierarchy of tonal functions within a diatonic context. *Journal of Experimental Psychology: Human Perception and Performance*, *5*(4), 579–594. doi: 10.1037/0096-1523.5.4.579

Küssner, M. B., & Eerola, T. (2019). The content and functions of vivid and soothing visual imagery during music listening: Findings from a survey study. *Psychomusicology: Music, Mind, and Brain*, *29*(2–3), 90–99. doi: 10.1037/pmu0000238

Laukka, P., Eerola, T., Thingujam, N. S., Yamasaki, T., & Beller, G. (2013). Universal and culture-specific factors in the recognition and performance of musical affect expressions. *Emotion*, *13*(3), 434–449. doi: 10.1037/a0031388

Loui, P., Patterson, S., Sachs, M. E., Leung, Y., Zeng, T., & Przysinda, E. (2017). White matter correlates of musical anhedonia: Implications for evolution of music. *Frontiers in Psychology*, *8*, 1664. doi: 10.3389/fpsyg.2017.01664

Loui, P., & Przysinda, E. (2019). Music in the brain: Areas and networks. In R. Ashley & T. Renee (Eds.). *The Routledge Companion to Music Cognition* (pp. 13–24). London: Routledge.

Loui, P., & Wessel, D. L. (2008). Learning and liking an artificial musical system: Effects of set size and repeated exposure. *Misicae Scientiae*, *12*(2), 1–19. doi: 10.1177/102986490801200202

Loui, P., Wessel, D. L., & Hudson Kam, C. L. (2010). Humans rapidly learn grammatical structure in a new musical scale. *Music Perception*, *27*(5), 377–388. doi: 10.1525/mp.2010.27.5.377

Macoir, J., Berubé-lalancette, S., Wilson, M. A., Hudon, C., Gravel, P., Potvin, O., … Laforce, R. (2016). When the Wedding March becomes sad: Semantic memory impairment for music in the semantic variant of primary progressive aphasia. *Neurocase*, *22*(6), 486–495. doi: 10.1080/13554794.2016.1257025

Margulis, E. H. (2017). An exploratory study of narrative experiences of music. *Music Perception*, *35*(2), 235–248. doi: 10.1525/MP.2017.35.2.235

Martínez-Molina, N., Mas-Herrero, E., Rodríguez-Fornells, A., Zatorre, R. J., & Marco-Pallarés, J. (2016). Neural correlates of specific musical anhedonia. *Proceedings of the National Academy of Sciences of the United States of America*, *113*(46), E7337–E7345. doi: 10.1073/PNAS.1611211113

Mas-Herrero, E., Dagher, A., & Zatorre, R. J. (2018). Modulating musical reward sensitivity up and down with transcranial magnetic stimulation. *Nature Human Behaviour*, *2*, 27–32. doi: 10.1038/s41562-017-0241-z

Mas-Herrero, E., Marco-Pallares, J., Lorenzo-Seva, U., Zatorre, R. J., & Rodriguez-Fornells, A. (2013). Individual differences in music reward experiences. *Music Perception*, *31*(2), 118–138. doi: 10.1525/mp.2013.31.2.118

Mas-Herrero, E., Zatorre, R. J., Rodriguez-Fornells, A., & Marco-Pallarés, J. (2014). Dissociation between musical and monetary reward responses in specific musical anhedonia. *Current Biology*, *24*(6), 699–704. doi: 10.1016/j.cub.2014.01.068

McDermott, J. H., Schultz, A. F., Undurraga, E. A., & Godoy, R. A. (2016). Indifference to dissonance in native Amazonians reveals cultural variation in music perception. *Nature*, *535*, 547–550. doi: 10.1038/nature18635

Meyer, L. B. (1956). *Emotion and meaning in music*. Chicago: University of Chicago Press.

Omigie, D. (2016). Basic, specific, mechanistic? Conceptualizing musical emotions in the brain. *The Journal of Comparative Neurology*, *524*(8), 1676–1686. doi: 10.1002/cne.23854

Palmer, S. E., Schloss, K. B., Xu, Z., & Prado-León, L. R. (2013). Music–color associations are mediated by emotion. *Proceedings of the National Academy of Sciences of the United States of America*, *110*(22), 8836–8841. doi: 10.1073/pnas.1212562110

Paquette, S., Takerkart, S., Saget, S., Peretz, I., & Belin, P. (2018). Cross-classification of musical and vocal emotions in the auditory cortex. *Annals of the New York Academy of Sciences*, *1423*(1), 329–337. doi: 10.1111/nyas.13666

Popescu, T., Neuser, M. P., Neuwirth, M., Bravo, F., Mende, W., Boneh, O., … Rohrmeier, M. (2019). The pleasantness of sensory dissonance is mediated by musical style and expertise. *Scientific Reports*, *9*, 1070. doi: 10.1038/s41598-018-35873-8

Pralus, A., Belfi, A., Hirel, C., Lévêque, Y., Fornoni, L., Bigand, E., Jung, J., Tranel, D., Nighoghossian, N., Tillmann, B., & Caclin, A. (2020). Recognition of musical emotions and their perceived intensity after unilateral brain damage. *Cortex*, *130*, 78–93. doi: 10.1016/j.cortex.2020.05.015

Reid, V. M., & Striano, T. (2008). N400 involvement in the processing of action sequences. *Neuroscience Letters*, *433*(2), 93–97. doi: 10.1016/j.neulet.2007.12.066

Rohrmeier, M., & Rebuschat, P. (2012). Implicit learning and acquisition of music. *Topics in Cognitive Science*, *4*(4), 525–553. doi: 10.1111/j.1756-8765.2012.01223.x

Roy, M., Shohamy, D., & Wager, T. D. (2012). Ventromedial prefrontal-subcortical systems and the generation of affective meaning. *Trends in Cognitive Sciences, 16*(3), 147–156. doi: 10.1016/j.tics.2012.01.005

Sachs, M. E., Habibi, A., Damasio, A., & Kaplan, J. T. (2018). Decoding the neural signatures of emotions expressed through sound. *NeuroImage, 174*, 1–10. doi: 10.1016/j.neuroimage.2018.02.058

Salimpoor, V. N., Benovoy, M., Larcher, K., Dagher, A., & Zatorre, R. J. (2011). Anatomically distinct dopamine release during anticipation and experience of peak emotion to music. *Nature Neuroscience, 14*, 257–262. doi: 10.1038/nn.2726

Salimpoor, V. N., van den Bosch, I., Kovacevic, N., McIntosh, A. R., Dagher, A., & Zatorre, R. J. (2013). Interactions between the nucleus accumbens and auditory cortices predict music reward value. *Science, 340*(6129), 216–219. doi: 10.1126/science.1231059

Sanfilippo, K. R. M., Spiro, N., Molina-Solana, M., & Lamont, A. (2020). Do the shuffle: Exploring reasons for music listening through shuffled play. *PLoS One, 15*(2), e0228457. doi: 10.1371%2Fjournal.pone.0228457

Särkämö, T., Tervaniemi, M., Soinila, S., Autti, T., Silvennoinen, H. M., Laine, M., & Hietanen, M. (2009). Cognitive deficits associated with acquired amusia after stroke: A neuropsychological follow-up study. *Neuropsychologia, 47*(12), 2642–2651. doi: 10.1016/j.neuropsychologia.2009.05.015

Satoh, M., Kato, N., Tabei, K. I., Nakano, C., Abe, M., Fujita, R., Kida, H., Tomimoto, H., & Kondo, K. (2016). A case of musical anhedonia due to right putaminal hemorrhage: A disconnection syndrome between the auditory cortex and insula. *Neurocase, 22*(6), 518–525. doi: 10.1080/13554794.2016.1264609

Satoh, M., Nakase, T., Nagata, K., & Tomimoto, H. (2011). Musical anhedonia: Selective loss of emotional experience in listening to music. *Neurocase, 17*(5), 410–417. doi: 10.1080/13554794.2010.532139

Schiavio, A., van der Schyff, D., Cespedes-Guevara, J., & Reybrouck, M. (2017). Enacting musical emotions. sense-making, dynamic systems, and the embodied mind. *Phenomenology and the Cognitive Sciences, 16*, 785–809. doi: 10.1007/s11097-016-9477-8

Schneider, B., & Koenigs, M. (2017). Human lesion studies of ventromedial prefrontal cortex. *Neuropsychologia, 107*, 84–93. doi: 10.1016/j.neuropsychologia.2017.09.035

Slevc, L. R. (2012). Language and music: Sound, structure, and meaning. *WIREs Cognitive Science, 3*(4), 483–492. doi: 10.1002/wcs.1186

Slevc, L. R., & Patel, A. D. (2011). Meaning in music and language: Three key differences: Comment on "Towards a neural basis of processing musical semantics" by Stefan Koelsch. *Physics of Life Reviews, 8*(2), 110–111. doi: 10.1016/j.plrev.2011.05.003

Steinbeis, N., & Koelsch, S. (2009). Understanding the intentions behind man-made products elicits neural activity in areas dedicated to mental state attribution. *Cerebral Cortex, 19*(3), 619–623. doi: 10.1093/cercor/bhn110

Taruffi, L., & Küssner, M. B. (2019). A review of music-evoked visual mental imagery: Conceptual issues, relation to emotion, and functional outcome. *Psychomusicology: Music, Mind, and Brain, 29*(2–3), 62–74. doi: 10.1037/pmu0000226

Terwogt, M. M., & Van Grinsven, F. (1988). Recognition of emotions in music by children and adults. *Perceptual and Motor Skills, 67*(3), 697–698. doi: 10.2466%2Fpms.1988.67.3.697

Vieillard, S., Peretz, I., Gosselin, N., Khalfa, S., Gagnon, L., & Bouchard, B. (2008). Happy, sad, scary and peaceful musical excerpts for research on emotions. *Cognition & Emotion, 22*(4), 720–752. doi: 10.1080/02699930701503567

Wang, Q. J., Woods, A. T., & Spence, C. (2015). "What's your taste in music?" A comparison of the effectiveness of various soundscapes in evoking specific tastes. *I-Perception, 6*(6), 1–23. doi: 10.1177/2041669515622001

Warrenburg, L. A. (2020). Comparing musical and psychological emotion theories. *Psychomusicology: Music, Mind, and Brain, 30*(1), 1–19. doi: 10.1037/pmu0000247

Whiteford, K. L., Schloss, K. B., Helwig, N. E., & Palmer, S. E. (2018). Color, music, and emotion: Bach to the blues. *I-Perception, 9*(6), 1–27. doi: 10.1177/2041669518808535

Zator, K., & Katz, A. N. (2017). The language used in describing autobiographical memories prompted by life period visually presented verbal cues, event-specific visually presented verbal cues and short musical clips of popular music. *Memory, 25*(6), 831–844. doi: 10.1080/09658211.2016.1224353

23

THE MEANING OF TOOLS

The pragmatic value of semantic knowledge

François Osiurak, Josselin Baumard, Catherine Merck, and Mathieu Lesourd

Introduction

Humans have accumulated techniques and tools that are too complex to be invented by a single individual, a phenomenon known as cumulative technological culture (Legare & Nielsen, 2015; Osiurak & Reynaud, 2020). One of the major outcomes of this phenomenon is that humans possess a large and diverse repertoire of tools. Understanding the neurocognitive bases of human tool use represents an enduringly fascinating question. An intuitive hypothesis is that human tool use is critically based on semantic knowledge: "I can use a hammer because I know that it is something that pounds nails" (Rothi et al., 1991; Roy & Square, 1985; van Elk et al., 2014). However, the semantic knowledge hypothesis of tool use has been subject to intense debate in neuropsychology on the grounds that patients with selective semantic memory deficits are frequently still able to use tools in a relatively appropriate manner (e.g., Buxbaum et al., 1997; Osiurak et al., 2008; Silveri & Ciccarelli, 2009). This finding has also led to speculation about the role of semantic knowledge in tool use. A potential limitation of the semantic knowledge hypothesis is that it views semantic knowledge as socially decontextualized, enabling understanding of the specific use of a familiar tool. However, a more coherent picture emerges when one considers semantic knowledge as cognitive processes providing *the socio-contextual information* that is sometimes needed to understand the specific use of a familiar tool. In other words, semantic knowledge might be more pragmatic than previously thought. This epistemological shift is perfectly in line with the neurosemiotic approach, which stresses that context-dependence effects are pervasive in everyday cognition (e.g., Adolfi et al., 2017; Ibáñez & Manes, 2012). In this chapter, we present a new analysis of the role of semantic knowledge in human tool use, which contributes to increasing interest in a neurosemiotic of tool use.

The neurosemiotic approach diverges from representationalist perspectives in at least two respects. First, it conceptualizes cognition (especially in language processes) as emerging from dynamic, enactive, and embodied processes, thus establishing a strong link between cognitive and motor components (García & Ibáñez, 2014a, 2014b, 2016; Ibáñez et al., 2013; for a review, see García & Ibáñez, 2017). Second, it stresses the key role of context-dependence effects on cognition (social cognition, in particular) processes (Adolfi et al., 2017; Ibáñez & Manes, 2012). The theoretical discussion initiated in this chapter extends this second aspect to the specific case of tool use, with the aim of showing some of the interests of the neurosemiotic approach to the study of tool use.

DOI: 10.4324/9781003051817-28

From semantic knowledge ...

The classical semantic knowledge hypothesis

Semantic memory can be defined as a system that processes, stores, and retrieves information about the meaning of words, concepts, facts, and persons (Warrington, 1975; for more recent accounts, see Chen et al., 2017; Lambon Ralph et al., 2017). In this frame, semantic knowledge regarding tools – or rather artifacts (see Box 23.1) – contains information about the objects with which familiar tools are commonly used (e.g., a nail for a hammer) or the typical location where they can be found (e.g., a workshop). For the sake of clarity, we will hereafter use the term "semantic knowledge" to refer to semantic knowledge about tools. This knowledge can be assessed by asking patients to name or describe the tools presented (e.g., the object commonly associated or its purpose) or with picture-matching tasks (e.g., target: corkscrew; choices: wine bottle, glass, or piece of wood; see Hodges et al., 2000). Imaging evidence indicates that semantic knowledge relies on the integrity of the temporal lobes (Goldenberg & Spatt, 2009).

Box 23.1 The multiple meanings of tools

Tool use can broadly be defined as the use of an external object to alter the condition of another object (Shumaker et al., 2011). Three main categories of tool use can be distinguished. First, *familiar tool use* refers to the use of familiar tools in a conventional way (e.g., pounding a nail with a hammer). Familiar tools can be viewed here as artifacts – that is, tools that have been made for a specific purpose (e.g., a hammer, a knife). For the sake of clarity, we will discuss only the results obtained from familiar tool use tasks in which only one tool is presented with its corresponding object. However, fully understanding the role of semantic knowledge in familiar tool use clearly requires a detailed examination of studies including a choice condition (i.e., choosing among several familiar tools the appropriate one before actually using it with the object presented – e.g., Baumard et al., 2016). Second, the term *unfamiliar tool use* refers to the use of familiar tools in an unconventional way (e.g., using a knife to drive a screw or the handle of a fork to eat yoghurt). Third, the term *novel tool use* refers to the use of a tool that has no specific purpose (e.g., using a stone to make a wooden spear or to pound a small nail, or using a wire to make a hook). These tools can be "natural" (e.g., stone) or manmade (e.g., wire).

These three categories correspond to cases of *real tool use*, in which the individual actually uses the tool with an object. No less interesting is the case of *single tool use*, which consists in asking patients to show the use of a familiar tool presented in isolation. The patient can grasp this familiar tool, but no mechanical action is expected, given that there is no additional object presented. Indeed, single tool use necessarily implies familiar tools because no specific use can be associated with a stone or a wire (as in novel tool use – see above). In addition, the use expected is the conventional use of the familiar tool presented. If the patient shows how to use a knife to drive a screw, the demonstration is considered erroneous (see below). Note that the distinction between real tool use and single tool use is rarely considered as providing important information in the literature. Yet such distinction is useful to understand the role of the different neurocognitive processes – and particularly of semantic knowledge – underlying human tool use.

Some brain-damaged patients can show severe difficulties when asked to select or actually use familiar tools in an appropriate manner.[1] For instance, the patient can attempt to pound a nail with a fork. These tool use disorders, also called apraxia of tool use,[2] have been subject to interpretation (e.g., Geschwind, 1975; Heilman et al., 1982; Liepmann, 1920; for a review, see Goldenberg, 2013). The first link between semantic memory and apraxia of tool use was proposed by Roy and Square (1985), who developed a two-stage model of apraxia consisting of a production system and a conceptual system. For them, apraxia of tool use reflects an impairment of the conceptual system, which contains semantic knowledge. A few years later, De Renzi and Lucchelli (1988) proposed the term "amnesic apraxia" to account for these difficulties. Finally, Rothi et al. (1991) capitalized on Roy and Square's model and formulated a now classical cognitive model of apraxia, according to which apraxia of tool use results from impaired semantic knowledge. To stress the conceptual nature of the disorder, they proposed the term "conceptual apraxia" (Ochipa et al., 1992). Since then, most cognitive models of apraxia have included a conceptual component corresponding to semantic knowledge (Buxbaum, 2001; Cubelli et al., 2000; van Elk et al., 2014).

No evidence for the classical semantic knowledge hypothesis

The classical semantic knowledge hypothesis described just above – hereafter called the classical hypothesis – posits that patients' difficulties in selecting and actually using tools appropriately (i.e., familiar tool use) are due to impaired semantic knowledge. Therefore, a first key prediction is that impairment in semantic memory tasks should systematically be associated with these difficulties (Prediction A; see Baumard et al., 2019). A second key prediction is that these difficulties should preferentially occur after damage to the temporal lobes, which is thought to be involved in the storage of semantic memory (Prediction B). Nonetheless, some patients can name or describe tools that they are unable to use (Fukutake, 2003; Heath et al., 2003; Moreaud et al., 1998; Motomura & Yamadori, 1994; see also Zangwill, 1960). The inverse pattern of performance has also been found (Bartolo et al., 2007; Buxbaum et al., 1997; Forde & Humphreys, 2000; Goldenberg & Spatt, 2009; Lauro-Grotto et al., 1997; Negri et al., 2007; Silveri & Ciccarelli, 2009). For example, Negri et al. (2007) reported the cases of two patients: D.L. with a probable semantic dementia and A.M. with an atypical onset of Alzheimer disease. Both patients had a selective loss of semantic knowledge, assessed with picture-matching tasks. By contrast, their ability to actually use tools with their corresponding objects (i.e., real tool use) was surprisingly preserved. These findings suggest that apraxia of tool use does not necessarily result from impaired semantic knowledge, thereby invalidating Prediction A. In addition, a significant body of literature has shown that apraxia of tool use is associated with damage to the left inferior parietal lobe and not the temporal lobes (e.g., Goldenberg & Spatt, 2009; for a review, see Osiurak et al., 2020, see also below). These findings invalidate Prediction B. To paraphrase Buxbaum et al. (1997), intact semantic knowledge is neither necessary nor sufficient to use tools.

... to technical reasoning

Epistemological consideration

Beyond the absence of systematic link between impaired semantic knowledge and apraxia of tool use, the classical hypothesis also suffers from epistemological limitations. As mentioned above, semantic knowledge is thought to encompass information about the objects with which familiar tools are commonly used or the typical location where they can be found. In other words, semantic knowledge concerns the specific purpose associated with artifacts (Box 23.1). From this perspective, semantic knowledge is useful, at best, for what we call familiar tool use – that is, the use of an artifact for its specific/canonical purpose (e.g., using a hammer to pound a nail). However, semantic knowledge becomes useless in contexts of novel tool use or unfamiliar tool use (Box 23.1). The fact that semantic knowledge is not critical for all tool use situations questions the evolutionary and anthropological value of the classical hypothesis. This hypothesis seems to only consider the context of modern humans, for whom a wide range of familiar tools is available. Thus, humans are seen as mere manipulators, facing the challenge of recognizing familiar tools through their specific purposes. However, if our ancestors had needed semantic knowledge to use familiar tools, they could have not initiated the shift from novel tool use to familiar tool use, which consists of assigning a specific purpose to a tool by using it repeatedly and crafting it so that the tool becomes "familiar." In sum, the classical hypothesis models how modern humans manipulate familiar tools for their specific purpose without considering the validity of such a scenario in a more comprehensive evolutionary and anthropological framework.

Proponents of the classical hypothesis have been aware of the aforementioned limitation. They have argued for the existence of a non-semantic route to action, which is critical when humans use novel tools or familiar tools in a non-conventional way[3] (i.e., novel tool use and unfamiliar tool use, respectively; see Humphreys, 2001; Riddoch et al., 1998; Rothi et al., 1991; Rumiati & Humphreys, 1998; for similar accounts, see Goldenberg & Hagmann, 1998; Hodges et al., 2000). This non-semantic route has been also viewed as a way of compensating for the loss of semantic knowledge, thereby allowing a patient with selective semantic deficits to use familiar tools in a conventional way (i.e., familiar tool use). Nevertheless, the semantic route remains the default option for familiar tool use. This is the multiple-routes-to-action hypothesis.

At a theoretical level, one may wonder why the classical hypothesis maintains that semantic knowledge is central even though another cognitive component (i.e., the non-semantic route) can deal with all tool use situations. This is all the more surprising given that familiar tool use is not deeply impaired following lesions of the temporal lobes, which are involved in semantic knowledge. In other words, the classical hypothesis posits that semantic knowledge is central to human tool use, whereas impaired semantic knowledge is not linked to difficulties in the different tool use situations (i.e., familiar tool use, unfamiliar tool use, and novel tool use).[4] In addition, the multiple-routes-to-action hypothesis raises the question of why the human brain would possess two cognitive systems able to support the same cognitive function. A more parsimonious account is that there is no redundancy in the brain. Different cognitive functions can be involved in the same behavior so that damage to these different functions can lead to disturb this behavior. The illusion may thus arise that such different cognitive functions support this behavior. However, if the behavior is studied more carefully, it is possible to identify the behavioral impairments associated with each function and, thus, to understand the specific roles of each.[5]

As discussed below, this is not to say that semantic knowledge is not involved at all in tool use situations. Nevertheless, to develop a new approach to semantic knowledge, two key assumptions have to be made. The first is that any cognitive model of human tool use must be viable at an evolutionary and anthropological level. Therefore, such a model must not focus just on familiar tool use; rather, it should account for all tool use situations, including unfamiliar tool use and novel tool use. In this respect, the non-semantic route proposed by classical cognitive models appears to be an appropriate candidate to explain how humans use tools. The second is that the human brain does not possess interchangeable routes to action. As mentioned, we do not deny that semantic knowledge can be involved in tool use situations. However, semantic knowledge does not, strictly speaking, support real tool use. So, if we intend to understand what its role exactly is, we must acknowledge that semantic knowledge serves another function. Before elaborating on this point, we will present some recent advances in our understanding of the so-called non-semantic route, allowing us to specify what semantic knowledge is not.

The technical reasoning hypothesis

The technical reasoning hypothesis has been developed as an alternative to the classical hypothesis (Osiurak et al., 2010; Osiurak & Badets, 2016; for similar accounts, see Goldenberg, 2013; Pinker, 2010; Vaesen, 2012) (see Figure 23.1). The main epistemological shift thus initiated has been to consider that the so-called non-semantic route is not the default route, while acknowledging key neurocognitive process that support the ability to use tools in all tool use situations[6] – that is, familiar, unfamiliar, and novel tool use. The core assumption is that people use tools to solve most of the mechanical problems they face daily. To do so, they reason at a technical level by using non-declarative

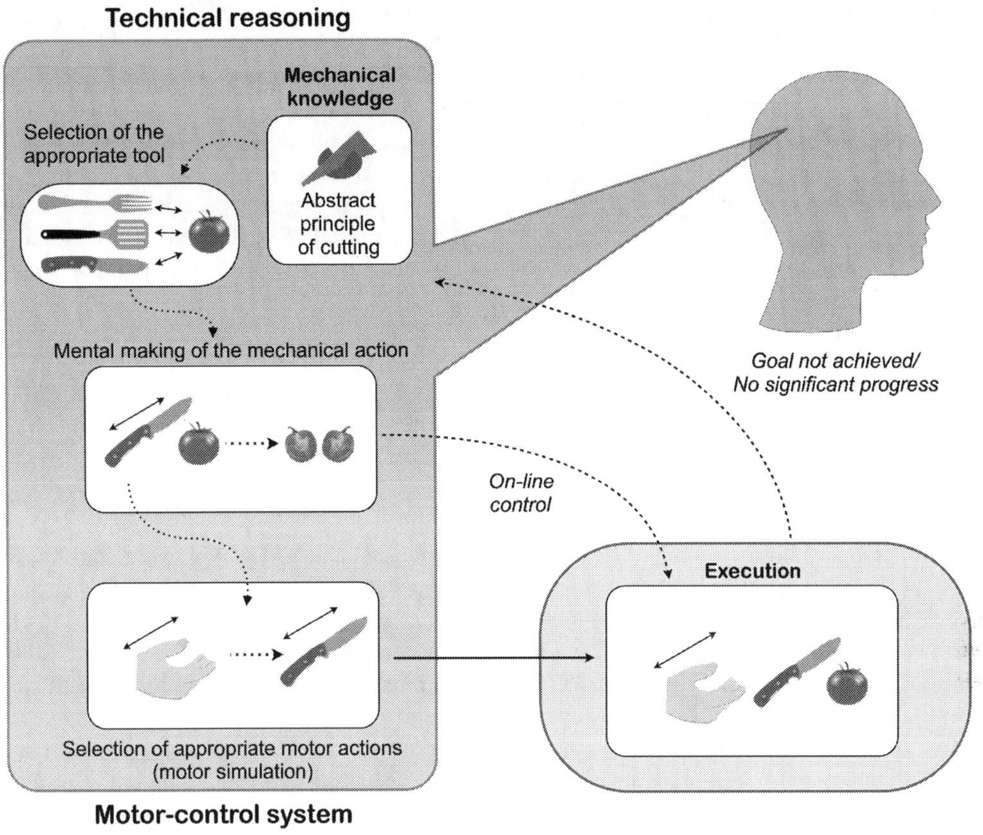

Figure 23.1 Technical reasoning and its interaction with the motor control system

This illustration is based on an instance of familiar tool use (i.e., a knife). However, technical reasoning is not specific to familiar tool use because it also concerns any situations in which it is necessary to solve a physical problem, such as when making tools or during construction behavior, or in any instances requiring the understanding of the mechanics of the physical world (e.g., novel tool use). The goal here is to cut a tomato. Three tools are present (spatula, fork, and knife). Technical reasoning consists in making correspondence between the abstract principle of cutting (mechanical knowledge) and the physical properties of the tools present in the environment. This reasoning allows the user to form a mental simulation of the appropriate mechanical action (i.e., mental making), which then biases the selection of appropriate motor actions (e.g., the knife is graspable and move-able with back-and-forth elbow movements) and motor simulation (i.e., simulation of movements to assess their energetic cost). The execution is then controlled online at a perceptual level with reference to the expected mechanical action. Finally, if the goal is not achieved or if the action appears to be ineffective, the process returns to technical reasoning to adapt the mental simulation of the mechanical action to the present situation (e.g., change of the point of percussion or orientation of the blade) or to select another tool, for instance. Technical reasoning is preferentially impaired after damage to the left inferior parietal lobe (particularly the left area PF – e.g., in stroke patients), whereas the motor-control system is preferentially impaired after damage to more superior parietal structures (particularly the intraparietal sulcus; e.g., in patients with cortico-basal degeneration). See e-book for a full-color version of this figure.

mechanical knowledge containing information about physical object properties (e.g., levering, cutting, hammering). The reasoning ends with the generation of a mental simulation of the mechanical action to be performed – that is, mental making, such as the motion of a knife on a tomato. This mental simulation then biases the selection of the appropriate motor actions in order to realize the mechanical action (i.e., motor-control system). The selection of the appropriate motor actions primarily involves the intraparietal sulcus within the posterior parietal cortex, whereas technical reasoning skills are mainly supported by the area PF (i.e., parietal area F) within the left inferior parietal lobe (Reynaud et al., 2016; Reynaud et al., 2019) (see below).

Evidence for the technical reasoning hypothesis has come from the study of brain-damaged patients with apraxia of tool use. Interestingly, these patients can show difficulties not only in using familiar tools in a conventional way (i.e., familiar tool use), but also in using them in a non-conventional way (i.e., unfamiliar tool use) or in using, selecting, and even making novel tools to solve mechanical problems (e.g., creating a hook by folding a wire – novel tool use) (Goldenberg & Hagmann, 1998; Goldenberg & Spatt, 2009; Heilman et al., 1997; Osiurak et al., 2009; for reviews, see Baumard, Osiurak, Lesourd, & Le Gall, 2014; Osiurak et al., 2020). These difficulties have been found in patients with damage to the left inferior parietal lobe (e.g., Goldenberg & Hagmann, 1998; Goldenberg & Spatt, 2009). Neuroimaging meta-analyses have also confirmed that the left area PF is preferentially activated when participants have to focus on the mechanical actions involving a tool and an object (Reynaud et al., 2016), as well as when participants watch other individuals using tools (Reynaud et al., 2019). This last finding is particularly interesting because it implies that technical reasoning enables humans to not only use tools but also learn how to use them through social transmission, which is critical for the emergence of cumulative technological culture (Osiurak & Reynaud, 2020; see also Osiurak et al., 2021a).

As mentioned above, the technical reasoning hypothesis posits that technical reasoning is exclusively in charge of solving mechanical problems in our everyday life, thereby implying that semantic knowledge cannot be concerned by this aspect. This contributes to explain why patients with selective semantic memory deficits can actually use novel tools as well as familiar tools in a conventional or non-conventional way. Put differently, it is one thing to know that early humans were able to make stone tools, and it is quite another to be able to actually make stone tools. While the former needs semantic knowledge, the latter requires the mastery of stone fracture,[7] as demonstrated in experimental archaeology studies (e.g., Bril et al., 2010). Technical reasoning is useful to solve the "mechanical constraint," raising the question of what constraint is solved by semantic knowledge (for discussion, see Osiurak, 2014).[8] In the following lines, we will elaborate on this point from a neurosemiotics stance, leading us to suggest that semantic knowledge might be more pragmatic than previously thought.

When are semantic knowledge and technical reasoning involved?

Real tool use

The working hypothesis defended here is that semantic knowledge provides socio-contextual information about the common purpose associated with familiar tools (Osiurak, 2014, 2017, 2020). The rationale is based on a significant body of findings that have shown patients with selective semantic memory deficits/temporal lobe lesions (e.g., semantic dementia) can sometimes encounter specific difficulties in single tool use tasks (Baumard et al., 2016; Corbett et al., 2015; Hodges et al., 2000; Silveri & Ciccarelli, 2009; Sirigu et al., 1991; Osiurak et al., 2008). The important question is why these patients are impaired when asked to show how to use tools in isolation (i.e., single tool use) and not when they have the opportunity to actually use them with their corresponding objects (i.e., real tool use), irrespective of whether the use is familiar, unfamiliar or novel.

First, note the semantic memory deficit is selective in these patients, suggesting that technical reasoning is spared. Therefore, the presentation of the tool and the object can allow them to use their technical reasoning skills to infer the potential mechanical actions to be performed. This explains why these patients are relatively unimpaired when asked to use familiar tools, as well as novel tools, to solve mechanical problems.[9] Indeed, making a hook with a wire to extract a target stuck in a box (novel tool use) or using a knife to cut bread (familiar tool use) both imply understanding the underlying physical principles. In both tasks, there is no need for semantic knowledge because there is no need to recognize the tools and objects presented.[10] More interestingly, in some cases the familiar tool use task can even become a novel tool use task. This is the case when the semantic memory deficits are so pronounced that the patients have severe difficulties in recognizing the familiar tools and the associated objects presented. Nevertheless, again even a patient with massive semantic memory deficits can be able to actually use a great number of familiar tools appropriately because the problem remains the same: reasoning at a technical level to find out the appropriate mechanical action to solve the task. Finally, it is noteworthy that semantic knowledge can play an indirect role in the performance of these patients, notably when the artifact presented is opaque. For instance, it is hard to know that a padlock possesses a hidden mechanical system merely by looking at it. In this case, semantic knowledge can be useful to provide the information that it is something commonly used to lock. Thus, without the information, an individual could grasp the key presented and attempt to insert it into the padlock without turning the key. This corresponds to the kind of "errors" that patients with selective semantic memory deficits can make when the artifacts presented are opaque (Baumard et al., 2016; for discussion about the role of semantic knowledge in tool use in normal aging, see Lesourd et al., 2017b). Regardless, this pattern strongly diverges from the one reported in left brain-damaged patients with apraxia of tool use, who can select inappropriate tools and be unable to perform appropriate mechanical actions (Lesourd et al., 2016; Osiurak et al., 2013).

Single tool use

Things are different for single tool use. The technical reasoning hypothesis assumes that technical reasoning is also needed in this task. Even if the object is absent, the patient needs to generate a potential mechanical action involving this absent object in order to show how to use the tool presented in isolation. A strong prediction is that impaired performance in real tool use is necessarily associated with impaired performance in single tool use. No evidence so far has invalidated this prediction. Nevertheless, the patient has to solve an additional problem, namely to imagine the absent object. To do so, technical reasoning is of no interest. Instead, we hypothesize that semantic knowledge is necessary to solve this problem, as it allows the patient to know the specific purpose of the familiar tool, the object commonly associated with it, or the context in which the tool is commonly used. Indeed, if a neuropsychologist shows you a key, semantic knowledge will indicate that it is something commonly used to open a padlock or a door. Thus, you can deduce that the neuropsychologist expects from you to demonstrate how to use this key to open a padlock or a door. Then you will reason technically to generate the mechanical action required, leading you to select the appropriate motor actions to perform the demonstration expected.

The important predictions derived from our hypothesis are that single tool use should be more severely impaired in patients with selective semantic memory deficits than real tool use (Prediction 1), and that the greater the semantic memory deficit, the worse the performance in single tool use (Prediction 2). As mentioned above, a significant body of evidence indicates that the performance of patients with selective semantic memory deficits is relatively spared in real tool use, contrasting with poor performance in single tool use and supporting Prediction 1. Furthermore, a link can be found between the loss of semantic knowledge and the performance in single tool use tasks, validating Prediction 2. For instance, Hodges et al. (2000) investigated nine patients with semantic dementia. As expected, the patients performed worse than healthy matched controls in both semantic picture-matching and single tool use tasks. Importantly, they also found a strong correlation between both (Figure 23.2) (for a more comprehensive review on this aspect, see Osiurak et al., 2021b).[11]

Although interesting, these findings do not provide a qualitative description of the behavior of patients with selective semantic memory deficits in single tool use tasks. Two single case studies are informative in this regard. Sirigu et al. (1991) reported the case of a patient, F.B., with bitemporal lobe lesions caused by herpetic encephalitis. F.B. had great difficulties recognizing the familiar tools presented in isolation. However, he was able to demonstrate alternative uses, which were nevertheless

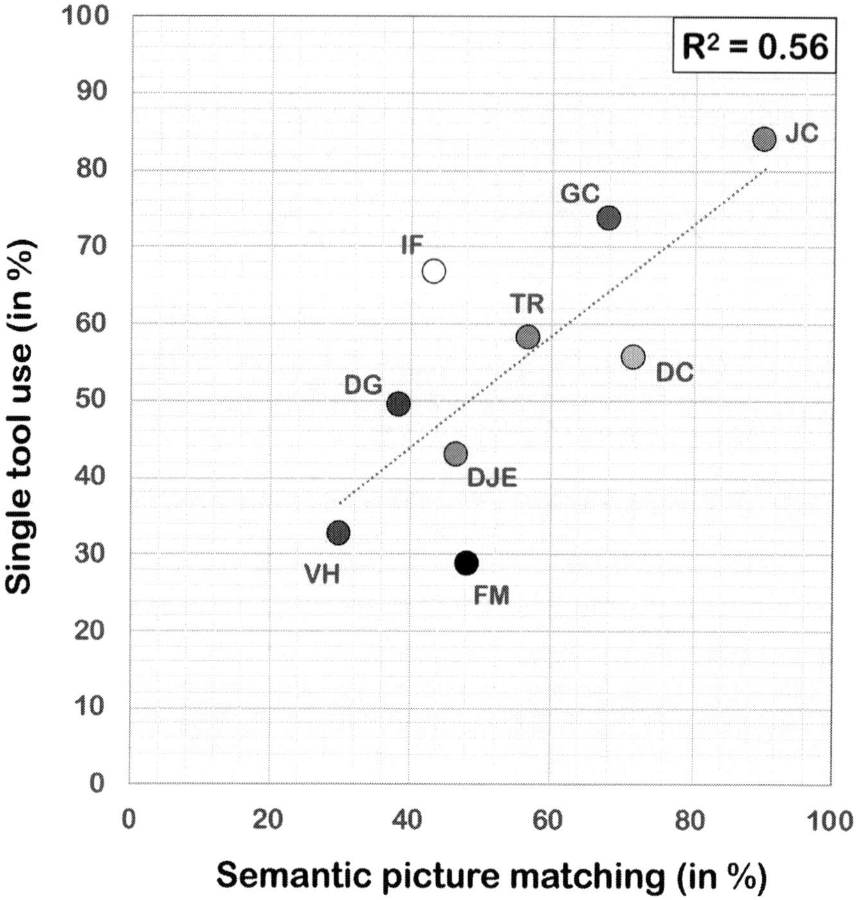

Figure 23.2 Relationship between semantic picture matching task and single tool use task

The score of semantic picture matching corresponds to the average on the three sub-tests employed by Hodges et al. (i.e., matching object to recipient, matching object to typical location, matching objects for shared purpose). We then converted this mean into percentages. The score of single tool use corresponds to the average on the three sub-scores used by Hodges et al. (i.e., hold, orientation, movement). We then converted this mean into percentages. As shown, a strong linear relationship is found between the two tasks. See e-book for a full-color version of this figure.

not associated with the specific purpose of the familiar tool. For example, when asked to recognize a nail clipper, he said: "It can attach several sheets of paper together. You turn the piece on the top and tip it back (makes the precise movement sequence). You press and it maintains them" (Sirigu et al., 1991: 2566). We also described a similar case, M.J.C., who had left temporal lobe lesions following a closed-head injury (Osiurak et al., 2008). Semantic knowledge was severely impaired. She could not name or recognize most of the familiar tools presented. Her performance in real tool use tasks was relatively intact when assessed with familiar and unfamiliar tool use tasks. By contrast, she had difficulties in demonstrating the use of familiar tools presented in isolation (i.e., single tool use). In a very similar way to F.B., she nevertheless proposed alternative uses, which were not those expected. She used a screwdriver as a gimlet, applying it perpendicularly to the desktop and performing clockwise and anticlockwise rotations with it. She added: "One can make a hole with it" (Osiurak et al., 2008: 178). She used the key to rub the edge of the wooden desk. The desktop had a hole to insert electrical wires. However, there was no electrical wire and a plastic cork closed it. M.J.C. used the bottle-opener as a lever to remove the plastic cork, again suggesting that this tool can be used to perform this action.

The two aforementioned case-studies help us to better understand the role of semantic knowledge in single tool use. First, both patients were able to demonstrate alternative uses that were viable at a mechanical level. This can be explained by the preservation of technical reasoning skills, which allowed them to generate mechanical actions involving the familiar tools and the physical environment of the clinical setting. This is corroborated at least by M.J.C., who had good performance in real tool use tasks. Second, the selective loss of semantic knowledge prevented them from determining what the specific purpose of the familiar tools presented was and, as a result, which was the absent object involved in the demonstration. Therefore, they exploited the different objects of the clinical setting to show alternative uses (e.g., sheets of paper, desktop, plastic cork). In a way, the single tool use task became a novel tool use task. Nevertheless, these alternative uses were not those expected, thereby stressing the ambiguity of the single tool use task that both patients did not resolve.

What is the role of semantic knowledge?

Semantic or pragmatic knowledge?

This leads us to raise the question: What is really measured in the single tool use task? The classical hypothesis suggests that it taps semantic knowledge in order to know how to use the familiar tool presented in isolation in the same way as in real tool use tasks. However, this view is decontextualized because it ignores that a single familiar tool can be involved in a multitude of mechanical actions. A newspaper, say, can be employed to light a fire or to clean a dirty floor. Nevertheless, if a neuropsychologist shows it to a patient, the demonstration expected is to open and pretend to read it, even if this patient never uses it in this manner. If a patient shows how to light a fire with it, the demonstration will be considered erroneous. Therefore, what the single tool use task really assesses is the patient's ability to show the common use of the familiar tool in a given society in order to satisfy the examiner's expectations. This leads to take into account a related aspect, which is also largely ignored to interpret the performance obtained in this task, namely the presence of the examiner. In real tool use tasks, this presence might have a lesser impact because the presentation of both the tool and the object guides the behavior toward a single possible solution. The real tool use task is clearly a close-ended problem. By contrast, the single tool use task can be viewed as an open-ended problem inasmuch as the patient has to decide which is the mechanical action expected among the potential ones. This decision needs to take into consideration the presence of examiners and their expectations, which are based on socially shared knowledge. In broad terms, solving this task needs to take the viewpoint of examiners and to infer what is the use they expect. Our hypothesis is that semantic knowledge is critical to resolve this aspect of single tool use, allowing the patients to access to socially shared knowledge about artifacts (Osiurak, 2014, 2020). In this way, semantic knowledge might be more pragmatic than previously thought.

Organizing the search within episodic memory

The observation of how patients with selective semantic memory deficits behave in single tool use is of great interest for understanding the role of semantic knowledge in tool use (Box 23.2). However, it is not viable at an evolutionary and anthropological level to consider that semantic knowledge is useful to demonstrate the use of single tools, namely a relatively artificial situation. The classical semantic knowledge hypothesis assumes that semantic knowledge supports the actual use of tools. Although, as discussed so far, evidence challenges this interpretation, the hypothesis provides an adaptive explanation of the role of semantic knowledge. The same theoretical effort thus needs to be made.

Box 23.2 Thematic versus taxonomic knowledge

Behavioral and neural evidence has supported the distinction between thematic and taxonomic knowledge (Schwartz et al., 2011; for a review, see Mirman et al., 2017; see also Rogers et al., 2004). Note that this distinction is not specific to tools. Thematic knowledge encompasses information about relations that are organized based on complementarity in events and brings together objects belonging to the same temporal and/or spatial context (e.g., dog-bone). By contrast, taxonomic knowledge refers relations that are organized based on similarity and objects that share features (e.g., visual features; dog-horse). The anterior portions of the temporal lobes and the temporo-parietal junction are particularly important for taxonomic knowledge and thematic knowledge, respectively (Mirman et al., 2017). Support for this neural dissociation has notably come from studies of semantic dementia, which is characterized by an atrophy of the anterior portions of the temporal lobes (Hodges et al., 1992). More specifically, these studies have found that taxonomic knowledge is impaired whereas thematic knowledge is relatively preserved in semantic dementia, corroborating the involvement of the anterior portions of the temporal lobes in the processing of taxonomic knowledge (Merck et al., 2019, 2020). Interestingly, these findings, taken together with the discussion initiated in this chapter, seem to indicate that the difficulties reported in patients with semantic dementia in single tool use tasks might be associated to a deficit in taxonomic knowledge but not in thematic knowledge. The important question is why that is so. We are not able to offer any insight into this potential relationship, thus explaining why we have not discussed this dissociation so far in this chapter. Nevertheless, we are convinced that this finding deserves further investigation.

We formulate the working hypothesis that semantic knowledge enables us to organize the search within episodic memory, allowing us to store and retrieve our tools and objects more easily (for more elaboration, see Osiurak, 2014, 2017, 2020). When someone meets a mechanical problem, all the tools and objects needed to perform the appropriate mechanical action – generated through technical reasoning – are not always directly available. So, the constraint we frequently face is to determine where they can be found (i.e., the space constraints; see Osiurak, 2014). Thus, storing semantic categories associated with our everyday life activities, such as eating or washing, is particularly useful to mentally travel in our episodic memory in the search of the potential appropriate tools and objects (for a similar interpretation, see Tulving, 1972). In some cases, even if we cannot remember precisely where the tool is (e.g., hammer), this semantic organization can help us to infer where we have a chance to find this tool (e.g., in the workshop or even at the supermarket). This semantic organization is also reinforced – or might emerge – from the mere fact that we are all concerned more or less by the same activities because of our belonging to the same species. Thus, most people possess at home a space dedicated to eating or washing activities, and this organization around these activities is visible at the societal level (e.g., the different kinds of shops associated with species activities: grocer's shop, butcher's shop, hairdressing salon). This is also visible in the different sections of a supermarket, which we can understand even when the supermarket is new. The outstanding question is whether these different semantic categories are learned through repeated experiences or based on natural predispositions. Be that as it may, the development of these semantic categories during our lifetime allows us not only to organize the search in our own episodic memory to retrieve tools and objects, but also to share knowledge with our conspecifics about what they may know about a specific familiar tool or object (as required in the single tool use task).

Conclusion

We hypothesized that semantic knowledge provides socio-contextual information that can be useful in some social interactions, including clinical settings. This rationale is based on the performance of patients with selective semantic memory deficits in single tool use. Such a task might require the patient to adopt the examiner's viewpoint to determine the use expected. In this respect, we drew a direct link between single tool use and socio-cognitive skills, which is perfectly consistent with the research developed in the field of neurosemiotics. Indeed, Ibáñez and Manes (2012) developed a social context network model to explain how humans take into account contextual cues to interpret information extracted from social interactions. This network comprises three main components, each associated with a specific brain region: contextual update and predictions (prefrontal areas); internal-external coordination (insular cortex); and value-based context-target associations (temporal regions). Although the role played by the temporal lobes discussed in this chapter does not fit exactly the function of the temporal regions proposed by this model, there is an agreement about the idea that temporal regions could participate in the socio-contextual interpretation of information extracted from social interactions. Interestingly, this model has been developed from the study of patients with the behavioral variant of frontotemporal dementia, whereas most of the cases of patients with selective semantic memory deficits discussed in this chapter had semantic dementia, another variant of frontotemporal dementia. This corroborates the view that a kind of semantic-executive fronto-insular-temporal network may be responsible for processing socio-contextual effects. If the link we draw here between single tool use and socio-cognitive skills is true, we could expect that patients with insular or frontal lobe lesions (as in the behavioral variant of the frontotemporal dementia) could also show difficulties in this kind of tasks, not because of their semantic impairment but because of their difficulties to take into account the examiner's viewpoint (i.e., the social context of the situation). Future research is needed to explore this interesting aspect of tool use.

As outlined in the introduction, the role of context-dependence effects is only one of the many facets of the neurosemiotic approach, which stresses the relevance of studying the relationships between semantic, pragmatics, motor systems, and language processes in order to improve our understanding of the links between culture, context, body, brain, and semantics. Admittedly, this chapter is far from revealing all the possibilities that the neurosemiotic approach offers to study human tool use. Nevertheless, we hope it contributes to illustrate how the neurosemiotic approach can be helpful to revise classical cognitive models.

Acknowledgments

This work was performed within the framework of the LABEX CORTEX (ANR-11-LABX-0042) of Université de Lyon, within the program "Investissements d'Avenir" (ANR-11- IDEX-0007) operated by the French National Research Agency (ANR).

Notes

1 Apraxia can be assessed by asking patients to show how to use a tool without holding the tool (pantomime of use), while holding the tool (single tool use) or by actually using it with the corresponding object (real tool use; see Box 23.1). Here we will focus on real tool use tasks, which are the closest to the patient's everyday experience. We will also discuss the interest of single tool use tasks in understanding the role of semantic knowledge in tool use. For the sake of clarity, we will not present the findings obtained with pantomime of use (for discussion, see Finkel et al., 2018; Goldenberg, 2013; Lesourd et al., 2017a).

2 We will employ the terms "apraxia of tool use" and "tool use disorders" interchangeably to describe the difficulties encountered by brain-damaged patients in real tool use tasks (i.e., when the patient is asked to *actually* perform a mechanical action involving a tool and an object).

3 The conceptual system developed by Roy and Square (1985) diverges from this perspective in assuming that semantic knowledge also contains information about the mechanical actions that can be performed when using tools. For them, this kind of knowledge is an integral part of the conceptual system and does not involve a non-semantic route.

4 A significant body of evidence has shown that novel and unfamiliar tool use is also relatively intact in patients with selective semantic memory deficits/temporal lobe lesions (e.g., Baumard et al., 2016; Bozeat et al., 2002; Goldenberg & Spatt, 2009; Hodges et al., 2000; Lesourd et al., 2016; Osiurak et al., 2008).

5 For instance, as discussed in more detail below, the single tool use task requires technical reasoning in order to generate appropriate mechanical actions and semantic knowledge to determine the specific purpose associated with the tool presented in isolation. As a result, a deficit in technical reasoning or in semantic knowledge can lead to impaired performance in this task, although the cognitive origins of the impairment differ.

6 As explained below, technical reasoning skills are critical to solve mechanical problems. These skills are involved not only in the use of physical tools but also in tool making (e.g., making a knife) or construction behavior (e.g., building a bridge) (Osiurak & Heinke, 2018).

7 The notion of know-how is sometimes employed to refer to this physical understanding (e.g., Pinker, 2010). This notion is very close to that of technical reasoning.

8 Neurophysiological findings have indicated the existence of three main pathways originating from the visual cortex to the superior parietal cortex/intraparietal sulcus (dorso-dorsal pathway), the inferior parietal cortex (ventro-dorsal pathway), and the temporal cortex (ventral pathway, e.g., see Rizzolatti & Matelli, 2003). This three-pathway framework has been developed from the initial distinction between the dorsal "where"/ "how?" pathway (vision for action) and the ventral "what" pathway (vision for action; Goodale & Milner, 1992; Ungerleider & Mishkin, 1982), which has been particularly useful to investigate the evolutionary link between action and language (Arbib, 2006, 2010, 2017). The technical reasoning hypothesis is also based on the three-pathway network (Osiurak et al., 2017): the motor-control system (dorso-dorsal pathway), technical reasoning (ventro-dorsal pathway), and semantic knowledge (ventral pathway). Thus, whereas the motor-control system and technical reasoning are viewed as oriented toward the action domain (motor actions for the motor-control system, and mechanical actions for technical reasoning), semantic knowledge is viewed as oriented toward the perception domain (i.e., recognition).

9 Lesourd et al. (2016) asked patients with semantic dementia (i.e., with a selective loss of semantic memory) to use novel tools to solve mechanical problems. Eight novel tools were presented for each mechanical problem. They observed that the patients could generally select and use the most appropriate tool to extract the target out from the box. Interestingly, they also reported the use of many non-necessary but relevant tools, consisting of using a shorter stick, for instance, when the target was close to the exit instead of extracting the target with the relevant longer stick needed to perform the correct mechanical action (e.g., a levering action). The proportion of use of non-necessary relevant tools was similar as the one found in healthy matched controls. More globally, patients with semantic dementia followed a strategy that was also very close to the one reported in healthy matched controls (e.g., exploration time, number of tools selected). These findings confirm the preservation of technical reasoning skills and the appetence for using them in patients with selective semantic memory deficits.

10 We are not saying here that healthy individuals do not recognize relatively spontaneously the tools and objects presented in familiar tool use tasks. Instead, we mean that this is of no need to use them appropriately.

11 More generally, patients with selective semantic memory deficits are expected to be impaired to demonstrate the use of a tool without actually using it with an object (i.e., in no real-tool use tasks). For the sake of clarity, we have restricted our discussion to single tool use tasks. However, patients with selective semantic memory deficits should also meet difficulties in pantomime of use tasks, in which it is required to demonstrate the use of a tool presented in isolation (as in single tool use tasks) without holding it (contrary to single tool use tasks). This prediction was recently confirmed, for instance, by Johnen et al. (2018), who found poor performance in patients with semantic memory deficits (semantic dementia or non-fluent primary progressive aphasia) in a pantomime of use task. They also reported a close link between the pantomime of use performance and the severity of the semantic deficit. In other words, it is likely that the involvement of semantic knowledge in single tool use could be extended more broadly to pantomime of use.

References

Adolfi, F., Couto, B., Richter, F., Decety, J., Lopez, J., Sigman, M., Manes, F., & Ibáñez, A. (2017). Convergence of interoception, emotion, and social cognition: A twofold fMRI meta-analysis and lesion approach. *Cortex, 88*, 124–142. doi: 10.1016/j.cortex.2016.12.019

Arbib, M. A. (2006). The mirror system hypothesis on the linkage of action and languages. In A. M. Arbib (Ed.), *From Action to Language Via the Mirror Neuron System*, (pp. 1–47). Cambridge: Cambridge University Press.

Arbib, M. A. (2010). Mirror system activity for action and language is embedded in the integration of dorsal and ventral pathways. *Brain & Language, 112*, 12–24. doi: 10.1016/j.bandl.2009.10.001

Arbib, M. A. (2017). Toward the language-ready brain: Biological evolution and primate comparisons. *Psychonomic Bulletin & Review, 24*, 142–150. doi: 10.3758/s13423-016-1098-2

Bartolo, A., Daumüller, M., Della Sala, S., & Goldenberg, G. (2007). Relationship between object-related gestures and the fractionated object knowledge system. *Behavioural Neurology, 18*, 143–147. doi: 10.1155/2007/241670

Baumard, J., Lesourd, M., Jarry, C., Merck, C., Etcharry-Bouyx, F., Chauviré, V., Belliard, S., Moreaud, O., Croisile, B., Osiurak, F., & Le Gall, D. (2016). Tool use disorders in neurodegenerative diseases. Roles of semantic memory and technical reasoning. *Cortex, 82*, 119–132. doi: 10.1016/j.cortex.2016.06.007

Baumard, J., Lesourd, M., Remigereau, C., Merck, C., Jarry, C., Etcharry-Bouyx, F., Chauviré, V., Belliard, S., Moreaud, O., Osiurak, F., & Le Gall, D. (2019). The – weak – role of memory in tool use: Evidence from neurodegenerative diseases. *Neuropsychologia, 129*, 117–132. doi: 10.1016/j.neuropsychologia.2019.03.008

Baumard, J., Osiurak, F., Lesourd, M., & Le Gall, D. (2014). Tool use disorders after left brain damage. *Frontiers in Psychology, 5*, 473. doi: 10.3389/fpsyg.2014.00473

Bozeat, S., Lambon Ralph, M. A., Patterson, K., & Hodges, J. R. (2002). When objects lose their meaning: What happens to their use? *Cognitive, Affective, and Behavioral Neurosciences, 2*, 236–251. doi: 10.3758/CABN.2.3.236

Bril, B., Rein, R., Nonaka, T., Wenban-Smith, F., & Dietrich, G. (2010). The role of expertise in tool use: Skill differences in functional action adaptations to task constraints. *Journal of Experimental Psychology: Human Perception and Performance, 36*, 825–839. doi: 10.1037/a0018171

Buxbaum, L. J. (2001). Ideomotor Apraxia: A call to action. *Neurocase*, 7, 445–448. doi: 10.1093/neucas/7.6.445

Buxbaum, L. J., Schwartz, M. F., & Carew, T. G. (1997). The role of memory in object use. *Cognitive Neuropsychology, 14*, 219–254. doi: 10.1080/026432997381565

Chen, L., Lambon Ralph, M. A., & Rogers, T. T. (2017). A unified model of human semantic knowledge and its disorders. *Nature Human Behavior, 1*, 39. doi: 10.1038/s41562-016-0039

Corbett, F., Jefferies, E., Burns, A., & Lambon Ralph, M. A. (2015). Deregulated semantic cognition contributes to object-use deficits in Alzheimer's disease: A comparison with semantic aphasia and semantic dementia. *Journal of Neuropsychology, 9*, 219–241. doi: 10.1111/jnp.12047

Cubelli, R., Marchetti, C., Boscolo, G., & Della Sala, S. (2000). Cognition in action: Testing a model of limb apraxia. *Brain and Cognition, 44*, 144–165. doi: 10.1006/brcg.2000.1226

De Renzi, E., & Lucchelli, F. (1988). Ideational apraxia. *Brain, 111*, 1173–1185. doi: 10.1093/brain/111.5.1173

Finkel, L., Hogrefe, K., Frey, S. H., Goldenberg, G., & Randerath, J. (2018). It takes two to pantomime: Communication meets motor cognition. *NeuroImage: Clinical, 19*, 1008–1017. doi: 10.1016/j.nicl.2018.06.019

Forde, E. M. E., & Humphreys, G. W. (2000). The role of semantic knowledge and working memory in everyday tasks. *Brain and Cognition, 44*, 214–252. doi: 10.1006/brcg.2000.1229

Fukutake, T. (2003). Apraxia of tool use: An autopsy case of biparietal infarction. *European Neurology, 49*, 45–52. doi: 10.1159/000067027

García, A. M., & Ibáñez, A. (2014a). Words in motion: Motor-language coupling in Parkinson's disease. *Translational Neuroscience, 5*, 152–159. doi: 10.2478/s13380-014-0218-6

García, A. M., & Ibáñez, A. (2014b). Two-person neuroscience and naturalistic social communication: The role of language and linguistic variables in brain-coupling research. *Frontiers in Psychiatry, 5*, 124. doi: 10.3389/fpsyt.2014.00124

García, A. M., & Ibáñez, A. (2016). Hand typing what hands do: Action-semantic integration dynamics throughout written verb production. *Cognition, 149*, 56–66. doi: 10.1016/j.cognition.2016.01.011

García, A. M., & Ibáñez, A. (2017). A touch with words: Dynamic synergies between manual actions and language. *Neuroscience & BioBehavioral Reviews, 68*, 59–95. doi: 10.1016/j.neubiorev.2016.04.022

Geschwind, N. (1975). The apraxias: Neural mechanisms of disorders of learned movement. *American Scientist, 63*, 188–195. doi: 10.1016/0093-934X(80)90151-0

Goldenberg, G. (2013). *Apraxia: The Cognitive Side of Motor Control.* Oxford: Oxford University Press.

Goldenberg, G., & Hagmann, S. (1998). Tool use and mechanical problem solving in apraxia. *Neuropsychologia, 36*, 581–589. doi: 10.1016/s0028-3932(97)00165-6

Goldenberg, G., & Spatt, J. (2009). The neural basis of tool use. *Brain, 132*, 1645–1655. doi: 10.1093/brain/awp080

Goodale, M. A., & Milner, D. (1992). Separate visual pathways for perception and action. *Trends in Neurosciences, 15*, 20–25. doi: 10.1016/0166-2236(92)90344-8

Heath, M., Almeida, Q. J., Roy, E. A., Black, S. E., & Westwood, D. (2003). Selective dysfunction of tool-use: A failure to integrate somatosensation and action. *Neurocase, 9*, 156–163. doi: 10.1076/neur.9.2.156.15072

Heilman, K. M., Maher, L. M., Greenwald, M. L., & Rothi, L. J. G. (1997). Conceptual apraxia from lateralized lesions. *Neurology, 49*, 457–464. doi: 10.1212/wnl.49.2.457

Heilman, K. M., Rothi, L. J., & Valenstein, E. (1982). Two forms of ideomotor apraxia. *Neurology, 32*, 342–346. doi: 10.1212/WNL.32.4.342

Hodges, J. R., Bozeat, S., Lambon Ralph, M. A., Patterson, K., & Spatt, J. (2000). The role of knowledge in object use: Evidence from semantic dementia. *Brain, 123*, 1913–1925. doi: 10.1093/brain/123.9.1913

Hodges, J. R., Patterson, K., Oxbury, S., & Funnell, E. (1992). Semantic dementia: Progressive fluent aphasia with temporal lobe atrophy. *Brain, 115*, 1783–1806. doi: 10.1093/brain/115.6.1783

Humphreys, G. W. (2001). Objects, affordances… action! *The Psychologist, 14*, 408–413.

Ibáñez, A., Cardona, J. F., Dos Santos, Y. V., Blenkmann, A., Aravena, P., Roca, M., Hurtado, E., Nerguizian, M., Amoruso, L., Gomez-Arevalo, G., Chade, A., Dubrovsky, A., Gershanik, O., Kochen, S., Glenberg, A., Manes, F., & Bekinschtein, T. (2013). Motor-language coupling: Direct evidence from early Parkinson's disease and intracranial cortical recordings. *Cortex, 49*, 968–984. doi: 10.1016/j.cortex.2012.02.014

Ibáñez, A., & Manes, F. (2012). Contextual social cognition and the behavioral variant of frontotemporal dementia. *Neurology, 78*, 1354–1362. doi: 10.1212/WNL.0b013e3182518375

Johnen, A., Reul, S., Wiendl, H., Meuth, S. G., & Duning, T. (2018). Apraxia profiles: A single cognitive marker to discriminate all variants of frontotemporal lobar degeneration and Alzheimer's disease. *Alzheimer's & Dementia: Diagnosis, Assessment & Disease Monitoring, 10*, 363–371. doi: 10.1016/j.dadm.2018.04.002

Lambon Ralph, M. A., Jefferies, E., Patterson, K., & Rogers, T. T. (2017). The neural and computational bases of semantic cognition. *Nature Reviews Neuroscience, 18*, 42–55. doi: 10.1038/nrn.2016.150

Lauro-Grotto, R., Piccini, C., & Shallice, T. (1997). Modality-specific operations in semantic dementia. *Cortex, 33*, 593–622. doi: 10.1016/s0010-9452(08)70720-2

Legare, C. H., & Nielsen, M. (2015). Imitation and innovation: The dual engines of cultural learning. *Trends in Cognitive Sciences, 19*, 688–699. doi: 10.1016/j.tics.2015.08.005

Lesourd, M., Baumard, J., Jarry, C., Etcharry-Bouyx, F., Belliard, S., Moreaud, O., Croisile, B., Chauviré, V., Granjon, M., Le Gall, D., & Osiurak, F. (2016). Mechanical problem-solving in Alzheimer's disease and semantic dementia. *Neuropsychology, 30*, 612–623. doi: 10.1037/neu0000241

Lesourd, M., Baumard, J., Jarry, C., Etcharry-Bouyx, F., Belliard, S., Moreaud, O., Croisile, B., Chauviré, V., Granjon, M., Le Gall, D., & Osiurak, F. (2017a). Rethinking the cognitive mechanisms underlying pantomime of tool use: Evidence from Alzheimer's disease and semantic dementia. *Journal of the International Neuropsychological Society, 23*, 128–138. doi: 10.1017/S1355617716000618

Lesourd, M., Baumard, J., Jarry, C., Le Gall, D., & Osiurak, F. (2017b). A cognitive-based model of tool use in normal aging. *Aging, Neuropsychology, & Cognition, 24*, 363–386.

Liepmann, H. (1920). Apraxie. *Ergebnisse der gesamten Medizin, 1*, 516–540. doi: 10.1080/13825585.2016.1218822

Merck, C., Noël, A., Jamet, E., Robert, M., Hou, C., Salmon, A., Belliard, S., & Kalénine, S. (2019). Identification of taxonomic and thematic relationships: Do the two semantic systems have the same status in semantic dementia. *Journal of Clinical and Experimental Neuropsychology, 41*, 946–964. doi: 10.1080/13803395.2019.1641186

Merck, C., Noël, A., Jamet, E., Robert, M., Salmon, A., Belliard, S., & Kalénine, S. (2020). Overreliance on thematic knowledge in semantic dementia: Evidence from an eye-tracking paradigm. *Neuropsychology, 34*, 331–349. doi: 10.1037/neu0000616

Mirman, D., Landrigan, J. F., & Britt, A. E. (2017). Taxonomic and thematic semantic systems. *Psychological Bulletin, 143*, 499–520. doi: 10.1037/bul0000092

Moreaud, O., Charnallet, A., & Pellat, J. (1998). Identification without manipulation: A study of the relations between object use and semantic memory. *Neuropsychologia, 36*, 1295–1301. doi: 10.1016/s0028-3932(98)00034-7

Motomura, N., & Yamadori, A. (1994). A case of ideational apraxia with impairment of object use and preservation of object pantomime. *Cortex, 30*, 167–170. doi: 10.1016/s0010-9452(13)80332-2

Negri, G. A., Lunardelli, A., Reverberi, C., Gigli, G. L., & Rumiati, R. I. (2007). Degraded semantic knowledge and accurate object use. *Cortex, 43*, 376–388. doi: 10.1016/s0010-9452(08)70463-5

Ochipa, C., Rothi, L. J. G., & Heilman, K. M. (1992). Conceptual apraxia in Alzheimer's disease. *Brain, 115*, 1061–1072. doi: 10.1093/brain/115.4.1061

Osiurak, F. (2014). What neuropsychology tells us about human tool use? The four constraints theory (4CT): Mechanics, space, time, and effort. *Neuropsychology Review, 24*, 88–115. doi: 10.1007/s11065-014-9260-y

Osiurak, F. (2017). Cognitive paleoanthropology and technology: Toward a parsimonious theory (PATH). *Review of General Psychology, 21*, 292–307. doi: 10.1037/gpr0000129

Osiurak, F. (2020). *The Tool Instinct*. Hoboken, NJ: Wiley.

Osiurak, F., Aubin, G., Allain, P., Jarry, C., Richard, I., & Le Gall, D. (2008). Object utilization versus object usage: A single-case study. *Neurocase, 14*, 169–183. doi: 10.1080/13554790802108372

Osiurak, F., & Badets, A. (2016). Tool use and affordance: Manipulation-based versus reasoning-based approaches. *Psychological Review*, *123*, 534–568. doi: 10.1037/rev0000027

Osiurak, F., Claidière, N., Bluet, A., Brogniart, J., Lasserre, S., Bonhoure, T., Di Rollo, L., Gorry, N., Polette, Y., Saude, A., Federico, G., Uomini, N., & Reynaud, E. (in press). Technical reasoning bolsters cumulative technological culture through convergent transformations. *Science Advances*.

Osiurak, F., & Heinke, D. (2018). Looking for Intoolligence: A unified framework for the cognitive study of human tool use and technology. *American Psychologist*, *73*, 169–185. doi: 10.1037/amp0000162

Osiurak, F., Jarry, C., Allain, P., Aubin, G., Etcharry-Bouyx, F., Richard, I., Bernard, I., & Le Gall, D. (2009). Unusual use of objects after unilateral brain damage: The technical reasoning model. *Cortex*, *45*, 769–783. doi: 10.1016/j.cortex.2008.06.013

Osiurak, F., Jarry, C., & Le Gall, D. (2010). Grasping the affordances, understanding the reasoning: Toward a dialectical theory of human tool use. *Psychological Review*, *117*, 517–540. doi: 10.1037/a0019004

Osiurak, F., Jarry, C., Lesourd, M., Baumard, J., & Le Gall, D. (2013). Mechanical problem-solving in left brain-damaged patients and apraxia of tool use. *Neuropsychologia*, *51*, 1964–1972. doi: 10.1016/j.neuropsychologia.2013.06.017

Osiurak, F., Lasserre, S., Arbanti, J., Brogniart, J., Bluet, A., Navarro, J., & Reynaud, E. (2021a). Technical reasoning is important for cumulative technological culture. *Nature Human Behaviour, 5*, 1643–1651. doi: 10.1038/s41562-021-01159-9

Osiurak, F., Lesourd, M., Navarro, J., & Reynaud, E. (2020). Technition: When tools come out of the closet. *Perspectives on Psychological Science*, *15*, 880–897. doi: 10.1177/1745691620902145

Osiurak, F., & Reynaud, E. (2020). The elephant in the China shop: When technical reasoning meets cumulative technological culture. *Behavioral and Brain Sciences*, *43*, e156. doi: 10.1017/S0140525X20000291

Osiurak, F., Reynaud, E., Baumard, J., Rossetti, Y., Bartolo, A., & Lesourd, M. (2021b). Pantomime of tool use: Looking beyond apraxia. *Brain Communications, 3*, facb263. doi: 10.1093/braincomms/fcab263

Osiurak, F., Rossetti, Y., & Badets, A. (2017). What is an affordance? 40 years later. *Neuroscience & BioBehavioral Reviews*, 77, 403–417. doi: 10.1016/j.neubiorev.2017.04.014

Pinker, S. (2010). The cognitive niche: Coevolution of intelligence, sociality, and language. *Proceedings of the National Academy of Science of the United States of America*, *107*, 8993–8999. doi: 10.1073/pnas.0914630107

Reynaud, E., Lesourd, M., Navarro, J., & Osiurak, F. (2016). On the neurocognitive origins of human tool use: A critical review of neuroimaging data. *Neuroscience & BioBehavioral Reviews*, *64*, 421–437. doi: 10.1016/j.neubiorev.2016.03.009

Reynaud, E., Navarro, J., Lesourd, M., & Osiurak, F. (2019). To watch is to work: A critical review of neuroimaging data on Tool use Observation Network (ToON). *Neuropsychology Review*, *29*, 484–497. doi: 10.1007/s11065-019-09418-3

Riddoch, M. J., Edwards, M. G., Humphreys, G. W., West, R., & Heafield, T. (1998). Visual affordances direct action: Neuropsychological evidence from manual interference. *Cognitive Neuropsychology*, *15*, 645–683. doi: 10.1080/026432998381041

Rizzolatti, G., & Matelli, M. (2003). Two different streams form the dorsal visual system: Anatomy and functions. *Experimental Brain Research*, *153*, 146–157. doi: 10.1007/s00221-003-1588-0

Rogers, T. T., Lambon Ralph, M. A., Garrard, P., Bozeat, S., McClelland, J. L., Hodges, J. R., & Patterson, K. (2004). Structure and deterioration of semantic memory: A neuropsychological and computational investigation. *Psychological Review*, *111*, 205–235. doi: 10.1037/0033-295X.111.1.205

Rothi, L. J. G., Ochipa, C., & Heilman, K. M. (1991). A cognitive neuropsychological model of limb praxis. *Cognitive Neuropsychology*, *8*, 443–458. doi: 10.1080/02643299108253382

Roy, E. A., & Square, P. A. (1985). Common considerations in the study of limb, verbal and oral apraxia. In E. A. Roy (Ed.), *Neuropsychological Studies of Apraxia and Related Disorders* (pp. 111–161). Amsterdam: Elsevier.

Rumiati, R. I., & Humphreys, G. W. (1998). Recognition by action: Dissociating visual and semantic routes to action in normal observers. *Journal of Experimental Psychology: Human Perception and Performance*, *24*, 631–647. doi: 10.1037//0096-1523.24.2.631

Schwartz, M., Kimberg, D. Y., Walker, G. M., Brecher, A., Faseyitan, O. K., Dell, G. S., Mirman, D., & Coslett, H. B. (2011). Neuroanatomical dissociation for taxonomic and thematic knowledge in the human brain. *Proceedings of the National Academy of Science of the United States of America*, *108*, 8520–8524. doi: 10.1073/pnas.1014935108

Shumaker, R. W., Walkup, K. R., & Beck, B. B. (2011). *Animal Tool Behavior.* Baltimore, MD: John Hopkins University Press.

Silveri, M. C., & Ciccarelli, N. (2009). Semantic memory in object use. *Neuropsychologia*, *47*, 2634–2641. doi: 10.1016/j.neuropsychologia.2009.05.013

Sirigu, A., Duhamel, J. R., & Poncet, M. (1991). The role of sensorimotor experience in object recognition. *Brain*, *114*, 2555–2573. doi: 10.1093/brain/114.6.2555

Tulving, E. (1972). Episodic and semantic memory. In E. Tulving & W. Donaldson (Eds.), *Organization of Memory* (pp. 381–403). New York: Academic Press.

Ungerleider, L. G., & Mishkin, M. (1982). Two cortical visual systems. In M. A. Goodale & R. J. W. Mansfield (Eds.), *Analysis of visual behavior* (pp. 549–586). Cambridge, MA: MIT Press.

Vaesen, K. (2012). The cognitive bases of human tool use. *Behavioral and Brain Sciences*, *35*, 203–218. doi: 10.1017/S0140525X11001452

van Elk, M., van Schie, H., & Bekkering, H. (2014). Action semantics: A unifying conceptual framework for the selective use of multimodal and modality-specific object knowledge. *Physics of Life Reviews*, *11*, 220–250. doi: 10.1016/j.plrev.2013.11.005

Warrington, E. K. (1975). The selective impairment of semantic memory. *Quarterly Journal of Experimental Psychology*, *27*, 635–657. doi: 10.1080/14640747508400525

Zangwill, O. L. (1960). Le problème de l'apraxie idéatoire. *Revue Neurologique*, *102*, 595–603. doi: 10.1016/S0010-9452(69)80036-5

24

INTERPRETING THE SIGNALS WITHIN

Meaning and prediction during interoception

Ryan Smith and Sahib S. Khalsa

Introduction

It is a common experience in everyday life to notice changes in hunger, thirst, heart rate, breathing, temperature, and other sensations in one's body. These sensations come about because the brain exchanges signals with the rest of the body, and it must use these signals to figure out what is happening in the body and why – which also informs decisions about what to do. For example, if temperature signals indicate that the body is too warm, and the brain can further infer that this is due to sun exposure, the decision can be made to move into the shade. Sometimes we can also infer these states in others, such as noticing that other people are perspiring and inferring that they must be feeling hot. Perceiving and interpreting events inside the body, such as in the examples above, is called interoception. This topic has garnered growing research attention in recent years, but it has not yet received thorough consideration from the perspective of neurosemiotics. In this chapter, we explore potential ways in which each of these fields might build on and inform the other.

The term "interoception" broadly refers to the process through which the nervous system senses, interprets, and integrates afferent signals carrying information about internal bodily states (Khalsa, Adolphs et al., 2018). This includes, but is not limited to, information about the state of the cardiovascular, respiratory, and gastrointestinal systems, as well as blood composition attributes such as levels of acidity, glucose, osmolality, inflammatory cytokines, and various hormones (also referred to as "neurohumoral"). When viewed from the perspective of neurosemiotics – and specifically its focus on how information is represented and signaled – these phenomena motivate major questions. How is interoceptive information signaled? How are these signals integrated and used by the nervous system? How does the brain (and the individual) interpret and derive meaning from these signals? How is the state of the body internally represented and at what levels of description? In what ways might internal bodily states be signaled to other individuals? How might these signaling and representation processes be compromised and contribute to disturbances of physical and mental health?

At present, many aspects of interoceptive processing remain poorly understood. However, in combination with classic work within peripheral neurophysiology, recent advances have begun to speak to them. In this chapter, we offer a selective review of work touching on these questions – with

DOI: 10.4324/9781003051817-29

the aim of equipping the reader with the necessary tools to further pursue the role of representation, meaning, and prediction from a neurosemiotic perspective in relation to interoception. Symmetrically, our discussion will also highlight how – by describing a previously under-considered class of signals and representations – interoception may in turn point toward new directions for work in neurosemiotics.

Afferent signaling, integration, and perceptual representation

The nervous system, composed of central (the brain and the spinal cord) and peripheral (autonomic and somatic) branches, has access to interoceptive signals arising from numerous sources (Benarroch, 1993; Berntson & Khalsa, 2021). From a temporal standpoint, a major division occurs between chemical and peripheral neuronal signaling sources. Chemical signaling, which unfolds along a slower timescale than neuronal signaling, involves direct points of contact between neural tissue and the internal milieu (defined as the non-neural components of the body) at specific sites – called circumventricular organs (CVOs) – that lack a typical blood-brain-barrier. There are about three such locations within the brainstem (e.g., area postrema) and subcortical levels of the brain (e.g., the subfornical organ, underneath the fornix, and the organum vasculosum of the lamina terminalis, near the hypothalamus) (Benarroch, 2011). At these sites, neurons of the CVO are selectively sensitive to changing blood levels of a range of substances, including circulating chemical indicators of cardiovascular and metabolic status, serum osmolarity, and levels of sodium and calcium (among others) – and drive regulatory reflexes and behaviors (e.g., vomiting, water and food intake, and metabolic and immune responses). In contrast to the slow timescale of chemical signaling, neural signals from the periphery are rapidly carried from several organ systems (e.g., cardiovascular, respiratory, gastrointestinal, urinary) via afferent axonal channels through nerves such as the vagus nerve as well as other autonomic (e.g., sympathetic and parasympathetic), spinal cord, and cranial nerve pathways. Neuronal signals from peripheral organ systems traverse several synaptic connections prior to reaching the central nervous system, typically within dedicated pathways (e.g., thinly myelinated slow-conducting vs. thickly myelinated fast-conducting nerve fibers) communicating specific sensory information. The first levels of central neural representation[1] occur within brainstem nuclei, with the nucleus of the solitary tract being a primary waypoint. This nucleus is spatially arranged to implement an organotopic mapping, with different sub-regions devoted to tracking changes in the state of different organs (i.e., housing distinct neurons with firing rates selectively covarying with the state of those organs). Cross-talk between these sub-regions at this level can begin to integrate information from multiple organ systems.

A notable feature of interoception is its integrative and hierarchical nature (Smith et al., 2017). For example, there appear to be several levels of processing above the brainstem, which progressively integrate interoceptive information with skeleto-motor, proprioceptive and somatosensory information, exteroceptive (e.g., visual, auditory) information, long-term memory, contextual information, and cognitive control processes. For example, interoceptive information appears to guide (1) the regulation of stereotyped behavioral responses within the periaqueductal gray (PAG) and hypothalamus (e.g., defensive freezing, shivering), (2) the generation of coordinated affective responses (with visceral, behavioral, and cognitive components) within the amygdala and related nuclei, and (3) the allocation of cognitive resources (e.g., selective attention) to metabolically relevant information within the insular and cingulate cortices. This progressive integration – with greater degrees of multimodality as one moves to higher hierarchical levels of processing – raises the possibility that some neurons or neuronal populations may encode/represent a type of conjunction of two or more sources of information that are expected to co-vary. These representations, as we now turn to, may be best understood as predictive.

The neurosciences in general have begun to converge on a conception of the brain as a type of "prediction machine" (Bastos et al., 2012; Friston, 2010; Smith, Badcock et al., 2020).[2] Briefly, a body of work now supports the idea that the signals or messages passed between neurons take the form of various types of predictions and prediction errors. One prominent variant of this broad notion is predictive coding (Friston, 2005), which suggests that brain regions are arranged with re-entrant reciprocal connections between many levels in a hierarchy, with each layer encoding particular hypotheses about the world (including the body), and relaying predictions about the patterns of sensory input (or lower-level representations) that would be consistent with those hypotheses. Upward messages, in turn, convey prediction error signals (encoding deviations from predictions based on current beliefs) that drive the system to revise beliefs until these error signals are minimized.

Multiple proposals (Barrett & Simmons, 2015; Paulus et al., 2019; Seth, 2013; Seth et al., 2011; Stephan et al., 2016), and emerging empirical evidence (Smith, Kuplicki et al., 2020), support the idea that this picture may also characterize interoceptive processing. Namely, that the hierarchical neural processing and integration of interoceptive signals can be understood as exchanges of prediction and prediction error signals. Most theories of this kind have focused on cortical processing, in which the posterior and mid insula plays a major role in encoding hypotheses about, and relaying predictive messages associated with, the subset of interoceptive variables that can, in some circumstances, be perceived consciously (e.g., cardiorespiratory, gastrointestinal, and genitourinary percepts). These regions of the insula putatively receive prediction error signals from the ventromedial posterior thalamic nucleus (Strigo & Craig, 2016), which in turn receive afferent information about bodily states from the brainstem.

Moving upward in this proposed hierarchy, it is suggested that interoceptive percepts are in turn shaped by higher-level predictions conveyed by agranular sectors of the anterior insular and cingulate cortices, which themselves integrate interoceptive information (e.g., about metabolic states and predicted demands) with higher-level cognitive processes (e.g., goals, context, working memory contents). The resulting processing allows predictive guidance over cognition and behavior so as to prioritize the maintenance of the body within the homeostatic visceral and environmental conditions consistent with continued survival. The overall picture of signaling and representation within interoception is thus hierarchical, predictive, and aimed in the service of adaptively regulating bodily states and behaviors. As one ascends this predictive hierarchy, integration may therefore take the form of encoding conditional probabilities. This is because, when a level of processing has access to multiple signal types, it can infer the probability of one thing based on information about another thing. For example, consider an individual walking down a path in the forest and encountering a bear. If a level of processing had access to information from both interoceptive and visual signals, it could infer the conditional probability of an elevated heart rate *given* the exteroceptive observation of a dangerous animal; or it could infer the probabilistic benefits of selectively attending to the length of a potential path of escape *given* current blood glucose levels (Park et al., 2014; Proffitt et al., 2003; Salomon et al., 2018; Salomon et al., 2016; Schnall et al., 2008; Witt et al., 2009; Witt & Proffitt, 2008; Witt et al., 2004).

Importantly, this predictive view of interoceptive representation (and representation more generally) is explicitly action-oriented (Clark, 2015). This connects with previous proposals that distinguish between carrying "information" (i.e., where the presence of a symbol carries information about [reduces uncertainty with respect to] the presence of its referent [Dretske, 1981]) and carrying meaning – where things mean something to an organism (or an organism *understands* something) because they predict the future actions an organism should take to achieve its goals, desires, or more basic biological imperatives (Macdonald & Papineau, 2006; Smith, 2014; 2016; 2017; Williams, 2018). As we turn to next, this vision of interoceptive representation may have important implications for neurosemiotics, and the specific way the brain interprets the *conceptual/semantic* (as opposed to perceptual) meaning and implications of interoceptive signals.

Interoceptive meaning-making and emotion

Predictive neural hierarchies do not stop with perceptual-level representation. Yet higher levels of representation involving conceptual/semantic content have been associated with cortical hubs of the "default network" – with primary examples being anterior temporal and medial prefrontal/parietal cortices (Binder et al., 2009). One widely studied example of this type of meaning-making corresponds to the recognition and awareness of one's own emotions (Barrett, 2017; Smith et al., 2018; Smith & Lane, 2015), where quantitative simulations of predictive hierarchical processing have been reported (Allen, et al., 2019; Hesp et al., 2020; Smith, Lane, et al., 2019; Smith et al., 2019). The basic premise here is that interoceptive percepts (e.g., a racing heart, shivering, changes in skin temperature) are a central aspect of emotional experience, but that they need to be recognized as such via a concept-level inference process (although note that emotion concepts can be primed unconsciously (Zemack-Rugar et al., 2007), so emotion concept representation should be seen as a necessary but not sufficient condition for reportable emotional experience). For example, when feeling a racing heart and tightness in one's chest, one could infer (1) that this is simply due to anxiety or (2) that it is due to a heart attack. These are two highly diverging ways of interpreting the meaning of bodily sensations, which entail very different predictions about the best course of (both skeletomotor and visceromotor) action – for example, practicing a relaxation technique in the former scenario versus going to the emergency department in the latter scenario.

Typically, disambiguating between alternative interpretations requires the acquisition and deployment of context-sensitive prior expectations within a predictive hierarchy. For example, one might be more prone to infer the presence of a heart attack given knowledge of a family history of cardiac disease. Alternatively, one might confidently interpret the bodily sensations as indicative of anxiety when preparing to give a public speech.

One potentially unique difficulty worth highlighting with this type of meaning-making in interoception arises from *incomplete access* and *poor perceptual specificity*. Incomplete access refers to the fact that some visceral variables, although tracked by the brain, are not directly accessible to the perceptual capacities of the individual. Some common examples include acid/base balance in the blood (i.e., blood pH), blood pressure, or peristaltic activity within the small intestine. There is no clear and direct percept available for such variables, which appears to correspond to the fact that neurons encoding them are not afforded the broad and selective influence across frontoparietal cortices associated with conscious perception (Dehaene, 2014). This contrasts with visceral variables such as the cardiac cycle, which, although not always consciously experienced, can be brought into perceptual awareness as a result of selective attention (Simmons et al., 2013) or perturbation outside of resting ranges – for example, pharmacologically-induced heart-rate elevations (Hassanpour et al., 2016).

Poor perceptual specificity refers to the fact that some interoceptive stimuli are only detectable indirectly (often requiring background knowledge to interpret or infer), or that they are perceptually symbolized in a vague manner that precludes clear interpretation. For example, low blood pressure can result in dizziness, concentration difficulty, nausea, blurry vision, or "seeing stars," which may require substantial medical knowledge to recognize as such, or prior familiarity with these symptoms. Other examples can be mentioned: deviations from standard blood pH values can result in headache, nausea, or fatigue; high levels of systemic inflammation can result in anhedonia, fatigue, and reduced motivation; visceral pain (pain due to internal organ injury) is often "referred" to other somatic bodily locations (e.g., myocardial ischemia producing pain experienced in the shoulder or jaw region). In each of these examples, current perceptual experience alone precludes accurate interpretation.

Lastly, it is important to recognize that, unlike other sensory modalities, interoception has less opportunity to benefit from what can be thought of as "cross-modal double checking." It is well known, for example, that vision and hearing can inform each other. For example, based on visually perceived lip movement, the same sound can be perceived as different phonemes. This is referred to as the McGurk effect, whereby, for example, one and the same syllable is perceived as either "ba" or "ga" depending on whether the speaker's lips close or remain open (Alsius et al., 2018). Other examples include the double-flash and rubber hand illusions. In the former, two fast auditory tones lead a single flash of light to be perceived as two consecutive flashes; in the latter, a rubber hand begins to feel like one's own when one sees that rubber hand being stroked while feeling coincident strokes on one's actual hand, which is out of sight (Bowen et al., 1987; Litwin, 2019). In contrast, potential inaccuracies in interoceptive representations have less opportunity to be refined by the other senses because these other senses do not carry as much potentially corrective information about visceral states. Each of these issues thus makes interpreting the meaning of interoceptive states especially challenging. From the perspective of neurosemiotics, the ambiguity inherent to the interpretation of interoceptive signals might result in a greater diversity of available conceptualizations, and at different levels of description (e.g., biological, psychological, cultural, or various combinations of each). For example, this might explain instances in which "butterflies in the stomach" can be variably interpreted as eager anticipation (e.g., falling in love) or alternatively, as different forms of dread (e.g., nausea, anxiety).

Social signaling of interoceptive states

A further question about the neurosemiotics of interoception pertains to how one's internal bodily states are communicated to others. Aside from explicit communication via language (e.g., "my heart is racing right now"), at first glance it may not be intuitively obvious how non-verbal signaling of one's interoceptive state could occur, as many interoceptive variables are not externally observable. However, it may not always be necessary to indicate one's interoceptive state to another at an explicit/verbal level. For example, it has been recently suggested that humans can perceive the heartbeat of another person based on cardiac-associated fluctuations of their visual appearance alone (Galvez-Pol et al., 2020). The question about interpersonal interoceptive signaling might also superficially seem quite distinct from the issues discussed previously; however, as we now discuss, it is in fact highly connected.

The primary link of interest returns to predictive, multimodal inference. Specifically, it draws on the fact that interoceptive, exteroceptive, and proprioceptive states have predictable co-variance relationships. This entails that, so long as an individual has learned these co-variance relations within themselves, they can be (fairly reliably) used to infer interoceptive states in others. As one simple example, when viewing another individual running rapidly on a treadmill, one can infer that they are feeling shortness of breath. More interestingly, when one individual has just been insulted, and a second individual perceives that the first is displaying signs of muscle tension and an "angry" facial expression, the second individual may reasonably infer that the first has experienced an elevation in heart rate or blood pressure (especially if their breathing rate is also visibly elevated). Other examples abound. Individuals are likely in states of low blood glucose if they are moving sluggishly and have not eaten for a lengthy period; an individual laying in a hammock smiling can be seen as indirectly signaling a pleasant, low arousal state, and so forth. Previous work has also suggested a type of "replicative interactive inference" in which one individual can automatically mimic the visible body states of another (e.g., their posture or movement) to better understand their interoceptive state, because this mimicry can engage similar interoceptive states (Quadt, 2017).

Interoceptive states can thus be signaled not only within the body of an individual, but also between individuals. That is, they can be indirectly signaled to other individuals through exteroceptive sensory (e.g., visual, auditory) channels. Crucially, the signal "sender" also has some control over what is communicated. For example, an individual might effortfully suppress outward expressions of anger to prevent signaling an elevated arousal state. A signal "receiver" can then in turn communicate social approval or disapproval of the sender's perceived state. A receiver might further attempt to change the sender's interoceptive state. For example, individuals often try to calm others down by conveying support after a tragic event. In some cases of maternal care, mothers also use skin-to-skin contact to regulate the body temperature their children (Nyqvist et al., 2010).

Other interesting examples come from an emerging literature on interpersonal autonomic synchrony, reviewed in Palumbo et al. (2017). This literature has shown that some interoceptive variables (e.g., cardiac and respiratory cycles) can become correlated or anticorrelated during specific types of social interactions. Although not fully understood, in some cases this may arise through the exchange of social signals that create a shared context with similar expected metabolic demands in both participating individuals. In each of these situations, interoceptive states can be conveyed indirectly to others (both intentionally and unintentionally) by drawing on a shared theory of mind reflecting the belief that there are reliable exteroceptively perceivable correlates of another's internal bodily state (Figure 24.1).

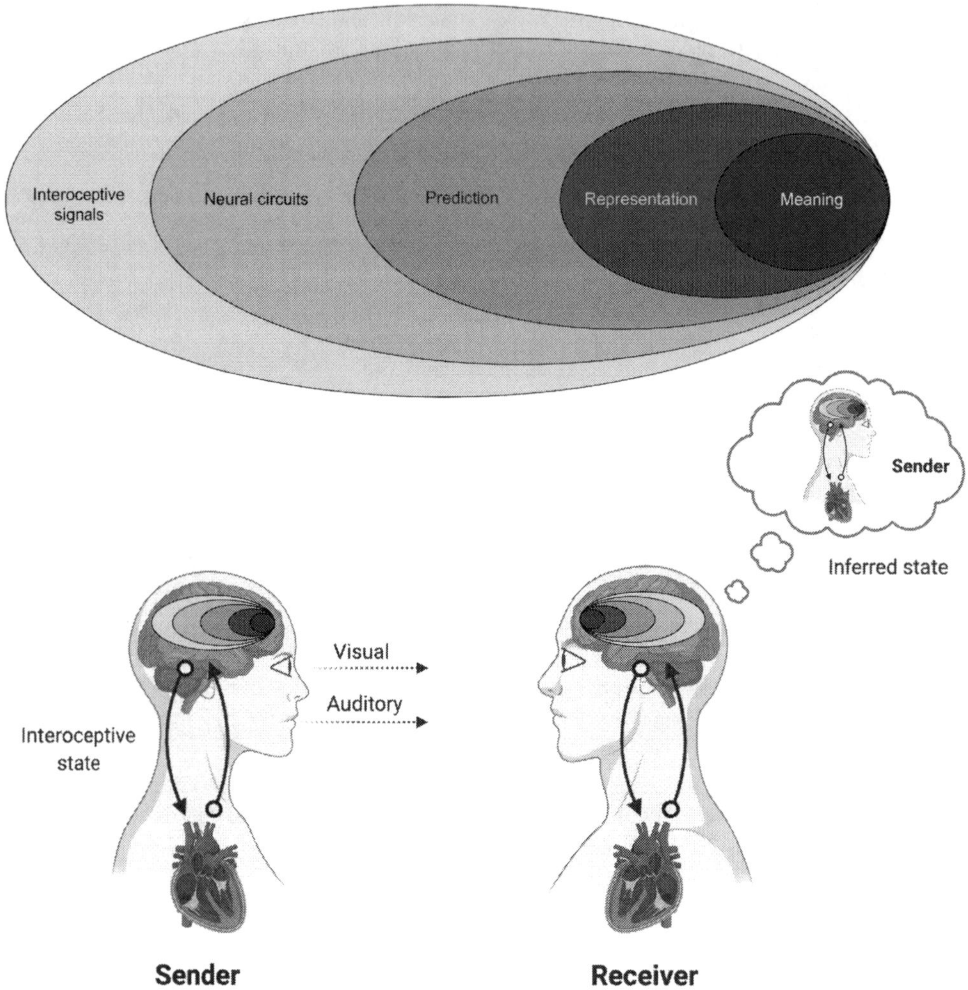

Figure 24.1 Neurosemiotics of interoception

Top: The neurosemiotics of interoception occurs via a layered process which progresses from discrete physiological constituents (e.g., cardiac, respiratory, gastrointestinal, genitourinary, chemical, humoral, and immune signals) to neural circuits (e.g., arousal, appetitive, cognitive, affective, social, nociceptive, thermoregulatory and threat) supporting abstract constituents involved in the representation, meaning, and prediction of the individual's internal and external environment. Bottom: Some interoceptive signals are emoted and can even be "sent" outside of the body and received by other individuals. Interpersonal communication can thus involve a third level of signaling, at the level of interoception, which provides implicit information regarding an individual's physiological state. In other words, interoceptive signals constantly carry information relevant to interpreting the internal state of the body ("within me") and this information is indirectly (i.e., via exteroceptive cues) accessible to interpretation by others in the outside world. Portions of the bottom figure were created with BioRender. See e-book for a full-color version of this figure.

Maladaptive interoceptive representation

Interoceptive experiences are often characterized by states of heightened physiological and psychological arousal, particularly when homeostatic deviations occur in response to threats – or potential threats – to the body. Disturbances of interoception have been increasingly linked to the expression of mental health disorders, particularly as a means of explaining certain symptoms, but also in regard to the underlying pathophysiology (Khalsa, Adolphs et al., 2018). So, what does it mean to have abnormal interoceptive representation? At a basic level, this refers to representations of interoceptive states that do not correspond to true interoceptive states. This can also involve inaccuracies in one's expectations about future interoceptive states – as well as how they relate to exteroceptive states. We have previously referred to a discrepancy between predicted and true interoceptive states as a "somatic error" with regard to anxiety (Khalsa & Feinstein, 2019).

Specifically, somatic errors refer to inadequate predictions about the current or future state of the body. When these inadequate predictions fail to be corrected over time, this can result in a sustained breakdown in adaptive brain–body interactions – reducing the brain's ability to (1) maintain current visceral states within adaptive ranges via visceromotor control, (2) select skeletomotor actions to prevent future deviations from adaptive visceral states, and (3) adaptively integrate interoceptive and exteroceptive signals to update higher-level (conceptual) beliefs about one's self and one's situation in the world.

It is likely that somatic errors are present in numerous mental health conditions beyond anxiety. For example, individuals with depression show blunted insular cortex activation during cardiac interoceptive attention (Avery et al., 2014), and differences in reward and interoceptive neurocircuitry depending on whether the depression is associated with an increased or decreased appetite (Simmons et al., 2016). Individuals with addiction show hyperreactive responses in interoceptive neurocircuitry during anticipation and receipt of salient (aversive and pleasant) stimuli (Berk et al., 2015; Stewart et al., 2015), but also show blunted insula activity during baseline (non-perturbation) states *despite* reporting amplified ratings of heart-related sensations (Stewart et al., 2019). Individuals with eating disorders report heightened interoceptive sensations during both endogenous (Lapidus et al., 2020) and exogenous (Khalsa et al., 2015) perturbations, and exhibit abnormal activity in the insular and cingulate cortices (Berner et al., 2017; Berner et al., 2019; Kerr et al., 2016), brain regions that are central to the representation and regulation of interoceptive signals. We also previously observed evidence for a heightened vulnerability to "visceral illusions" (i.e., self-reported changes in cardiorespiratory activity in the absence of objective changes) in anorexia nervosa (Khalsa et al., 2015), which localizes in specific body regions – for example, the chest (Khalsa et al., 2018).

The aforementioned studies collectively illustrate how aberrant interoceptive representation plays out in the brain and body. But what of the maladaptive consequences of a failure to accurately represent the relationship between interoceptive states and the environment external to the body? A persistent deviation between interoceptive representations and true bodily states is thought to put a strain on the homeostatic reflexes involved in maintaining the body within adaptive states and returning it to adaptive states after perturbation. If the body's recovery mechanisms are unable to restore the body to homeostatic ranges (i.e., ranges of values for physiological variables consistent with long-term survival), the ensuing response may lead to a shift in homeostatic setpoints (i.e., target values for physiological variables during visceral regulation) through the process of allostasis – where bodily states are adjusted pre-emptively due to anticipated future deviations involving novel or potentially threatening experiences (McEwen, 1998, 2017; Sterling, 2012).

Allostasis can adaptively adjust homeostatic setpoints in the context of continual predictions of future deviations in body state, whereas allostatic dysfunction can occur when the brain makes continual predictions of future deviations that never occur (i.e., such that setpoints remain adjusted out of adaptive ranges). Key signals involved in the implementation of allostasis include adrenaline, cortisol, metabolic hormones, and pro- and anti-inflammatory cytokines (McEwen, 2017), which have both peripheral and central influences at the neural and chemohumoral levels, at both short and long timescales. Allostatic dysfunction has been linked to a diversity of conditions, via an inability to adjust uncertainty estimates over predicted bodily outcomes (Peters et al., 2017). Thus, the machinery involved in adapting to bodily stress relies fundamentally on interoceptive processing, and dysregulation of this machinery appears to contribute to imbalances of physical and mental health.

This inability to adaptively enact allostasis is a central component of interoceptive models of psychopathology (Barrett et al., 2016; Harshaw, 2015). Delineating the mechanisms underlying these interoceptive processes will likely require the combination of advanced approaches – for example, computational modeling (Petzschner et al., 2021; Stephan et al., 2016; Tschantz et al., 2021) – and the development of new methodologies capable of illuminating the manner in which interoceptive signals traverse the nervous system during neurosemiosis, as discussed in the next section.

Neurosemiotics of interoception: theoretical, methodological, and epistemological implications

In the preceding sections, we addressed several questions aiming to integrate interoception and neurosemiotics. At the most basic level, any comprehensive approach to neurosemiotics will be incomplete without incorporating interoception – because the neural systems supporting interoception are integral to all other systems in the brain. They provide key information to other neural systems about the metabolic/visceral state of the body and guide cognition and behavior – including social behavior – toward maintaining the body in conditions consistent with survival. As we have seen, interoceptive states can also be indirectly signaled to others – playing an important role in interpersonal communication and social cognition. One important future direction for neurosemiotics, suggested by the work reviewed here, will be to further explore the detailed way in which interpersonal interoceptive signaling contributes to social communication. It appears plausible that such signals could influence communication in subtle ways, some of which may escape awareness.

As a first step toward a neurosemiotics of interoception, we have offered tentative (but necessarily incomplete) answers to the six questions posed in the introduction. Specifically, we have highlighted afferent pathways by which different organ systems can provide ongoing information about the state of the body. We have introduced prediction-based neurocomputational models of interoception suggesting that afferent signals are integrated with the brain's overall model of the world by eliciting prediction errors that provide corrective information relative to prior beliefs about bodily states. We have described how hierarchical processing can integrate interoceptive information with signals from other sensory channels as well as from memory, allowing the brain to generate explanations of the causes of patterns in these combined signals – ultimately allowing the brain to infer their most likely conceptual/semantic interpretation. Finally, we have highlighted a range of pathways by which interoceptive states can be interpersonally signaled, and how all the above-mentioned processes can break down in clinical contexts.

As our answers to these questions make clear, interoception is now recognized as a neural process that is inherently integrative with respect to a major subset of sensory signaling occurring within the body, ranging from molecular sensors to circuitry contributing to perceptual awareness. In contrast with more circumscribed approaches for studying single mechanisms, this updated conceptualization facilitates a more holistic and organismal viewpoint that (1) uses multidimensional measurement approaches for characterizing distinct levels of processing, and (2) integrates multiple levels and types of interoceptive processing into an overarching framework. It thus embraces the complexity involved in understanding the interactions between multiple biological systems.

The neurosemiotics of interoception offers additional layers of complexity (as outlined in Figure 24.1), which afford a broader perspective on information integration. This perspective provides a way to understand how the intersecting streams of information from within our brains and bodies can be meaningfully interpreted in relation to the brains and bodies of others with which we interact.

This dyadic dynamic is grounded in a biological framework that has the advantage of considering the physical characteristics of self-processing without denying the importance of the phenomenological characteristics that accompany feelings. It may also allow the study of additional layers of complexity, such as the interactions between family units, social groupings, and eventually societal and cultural influences, which have been a major focus of traditional semiotic perspectives.

However, the contribution of interoception to this larger project is limited on its own. These limits are eloquently articulated by Antonio Damasio (2019: 218) as follows:

> Basic homeostasis remains a somewhat parochial affair, focused on the temple that human subjectivity has designed and erected – the self. It can be extended with more or less effort to the family and the small group. It can be extended further out, to larger groups, on the basis of circumstances and negotiations in which the prospects of general benefits and power are well balanced. But homeostasis, as found in each of our individual organisms, is not *spontaneously* concerned with very large groups, especially heterogenous groups, let alone with cultures or civilizations as a whole.

Thus, without relying on additional perspectives, which are the domains of fields such as cognitive science, the social sciences, experimental psychology, linguistics, social studies, history, and philosophy, among others, insights derived from the neurosemiotics of interoception are likely to be circumscribed and contribute to only some parts of the whole picture.

Conclusion

In this chapter, we have showcased the way current work in interoception research can be used to address questions that would be central to neurosemiotics. This includes work showing what is known about the way information regarding the body is signaled to the brain, how it is represented, how its meaning is inferred, and how it may even be signaled to others. We also briefly considered how interoceptive signaling and representation processes may break down in certain physical and mental health conditions. A general theme that can be brought out by the example work we have described is that, for any complete biological account of semiotics, signals from inside the body and the way they are represented will need to be incorporated. An account solely focused on explaining signal encoding and communication outside the body will miss an important part of the complete picture. Interoception research can therefore inform and advance neurosemiotics. In a parallel fashion, the questions motivated by neurosemiotics, when applied to interoception, can guide thinking and motivate research in fruitful ways.

Due to the centrality of interoception in driving the focus of cognition and behavior towards meeting the biological imperatives of the organism, it necessarily plays a multi-modal, integrative role in the broader signaling processes that occur both within and between individuals to meet those imperatives – offering a more holistic account of both intra- and inter-personal communication that, through collaboration with other fields of study, promises to advance our understanding of semiotic processes more generally. We look forward to synergistic, bidirectional interactions between these fields of study.

Notes

1 We recognize that the term "representation" is associated with a notable amount of controversy and can be used in multiple ways, and that our usage should be clarified here. In this context, because we appeal to predictive processing models of the brain throughout this chapter, it is worth noting the common conceptions of representation in these models. While arguments have been made for a number of specific positions, most appeal in some way to what an internal state predicts and to how it guides action. As one example, Williams has

defended the position that representations in predictive processing are resemblance-based, organism-relative, and aimed at pragmatic success as opposed to veridicality (Williams, 2018); also see (Clark, 2015). However, while we draw on predictive processing models of brain function, nothing argued here depends on strong commitments to any specific theory of representation. In the context of interoceptive processing, it is sufficient to consider our use of the term "representation" as denoting particular internal states (i.e., patterns and locations of neural activity) that are, under normal conditions, selectively sensitive to specific changes in the internal state of the body, and which convey information about those changes appropriately to other systems in the brain.

2 For a review of historical and recent conceptualizations of the brain as a machine, see Cobb (2020).

References

Allen, M., Levy, A., Parr, T., & Friston, K. J. (2019). In the body's eye: The computational anatomy of interoceptive inference. *BioRxiv, 603928*. doi: 10.1101/603928

Alsius, A., Pare, M., & Munhall, K. G. (2018). Forty years after hearing lips and seeing voices: The McGurk effect revisited. *Multisensory Research, 31*(1–2), 111–144. doi: 10.1163/22134808-00002565

Avery, J. A., Drevets, W. C., Moseman, S. E., Bodurka, J., Barcalow, J. C., & Simmons, W. K. (2014). Major depressive disorder is associated with abnormal interoceptive activity and functional connectivity in the insula. *Biological Psychiatry, 76*(3), 258–266. doi: 10.1016/j.biopsych.2013.11.027

Barrett, L. (2017). *How Emotions are Made: The Secret Life of the Brain*. Boston: Houghton Mifflin Harcourt.

Barrett, L. F., Quigley, K. S., & Hamilton, P. (2016). An active inference theory of allostasis and interoception in depression. *Philosophical Transactions of the Royal Society B: Biological Sciences, 371*(1708). doi: 10.1098/rstb.2016.0011

Barrett, L., & Simmons, W. (2015). Interoceptive predictions in the brain. *Nature Reviews Neuroscience, 16*, 419–429. doi: 10.1038/nrn3950

Bastos, A., Usrey, W., Adams, R., Mangun, G., Fries, P., & Friston, K. (2012). Canonical microcircuits for predictive coding. *Neuron, 76*, 695–711. doi: 10.1016/j.neuron.2012.10.038

Benarroch, E. E. (1993). The central autonomic network: Functional organization, dysfunction, and perspective. *Mayo Clinic Proceedings, 68*, 988–1001. doi: 10.1016/s0025-6196(12)62272-1.

Benarroch, E. E. (2011). Circumventricular organs: receptive and homeostatic functions and clinical implications. *Neurology*, 77(12), 1198–1204. doi: 10.1212/WNL.0b013e31822f04a0

Berk, L., Stewart, J. L., May, A. C., Wiers, R. W., Davenport, P. W., Paulus, M. P., & Tapert, S. F. (2015). Under pressure: Adolescent substance users show exaggerated neural processing of aversive interoceptive stimuli, *Addiction*, 110(12), 2025–2036. doi: 10.1111/add.13090

Berner, L. A., Simmons, A. N., Wierenga, C. E., Bischoff-Grethe, A., Paulus, M. P., Bailer, U. F., & Kaye, W. H. (2019). Altered anticipation and processing of aversive interoceptive experience among women remitted from bulimia nervosa. *Neuropsychopharmacology, 44*(7), 1265–1273. doi: 10.1038/s41386-019-0361-4

Berner, L. A., Simmons, A. N., Wierenga, C. E., Bischoff-Grethe, A., Paulus, M. P., Bailer, U. F., Kaye, W. H. (2017). Altered interoceptive activation before, during, and after aversive breathing load in women remitted from anorexia nervosa. *Psychological Medicine*, 48(1), 148–154. doi: 10.1017/S0033291717001635

Berntson, G. G., & Khalsa, S. S. (2021). Neural circuits of interoception. *Trends in Neurosciences, 44*(1), 17–28. doi: 10.1016/j.tins.2020.09.011.

Binder, J., Desai, R., Graves, W., & Conant, L. (2009). Where is the semantic system? A critical review and meta-analysis of 120 functional neuroimaging studies. *Cerebral Cortex, 19*, 2767–2796. doi: 10.1093/cercor/bhp055

Bowen, R. W., Mallow, J. V., & Harder, P. J. (1987). Some properties of the double-flash illusion. *Journal of the Optical Society of America*, 4(4), 746–755. doi: 10.1364/josaa.4.000746

Clark, A. (2015). *Surfing Uncertainty: Prediction, Action, and the Embodied Mind*. New York: Oxford University Press.

Cobb, M. (2020). *The Idea of the Brain: The Past and Future of Neuroscience*. New York: Basic Books.

Damasio, A. (2019). *The Strange Order of Things: Life, Feeling, and the Making of Cultures*. New York: Pantheon.

Dehaene, S. (2014). *Consciousness and the Brain*. New York: Viking.

Dretske, F. (1981). *Knowledge and the Flow of Information*. Cambridge, MA: MIT Press.

Friston, K. (2005). A theory of cortical responses. *Philosophical Transactions of the Royal Society of London. Series B, Biological Sciences, 360*, 815–836. doi: 10.1098/rstb.2005.1622

Friston, K. (2010). The free-energy principle: A unified brain theory? *Nature Reviews Neuroscience, 11*, 127–138. doi: 10.1038/nrn2787

Galvez-Pol, A., Salome, A., Li, C., & Kilner, J. M. (2020). Direct perception of other people's heart rate. *PsyArXiv*. doi: 10.31234/osf.io/7f9pq.

Harshaw, C. (2015). Interoceptive dysfunction: toward an integrated framework for understanding somatic and affective disturbance in depression. *Psychological Bulletin, 141*(2), 311–363. doi: 10.1037/a0038101

Hassanpour, M. S., Yan, L., Wang, D. J., Lapidus, R. C., Arevian, A. C., Simmons, W. K., Feusner, J. D., & Khalsa, S. S. (2016). How the heart speaks to the brain: Neural activity during cardiorespiratory interoceptive stimulation. *Philosophical Transactions of the Royal Society B: Biological Sciences, 371*(1708). doi: 10.1098/rstb.2016.0017

Hesp, C., Smith, R., Allen, M., Friston, K. J., & Ramstead, M. J. D. (2020). Deeply felt affect: The emergence of valence in deep active inference. *Neural Computation*, 1–49. doi: 10.1162/neco_a_01341

Kerr, K. L., Moseman, S. E., Avery, J. A., Bodurka, J., Zucker, N. L., & Simmons, W. K. (2016). Altered insula activity during visceral interoception in weight-restored patients with anorexia nervosa. *Neuropsychopharmacology, 41*(2), 521–528. doi: 10.1038/npp.2015.174

Khalsa, S. S., Adolphs, R., Cameron, O. G., Critchley, H. D., Davenport, P. W., Feinstein, J. S., Feusner, J. D., Garfinkel, S. N., Lane, R. D., Mehling, W. E., Meuret, A. E., Nemeroff, C. B., Oppenheimer, S., Petzschner, F. H., Pollatos, O., Rhudy, J. L., Schramm, L. P., Simmons, W. K., Stein, M. B., … Interoception Summit. (2018). Interoception and mental health: A roadmap. *Biological Psychiatry: Cognitive Neuroscience and Neuroimaging, 3*(6), 501–513. doi: 10.1016/j.bpsc.2017.12.004

Khalsa, S. S., Craske, M. G., Li, W., Vangala, S., Strober, M., & Feusner, J. D. (2015). Altered interoceptive awareness in anorexia nervosa: effects of meal anticipation, consumption and bodily arousal. *International Journal of Eating Disorders, 48*(7), 889–897. doi: 10.1002/eat.22387

Khalsa, S. S., & Feinstein, J. S. (2019). *The somatic error hypothesis of anxiety*. New York: Oxford University Press.

Khalsa, S. S., Hassanpour, M. S., Strober, M., Craske, M. G., Arevian, A. C., & Feusner, J. D. (2018). Interoceptive anxiety and body representation in anorexia nervosa. *Front Psychiatry, 9*, 444. doi: 10.3389/fpsyt.2018.00444

Lapidus, R. C., Puhl, M., Kuplicki, R., Stewart, J. L., Paulus, M. P., Rhudy, J. L., Feinstein, J. S., Khalsa, S. S., & Tulsa, I. (2020). Heightened affective response to perturbation of respiratory but not pain signals in eating, mood, and anxiety disorders. *PLoS One, 15*(7), e0235346. doi: 10.1371/journal.pone.0235346

Litwin, P. (2019). Extending Bayesian models of the rubber hand illusion. *Multisensory Research*, 1–34. doi: 10.1163/22134808-20191440

Macdonald, G., & Papineau, D. (2006). *Teleosemantics*. Oxford: Oxford University Press.

McEwen, B. S. (1998). Stress, adaptation, and disease: Allostasis and allostatic load. *Annals of the New York Academy of Sciences, 840*, 33–44. doi: 10.1111/j.1749-6632.1998.tb09546.x

McEwen, B. S. (2017). Allostasis and the epigenetics of brain and body health over the life course: The brain on stress. *JAMA Psychiatry, 74*(6), 551–552. doi: 10.1001/jamapsychiatry.2017.0270

Nyqvist, K. H., Anderson, G. C., Bergman, N., Cattaneo, A., Charpak, N., Davanzo, R., Ewald, U., Ibe, O., Ludington-Hoc, S., Mendoza, S., Pallás-Allonso, C., Ruiz, J. G., Sizun, J., & Widström, A-M. (2010). Towards universal Kangaroo Mother Care: recommendations and report from the First European conference and Seventh International Workshop on Kangaroo Mother Care. *Acta Paediatrica, 99*(6), 820–826. doi: 10.1111/j.1651-2227.2010.01787.x

Palumbo, R. V., Marraccini, M. E., Weyandt, L. L., Wilder-Smith, O., McGee, H. A., Liu, S., & Goodwin, M. S. (2017). Interpersonal autonomic physiology: A systematic review of the literature. *Personality and Social Psychology Review, 21*(2), 99–141. doi: 10.1177/1088868316628405

Park, H. D., Correia, S., Ducorps, A., & Tallon-Baudry, C. (2014). Spontaneous fluctuations in neural responses to heartbeats predict visual detection. *Nature Neuroscience, 17*(4), 612–618. doi: 10.1038/nn.3671

Paulus, M. P., Feinstein, J. S., & Khalsa, S. S. (2019). An active inference approach to interoceptive psychopathology. *Annual Review of Clinical Psychology, 15*, 97–122. doi: 10.1146/annurev-clinpsy-050718-095617

Peters, A., McEwen, B. S., & Friston, K. (2017). Uncertainty and stress: Why it causes diseases and how it is mastered by the brain. *Progress in Neurobiology*. doi: 10.1016/j.pneurobio.2017.05.004

Petzschner, F. H., Garfinkel, S. N., Paulus, M. P., Koch, C., & S.S., K. (2021). Computational models of interoception and body regulation. *Trends in Neurosciences, 44*(1), 63–76. doi: 10.1016/j.tins.2020.09.012.

Proffitt, D., Stefanucci, J., Banton, T., & Epstein, W. (2003). The role of effort in perceiving distance. *Psychological Science, 14*, 106–112. doi: 10.1111/1467-9280.t01-1-01427

Quadt, L. A. (2017). Action-oriented predictive processing and social cognition. In T. K. Metzinger, & W. Wiese (Eds.), *Philosophy and Predictive processing*. Midtjylland: MIND Group.

Salomon, R., Ronchi, R., Donz, J., Bello-Ruiz, J., Herbelin, B., Martet, R., Faivre, N., Schaller, K., & Blanke, O. (2016). The insula mediates access to awareness of visual stimuli presented synchronously to the heartbeat. *Journal of Neuroscience, 36*(18), 5115–5127. doi: 10.1523/JNEUROSCI.4262-15.2016

Salomon, R., Ronchi, R., Donz, J., Bello-Ruiz, J., Herbelin, B., Faivre, N., Schaller, K., & Blanke, O. (2018). Insula mediates heartbeat related effects on visual consciousness. *Cortex, 101*, 87–95. doi: 10.1016/j.cortex.2018.01.005

Schnall, S., Harber, K., Stefanucci, J., & Proffitt, D. (2008). Social support and the perception of geographical slant. *Journal of Experimental Social Psychology, 44*, 1246–1255. doi: 10.1016/j.jesp.2008.04.011

Seth, A. K. (2013). Interoceptive inference, emotion, and the embodied self. *Trends in Cognitive Sciences*, *17*(11), 565–573. doi: 10.1016/j.tics.2013.09.007

Seth, A. K., Suzuki, K., & Critchley, H. D. (2011). An interoceptive predictive coding model of conscious presence. *Frontiers in Psychology*, *2*, 395. doi: 10.3389/fpsyg.2011.00395

Simmons, W. K., Avery, J. A., Barcalow, J. C., Bodurka, J., Drevets, W. C., & Bellgowan, P. (2013). Keeping the body in mind: Insula functional organization and functional connectivity integrate interoceptive, exteroceptive, and emotional awareness. *Human Brain Mapping*, *34*(11), 2944–2958. doi: 10.1002/hbm.22113

Simmons, W. K., Burrows, K., Avery, J. A., Kerr, K. L., Bodurka, J., Savage, C. R., & Drevets, W. C. (2016). Depression-related increases and decreases in appetite: Dissociable patterns of aberrant activity in reward and interoceptive neurocircuitry. *The American Journal of Psychiatry*, *173*(4), 418–428. doi: 10.1176/appi.ajp.2015.15020162

Smith, R. (2014). Explanation, understanding, and control. *Synthese*, *191*(17), 4169–4200. doi: 10.1007/s11229-014-0521-3

Smith, R. (2016). The relationship between consciousness, understanding, and rationality. *Philosophical Psychology*, 29(7), 943–957. doi: 10.1080/09515089.2016.1172700

Smith, R. (2017). A neuro-cognitive defense of the unified self. *Consciousness and Cognition*, *48*, 21–39. doi: 10.1016/j.concog.2016.10.007

Smith, R., Badcock, P. B., & Friston, K. J. (2020). Recent advances in the application of predictive coding and active inference models within clinical neuroscience. *Psychiatry and Clinical Neurosciences*, *75*(1), 3–13. doi: 10.1111/pcn.13138

Smith, R., Killgore, W. D. S., & Lane, R. (2018). The structure of emotional experience and its relation to trait emotional awareness: A theoretical review. *Emotion*, *18*(5), 670–692. doi: 10.1037/emo0000376

Smith, R., Kuplicki, R., Feinstein, J., Forthman, K. L., Stewart, J. L., Paulus, M. P., & Khalsa, S. S. (2020). A Bayesian computational model reveals a failure to adapt interoceptive precision estimates across depression, anxiety, eating, and substance use disorders. *medRxiv*. doi: 10.1101/2020.06.03.20121343

Smith, R., Lane, R., Parr, T., & Friston, K. J. (2019). Neurocomputational mechanisms underlying emotional awareness: Insights afforded by deep active inference and their potential clinical relevance. *Neuroscience & Biobehavioral Reviews*, *107*, 473–491. doi: 10.1016/j.neubiorev.2019.09.002

Smith, R., & Lane, R. D. (2015). The neural basis of one's own conscious and unconscious emotional states. *Neuroscience & Biobehavioral Reviews*, *57*, 1–29. doi: 10.1016/j.neubiorev.2015.08.003

Smith, R., Parr, T., & Friston, K. J. (2019). Simulating emotions: An active inference model of emotional state inference and emotion concept learning. *Frontiers in Psychology*, *10*, 2844. doi: 10.3389/fpsyg.2019.02844

Smith, R., Thayer, J. F., Khalsa, S. S., & Lane, R. D. (2017). The hierarchical basis of neurovisceral integration. *Neuroscience & Biobehavioral Reviews*, *75*, 274–296. doi: 10.1016/j.neubiorev.2017.02.003

Stephan, K., Manjaly, Z., Mathys, C., Weber, L., Paliwal, S., Gard, T., Tittgemeyer, M., Fleming, S. M., Haker, H., Seth, A. K., & Petzschner, F. (2016). Allostatic self-efficacy: A metacognitive theory of dyshomeostasis-induced fatigue and depression. *Frontiers in Human Neuroscience*, *10*, 550. doi: 10.3389/fnhum.2016.00550

Sterling, P. (2012). Allostasis: A model of predictive regulation. *Physiology & Behavior*, 106(1), 5–15. doi: 10.1016/j.physbeh.2011.06.004

Stewart, J. L., Khalsa, S. S., Kuplicki, R., Puhl, M., Investigators, T., & Paulus, M. P. (2019). Interoceptive attention in opioid and stimulant use disorder. *Addiction Biology*, e12831. doi: 10.1111/adb.12831

Stewart, J. L., May, A. C., Tapert, S. F., & Paulus, M. P. (2015). Hyperactivation to pleasant interoceptive stimuli characterizes the transition to stimulant addiction. *Drug and Alcohol Dependence*, *154*, 264–270. doi: 10.1016/j.drugalcdep.2015.07.009

Strigo, I. A., & Craig, A. D. (2016). Interoception, homeostatic emotions and sympathovagal balance. *Philosophical Transactions of the Royal Society B: Biological Sciences*, *371*(1708). doi: 10.1098/rstb.2016.0010

Tschantz, A., Barca, L., Maisto, D., Buckley, C. L., Seth, A. K., & Pezzulo, G. (2021). Simulating homeostatic, allostatic and goal-directed forms of interoceptive control using Active Inference. *bioRxiv*. doi: 10.1101/2021.02.16.431365

Williams, D. (2018). Predictive processing and the representation wars. *Minds and Machines*, *28*(1), 141–172. doi: 10.1007/s11023-017-9441-6

Witt, J., Linkenauger, S., Bakdash, J., Augustyn, J., Cook, A., & Proffitt, D. (2009). The long road of pain: Chronic pain increases perceived distance. *Experimental Brain Research*, *192*, 145–148. doi: 10.1007/s00221-008-1594-3

Witt, J., & Proffitt, D. (2008). Action-specific influences on distance perception: A role for motor simulation. *Journal of Experimental Psychology. Human Perception and Performance*, *34*, 1479–1492. doi: 10.1037/a0010781

Witt, J., Proffitt, D., & Epstein, W. (2004). Perceiving distance: A role of effort and intent. *Perception*, *33*, 577–590. doi: 10.1068/p5090

Zemack-Rugar, Y., Bettman, J., & Fitzsimons, G. (2007). The effects of nonconsciously priming emotion concepts on behavior. *Journal of Personality and Social Psychology*, *93*, 927–939. doi: 10.1037/0022-3514.93.6.927

25

THE HIERARCHICAL SEMANTICS OF SELF

Georg Northoff and Diego Gorini

Introduction

The self is a basic phenomenon of our life and existence. While the concept of self has been discussed extensively in philosophy over the last three centuries, its presence in psychology and neuroscience is more recent. Various studies have shown complex psychological (Sui & Humphreys, 2015) and neural (Apps & Tsakiris, 2014; Frewen et al., 2020; Northoff et al., 2006; Qin et al., 2020; Tsakiris, 2016, 2017; van den Meer et al., 2010) correlates of the self; yet, a crucial neurosemiotic question remains unanswered: How are these signatures and their psychological manifestation related to semantics? Is there correspondence – if not a convergence – between the neural hierarchies of the self and those of semantic systems? And if so, what enables such a convergence?

Neurosemiotics investigates signs and their intersubjective manifestations by bridging neurobiological levels with explanations of "psychological" phenomena such as cognition, intentionality, and meaning. Across multiple levels of interactions, semantics is one of the semiotic dimensions more critically related to meaning. In this chapter, we use a tool of neurosemiotics to forge interdisciplinary links between the self and semantics. We will focus on semantic analogies among neural hierarchies of the self and semantic hierarchies, as well as their respective and convergent timescales. We will enrich our proposals by providing insight from a computational model of vector semantic space operating on a temporal continuum of long and short timescales. Briefly, we aim to address vital questions about the self and semantics, charting their connections with a neurosemiotic approach.

Hierarchical layers of self

Contemporary research on the self spans diverse psychological, neural, and conceptual levels. Psychologically, the self impacts functions such as perception (Sui et al., 2012), reward (deGreck et al., 2008; Yankoskaya et al., 2020), action (Frings & Wentura, 2014), emotion (Northoff et al., 2009), attention (Sui et al. 2013), and decision-making (Nakao et al., 2016, 2019). Neurally, the self (as well as these functions) has been associated with multiple brain regions, including cortical midline structures (Northoff et al., 2006), premotor and motor cortices (Hu et al., 2016; Qin et al., 2020), the insula (Enzi et al., 2009), the temporo-parietal junction (Qin et al., 2016, 2020), and the anterior cingulate cortex (Qin et al., 2016, 2020), as well as subcortical regions such as the amygdala, the ventral tegmental area, and the midbrain (deGreck et al., 2008). These findings have inspired specific conceptualizations of

DOI: 10.4324/9781003051817-30

the self. Following Mesulam (1998) and others, including McLean (1990) and Panksepp (1998), the brain's cortical organization has been conceived in a layer-based way as in terms of radial-concentric organization. The radial-concentric approach is also reflected in the three-layer model by Feinberg and Northoff (Northoff et al., 2011), the assumption of a dynamic core (DePasquale et al., 2018), and the core–periphery hierarchy with a sensory-transmodal gradient (Margulies et al., 2016).

Despite some differences, these radial-concentric models share the assumption of gradient patterns – that is, a continuum of different processes, regions, and functions. Gradient patterns can be conceived as hallmark features of neural hierarchies (Huntenberg et al., 2018; Margulies et al., 2016). Following these developments, we propose an analogous hierarchy of the self, equally typified by gradient patterns (Qin et al., 2020). Such a hierarchical model of the self integrates and unifies different neural, psychological, and conceptual correlates by assuming a gradient pattern of different layers of self-processing – that is, self-related, self-predictive, and self-referential processing (Northoff, 2007, 2016). This view offers fruitful foundations to examine the key question tackled herein.

From the hierarchy of self to semantic similarity and relatedness

Do these layers of self-specificity converge with analogous semantic layers? Our main assumption is that the hierarchy of self converges with a semantic hierarchy of semantic similarity and relatedness. This, as we demonstrate, is possible through shared time windows. While the different layers of self can be distinguished by their different timescales (from short to long), semantic similarity and relatedness (see below for definition) are also mediated by short and long timescales, respectively.

Therefore, we propose that timescales provide the link, if not the "common currency" (Northoff et al., 2020), of self and semantics, as both are mediated by the co-occurrence of short and long timescales. Our proposal lies at the interface between semantics, semiotics, and neuroscience. It is semantic in that we are concerned with meaning and how it is constructed. For that, we assume that timescales are key in constructing meaning, thus adopting a temporal view of semantics. Such a view invites semiotic insights, as the self deploys acts and objects that take on the role of "signs" through their integration within the timescales of the self. This touches upon neurosemiotics, as we assume these timescales are yielded by and based on the brain, as the most basic features of our self.

These three layers of self-specificity constitute the core proposal to trace neurosemiotic links between the self and semantics, as discussed in the first and second parts. Drawing on structuralist research, we distinguish between semantic similarity and relatedness. After establishing these concepts, we derive further insights from a recent computational model of vector semantic space that associates semantic relatedness and similarity with different timescales, long and short. That, as outlined in the third part, provides the link to the self, which also operates on a temporal continuum of long and short timescales. Specifically, we postulate that the three layers of self (self-related, self-predictive, and self-referential) mediate the temporal continuum of semantic similarity and relatedness with their short and long-time windows.

Neural hierarchy of self: Different layers of self-processing

Layers and neural hierarchy of self

A recent large-scale meta-analysis on healthy subjects (Qin et al., 2020) integrated imaging studies that focused on different aspects of the self, namely inner body (interoceptive processes), outer body (extero-proprioceptive processes), and reflections on one's own mental states. Different regions were associated with each of the three layers, and the regions of the lower layer were included within the next upper layer (see below for details). Together, this amounts to a spatial multi-layered nested hierarchical model of self (Qin et al., 2020), including an intero-exteroceptive self, an extero-proprioceptive/cognitive self, and a higher-order reflective or mental self.

The interoceptive self (i.e., how the brain processes and perceives the body's inner organs and their input) was investigated through fMRI studies that measured interoceptive awareness, including cardiorespiratory, urogenital, and gastrointestinal awareness. That was complemented by fMRI studies on the extero-proprioceptive self, focusing on external bodily inputs, such as facial or proprioceptive input signals. Finally, studies were included that tapped on more cognitive aspects of self, employing trait adjectives or other stimuli so that subjects became aware of their own self as distinct from others (Figure 25.1).

The intero-exteroceptive self: Self-related processing

Based on the interoceptive studies, there is a more basic or lower layer of self, an interoceptive self that is related to regions that mostly process interoceptive signals –for example, the bilateral insula, the dorsal anterior cingulate cortex, the thalamus, and the parahippocampus, thus including mainly regions of the salience network (Menon, 2011; Qin et al., 2020). The fact that these regions were shared among the different kinds of interoceptive awareness (i.e., cardiorespiratory, urogenital, and gastrointestinal) speaks to their role in integrating different interoceptive inputs from various inner-body organs (Craig, 2009). One can thus identify an "interoceptive or vegetative self" (Azzalini et al. 2019); Tsakiris, 2017), "bodily self" or "proto-self" (Panksepp, 1998) as the most basic and fundamental layer of self. However, subcortical and cortical regions, such as the thalamus and the insula, don't just process interoceptive inputs from the inner body. They also process exteroceptive stimuli from the outer environment (Craig, 2009). Given such intero-exteroceptive convergence, we characterize this level of self as self-related processing (SLP) and an intero-exteroceptive self.

To better understand SLP, we need to distinguish between intrinsic and extrinsic self-specificity. Self-specificity does not come with the stimuli themselves – it is not an intrinsic feature. For instance, even our name is not intrinsic to our self as our parents could have named us otherwise. The same is true of our face, which due to changes by external events or over the course of life, can change in major ways without affecting our self – it is still my face despite all the changes. Therefore, self-specificity is an extrinsic rather than intrinsic feature of stimuli or contents.

A typical example is the rubber hand illusion. We can conceive another person's hand or arm as our own body's hand or arm – this means that our own body's hand is not an intrinsic feature of our self as my body's own hand can also be related with a hand from another body (Tsakiris, 2017). This may be due mostly to complex processes that integrate the multiple interoceptive input streams with the extero- and proprioceptive input streams (Tsakiris, 2017) in a seemingly purely stochastic way (Apps & Tsakiris, 2014), independent of their respective origin (Northoff, 2016). This results in an intero-exteroceptive self that endows self-specificity to interoceptive and exteroceptive inputs by integrating them in ways that are specific for the respective person (that is, his/her self). The intero-exteroceptive self is thus, in its most basic way, an integrative self (Sui & Humphreys, 2015).

Predictive or cognitive self: Self-predictive processing

The next or middle layer of self includes what Qin et al. (2020) describe as proprioceptive or exteroceptive self. This can also be taken as a first instance of a cognitive self. FMRI studies focusing on external bodily-related inputs, such as facial or proprioceptive inputs, implicate regions like the bilateral insula, the inferior frontal gyrus, the premotor cortex, the temporo-parietal junction (TPJ), and the medial prefrontal cortex (MPFC). As these regions process inputs from different sensory modalities, they may be key not only for integrating extero- and proprioceptive modalities, but also different exteroceptive sensory modalities – that is, cross-modal integration. Despite their differences, these regions share the processing of proprioceptive inputs related to one's own body – one can thus speak of a "proprio- or exteroceptive self, or embodied self" (Panksepp, 1998; Tsakiris, 2017). This

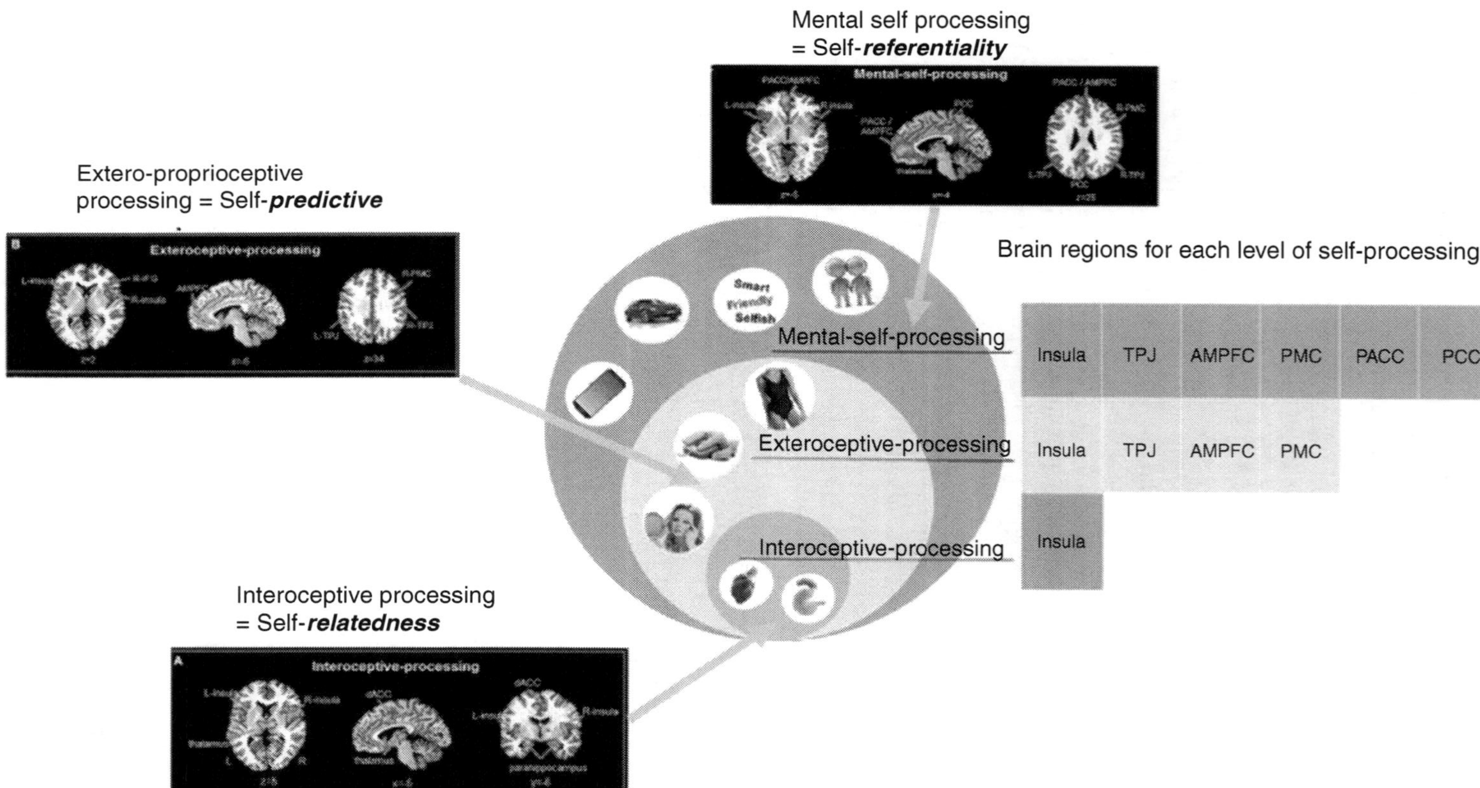

Figure 25.1 Hierarchy of self

This model is presented as obtained in a large-scale meta-analysis of self by Qin et al. (2020). The black boxes show the regions obtained for each layer of self-processing, while the middle blue-free circles show the nested hierarchy with the regions of the lower layer resurfacing and nesting within the next more extended layer and so forth. See e-book for a full-color version of this figure.

may be conceived as the most basic instance of prediction, and thus of cognition. We therefore characterize this level of self as self-predictive processing (SPP) or cognitive self.

SPP implies that self-specific contents can serve to predict or anticipate future stimuli and their respective contents. More specifically, self-specific contents serve as predicted inputs which are then compared with the actual inputs from the body and/or the world. SPP has been mainly examined in paradigms involving either parts of the body, like faces (see Hu et al., 2016, for meta-analysis of self-face paradigms) and arms (as in the rubber hand illusion; Apps & Tsakiris, 2014); or, alternatively, the whole body (Blanke et al., 2015).

This concerns mainly the proprioceptive and exteroceptive stimuli/contents of the body. SPP is based on the theory of predictive coding (Friston, 2010) as applied to the self (Apps & Tsakiris, 2014). Predictive coding claims that the degree of matching or difference between the predicted input and the actual input determines further processing and subsequent behavior (Friston, 2010, 2018; Apps & Tsakiris, 2014).

Applied to the specific case of the self, this results in the following: if the stimulus (i.e., the actual input) is different from the self-specific content that is the predicted input, then there will be a large prediction error indicating a discrepancy between the self-specific content and the stimulus – the actual stimulus will then be endowed with a low degree of self-relatedness. If, in contrast, the self-specific content as predicted input matches strongly with the input stimulus, this results in a small prediction error with a high degree of self-specificity attributed to the stimulus. The underlying mechanism here is that the brain can predict the self based on multisensory integration and a probabilistic representation of the self – that is, self-contents (Apps & Tsakiris, 2014).

The predictive relation in SPP is based on the stochastic properties of the self as predicted input and the actual input. This is so because predictive coding and SPP are based on a stochastically based active inference from its present self-specific content as predicted input to actual inputs – e.g., future stimuli (Seth, 2013; Friston, 2018; Moutoussis et al., 2014; Apps & Tsakiris, 2014). That also entails a rather lower-order processing mode, as such stochastically based inference and matching can well operate in at least a partially implicit and involuntary mode. That distinguishes SPP from the more explicit level of higher-order reflective or mental self-processing, self-referential processing as we will discuss in the next section.

Higher-order reflective or mental self: Self-referential processing

Finally, the highest layer of self (Qin et al., 2020) has been related to typical midline regions of the default mode network (DMN), like the medial prefrontal and the posterior cingulate cortices as well as the regions included in the second level (most notably, the bilateral TPJ) and the first level (the bilateral insula and thalamus). These regions seem to be recruited when one needs to represent one's own self in mental states – one can therefore also speak of a "mental or cognitive self" (Qin et al, 2020) or "extended self" (Damasio, 2010).

Self-specific stimuli in these paradigms usually involve the subjects' own name, his/her face, or personally related trait adjectives (see above). Importantly, the self-specificity of these stimuli is given and presupposed and thus pre-existing (or ready-made): these experimental paradigms do not focus so much on the stimuli themselves but rather on the psychological content of the stimuli and how the subject refers to self- and non-self-specific stimuli. These paradigms thus test for the difference between the subjects' referring to self- and non-self-specific stimuli – the underlying processing mode is therefore described as self-referential processing (SRP) (Sui & Humphreys, 2015; Sui et al., 2012).

On the psychological level, SRP involves a variety of different psychological functions. Several self-paradigms require subjects to focus their attention on self-specific stimuli vs. non-self-stimuli (Sui et al., 2012; Sui & Humphreys, 2015). Since self- and non-self-specific stimuli lead to different recruitment of attentional resources (Sui et al. 2013; Sui & Humphreys, 2015), attention may need to be considered yet another important cognitive feature required by self-reference. Moreover, other cognitive self-paradigms require subjects to imagine self-specific contents versus non-self-specific contents in past, present, and future (d'Argembeau et al., 2010) – self-reference here involves imagination of future and past, described as episodic simulation (Schacter et al., 2012).

Taken together, SRP can be characterized by the subjects' reference to self-specific contents, hence the name self-*referential*. SRP is usually coined self-reflection (Hu et al., 2016;, Sui and Humphreys, 2015, Northoff, 2016), as one reflects upon one's own self and its self-specific contents by recruiting various cognitive functions. Other related concepts include self-certainty, self-recognition, and self-insight (see Philippi & Koenigs, 2014). While somewhat distinct, these terms are nevertheless unified by the fact that they all describe the subjects' reference to self-specific psychological contents in a higher-order reflective or mental way.

Nested hierarchy of self: Different spatial and temporal scales are integrated

Together, these findings point to what Qin et al. (2020) describe as a "nested hierarchy of self": regions of the lower level were included in the next higher level, where they were complemented by additional regions, and so forth. For instance, the bilateral insula was present on the most basic level (i.e., the interoceptive self) and resurfaced, in completely independent imaging studies, in both second (i.e., proprioceptive self) and third (i.e., mental self) levels. The same holds true for the bilateral TPJ, which first showed in the intermediate layer of the proprioceptive self and resurfaced again in the third level of the mental self. Accordingly, each of the hierarchical levels of self recruits both overlapping and separate regions compared to other levels amounting to spatial nestedness with a spatially nested hierarchy of self.

This conforms to nestedness as a spatial hierarchy of self: the lower layer regions are integrated within the more extended regions of the next upper layer and so forth. That conforms to an analogous nestedness of different layers of self-processing: self-related processing is integrated and resurfaces within SPP which, in turn, is integrated within SRP. Finally, on the more psychological level, this means that the intero-exteroceptive self is integrated and nested within the predictive self and that, in turn, it resurfaces within the higher-order cognitive reflective or mental self.

It shall also be noted that the spatial hierarchy of self in the brain is accompanied by a corresponding temporal hierarchy. The regions' neural activity displays different timescales – that is, intrinsic neural timescales (INT), which can be measured by the autocorrelation window (ACW). The upper layer regions, like the DMN, and midline structures show the longest ACW with long time windows optimally suited for temporal integration (Golesorkhi et al., 2021). While the intero- and exteroceptive regions exhibit much shorter ACW – the temporal windows of their neural activity are thus better suited for temporal segregation than temporal integration (Golesorkhi et al., 2021).

Recent studies also associate the self with the brain's INT. The higher the degree of self-specificity on the mental level, the longer the ACW and thus the higher the degrees of possible temporal integration (Huang et al., 2016; Kolvoort et al., 2020). This strongly suggests that the three layers of self-specific processing (self-relatedness, self-prediction, and self-reference) can also be distinguished in their temporal hierarchy: self-related processing involves shorter timescales which are nested and contained within the longer ones of SPP and ultimately within the longest ones of SRP. We are now ready to turn to semantics. We will see that semantics may also be viewed in terms of its timescales, which may provide an intrinsic connection between language/meaning, brain, and self.

Self meets language: Semantic similarity and semantic relatedness

Semantic relatedness versus semantic similarity

For creatures living in the midst of a continuous flux of information, categorical perception is a fundamental surviving skill that has been carefully studied by psychology and the cognitive sciences

(Harnad, 2003). In fact, determining that two things are identical, similar, or simply related is a complex cognitive ability that has proven difficult to formalize in semantics (McRae et al., 2012; Schulte im Walde, 2020).

Take, for example, the pairs of words *cup* and *coffee*, and *cup* and *mug*. Which of these pairs has the stronger semantic similarity? We certainly employ the former pair in close proximity much more often than the latter pair, and the word *cup* primes the word *coffee* more strongly than the word *mug*. Thus, we are tempted to say that *cup* and *coffee* are similar words. Yet, cups and coffees are not at all similar, beyond the fact that they are both concrete entities. Cups and mugs, on the other hand, commonly share many attributes, such as shape, material, and function.

More precisely, semantic similarity between words *A* and *B* is commonly defined as having a high degree of substitutability, which usually entails that referents A and B share many attributes (Miller & Charles, 1991; Rapp, 2002; Schütze & Pedersen, 1993). Quite trivially, this explains why one can substitute some words with their synonym: synonyms are very similar words. On the other hand, words *cup* and *coffee* are said to be merely semantically related (rather than being similar), which usually entails that cups and coffees tend to co-occur in space and time. Again, this trivially explains the priming effect that word *cup* has on word *coffee*: one tends to perceive or interact with the referents within the same space-time window (Figure 25.2).

It is tempting to suppose that the distinction between *true similarity* and *simple relatedness* subsists only at the lexical level – that is, as relations between words. However, this semantic distinction extrapolates up to the behavioral and neural sciences, in the distinction between taxonomic versus thematic knowledge (Merck et al., 2019; Mirman et al., 2017; Schwartz et al., 2011). For example, given task X, you could determine that tools A and B are similar enough to be substitutable in the performing of that task. Knowing that tool A may substitute tool B maps semantic similarity to taxonomic knowledge, while knowing that both A and B relate to task X maps semantic relatedness to thematic knowledge. Alternatively, from a logical view, one could decide to adopt either a dog or a

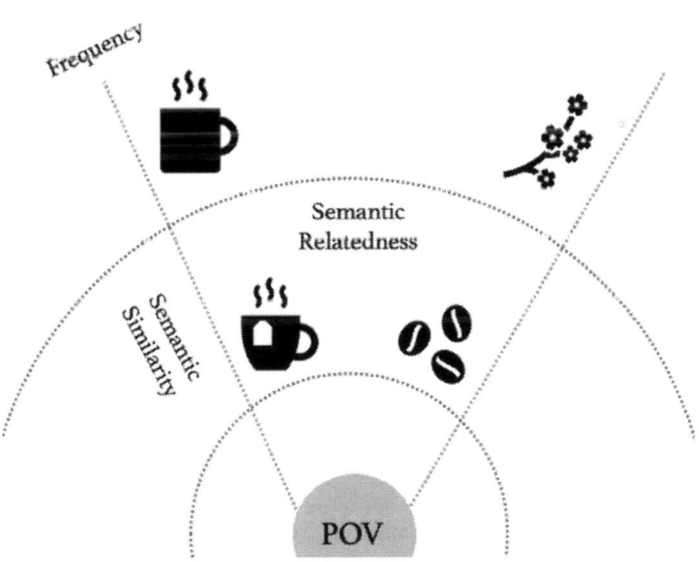

Figure 25.2 2D semantic map

This figure shows four objects (cup, mug, coffee, tea) from a single point of view (POV). Things along the semantic relatedness axis (blue) tend to *co-occur* within the same spatiotemporal window. Things along the semantic similarity axis (orange) tend to share many attributes and functions, hence the possibility of *substitution*. The radial distance from the POV alludes to the likelihood of each object given the respective context. See e-book for a full-color version of this figure.

cat for home; in this case, semantic similarity (and substitutability) maps to the logical operator OR, and semantic relatedness (and co-occurrence) maps to AND, as in $(cat \wedge home) \vee (dog \wedge home)$. A more general cognitive-semiotic process may be found underlying these mechanisms helping us make sense of the world along the distinction of semantic relatedness and similarity.

Finally, the distinction of semantic relatedness versus semantic similarity can also be viewed within the larger context of the self. The self provides references or a standard against or relative to how both semantic relatedness and semantic similarity are perceived. For instance, the self of a coffee addict will certainly draw an extremely close semantic relationship between coffee and cup. In contrast, the self of somebody who hates and does not drink coffee at all but tea may rather draw close semantic relation of the cup with the tea while, at the same time, perceiving a large semantic distance – that is, low relatedness of cup and coffee. Hence, the degrees of semantic relatedness and, ultimately, also of semantic similarity, strongly depend upon the context like on the self in which they operate.

Isomorphism of structural and semantic relations

Back to lexical semantics, the first step in this direction is to consider similarity and relatedness from the structural point of view (Erk, 2016; Peirsman, 2008; Sahlgren, 2008; Schulte im Walde, 2020). A bit like they are in mathematics, structural relationships in semantics should be understood as those relationships between words that occur by virtue of their *position* in a certain phrase or context, regardless of their content or referent. Studying word meaning without taking into account their referent may seem like a difficult task, but it turns out to be the essential requirement for machines to understand natural language, as we will see later. An example should suffice to clarify this point. A common task in many tests of second-language proficiency is for participants to be asked to guess ("fill in the blank") the most suitable word given a certain context (Landauer & Dumais, 1997). In English, sentences follow the structure subject–verb–object (SVO). So, if given the following sentence:

> "My grandfather ____ a successful lawyer,"
>
> the verbs *was*, *is*, and *will be* would surely come to mind, although, with less probability, other verbs are also possible, such as *met* and *saw*. Notably, this prediction is based entirely on the structural properties of the sentence. In fact, we could replace all of its words and the prediction would remain the same:
>
> "Her grandpa ____ an unsuccessful doctor."
>
> Clearly, the "horizontal" SVO structure allows for this kind of "vertical" substitution. However, finer-grained, nested structures also preserve this lexical property. The words *was*, *is*, and *will be* are merely conjugations of the verb *to be*, and conjugation is a typical example of vertical substitution. Other examples include pronouns (*my*, *her*), and semantic classes such as synonyms (*grandfather*, *grandpa*), co-hyponyms (*lawyer*, *doctor*), and antonyms (*successful*, *unsuccessful*).

More precisely, words having this "vertical" relationship within a linguistic structure are said to be paradigmatic parallels or to have a paradigmatic relation. Conversely, words having a "horizontal" relationship within a linguistic structure are said to be syntagmatic associates or to have a syntagmatic relation. And now we can better understand the distinction between true semantic similarity and simple relatedness: Similar words imply an underlying vertical, exclusive, paradigmatic relation, and hence the possibility of substitution. Likewise, related words imply an underlying horizontal, inclusive, syntagmatic relation, and hence the spatiotemporal co-occurrence. Together, one can speak of isomorphism of structural and semantic relations (Figure 25.3).

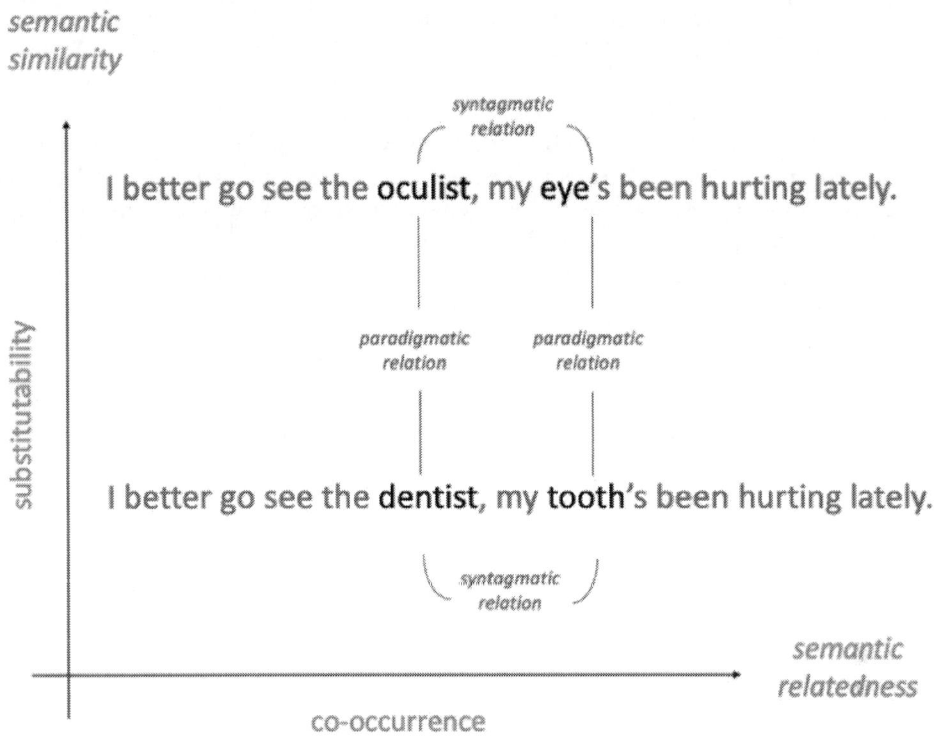

Figure 25.3 Structural and semantic relations along the same linguistic plane

Similar words have a "vertical" relation of substitutability because they are in a paradigmatic relation. Conversely, related words have a "horizontal" relation of co-occurrence because they are in a syntagmatic relation. The words in gray make clear that one and the same linguistic structure can serve as context to several similar *and* related words. See e-book for a full color version of this figure.

From isomorphism to structuralism: The self is part of sociocultural structure

Isomorphism of meaning and structure has only recently been the subject of study (Erk, 2016; Jezek, 2016; Peirsman, 2008; Sahlgren, 2008; Schulte im Walde, 2020). Its historical origins can be traced to Ferdinand de Saussure's linguistic structuralism (de Saussure, 1922), Wittgenstein's idea of word meaning as usage (Wittgenstein, 1953), and especially to the so-called distributional hypothesis developed by Harris (1954).

In a nutshell, this hypothesis attempts to explain the meaning of words (i.e., semantics) as a function of context (i.e., structure), and has been stated and restated in various ways over time: "Difference of meaning correlates with difference of distribution," "You shall know a word by the company it keeps," "Words which are similar in meaning occur in similar contexts,", and so on. The idea is that you do not necessarily need to know the content or referent of a word to infer its meaning, so as long as you know the context (or "company") it is usually found in. For example, maybe you have never seen an aardvark, but if you read the following sentences:[1]

> "The long-eared aardvark slept all day and ate insects all night."
>
> "With its rabbit-like ears and pig-like snout, the aardvark is an interesting looking animal."
>
> "Though it is a small mammal, the ant-eating aardvark finds its closest relative in the elephant."

You could probably guess that an aardvark is an animal similar to an anteater but with long ears – example adapted from Lenci (2008). In fact, the distributional hypothesis may explain the fast rate at which we are able to learn new words simply by reading (Landauer & Dumais, 1997). Moreover, acquiring semantic knowledge from distributional information may be particularly important in the case of abstract words, for which no external referent exists (Frassinelli et al., 2017). One can see that linguistic structuralism converges here more or less with what is described as distributional semantics, opening new avenues for the mathematical and computational formalization of semantic similarity and relatedness. These will be exploited in the next part.

This view of semantic relatedness and similarity carries important consequences for conceiving the relationship between language and the self. Structuralism conceives semantic relatedness and similarity according to their context, the spatiotemporal features of which are key in especially determining the network of semantic relatedness. The self is, by itself, part of that context; importantly, though, it is not to be identified or equated with the context. The self provides a perspectival view of that context while being itself only part or one aspect of that context. Hence, the above figure may need to be enlarged by drawing the context in which the relation of self to semantic relatedness and similarity occurs.

Back to our example with the coffee and tea drinker, now imagine that the coffee addict is a Chinese man having grown up in a predominant tea culture; this will certainly affect both his self (Han & Northoff, 2008) and how he perceives the semantic relatedness of the cup to both coffee and tea. One may guess that this will be different by his counterpart in, for instance, Italy, where coffee is much more often drunk than in China. The same, conversely, applies to the tea lover. Also, an Italian in China may want to drink coffee from a *gaiwan* or a *chawan* (both of which are typical Chinese bowls for preparing and drinking tea) because of the perceived semantic similarity to a coffee cup in Italy. In contrast, one cannot really imagine that a Chinese would associate such semantic similarity with a coffee cup since they relate *gaiwan* and *chawan* exclusively to tea drinking.

Accordingly, in addition to the self, the introduction of structuralism allows consideration of the self by itself as part of the more general and larger structure of the environment, a spatiotemporal structure. The latter, in turn, provides the ground or condition for establishing and constituting different degrees of semantic relatedness and similarity. The self, as discussed in the first part, may then be conceived primarily in terms of those structural relations or networks. It is primarily spatiotemporal, constituting and interweaving itself within the complex network of semantic relatedness and similarity of the respective cultural, social, and environmental contexts.

Computational mechanisms: Vector semantic space

A most interesting aspect of linguistic structuralism in the distributional hypothesis is that it can be, and has been, very successfully operationalized using relatively modest mathematical and computational means (Erk, 2012; Landauer & Dumais, 1997; Lenci, 2018; Turney & Pantel, 2010). This has made it possible to empirically test the capacity of the distributional hypothesis to model word meaning, and the semantic relations of similarity and relatedness, as well as other finer-grained semantic relations. The main idea behind these models is to map the semantic space of natural language to a mathematical vector space, so that to each word a corresponds an N-dimensional vector $\vec{a}$ encoding its meaning in a distributed fashion. Ideally, each dimension of the semantic vector space should encode some feature of word meaning (e.g., abstractness, concreteness). Although in practice it is not possible to be sure that that is what actually happens, semantic vector spaces do offer a clear semantic interpretation: vectors representing similar words are close in space. In other words, in a vector space, the semantic similarity of words i and j is a function of the distance between word vectors $\vec{i}$ and $\vec{j}$:

$$similarity(i, j) = \frac{1}{distance(\vec{i}, \vec{j})}$$

The most commonly used distance metric is cosine, and a typical application consists in finding the *k*-nearest neighbors of a given word. For example, the five nearest neighbors of the noun *lawyer* in this[2] vector semantic space (Kutuzov et al., 2017) are (in order of descending cosine score): *attorney, jurist, barrister, solicitor,* and *politician*. However, keep in mind that the *k*-nearest neighbors of a word are not necessarily those words that could be considered the most similar by human judgment. Rather, the *k*-nearest neighbors are those words with which the target word maintains the strongest paradigmatic relation, and that therefore could reasonably substitute it in a given sentence. This is perfectly in line with the idea that distributional semantics regards words simply as positions in a structure, and thus the vectors encode word meaning (or content) as a function of distributional (or structural) information. But where does that information come from? (Figure 25.4).

Vector semantic models are created from large collections of texts (in the order of billions of words) using either of two methods: by counting co-occurrence frequencies (Landauer & Dumais, 1997; Lenci, 2018; Turney & Pantel, 2010), or by training a neural network to predict masked words in a sentence (Collobert & Weston, 2008; Devlin et al., 2018; Mikolov et al., 2013; Pennington et al., 2014). Despite some negligible differences in performance (Baroni et al., 2014; Lenci, 2018), both methods are based on the same principle (e.g., the distributional hypothesis), and have been proven to be mathematically equivalent (Levy & Goldberg, 2014; Levy et al., 2015) – that is, either an explicit (counting models) or implicit (predictive models) factorization of a matrix of co-occurrence frequencies. For simplicity, here we will only deal with "predictive" models.

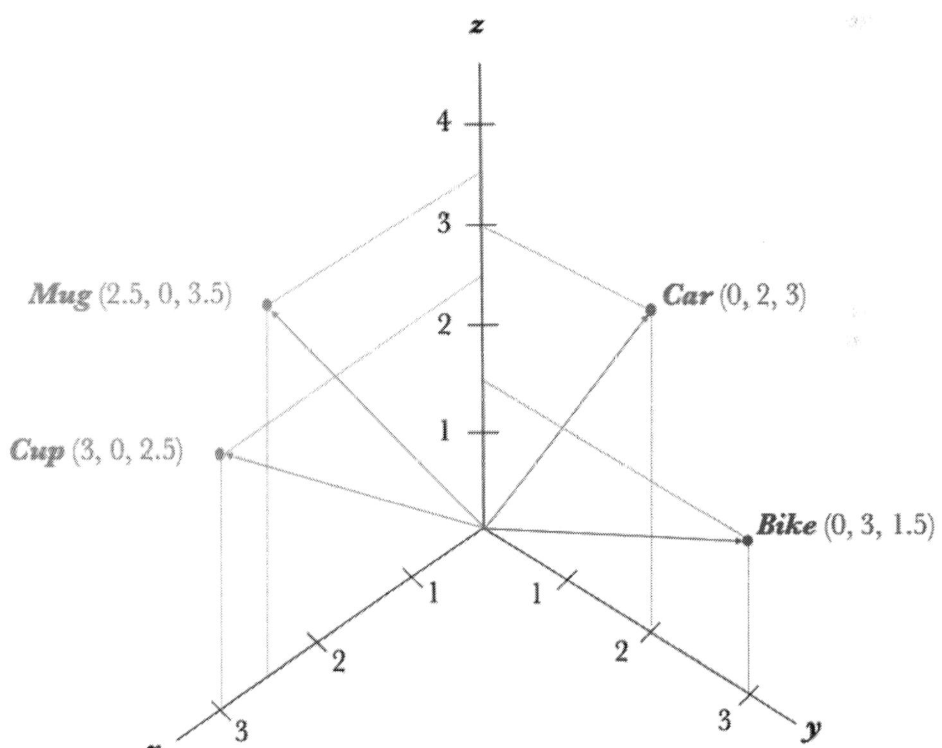

Figure 25.4 3D semantic vector space

Similar words (*mug* and *cup*, *car* and *bike*) tend to be close to each other in space. One may interpret the k-nearest neighbors of a word as a cluster representing a semantic family of some kind. Keep in mind that real semantic vector spaces have hundreds of dimensions (typically 100 or 300), so words can be close and further from each other along dimensions hard to interpret. See e-book for a full-color version of this figure.

Converging semantics, brain, and self through their timescales

Vector semantic space: Short- and long-time relations shape similarity and relatedness

We are now confronting the hardest part: taking into view the link between self and semantics. For that, we first go back to the semantic vector space itself and how it can be trained to yield semantic similarity and relatedness. Training a distributional model is a self-supervised task. Simplifying it quite a bit, a large collection of text is randomly segmented into training examples according to a so-called context window, the size of which ($1 \leq N$) determines the length of the training examples ($2N + 1$). For each training example, the distributional model learns to predict the word at the center, which is masked, based on the surrounding words – that is, based on the context. Essentially, the task is very similar to the "fill in the blank" exercise that was presented above, except that here the model can take into account only N number of words to the left and to the right of the mask (rather than the entire sentence); that is, it can only "see" the context window around the target word (Figure 25.5).

Intuitively, you could think that a longer context window would yield more accurate predictions, and consequently better semantic vector spaces. Note that semantic vector spaces refer primarily to positional distance in space which, as one can assume, translate into temporal distances in speed: the more distant two words are "located" from each in the semantic vector space, the more distant their respective positions in time. Hence, the spatial distances in the semantic vector space may translate into corresponding distances in time – see also Golesorkhi et al. (2021) for an analogous example of temporal and spatial convergence in brain topography. The concept of window, as used in the following sections, can thus be conceived in both spatial and temporal terms.

Extensive experimentation has shown that the size N of the context window actually determines the type of structural information that the model is able to capture (Agirre et al., 2009; Kiela & Clark, 2014; Kiela et al., 2015; Lapesa et al., 2014; Lapesa & Evert, 2017; Levy & Goldberg, 2014; Turney, 2012). Models trained on smaller windows ($N = 1, 2$) produce semantic vector spaces that capture or encode the paradigmatic relations between words and thus perform best on semantic similarity tasks (in which, clearly, human judgment is the gold standard). Conversely, models trained on larger windows produce semantic vector spaces encoding syntagmatic relations and thus perform best on semantic relatedness tasks. This result is important not only because it allows to distinctly model

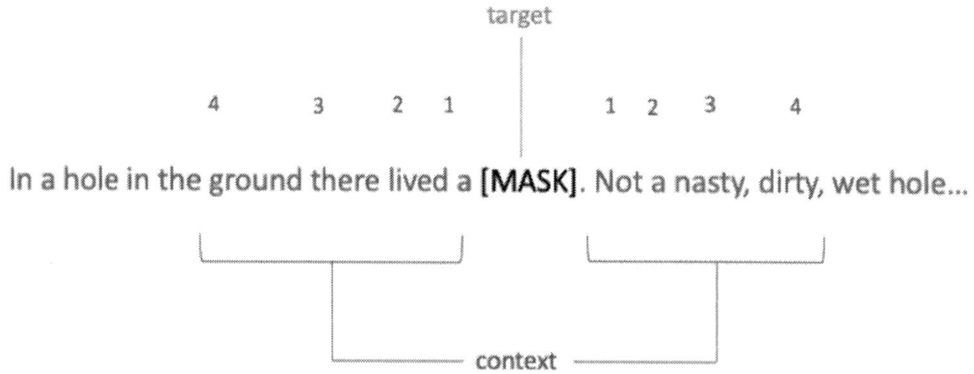

Figure 25.5 Example of a context window

This figure shows a context window of size n equals 4 around a masked word (*hobbit*) in a sentence. Keep in mind, though, that a real training example consists only of the words within the context window, and that training examples are kept within sentence boundaries, such as full stops in English. See e-book for a full-color version of this figure.

semantic similarity and semantic relatedness in a principled manner, but also because it points towards continuity of the semantic space rather than strict polarity, in which semantic similarity appears to be a constrained or "distilled" form of semantic relatedness.

The precise reason for this strong correlation of the size of the context window with the type of structural (and semantic) information encoded in the vector spaces remains unknown. It could be partly explained by the fact that small windows best capture the immediate syntactic function of a word in a certain linguistic context, whilst larger windows tend to associate words by topic (Erk, 2016).

However, even if distributional models were able to overcome the noise produced by the long-range syntactic dependencies commonly found in language, this explanation induces a gratuitous linguistic bias into the hypothesis, which does not allow for the extrapolation of the structural approach beyond word meaning. After all, semantic knowledge in humans is grounded on much more than just syntactic, combinatorial, or distributional schemes (Andrews et al., 2009; Carota et al., 2017; Pulvermüller, 2018; Vigliocco et al., 2004, 2009). So, the fact that vector spaces are able to model semantic knowledge only from a structural proxy of language demands deeper analysis and suggests that meaning may actually emerge from structure itself, while the strong correlation of window size with the type of structural relation suggests that detecting nested structures requires a variety of information processing windows.

Self, brain, and environment are predispositions of semantics

Together, the semantic vector space seems to provide a continuum of semantic relatedness and similarity (as distinguished from their polarity or dualism). Yet, where and how is such continuum coming from? What is the context for such continuum? This leads us back to the self and its respective environmental context.

The self provides a perspectival context for semantic relatedness and similarity: the continuum of semantic relatedness and similarity is viewed from and within a particular perspective, the perspective of the self as a particular person. That introduces differences in how the continuum of semantic relatedness and similarity is viewed: depending on the angle or perspective, the same two words, like *cup* and *coffee*, can be viewed to stand in different degrees of semantic closeness or distance in their semantic relatedness.

The self thus provides a perspectival context for the continuum of semantic relatedness and similarity. Yet where is the context itself, independent of its perspectival nature, coming from? This leads us to the environment – the cultural, ecological, and social context. We already argued that the coffee and tea lovers may view the degree of semantic relatedness of cup, tea, and coffee depending on their respective cultural context. Hence, it is ultimately the relationship of the self to its respective environmental context that determines the perspectival context as a setting for the continuum of semantic relatedness and similarity.

The semantic structure (i.e., the continuum of semantic relatedness and similarity) is in itself deeply embedded and anchored within the structural relation of self and environment. That structural relation of self–environment can, by itself, be traced to the relation of the brain and environment as the brain provides the basis for the self. The brain–environment relation as a basis for the self–environment relation is determined in spatiotemporal terms: the timescales of the world/environment relate to the timescales of the brain and ultimately the self. The self's timescales, in turn, may provide the temporal windows that map semantic relatedness and similarity on a temporal continuum of short and long windows.

In sum, we can now see how the vector- and window-based temporal determination of the continuum of semantic relatedness and similarity is related to the self and its own brain-based intrinsic temporal relationship with the environmental context. Like the self and the brain by themselves

(Northoff et al., 2020), semantic relatedness and similarity are intrinsically linked to the timescales of the environment as mediated through self and brain. It is because of such primarily temporal nature of our semantics that we can ascertain meaning (i.e., semantics) to words in terms of their similarity and relatedness.

Losing such context (i.e., our sense of self or the environment) means losing the temporal structure of semantics. This is what we mean when we say that the intrinsically temporal nature of self, brain, and environment provides a necessary condition or predisposition for semantics featured by the long and short windows of semantic relatedness and similarity.

From the hierarchy of self to the temporal continuum of semantic similarity and relatedness

We have so far treated the self as homogenous in the context of semantics. Yet that is not supported by the empirical data described in the first section. We differentiated self-related, self-predictive, and self-referential processes, each associated with different functions (intero-exteroception, cognitive, and higher-order-reflective dimensions, respectively). This raises the question of how these layers of self are related to the temporal continuum of semantic relatedness and similarity.

The three layers of self can be distinguished on spatial and temporal grounds. Following the meta-analysis by Qin et al. (2020), the lowest layer, interoceptive and self-related processing, is spatially restricted to subcortical regions and insula as cortical region; this means the spatial extension of the neural processing of interoceptive inputs is rather restricted to a small set of regions. The same applies temporally as the timescales are rather short here – that is short-time windows as reflected in the short ACW of these regions.

What does the spatial and temporal restriction of the lowest layer of self imply for its semantic processing? We saw that semantic similarity is related mainly to short spatial, and thereby temporal, windows in computational models. Short-time windows allow for temporal precision, which is exactly what is needed when determining semantic similarity: two different words need to be precisely compared and mapped onto each other, which requires the temporal precision provided by short-time windows. Albeit tentatively, we can see that short-time windows of the intero-exteroceptive layer of self-related processing may be ideally suited to allow for semantic similarity.

How about semantic relatedness? This requires longer-time windows. Those longer-time windows, as well as more spatial extension, are more prevalent at the opposite end of the hierarchy of self, the mental self with its self-referential processing recruiting longer timescales and large parts of cortical regions, the DMN. Given such especially temporal expansion, we assume that the longer timescales of the mental self and its self-referential processing are ideally suited to mediate semantic relatedness as that, per vector space, require longer-time windows.

Together, albeit tentatively, we assume that the brain's temporal (and spatial) hierarchy of self is related to the structural relation of semantic relatedness and similarity. Lower layers of the hierarchy of self with this more bodily-based self are more suited to process semantic similarity, while an increasing degree of semantic relatedness may be taken into view in the higher layers of the hierarchy of self, the mental self.

Importantly, what mediates the relationship of self and semantics is the temporal scale (and spatial ranges) with the transition of the self's short and long timescales providing the brain-based temporal continuum of semantic similarity and relatedness. The different durations of the timescales on the three layers of self allow for the integration of different signs by means of which distinct meanings are constructed. We can thus see how semantics, which focuses on meaning, converges here with neurosemiotics, the neural basis of signs, through the timescales of our brain-based self (Figure 25.6).

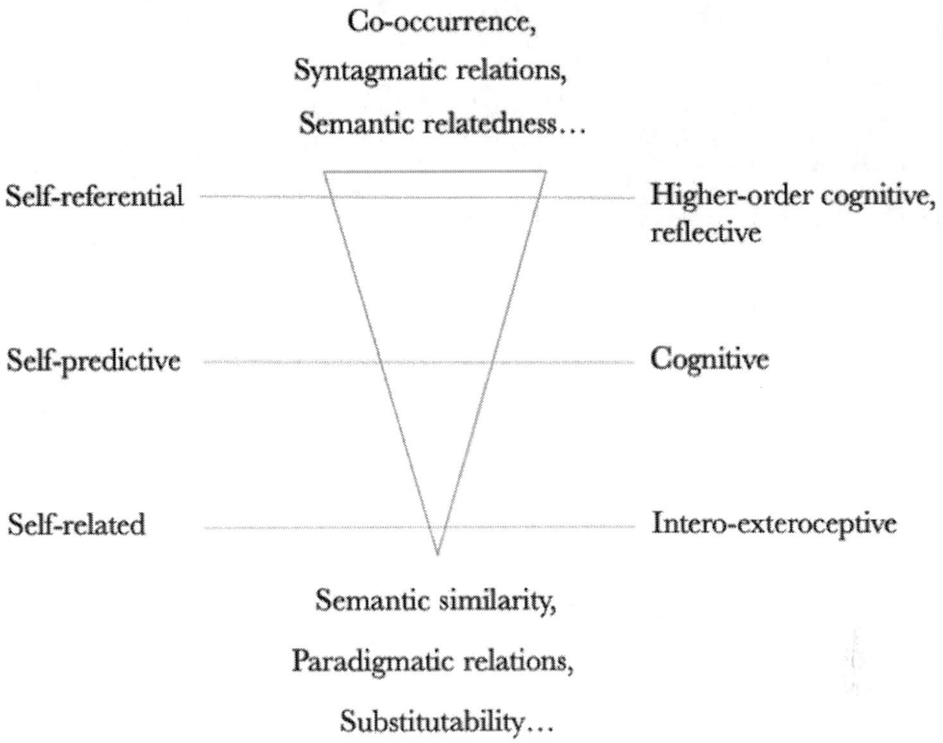

Figure 25.6 Layers of self

Layers of self (left and right) are related to the temporal continuum of semantic similarity and relatedness (middle cone). The conical shape recalls the radial perception in Figure 25.2. Semantically, it represents the fact that as the context window increases, the perception of semantic relatedness also increases. Concerning the self, it represents the fact that longer timescales mediate the more mental self, which is semantically related to semantic relatedness rather than semantic similarity.

Conclusion

We are confronted with an enormous psychological, neural, and conceptual diversity of self in current neuroscience and psychology. We here extend the previously proposed "Basis Model of Self-specificity" (Northoff, 2016) in a hierarchical way by assuming different layers of self-specific processing including self-related, self-predictive, and self-referential processing. Considering recent results in semantics, we postulate that the hierarchy of self is related to a more or less corresponding hierarchy of semantics along the lines of semantic similarity and relatedness.

Importantly, what mediates the self-semantic relation, as we postulate, are temporal features: lower layers of self are mediated by the brain's short timescales, which are ideal for yielding semantic similarity, while higher layers of self exhibit longer timescales that process semantic relatedness. Accordingly, we assume convergence of the brain-based self with semantics: through the active deployment of the self's neural timescales, different linguistic inputs are integrated into different meaningful wholes. What connects brain, self, semantics, and semiotics are, thus, their timescales –a potential "common currency" between them (Northoff et al., 2020).

Notes

1 https://wordsinasentence.com/aardvark-in-a-sentence
2 http://vectors.nlpl.eu/explore/embeddings/en

References

Agirre, E., Alfonseca, E., Hall, K., Kravalová, J., Pasca, M., & Soroa, A. (2009). A study on similarity and relatedness using distributional and wordnet-based approaches. In M. Ostendorf, M. Collins, S. Narayanan, D. W. Oard, & L. Vanderwende (Eds.), *Proceedings of Human Language Technologies: The 2009 Annual Conference of the North American Chapter of the Association for Computational Linguistics* (pp. 19–27). Boulder, CO: Association for Computational Linguistics.

Andrews, M., Vigliocco, G., & Vinson, D. (2009). Integrating experiential and distributional data to learn semantic representations. *Psychological Review, 116*(3), 463–498. doi: 10.1037/a0016261

Apps, M. A., & Tsakiris, M. (2014). The free-energy self: A predictive coding account of self-recognition. *Neuroscience & Biobehavioral Reviews, 41*, 85–97. doi: 10.1016/j.neubiorev.2013.01.029

Azzalini, D., Rebollo, I., & Tallon-Baudry, C. (2019). Visceral signals shape brain dynamics and cognition. *Trends in Cognitive* Sciences, 23(6), 488–509. doi: 10.1016/j.tics.2019.03.007

Baroni, M., Dinu, G., & Kruszewski, G. (2014). Don't count, predict! A systematic comparison of context-counting vs. context-predicting semantic vectors. In K. Toutanova, & H. Wu (Eds.), *Proceedings of the 52nd Annual Meeting of the Association for Computational Linguistics (Volume 1: Long papers)* (pp. 238–247). Baltimore, MD: Association for Computational Linguistics.

Blanke, O., Slater, M., & Serino, A. (2015). Behavioral, neural, and computational principles of bodily self-consciousness. *Neuron, 88*(1), 145–166. doi: 10.1016/j.neuron.2015.09.029

Carota, F., Kriegeskorte, N., Nili, H., & Pulvermüller, F. (2017). Representational similarity mapping of distributional semantics in left inferior frontal, middle temporal, and motor cortex. *Cerebral Cortex, 27*(1), 294–309. doi: 10.1093/cercor/bhw379

Collobert, R., & Weston, J. (2008). A unified architecture for natural language processing: Deep neural networks with multitask learning. In A. McCallum, & S. Roweis (Eds.), *Proceedings of the 25th international conference on Machine learning* (pp. 160–167). New York: Association for Computing Machinery.

Craig, A. D. (2009). How do you feel – now? The anterior insula and human awareness. *Nature Reviews Neuroscience, 10*(1), 59–70. doi: 10.1038/nrn2555

D'Argembeau, A., Stawarczyk, D., Majerus, S., Collette, F., Van der Linden, M., Feyers, D., Maquet, P., & Salmon, E. (2010). The neural basis of personal goal processing when envisioning future events. *Journal of Cognitive Neuroscience, 22*(8), 1701–1713. doi: 10.1162/jocn.2009.21314.

Damasio, A. (2010). *Y el cerebro creó al hombre*. Madrid: Destino.

de Greck, M., Rotte, M., Paus, R., Moritz, D., Thiemann, R., Proesch, U., Bruer, U., Moerth, S., Tempelmann, C., Bogerts, B., & Northoff, G. (2008). Is our self based on reward? Self-relatedness recruits neural activity in the reward system. *NeuroImage, 39*(4), 2066–2075. doi: 10.1016/j.neuroimage.2007.11.006

de Pasquale, F., Corbetta, M., Betti, V., & Della Penna, S. (2018). Cortical cores in network dynamics. *NeuroImage, 180*(Part B), 370–382. doi: 10.1016/j.neuroimage.2017.09.063

de Saussure, F. (1922). *Cours de linguistique generale* (C. Bally, A. Sechelaye, & A. Riedlinger, Eds., W. Baskin, Trans.). New York: McGraw-Hill.

Devlin, J., Chang, M. W., Lee, K., & Toutanova, K. (2018). BERT: Pre-training of deep bidirectional transformers for language understanding. In *Proceedings of the 2019 Conference of the North American Chapter of the Association for Computational Linguistics: Human Language Technologies, Volume 1 arXiv*, https://aclanthology.org/N19-1423

Enzi, B., de Greck, M., Prösch, U., Tempelmann, C., Northoff, G. (2009). Is our self nothing but reward? Neuronal overlap and distinction between reward and personal relevance and its relation to human personality. *PLoS One, 4*(12), e8429. doi: 10.1371/journal.pone.0008429

Erk, K. (2012). Vector space models of word meaning and phrase meaning: A survey. *Language and Linguistics Compass, 6*(10), 635–653. doi: 10.1002/lnco.362

Erk, K. (2016). What do you know about an alligator when you know the company it keeps? *Semantics and Pragmatics, 9*, 1–63. doi: 10.3765/sp.9.17

Frassinelli, D., Naumann, D., Utt, J., & m Walde, S. S. (2017). Contextual characteristics of concrete and abstract words. In C. Gardent, & C. Retoré (Eds.), *IWCS 2017 – 12th International Conference on Computational Semantics – Short papers* (Paper 10). Stroudsburg: Association for Computational Linguistics.

Frewen, P., Schroeter, M. L., Riva, G., Cipresso, P., Fairfield, B., Padulo, C., Kemp, A. H., Palaniyappan, L., Owolabi, M., Kusi-Mensah, K., Polyakova, M., Fehertoi, N., D'Andrea, W., Lowe, L., & Northoff, G. (2020). Neuroimaging the consciousness of self: Review, and conceptual-methodological framework. *Neuroscience & Biobehavioral Reviews, 112*, 164–212. doi: 10.1016/j.neubiorev.2020.01.023

Frings, C., & Wentura, D. (2014). Self-prioritization processes in action and perception. *Journal of Experimental Psychology: Human Perception and Performance, 40*(5), 1737–1740. doi: 10.1037/a0037376

Friston, K. (2010). The free-energy principle: A unified brain theory? *Nature Reviews Neuroscience, 11*, 127–138. doi: 10.1038/nrn2787

Friston, K. (2018). Am I self-conscious? (Or does self-organization entail self-consciousness?). *Frontiers in Psychology*, April 24. doi: 10.3389/fpsyg.2018.00579

Golesorkhi, M., Gomez-Pilar, J., Zilio, F., Berberian, N., Wolff, A., Yagoub, M. C. E., & Northoff, G. (2021). The brain and its time: Intrinsic neural timescales are key for input processing. *Communications Biology*, *470*, 970. doi: 10.1038/s42003-021-02483-6.

Han, S., & Northoff, G. (2008). Culture-sensitive neural substrates of human cognition: A transcultural neuroimaging approach. *Nature Reviews Neuroscience*, *9*, 646–654. doi: 10.1038/nrn2456

Harris, Z. S. (1954). Distributional structure. *Word*, *10*(2–3), 146–162. doi: 10.1080/00437956.1954.11659520

Harnad, S. (2003). Categorical perception. In L. Nadel (Ed.), *Encyclopedia of Cognitive Science* (pp. 169–177). London: Nature.

Hu, C., Di, X., Eickhoff, S. B., Zhang, M., Peng, K., Guo, H., & Sui, J. (2016). Distinct and common aspects of physical and psychological self-representation in the brain: A meta-analysis of self-bias in facial and self-referential judgements. *Neuroscience & Biobehavioral Reviews*, *61*, 197–207. doi: 10.1016/j.neubiorev.2015.12.003

Huang, Z., Obara, N., Davis, H. H., Pokorny, J., & Northoff, G. (2016). The temporal structure of resting-state brain activity in the medial prefrontal cortex predicts self-consciousness. *Neuropsychologia*, *82*, 161–170. doi: 10.1016/j.neuropsychologia.2016.01.025

Huntenburg, J. M., Bazin, P. L., & Margulies, D. S. (2018). Large-scale gradients in human cortical organization. *Trends in Cognitive Sciences*, *22*(1), 21–31. doi: 10.1016/j.tics.2017.11.002

Ježek, E. (2016). *The Lexicon: An Introduction*. Oxford: Oxford University Press.

Kiela, D., & Clark, S. (2014). A systematic study of semantic vector space model parameters. In A. Allauzen, R. Bernardi, E. Grefenstette, H. Larochelle, C. Manning, & S. Wen-tau Yi (Eds.), *Proceedings of the 2nd Workshop on Continuous Vector Space Models and Their Compositionality (CVSC)* (pp. 21–30). Gothenburg: Association for Computational Linguistics.

Kiela, D., Hill, F., & Clark, S. (2015). Specializing word embeddings for similarity or relatedness. In Ll. Màrquez, C. Callison-Burch, & J. Su (Eds.), *Proceedings of the 2015 Conference on Empirical Methods in Natural Language Processing* (pp. 2044–2048). Lisbon: Association for Computational Linguistics.

Kolvoort, I. R., Wainio-Theberge, S., Wolff, A., & Northoff, G. (2020). Temporal integration as "common currency" of brain and self-scale-free activity in resting-state EEG correlates with temporal delay effects on self-relatedness. *Human Brain Mapping*, *41*(15), 4355–4374. doi: 10.1002/hbm.25129

Kutuzov, A., Fares, M., Oepen, S., & Velldal, E. (2017). Word vectors, reuse, and replicability: Towards a community repository of large-text resources. In M. Jonsson (Ed.), *Proceedings of the 58th Conference on Simulation and Modelling* (pp. 271–276). Reykjavik: Linköping University Electronic Press.

Landauer, T. K., & Dumais, S. T. (1997). A solution to Plato's problem: The latent semantic analysis theory of acquisition, induction, and representation of knowledge. *Psychological Review*, *104*(2), 211–240. doi: 10.1037/0033-295X.104.2.211

Lapesa, G., & Evert, S. (2014). A large scale evaluation of distributional semantic models: Parameters, interactions and model selection. *Transactions of the Association for Computational Linguistics*, *2*, 531–546. doi: 10.1162/tacl_a_00201

Lapesa, G., & Evert, S. (2017). Large-scale evaluation of dependency-based DSMs. Are they worth the effort? In M. Lapata, P. Blunsom, & A. Koller (Eds.), *Proceedings of the 15th conference of the European chapter of the Association for computational linguistics: Volume 2, short papers* (pp. 394–400). Valencia: Association for Computational Linguistics.

Lenci, A. (2008). Distributional semantics in linguistic and cognitive research. *Italian Journal of Linguistics*, *20*(1), 1–31.

Lenci, A. (2018). Distributional models of word meaning. *Annual Review of Linguistics*, *4*, 151–171. doi: 10.1146/annurev-linguistics-030514-125254

Levy, O., & Goldberg, Y. (2014). Neural word embedding as implicit matrix factorization. *Advances in Neural Information Processing Systems*, *27*, 2177–2185.

Levy, O., Goldberg, Y., & Dagan, I. (2015). Improving distributional similarity with lessons learned from word embeddings. *Transactions of the Association for Computational Linguistics*, *3*, 211–225. doi: 10.1162/tacl_a_00134

MacLean, P. (1990). *The Triune Brain in Evolution*. New York: Plenum Press.

Margulies, D. S., Ghosh, S. S., Goulas, A., Falkiewicz, M., Huntenburg, J. M., Langs, G., Bezgin, G., Eickhoff, S. B., Castellanos, F. X., Petrides, M., Jefferies, E., & Smallwood, J. (2016). Situating the default-mode network along a principal gradient of macroscale cortical organization. *Proceedings of the National Academy of Sciences of the United States of America*, *113*(44), 12574–12579. doi: 10.1073/pnas.1608282113

McRae, K., Khalkhali, S., & Hare, M. (2012). Semantic and associative relations in adolescents and young adults: Examining a tenuous dichotomy. In V. F. Reyna, S. B. Chapman, M. R. Dougherty, & J. Confrey (Eds.), *The Adolescent Brain: Learning, Reasoning, and Decision Making* (pp. 39–66). Washington, DC: American Psychological Association.

Merck, C., Noël, A., Jamet, E., Robert, M., Hou, C., Salmon, A., Belliard, S., & Kalénine, S. (2019). Identification of taxonomic and thematic relationships: Do the two semantic systems have the same status in semantic dementia. *Journal of Clinical and Experimental Neuropsychology, 41*(9), 946–964. doi: 10.1080/13803395.2019.1641186

Menon, V. (2011). Large-scale brain networks and psychopathology: A unifying triple network model. *Trends in Cognitive Sciences, 15*(10), 483–506. doi: 10.1016/j.tics.2011.08.003

Mesulam, M. M. (1998). From sensation to cognition. *Brain, 121*(6), 1013–1052. doi: 10.1093/brain/121.6.1013

Mikolov, T., Sutskever, I., Chen, K., Corrado, G., & Dean, J. (2013). Distributed representations of words and phrases and their compositionality. *arXiv.* doi: https://doi.org/10.48550/arXiv.1310.4546

Miller, G. A., & Charles, W. G. (1991). Contextual correlates of semantic similarity. *Language and Cognitive Processes, 6*(1), 1–28. doi: 10.1080/01690969108406936

Mirman, D., Landrigan, J. F., & Britt, A. E. (2017). Taxonomic and thematic semantic systems. *Psychological Bulletin, 143*(5), 499–520. doi: 10.1037/bul0000092

Morel, N., Villain, N., Rauchs, G., Gaubert, M., Piolino, P., Landeau, B., Mézenge, F., Desgranges, B., Eustache, F., & Chételat, G. (2014). Brain activity and functional coupling changes associated with self-reference effect during both encoding and retrieval. *PLoS One, 9*(3), e90488.

Moutoussid, M., Fearon, P., El-Deredy, W., Dolan, R. J., & Fiston, K. (2014). Bayesian inferences about the self (and others): A review. *Conscious Cognition*, 25(100), 67–76. doi: 10.1016/j.concog.2014.01.00910.1371/journal.pone.0090488

Nakao, T., Miyagi, M., Hiramoto, R., Wolff, A., Gomez-Pilar, J., Miyatani, M., & Northoff, G. (2019). From neuronal to psychological noise: Long-range temporal correlations in EEG intrinsic activity reduce noise in internally-guided decision making. *NeuroImage, 201*, 116015. doi: 10.1016/j.neuroimage.2019.116015

Northoff, G. (2007). Psychopathology and pathophysiology of the self in depression – neuropsychiatric hypothesis. *Journal of Affective Disorders, 104*(1–3), 1–14. doi: 10.1016/j.jad.2007.02.012

Northoff, G. (2009). What are the subjective processes in our brain? Empirical and ethical implications of a relational concept of the brain. *American Journal of Bioethics, 9*(9), 27–28. doi: 10.1080/15265160903098390

Northoff, G. (2016). Is the self a higher-order or fundamental function of the brain? The "basis model of self-specificity" and its encoding by the brain's spontaneous activity. *Cognitive Neuroscience*, 7(1–4), 203–222. doi: 10.1080/17588928.2015.1111868

Northoff, G., Heinzel, A., de Greck, M., Bermpohl, F., Dobrowolny, H., & Panksepp, J. (2006). Self-referential processing in our brain: A meta-analysis of imaging studies on the self. *NeuroImage, 31*(1), 440–457. doi: 10.1016/j.neuroimage.2005.12.002

Northoff, G., Wainio-Theberge, S., & Evers, K. (2020). Is temporo-spatial dynamics the "common currency" of brain and mind? In Quest of "Spatiotemporal Neuroscience." *Physics of Life Reviews, 33*, 34–54. doi: 10.1016/j.plrev.2019.05.002

Northoff, G., Wiebking, C., Feinberg, T., & Panksepp, J. (2011). The "resting-state hypothesis" of major depressive disorder: A translational subcortical-cortical framework for a system disorder. *Neuroscience & Biobehavioral Reviews, 35*(9), 1929–1945. doi: 10.1016/j.neubiorev.2010.12.007

Panksepp, J. (1998). *Affective Neuroscience.* Oxford: Oxford University Press.

Peirsman, Y. (2008). Word space models of semantic similarity and relatedness. In K. Balogh (Ed.), *Proceedings of the 13th ESSLLI student session* (pp. 143–152). Hamburg: Freie und Hansestadt Hamburg.

Pennington, J., Socher, R., & Manning, C. D. (2014). Glove: Global vectors for word representation. In A. Moschitti, B. Pang, & W. Daelemans (Eds.), *Proceedings of the 2014 Conference on Empirical Methods in Natural Language Processing (EMNLP)* (pp. 1532–1543). Doha: Association for Computational Linguistics.

Philippi, C. L., & Koenigs, M. (2014). The neuropsychology of self-reflection in psychiatric illness. *Journal of Psychiatric Research, 54*, 55–63. doi: 0.1016/j.jpsychires.2014.03.004

Pulvermüller, F. (2018). The case of CAUSE: neurobiological mechanisms for grounding an abstract concept. *Philosophical Transactions of the Royal Society B: Biological Sciences, 373*(1752), 20170129. doi: 10.1098/rstb.2017.0129

Qin, P., Grimm, S., Duncan, N. W., Fan, Y., Huang, Z., Lane, T., Weng, X., Bajbouj, M., & Northoff, G. (2016). Spontaneous activity in default-mode network predicts ascription of self-relatedness to stimuli. *Social Cognitive and Affective Neuroscience, 11*(4), 693–702. doi: 10.1093/scan/nsw008

Qin, P., Wang, M., & Northoff, G. (2020). Linking bodily, environmental and mental states in the self-A three-level model based on a meta-analysis. *Neuroscience & Biobehavioral Reviews, 115*, 77–95. doi: 10.1016/j.neubiorev.2020.05.004

Rapp, R. (2002). The computation of word associations: Comparing syntagmatic and paradigmatic approaches. In *COLING 2002: The 19th International Conference on Computational Linguistics*. Stroudsburg: Association for Computational Linguistics.

Sahlgren, M. (2008). The distributional hypothesis. *Italian Journal of Disability Studies, 20*, 33–54.

Schacter, D. L., Addis, D. R., Hassabis, D., Martin, V. C., Spreng, R. N., & Szpunar, K. K. (2012). The future of memory: Remembering, imagining, and the brain. *Neuron*, *76*(4), 677–694. doi: 10.1016/j.neuron.2012.11.001

Schulte Im Walde, S. (2020). Distinguishing between paradigmatic semantic relations across word classes: human ratings and distributional similarity. *Journal of Language Modelling*, *8*(1), 53–101. doi: 10.15398/jlm.v8i1.199

Schütze, H., & Pedersen, J. (1993). A vector model for syntagmatic and paradigmatic relatedness. In *Proceedings of the 9th annual conference of the UW Centre for the new OED and text research* (pp. 104–113). Oxford: Oxford University Press.

Schwartz, M., Kimberg, D. Y., Walker, G. M., Brecher, A., Faseyitan, O. K., Dell, G. S., Mirman, D., & Coslett, H. B. (2011). Neuroanatomical dissociation for taxonomic and thematic knowledge in the human brain. *Proceedings of the National Academy of Science of the United States of America*, *108*(20), 8520–8524. doi: 10.1073/pnas.1014935108

Sui, J., He, X., Humphreys G. W. (2012). Perceptual effects of social salience: Evidence from self-prioritization effects on perceptual matching. *Journal of Experimental Psychology: Human Perception and Performance*, *38*(5), 1105–1117. doi: 10.1037/a0029792

Sui, J., & Humphreys, G. W. (2015). The integrative self: How self-reference integrates perception and memory. *Trends in Cognitive Sciences*, *19*(12), 719–728. doi: 10.1016/j.tics.2015.08.015

Sui, J., Rotshtein, P., & Humphreys, G. W. (2013). Coupling social attention to the self forms a network for personal significance. *Proceedings of the National Academy of Sciences of the United States of America*, *110*(19), 7607–7612. doi: 10.1073/pnas.1221862110

Tsakiris, M. (2017). The multisensory basis of the self: From body to identity to others. *Quarterly Journal of Experimental Psychology*, *70*(4), 597–609. doi: 10.1080/17470218.2016.1181768

Tsakiris, M., & Critchley, H. (2016). Interoception beyond homeostasis: Affect, cognition and mental health. *Philosophical Transactions of the Royal Society B: Biological Sciences*, *371*(1708), 20160002. doi: 10.1098/rstb.2016.0002

Turney, P. D. (2012). Domain and function: A dual-space model of semantic relations and compositions. *Journal of Artificial Intelligence Research*, *44*, 533–585. doi: 10.1613/jair.3640

Turney, P. D., & Pantel, P. (2010). From frequency to meaning: Vector space models of semantics. *Journal of Artificial Intelligence Research*, *37*, 141–188. doi: 10.1613/jair.2934

van der Meer, L., Costafreda, S., Aleman, A., & David, A. S. (2010). Self-reflection and the brain: A theoretical review and meta-analysis of neuroimaging studies with implications for schizophrenia. *Neuroscience & Biobehavioral Reviews*, *34*(6), 935–946. doi: 10.1016/j.neubiorev.2009.12.004

Vigliocco, G., Meteyard, L., Andrews, M., & Kousta, S. (2009). Toward a theory of semantic representation. *Language and Cognition*, *1*(2), 219–247. doi: 10.1515/LANGCOG.2009.011

Vigliocco, G., Vinson, D. P., Lewis, W., & Garrett, M. F. (2004). Representing the meanings of object and action words: The featural and unitary semantic space hypothesis. *Cognitive Psychology*, *48*(4), 422–488. doi: 10.1016/j.cogpsych.2003.09.001

Wittgenstein, L. (1953). *Investigaciones filosóficas (Philosophische Untersuchungen)*. London: Kegan Paul.

Yankouskaya, A., Bührle, R., Lugt, E., Stolte, M., & Sui, J. (2020). Intertwining personal and reward relevance: Evidence from the drift-diffusion model. *Psychological Research*, *84*, 32–50. doi: 10.1007/s00426-018-0979-6

INDEX